The Behavioral Neurology of Dementia

The Behavioral Neurology of Dementia

Edited by

Bruce L. Miller
University of California, San Francisco, USA

and

Bradley F. Boeve
The Mayo Clinic, Rochester, USA

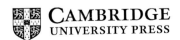

CAMBRIDGE
UNIVERSITY PRESS

University Printing House, Cambridge CB2 8BS, United Kingdom

Published in the United States of America by Cambridge University Press, New York

Cambridge University Press is part of the University of Cambridge.

It furthers the University's mission by disseminating knowledge in the pursuit of education, learning and research at the highest international levels of excellence.

www.cambridge.org
Information on this title: www.cambridge.org/9781107629998

© Cambridge University Press 2009

First published 2009
First paperback edition 2011
4th printing 2013

A catalogue record for this publication is available from the British Library

Library of Congress Cataloguing in Publication data
The behavioral neurology of dementia / edited by Bruce L. Miller and Bradley F. Boeve.
    p. ; cm.
  Includes bibliographical references and index.
  ISBN 978-0-521-85395-8 (hardback)
1. Dementia. 2. Clinical neuropsychology. I. Miller, Bruce L., 1949–
II. Boeve, Bradley F. III. Title.
  [DNLM: 1. Dementia. 2. Cognition Disorders. 3. Dementia–diagnosis. 4. Neurobehavioral Manifestations. WM 220 B4188 2009]
  RC521.B44 2009
  616.8'3–dc22

                                2008054302

ISBN 978-0-521-85395-8 Hardback
ISBN 978-1-107-62999-8 Paperback

....

Contents

Contributors

Deborah E. Barnes
Department of Psychiatry
University of California at San Francisco and Mental
Health Research Service
San Francisco VA Medical Center
San Francisco, CA, USA

Luis Bataller
Department of Neurology
University Hospital La Fe
Valencia, Spain

Bradley F. Boeve
Divisions of Behavioral Neurology and Movement
Disorders, Department of Neurology
Mayo Clinic
Rochester, MN, USA

Adam L. Boxer
UCSF Memory & Aging Center
Department of Neurology
University of California at San Francisco School of
Medicine
San Francisco, CA, USA

Thea Brennan-Krohn
Department of Neuropathology
Stanford Medical School
Palo Alto, CA, USA

María M. Corrada
Institute for Brain Aging and Dementia
Department of Neurology
University of California at Irvine
Irvine, CA, USA

Stephen Correia
Department of Psychiatry and Human Behavior
Warren Alpert Medical School of Brown University
Providence, RI, USA

Jeffrey L. Cummings
Departments of Neurology and Psychiatry and
Biobehavioral Sciences
Mary S. Easton Center for Alzheimer's Disease
Research and

Deane F. Johnson
Center for Neurotherapeutics
David Geffen School of Medicine at University of
California at Los Angeles
Los Angeles, CA, USA

Josep Dalmau
Division of Neuro-oncology
Department of Neurology, University of
Pennsylvania
Philadelphia, PA, USA

R. Rhys Davies
University Department of Neurology
Addenbrooke's Hospital, Cambridge, UK

Charles DeCarli
Alzheimer's Disease Center and Imaging of Dementia
and Aging (IDeA) Laboratory
Department of Neurology
Center for Neuroscience
University of California at Davis
Davis, CA, USA

Suzanne delaMonte
Department of Pathology
Warren Alpert Medical School of Brown
University
Providence, RI, USA

Michael D. Geschwind
UCSF Memory & Aging Center
Department of Neurology
University of California at San Francisco School of
Medicine
San Francisco, CA, USA

Maria Luisa Gorno-Tempini
UCSF Memory & Aging Center
Department of Neurology
University of California at San Francisco School of
Medicine
San Francisco, CA, USA

Aissa Haman
UCSF Memory & Aging Center
Department of Neurology
University of California at San Francisco School of
Medicine
San Francisco, CA, USA

John R. Hodges
MRC Brain and Cognitive Sciences Unit and University
Department of Neurology,
Cambridge, UK

Jee H. Jeong
Department of Neurology
Ewha Womans University Mokdong Hospital
Ewha Womans University School of Medicine
Seoul, Korea

Julene K. Johnson
UCSF Memory & Aging Center
Department of Neurology
University of California at San Francisco School
of Medicine
San Francisco, CA, USA

S. Andrew Josephson
UCSF Memory & Aging Center
Department of Neurology
University of California at San Francisco School
of Medicine
San Francisco, CA, USA

Kristin Kahle-Wrobleski
Eli Lilly and Company
Indianapolis, IN, USA

Aimee W. Kao
UCSF Memory & Aging Center
Department of Neurology
University of California at San Francisco School
of Medicine
San Francisco, CA, USA

Claudia H. Kawas
Institute for Brain Aging and Dementia
Department of Neurology and Department of
Neurobiology and Behavior
University of California at Irvine
Irvine, CA, USA

Brendan J. Kelley
Mayo Alzheimer's Disease Research Center
Department of Neurology
Mayo Clinic College of Medicine,
Rochester, MN, USA

Andrew Kertesz
Department of Cognitive Neurology
St Joseph's Hospital
London, Ontario, Canada

Eun-Joo Kim
Department of Neurology
Pusan National University Hospital
Pusan National University School of Medicine
Busan, Korea

Joel H. Kramer
UCSF Memory & Aging Center
Department of Neurology
University of California at San Francisco School of
Medicine
San Francisco, CA, USA

Casey E. Krueger
UCSF Memory & Aging Center
Department of Neurology
University of California at San Francisco School of
Medicine
San Francisco, CA, USA

Marcelo N. Macedo
Department of Neurology
University of California at San Francisco School of
Medicine
San Francisco, CA, USA

Gad A. Marshall
Memory Disorders Unit
Department of Neurology, Brigham and Women's
Hospital and
Massachusetts General Hospital
Harvard Medical School
Boston, MA, USA

Brandy R. Matthews
Department of Neurology
Indiana University School of Medicine
Indiana Alzheimer's Disease Center
Indianapolis, IN, USA

Adriane Votaw Mayda
Center for Neuroscience
University of California at Davis
Davis, CA, USA

Paul McMonagle
Department of Neurology
Royal Victoria Hospital
Belfast, Northern Ireland

Michelle Mellion
Department of Clinical Neurosciences
Warren Alpert Medical School of Brown University
Providence, RI, USA

Bruce L. Miller
UCSF Memory & Aging Center
Department of Neurology
University of California at San Francisco School of
Medicine
San Francisco, CA, USA

Duk L. Na
Department of Neurology
Samsung Medical Center
Sungkyunkwan University School of Medicine
Seoul, Korea

Christine Wu Nordahl
MIND Institute
University of California at Davis, Davis
CA, USA

Jennifer Ogar
UCSF Memory & Aging Center
Department of Neurology
University of California at San Francisco School of
Medicine
San Francisco, CA, USA

Karalyn Patterson
MRC Cognition and Brain Sciences Unit
Cambridge, UK

Ronald C. Petersen
Mayo Alzheimer's Disease Research Center
Department of Neurology
Mayo Clinic College of Medicine
Rochester, MN, USA

Caroline A. Racine
UCSF Memory & Aging Center
Department of Neurology
University of California at San Francisco School of
Medicine
San Francisco, CA, USA

Erik D. Roberson
Gladstone Institute of Neurological Disease and
UCSF Memory & Aging Center
Department of Neurology
University of California at San Francisco School of
Medicine
San Francisco, CA, USA

Howard Rosen
UCSF Memory & Aging Center
Department of Neurology
University of California at San Francisco School of
Medicine
San Francisco, CA, USA

Stephen Salloway
Departments of Clinical Neurosciences and
Psychiatry & Human Behavior
Warren Alpert Medical School of Brown
University
Providence, RI, USA

William W. Seeley
UCSF Memory & Aging Center
Department of Neurology
University of California at San Francisco School of
Medicine
San Francisco, CA, USA

Sang Won Seo
Department of Neurology
Samsung Medical Center, Sungkyunkwan University
School of Medicine
Seoul, Korea

Huidy Shu
UCSF Memory & Aging Center
Department of Neurology
University of California at San Francisco School of
Medicine
San Francisco, CA, USA

Maria Carmela Tartaglia
UCSF Memory & Aging Center
Department of Neurology
University of California at San Francisco School of
Medicine
San Francisco, CA, USA

Edmond Teng
Neurobehavior Unit, Veteran's Affairs Greater Los
Angeles Healthcare System and
Department of Neurology, David Geffen School of
Medicine at
University of California at Los Angeles
Los Angeles, CA, USA

Indre V. Viskontas
UCSF Memory & Aging Center
Department of Neurology
University of California at San Francisco School of
Medicine
San Francisco, CA, USA

Kristine Yaffe
Department of Psychiatry, Neurology and
Epidemiology
University of California at San Francisco and
Memory Disorders Clinic
San Francisco VA Medical Center
San Francisco, CA, USA

Introduction

Basic clinical approaches to diagnosis

Bruce L. Miller

There are few areas in all of medicine that are more difficult, yet gratifying, than the assessment, diagnosis and treatment of patients with cognitive complaints. Since the mid 1990s there have been dramatic changes in the accuracy of dementia diagnosis with improvements seen not only for Alzheimer's disease (AD), but also many of the other non-AD conditions including frontotemporal dementia (FTD), dementia with Lewy bodies (DLB), vascular dementia and Jakob–Creutzfeldt disease (CJD). Simultaneously, better detection and differential diagnosis of mild cognitive impairment (MCI), a condition that often represents an early stage of a specific degenerative or cerebrovascular condition, is now possible. One of the major reasons for these improvements is that research is helping to reveal specific roadmaps for the detection of each of these conditions, while simultaneously devising systematic approaches to rule out potentially treatable non-degenerative etiologies for cognitive impairment.

In this chapter, a simple approach to dementia at the bedside is described and clinical diagnosis is outlined with regards to the following categories:

- the history
- the examination including cognitive, behavioral, medical and neurological findings
- laboratory testing including genetic testing and brain imaging.

Additionally, a simple approach to treatment of the varied dementing conditions is described. With the approaches outlined in this chapter, a clinician can make highly accurate diagnoses for all of the major degenerative and vascular dementias and MCI, while simultaneously generating appropriate treatments once a diagnosis has been made. Although the features of all of these neurodegenerative disorders is described in a more comprehensive fashion throughout the

book, this chapter is meant to serve as an introduction to dementia, emphasizing a simple approach to diagnosis and treatment.

The history

No component of the diagnostic process is more important than is the history. Beyond its value for diagnosis, the historical features of the illness allow the clinician to quantify the burden of the disorder upon the caregiver, and define an approach to the treatment of both the dementia and the associated medical and psychiatric conditions. Additionally, the history offers important insights into whether or not non-standard laboratory testing such as genetic testing will be needed. For the primary care physician, the history is the primary guide as to whether or not a referral to a specialist will be necessary.

The history begins with determination of the first symptoms and with tracking of symptom progression. When a history is precisely taken, the clinician should be able to describe in vivid detail specific episodes that show a change from prior levels of function, and define a linear picture of how the disorder has progressed and fluctuated. The greater the specificity in the history, the greater is the likelihood that the clinician will be able to derive an accurate diagnosis. Ideally, the patient's history should be recorded like a script in a documentary movie, with a detailed story-line that is agreed upon by the patient and the historian(s). Many patients with dementing conditions are unable to track the symptoms of their illness accurately and, therefore, primary and collateral sources should always be sought. Defining the first symptoms and those that follow the initial complaints will help to determine where in the brain the dementia begins and to where it has spread. Often, in the more advanced stages of dementia, whatever the etiology, the pathology has spread diffusely making diagnosis difficult based upon current symptoms or findings. Therefore, even in advanced cases, focusing upon first symptoms will be the key to diagnosis.

The Behavioral Neurology of Dementia, eds. Bruce L. Miller and Bradley F. Boeve. Published by Cambridge University Press.
© Cambridge University Press 2009.

Patients with AD usually begin with forgetfulness because in this disorder pathology typically starts in the hippocampus. If progressive problems with speech or language are the first symptoms, an FTD-related condition such as non-fluent aphasia or semantic dementia is the major consideration. Prominent behavioral or personality changes such as disinhibition, apathy, compulsions, overeating, loss of sympathy and empathy for others suggest FTD, while visual deficits as an early feature suggest posterior cortical atrophy. Visual hallucinations or delusional mis-identification syndromes as early features of a dementia usually point to DLB. The presence of motor symptoms should be queried. Frequent falls are characteristic of progressive supranuclear palsy (PSP), or sometimes vascular dementia. Early movement abnormalities suggest the possibility of parkinsonian-dementia syndromes, such as DLB, PSP or corticobasal degeneration (CBD). Vascular dementia and CBD can begin with asymmetric motor findings.

Most of the degenerative dementias follow a slowly progressive and non-fluctuating course. In patients in whom symptoms vary from moment to moment or day to day, DLB and vascular dementia should be considered. Conversely, in patients who progress rapidly, an entirely different set of disorders must be considered including CJD, paraneoplastic syndromes, encephalitis, vasculitis, and metabolic disorders. Because patients with DLB are delirium prone, this disorder sometimes begins in an acute or subacute fashion.

A functional assessment of the patient is critical for the determination of the level of cognitive impairment and for helping to guide the family on management and outcome. Patients with mild cognitive impairment should have relatively normal day-to-day function, while completely normal day-to-day activities are more typical of individuals in whom cognition is normal.

The psychiatric history is not only critically important for differential diagnosis but also helps the clinician to target symptoms and behaviors with specific medications. Symptoms suggestive of depression, psychosis or anxiety should be sought and are typical of subcortical disorders but occur to a limited degree with all neurodegenerative conditions. Simple statements that a patient is depressed should not be accepted at face value. Apathy is common in dementia and does not necessarily represent depression. Pseudo-dementia due to depression is relatively rare in AD but the co-occurrence of dementia and depression is common. REM sleep-behavior syndrome is a characteristic of synuclein-related disorders including DLB, Parkinson's disease (PD) and multi-system atrophy, while sleep apnea can greatly exacerbate cognitive deficits. Understanding the nature and severity of psychiatric disturbances can be facilitated with questionnaires like the Neuropsychiatric Inventory or Geriatric Depression Scale. One of the major responsibilities of the clinician is to make sure that the caregiver is coping with the illness, and referrals of the caregiver for psychiatric care should always be considered.

Past illnesses and medications are a key component of the history. Anxiolytics, anticholinergic and anti-psychotic compounds can have profoundly negative influences upon the behavioral and cognitive status of patients, and current and past medications need to be reviewed carefully. Similarly, an acute change in cognitive status should trigger the search for toxic, metabolic or infectious diseases.

Mental status testing

Mental status testing is helpful for staging the dementia, for differentiating one dementia from another and for understanding how the cognitive deficits influence day-to-day behaviors. A variety of screening tools are available to help the clinician to search for cognitive deficits, but it is critically important that the strengths and limitations of these screening tools are understood. The Mini-Mental State Examination (MMSE) is an excellent tool for following AD, FTD, DLB and many other dementias once a diagnosis has been made. Additionally, the dementing conditions tend to show somewhat distinctive patterns on the MMSE. Patients with AD tend to fail on orientation, recall and sometimes the intersecting pentagons; patients with FTD often have trouble with "world" backwards and patients with DLB have particular difficulty correctly drawing the intersecting pentagons and spelling "world" backwards. A shaky tremulous drawing or micrographia on the sentence or the copy of the pentagons suggest a parkinsonian disorder. Similarly, the copy should be analyzed for evidence of neglect, a sign of vascular dementia or CBD. It is important to realize that the MMSE is not sensitive to early dementing conditions of any kind, and tends to underestimate the severity of dementia in patients with frontosubcortical disorders such as FTD, PSP or Huntington's disease.

More extensive neuropsychological testing than the MMSE is necessary for patients with mild disease and to help with differential diagnosis. At the University of California at San Francisco (UCSF), we have constructed a bedside cognitive battery that probes working and episodic memory, animal and "d" word generation, alternating sequences, inhibition, drawing, language fluency, comprehension, naming, repetition and emotion recognition. The numbers generated from this battery prove valuable for determining whether or not there are longitudinal changes in cognition, either positive or negative. Also, this battery helps to define patterns of deficits, data that are critically valuable in differential diagnosis. Typical AD patients show problems with episodic visual and verbal memory, animal generation and sometimes drawing, with relative sparing of language and emotion recognition. There is a very different pattern in FTD, with poor performance in executive functions including working memory, "d" generation, alternating sequences and emotion recognition, with relative sparing of drawing and episodic memory. In progressive non-fluent aphasia (PNFA), cognitive performance is remarkably normal with the exception of word fluency, "d" generation and sometimes alternating sequence speed. Patients with semantic dementia show profound deficits in naming that are not improved by clues, along with deficits with episodic verbal memory and animal generation, while DLB is characterized by abnormalities in drawing and sometimes executive function.

The quality of cognitive testing and interpretation is extremely variable and the clinician should be able to perform their own cognitive testing and interpret reports from others. Normal performance on difficult mental status tasks is reassuring but when patients have persistent complaints, repeat testing may be indicated. Having a quantitative measure is particularly helpful in determining whether or not a patient has progressed over time.

Psychiatric and behavioral observations

Good clinicians understand the importance of bedside observations for differential diagnosis of dementia. Most patients with MCI, AD and PNFA are well behaved and socially correct. In contrast, in FTD, patients may come to their appointments inappropriately dressed, poorly groomed or exhibit inappropriate behaviors including grandiose comments, undue familiarity, repetitive motor behaviors, inappropriate staring or aversion of eye gaze. The absence of a smile, averted eye gaze, a soft voice that trails off and crying are features of a major depression. Similarly, paranoia, psychosis and hallucinations are often apparent in the interview with the patient. Not only are these symptoms helpful for differential diagnosis but they also aid in the targeting of specific behaviors with medications.

The medical and neurological examination

The general examination should be performed to search for evidence of hypertension, cardiac arrhythmias, heart failure, skin infections or bruises, pulmonary disease, anemia, jaundice or other evidence for systemic illness. Medical illnesses can cause cognitive impairment and can exacerbate or worsen subtle cognitive disorders caused by an underlying degenerative disorder. It should be noted that cerebrovascular risk factors predispose to both vascular dementia and to AD. As the degenerative disorders worsen, patients become less able to describe symptoms of medical illnesses, including pain. This makes it particularly important for the clinician to look carefully for medical conditions that might be exacerbating cognitive or behavioral symptoms.

The neurological examination is central to differential diagnosis. With classical AD, the neurological examination remains normal until the late stages of the illness. Therefore, features of parkinsonism in patients with mild dementia should suggest other disorders such as DLB, PSP or CBD. The DLB parkinsonian features are often slightly atypical but can include facial bradykinesia, a soft festinating voice, cogwheel rigidity, tremor, slowing of movement, micrographia and stooped posture with a festinating gait; these should suggest DLB. Axial rigidity, a stare, vertical gaze disturbance, square wave jerks of the eyes and frequent falls typify PSP, and asymmetric parkinsonism, ocular apraxia, dystonia and alien limb occur with CBD. Prominent autonomic symptoms such as orthostatic hypotension can occur with DLB but reflect multisystem atrophy. Pseudobulbar affect, uncontrollable laughter and crying associated with a brisk jaw jerk, is seen with amyotrophic lateral sclerosis (ALS), PSP and vascular dementia. Asymmetric pyramidal deficits are seen with cerebrovascular disease. Rapidly progressive dementia with parkinsonism brings up the possibility of CJD.

3

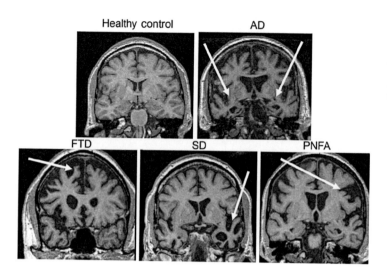

Fig. 1.1. Atrophy patterns in dementia. Patients showing different patterns of atrophy in T_1-weighted MRI images of healthy age-matched control. AD, Alzheimer's disease; FTD, frontotemporal dementia; SD, semantic dementia; PNFA, progressive non-fluent aphasia.

Laboratory testing and neuroimaging

The American Academy of Neurology has recommended a complete blood count, electrolytes, blood urea nitrogen (BUN) and serum glucose as part of the work-up for patients with memory complaints. Beyond these simple measures the clinician should remain flexible and adapt the evaluation to the conditions that are suggested by the patient's clinical syndrome. Elevations of serum calcium and phosphorus should be sought if there is a history of cancer, somnolence or bone pain. Liver failure should be considered in patients with dementia in whom chronic hepatitis or alcoholism is present. Neurosyphilis is exceedingly rare, and false positives are common with current screening techniques. For this reason, the rapid plasma reagin (RPR) test is no longer recommended for routine measurement. An electroencephalograph (EEG) is important in patients with spells, or fluctuating alertness. Lumbar puncture should be considered in patients with chronic headache, rapidly progressive changes or exposure to Lyme disease, human immunodeficiency virus (HIV) or syphilis.

Genetic testing should be considered in patients with autosomal dominant patterns of dementia. When genetic testing is performed, it should be done in conjunction with formal genetic counseling so that the patient is truly informed regarding the potential good and harm that can accompany this process. Presenilin 1 is the most common mutation for early-age-of-onset AD, while tau and progranulin mutations account for the vast majority of mutations linked to FTD. It is generally accepted that apolipoprotein polymorphisms should not be tested as their presence does not rule in or rule out AD.

Some sort of structural image should be performed in all patients with suspected dementia. Magnetic resonance imaging (MRI) is almost always preferable to computed tomography (CT) owing to its better resolution of tissue contrast. The presence of stroke, subdural hematoma, tumor, small bleeds caused by amyloid angiopathy, or excessive basal ganglia mineralization should be sought. Use of MRI is valuable for differential diagnosis of dementing conditions. Patients with AD show hippocampal and posterior parietal atrophy, white FTD is associated with anterior cingulate, orbitofrontal, insular and usually dorsolateral prefrontal atrophy (Fig. 1.1). In addition, the caudate and putamen often show atrophy. In CBD, frontally predominant and basal ganglia atrophy is common, while in PSP the frontal lobes tend to be spared but the midbrain is often atrophied. Changes in DLB are more variable but atrophy tends to be more posterior than in AD. CJD is associated with cortical ribboning and basal ganglia hyperintensities on fluid-attenuated inversion recovery (FLAIR) MRI, which demonstrate decrease diffusion of water molecules on diffusion-weighted imaging (DWI). This pattern reliably differentiates CJD from the other degenerative disorders. Often it is difficult to decide whether or not the vascular changes on an MRI are responsible for the cognitive syndrome. There is no hard rule to follow but the larger number of basal ganglia infarctions and white matter hyperintensities, the greater the likelihood that vascular disease accounts

Table 1.1. Clinical features of the major dementing conditions

Dementia	First symptom	Cognitive pattern	Neurology examination	Neuroimaging	Treatment
AD	Memory loss	Amnesia, word fluency	Normal till late	Posterior temporal/parietal, PIB positive	Cholinesterase inhibition, NMDA antagonist
FTD	Behavior-apathy, disinhibition, overeating	Loss of executive control	Normal (look for PSP, CBD, ALS)	Anterior frontotemporal insular, basal ganglia	SSRI, NMDA antagonist?
PNFA	Speech, word finding	Non-fluent, dysarthric, apractic speech	Sometimes asymmetric parkinsonism, axial rigidity	Left frontoinsular, basal ganglia	Speech therapy, treat parkinsonism, depression
DLB	Hallucinations, parkinsonism, delirium	Visuospatial, attentional	PD (can be normal at first)	Posterior inferior, Some are PIB positive	Cholinesterase inhibition, carbidopa-levodopa
SD	Word finding, loss of word meaning	Semantic loss, anomia	Normal till later	Anterior temporal	Consider cholinesterase inhibition
Vascular	Variable	Variable, subcortical lesions cause frontal syndrome	Variable, asymmetric, pyramidal deficits	Multiple strokes and/or subcortical white matter lesions	Stroke prevention, consider cholinesterase inhibition
CBD	Asymmetric parkinsonism, PNFA or behavioral	Like FTD or PNFA, sometimes parietal	Asymmetric PD, dystonia, ocular apraxia; alien hand	Frontal, basal ganglia, sometimes parietal	Exercise, treat parkinsonism, treat depression
PSP	Falls, PNFA, behavior	Loss of executive control	Supranuclear gaze palsy, axial rigidity	Midbrain atrophy (variable)	Exercise, treat PD
CJD	Rapid dementia, parkinsonism	Variable	PD, variable	Cortical ribbon, basal ganglia hyperintensity	None

Notes:
SSRI, selective serotonin-reuptake inhibitor; NMDA, *N*-methyl-D-aspartate; other abbreviations as in text.

Table 1.2. Underlying biology of the dementias

Dementia	Histology	Genes for	Molecules	Topography
AD	Amyloid plaques, neurofibrillary tangles	Causal: APP, PS1, PS2 Susceptibility: ApoE4, SIRT-1	Aβ-42, tau	Posterior temporal/parietal
FTD	Gliosis, spongiosus, Pick bodies, ubiquitin-TDP-43	Causal: progranulin, tau VCP, CHMP2B	Tau or TDP-43	Anterior frontotemporal insular, basal ganglia
PNFA	Gliosis, CBD or PSP pathology (see below)	Causal: progranulin, rarely tau, often sporadic	Tau	Left frontoinsular, basal ganglia
DLB	Lewy bodies, nigral loss, often amyloid plaques	Causal: rarely α-synuclein, often sporadic	α-Synuclein, often comorbid; Aβ-42	Posterior parietal, amygdala, basal ganglia, brainstem
SD	Gliosis, ubiquitin-TDP-43	Causal: rarely progranulin, tau, often sporadic	TDP-43	Anterior temporal, amygdala, eventually basal ganglia
Vascular	Infarctions, hyalinization of blood vessels	No specific causal genes	No	Subcortical white matter vulnerable with aging
CBD	Gliosis (cortical, subcortical) coiled tangles, astrocytic plaques	Progranulin, tau, susceptibility polymorphism is H1/H1 tau	Tau	Frontal, basal ganglia, sometimes parietal
PSP	Globose tangles, tufted astrocytes, neurofibrillary tangles	Rarely tau susceptibility polymorphism is H1/H1 tau	Tau	Midbrain, caudate, putamen, brainstem, cerebellum, some frontal
CJD	Astrocytosis, spongiosus	Prion gene mutations	Prion	Cortical, basal ganglia, cerebellum

Notes:
APP, amyloid precursor protein; Aβ-42, amyloid β-42; ApoE, apoprotein E; TDP-43, *TAR DNA*-binding protein 43; PSI, presenilin; CHMP2B, charged multivesicular body protein 2B; VCP, valosin-containing protein; other abbreviations as in text.

for at least some of the patient's cognitive symptoms. These lesions are cumulative and tend to cause deficits in frontal executive control as well as cognitive and motor slowing.

The role of nuclear imaging techniques such as single-photon emission computed tomography (SPECT) and positron emission tomography (PET) is debated. Although some suggest that SPECT and PET improve differentiation between AD and FTD, these techniques may not offer much beyond careful inspection of the atrophy patterns of MRI. Molecular imaging is emerging as an exciting adjunct to differential diagnosis. Amyloid imaging, particularly the Pittsburgh compound B (PIB), is already proving valuable in the differential diagnosis of AD from FTD. It is still too early to know what role that new MRI techniques including perfusion, diffusion tensor and functional MRI (fMRI) will play in dementia detection and differential diagnosis.

Summary

The diagnosis of degenerative disorders remains a clinical exercise that is largely determined after the taking of a careful history. Table 1.1 emphasizes the clinical features that differentiate the major dementing conditions. Fig. 1.1 shows the typical MRI patterns of the major dementias, while Table 1.2 emphasizes the underlying biology of the various dementias.

Chapter

2

Dementia with Lewy bodies

Caroline A. Racine

Introduction

Dementia with Lewy bodies (DLB) is clinical syndrome characterized by progressive dementia, parkinsonism and neuropsychiatric symptoms (McKeith *et al.*, 2004a). Pathologically, DLB is a synuclein disorder with widespread Lewy body pathology in the brainstem and cerebral cortex. Research has suggested that in individuals over 75 years, DLB is the second most common type of neurodegenerative dementia after Alzheimer's disease (AD). Although prevalent, our understanding of this complex disorder is in its relative infancy. The accurate diagnosis of DLB can be difficult owing to its frequent co-occurrence with AD and perceived similarity to other motor disorders such as Parkinson's disease (PD). However, the identification of individuals with DLB is extremely important because of the potential for life-threatening reactions to neuroleptic medications, and more encouraging, their ability to benefit greatly from treatment with anticholinesterase (AChEI) therapies.

Epidemiology

Epidemiological estimates have suggested that after AD, DLB is the second most common dementia in individuals over 75, with a prevalence rate of approximately 22% (Rahkonen *et al.*, 2003). Similarly, estimates of prevalence based on pathological data have suggested that DLB may represent between 15–35% of all dementia cases (Zaccai *et al.*, 2005), while population-based studies have estimated that DLB accounts for 5% of the population (Rahkonen *et al.*, 2003). In a pathologically confirmed sample, Williams *et al.* (2006) found that DLB was associated with increased mortality rates compared with AD (hazard ratio = 1.88), with a median survival of 78 years in DLB and 85 years in AD. However, rates of institutionalization and survival

in long-term care facilities did not differ significantly. A study from Sweden found that patients with DLB utilized twice the monetary resources needed for AD patients, which is strongly linked to a higher need for assistance with activities of daily living and subsequent assisted living placement (Bostrom *et al.*, 2006). Interestingly, in this study, increased monetary resources in DLB were not correlated with cognition (i.e. Mini-Mental Scale Examination [MMSE]) or level of neuropsychiatric symptoms (i.e. Neuropsychiatric Inventory [NPI]), which is more suggestive of placement secondary to motor difficulties. Indeed, other studies have found that motor impairment in DLB is a strong predictor of decreased functional abilities (Murman *et al.*, 2003.) Rapidity of progression has been found to be similar to that of AD (Stavitsky *et al.*, 2006). In summary, DLB is the second-most common form of dementia in individuals older than 75 and, relative to AD, is associated with increased functional impairment owing to motor deficits and a higher risk of mortality.

Clinical features
Diagnostic criteria

Diagnostic criteria for DLB were originally developed by a consensus workgroup (McKeith *et al.*, 1996) and have undergone subsequent revisions, with the most recent criteria being published in 2005 (McKeith *et al.*, 2005). As can be seen in Table 2.1, a central required feature for the diagnosis of DLB is the presence of dementia. 'Core' features of DLB include fluctuations in attention, visual hallucinations and parkinsonism. Additional supportive features include falls, syncope, neuroleptic sensitivity, REM sleep-behavior disorder (RBD), depression and delusions, amongst others. When dementia occurs in the context of well-established parkinsonism (> 1 year), a diagnosis of PD with dementia (PDD) is made. Exclusive of the temporal difference in symptom onset, DLB and PDD have overlapping clinical and pathological features and

The Behavioral Neurology of Dementia, eds. Bruce L. Miller and Bradley F. Boeve. Published by Cambridge University Press. © Cambridge University Press 2009.

7

Table 2.1. Research criteria for the diagnosis of dementia with Lewy bodies[a]

Features	Specific symptoms
Central feature	Presence of dementia (cognitive decline substantial enough to interfere with daily function)
Core features	Fluctuations in attention, recurrent visual hallucinations, parkinsonism
Suggestive features	REM sleep-behavior disorder, severe neuroleptic sensitivity, low dopamine transporter uptake in basal ganglia on SPECT/PET
Supportive features	Repeated falls/syncope, transient unexplained loss of consciousness, severe autonomic dysfunction, hallucinations in other modalities, delusions, depression, relative preservation of medial temporal lobe structure on CT/MRI, occipital hypoperfusion on SPECT/PET, abnormal MIBG myocardial scintigraphy, prominent slow-wave activity on EEG with temporal lobe transient sharp waves

Notes:
SPECT, single-photon emission computed tomography; PET, positron emission tomography; CT, computed tomography; MRI, magnetic resonance imaging; EEG, electroencephalography; MIBG, *meta*-iodobenzylguanidine.
[a]A diagnosis of dementia with Lewy bodies (DLB) requires the presence of the core feature of dementia. A diagnosis of probable DLB requires the presence of 2/3 core features, or the presence of one core and one suggestive feature. A diagnosis of possible DLB can be made with one core feature, and/or one or more suggestive features in the absence of any core features. Supportive features are frequently associated with DLB but are not part of the diagnostic criteria.
Source: From McKeith *et al.* (2005).

are largely felt to reflect the same underlying disorder (Galvin *et al.*, 2006; Lippa *et al.*, 2007).

Although the diagnosis of DLB has certainly become more standardized through the development of specific diagnostic criteria (e.g. McKeith *et al.*, 1996, 2000a, 2005), studies suggest that the accuracy of a clinical diagnosis of DLB ranges between 34 and 65% (Litvan *et al.*, 1998; Lopez *et al.*, 2002; Merdes *et al.*, 2003) although some studies have found accuracy rates as high as 83% (McKeith *et al.*, 2000a). As will be discussed below, the clinical correlates of DLB are often altered by concomitant AD pathology, which can make accurate diagnosis particularly difficult. Specific clinical features typically associated with DLB are described in more detail below.

Fluctuations in attention

Caregivers frequently report that patients with dementia experience fluctuations in cognitive abilities (e.g. "good days and bad days"). However, research has suggested that, in comparison to other diagnostic groups, patients with DLB show marked differences in attention and awareness, which may fluctuate over the course of minutes or hours. These transient episodes are often associated with altered levels of alertness (e.g. drowsiness) and may take on a confabulatory or delusional quality at times. Although fluctuations in attention are one of the core criteria for the diagnosis of DLB, no operational definition of "fluctuation" has been developed, making it difficult for clinicians to accurately use this feature for diagnosis.

Two measures have been developed to assess fluctuations in cognition via informant interview, the Clinician Assessment of Fluctuation and the One Day Fluctuation Assessment Scale (Walker *et al.*, 2000a). Increased scores on these scales were correlated with increased fluctuations in awareness as measured by neuropsychological testing and electroencephalography (EEG) (i.e. variability in theta rhythm). In addition, the scales were found to be effective in the differential diagnosis of DLB from both AD and vascular disease (DLB versus AD: sensitivity 81%, specificity 92%; DLB versus vascular disease: sensitivity 81%, specificity 82%) (Walker *et al.*, 2000b). A study by Ferman *et al.* (2004) examined normal elderly, patients with DLB and patients with AD and compared informants' responses on a 19-item questionnaire about fluctuations symptoms. They found that four symptoms reliably distinguished DLB from AD: daytime drowsiness and lethargy, daytime sleep of > 2 hours, staring into space for long periods of time, and episodes of disorganized speech. A study by Bradshaw *et al.* (2004), suggested that the qualitative features of fluctuations may be particularly helpful in the differential diagnosis of DLB. An examination of caregiver responses' on the Clinician Assessment of Fluctuation and the One Day Fluctuation Assessment Scale found that patients with DLB tend to show spontaneous transient fluctuations in awareness, with return to near-normal levels of cognition. These fluctuations tend to be independent of the environment and often have no discernible triggers. Most notably, the degree of variation in awareness can be extreme (e.g. can balance the checkbook one day but not hold a conversation other days). Consequently, one of the most sensitive clinical measures of fluctuation in DLB may be the amplitude of change between best and worst performance (McKeith, 2002). In contrast, patients with AD tend to show contextually dependent periods of increased confusion (e.g. conditions with high memory requirements, novel environments).

Quantitative measures have also shown significant abnormalities in attention in DLB. For example, a study by Ballard et al. (2002) found that on a battery of continuous performance tasks, patients with DLB or PDD showed similar levels of impairment in vigilance, reaction time and fluctuating choice reaction times. In contrast, patients with PD demonstrated decreased reaction times, but no fluctuations in attention, while patients with AD showed an intermediate pattern of increased reaction times and fluctuations (Ballard et al., 2002). Measures of brain activity have also shown abnormalities in attention. Using auditory-evoked potentials, DLB patients have been found to have deficits in prepulse inhibition, suggesting decreased ability to filter out irrelevant sensory information (Perriol et al., 2005). Studies with EEG have also demonstrated significant abnormalities in DLB, including diffuse slow-wave theta activity and periodic spike-wave complexes (Yamamoto and Imai, 1988; Doran et al., 2004). A study of EEG in 14 pathologically confirmed cases of DLB found loss of alpha activity and slow-wave transient activity in the temporal lobes (Briel et al., 1999). Thus, in addition to clinically observed features of fluctuating awareness, patients with DLB also show marked abnormalities on quantitative measures of attention abilities.

Overall, although fluctuations in attention may be difficult to define, a significant amount of research suggests that patients with DLB exhibit spontaneous transient alterations in consciousness. These fluctuations have been hypothesized to reflect a decline in acetylcholine (ACh) and/or brainstem dysfunction; however, additional research is needed to further understand this complex symptom and its underlying etiology.

Parkinsonism

Another key feature of DLB is the presence of parkinsonism. In contrast to classic PD, patients with, DLB/PDD tend to have a slightly different constellation of motor symptoms, with greater rigidity, less-frequent resting tremor and more symmetric presentation (Gnanalingham et al., 1997; Del Ser et al., 2000). Additionally, patients with DLB/PDD tend to fall into the postural instability-gait difficulty (PIGD) subtype of extrapyramidal dysfunction, as compared with the tremor dominant (TD) subtype associated with classic PD. In a study by Burn et al. (2003), patients with DLB and PDD were found to be more likely to have the PIGD subtype (PDD, 88%; DLB, 69%), while PD subjects were more evenly distributed between PIGD (38%) and TD (62%). A follow-up study by this group found that 25% of the PD patients with PIGD subtype developed dementia over 2 years, compared with none of the TD subtype. Therefore, the presence of PIGD motor subtype may be associated with an increased risk of developing dementia in the context of parkinsonism. Additionally, the PIGD subtype is thought to be less dopamine-dependent than TD and may be linked with cholinergic deficits observed in DLB/PDD (Jankovic et al., 1990). The presence of a gait disturbance may also assist with the differentiation of AD from non-AD dementias, including DLB/PDD. In particular, Allan et al. (2005) found that the presence of a parkinsonian gait was found in 93% of patients with PDD and 75% of patients with DLB and that these individuals were at a greater risk for falls (odds risk = 2.3). The presence of parkinsonian gait was able to identify patients with DLB/PDD from those with AD with 87% sensitivity and 84% specificity. Motor symptoms in DLB tend to be less responsive to treatment with levodopa compared with PD and PDD (Molloy et al., 2006; see Treatment/Management section for additional information).

In summary, parkinsonism is a key feature of DLB/PDD; however, the constellation of symptoms differs from classic PD, with increased gait difficulty and rigidity, symmetry of presentation and less-frequent resting tremor. These symptoms are less responsive to dopaminergic agonists and may reflect underlying cholinergic deficits in addition to alterations in dopamine.

REM sleep-behavior disorder

The REM sleep-behavior disorder is a parasomnia characterized by loss of muscle atonia during REM sleep, with resultant complex motor activity during dreaming (Schenck and Mahowald, 2002). Patients with RBD are at an increased risk for injuring themselves and their bed partners during these events, as they tend to "act out" dreams of being chased and/or attacked, and thus may punch, kick or perform other harmful behaviors during sleep. The condition is more prevalent in men and has a mean age of onset in the mid sixties (Olson *et al.*, 2000). It also appears to be a risk factor for developing a synuclein disorder (Boeve *et al.*, 1998, 2001), with some studies suggesting that up to 65% of individuals with RBD develop parkinsonism and/or dementia when followed longitudinally (Boeve *et al.*, 2003). The presence of RBD may herald the onset of a neurodegenerative condition by 10 or more years before the development of clinical symptoms (Tan *et al.*, 1996; Ferman *et al.*, 1999; Schenck *et al.*, 2002). Frequency estimates suggest that as many as 50% of patients with DLB exhibit RBD at some point, with the presence and severity of the RBD fluctuating over the clinical course (Boeve *et al.*, 2004). Occurrence of RBD is known to affect sleep quality, with qualitative ratings suggesting greater overall sleep disturbance in DLB and increased daytime sleepiness relative to AD (Grace *et al.*, 2000; Boddy *et al.*, 2007); however, the daytime sleepiness finding likely overlaps in part with the fluctuations in attention and awareness seen in DLB.

Pathologically, RBD has been associated with Lewy bodies in the brainstem (see Boeve *et al.*, 2004). Specifically, RBD has been associated with pathology in the pedunculopontine nucleus (PPN) and the locus coeruleus (LC), which involve both cholinergic and noradrenergic neurons. Consistent with RBD being one of the earliest symptoms of a potential underlying synuclein disorder, there is evidence for early Lewy body pathology in the lower brainstem nuclei in DLB (Braak *et al.*, 2003; see Boeve *et al.* [2007] for review). In summary, RBD is a frequently observed symptom in DLB that reflects a complex interaction between Lewy body pathology in the brainstem and neurotransmitter deficits, particularly in ACh. Occurrence of RBD often precedes DLB by 10 or more years, and thus may serve as one of the earliest hallmarks of the disorder.

Autonomic function

Autonomic dysfunction is also a prevalent feature of DLB (Horimoto *et al.*, 2003). When compared with other synuclein disorders, the degree of autonomic dysfunction in DLB is moderate, falling between the severe autonomic dysfunction seen in multisystem atrophy and the mild autonomic dysfunction observed in PD (Thaisetthawatkul *et al.*, 2004). Thaisetthawatkul *et al.* (2004) examined a sample of 20 patients with DLB and found that 95% had autonomic symptoms, with the most common symptoms being orthostatic intolerance (85%), orthostatic hypotension (50%),

adrenergic dysfunction (85%), distal anhidrosis (54%) and urinary symptoms (35%). Another study found that lower urinary tract dysfunction was found in all DLB patients studied (11/11), with the most common symptoms being urinary incontinence (91%), increased night-time frequency (82%), urgency (73%), increased daytime frequency (55%) and difficulty voiding (55%) (Sakakibara *et al.*, 2005). Urinary symptoms in particular are thought to be caused by an altered spino-bulbo-spinal micturition reflex that is dependent on both the cholinergic and dopaminergic pathways, as well as alterations at the level of the autonomic ganglia.

Although orthostatic hypotension and urinary incontinence are common in DLB, these symptoms typically do not appear within the first year of disease onset (Wenning *et al.*, 1999); however, case studies with autonomic symptoms as a presenting feature have been described (Kaufmann *et al.*, 2004). The appearance of autonomic dysfunction can occur prior to, concurrent with or after the onset of parkinsonism and cognitive difficulties (Sakakibara *et al.*, 2005). The presence of autonomic symptoms can assist with differential diagnosis, as patients with DLB and PDD have been found to show greater autonomic dysfunction than those with AD or vascular dementia, with some suggestion of greater dysfunction in PDD relative to DLB (Allan *et al.*, 2007). Importantly, the autonomic features observed in DLB/PDD are associated with poorer outcomes on measures of physical activity, activities of daily living, depression and quality of life (Allan *et al.*, 2006).

In particular, research using *meta*-iodoenzylguanidine (MIBG) cardiac scintigraphy has suggested early autonomic dysfunction in DLB. This compound is a physiologic analogue of norepinephrine and MIBG cardiac scintigraphy is a non-invasive tool for estimating local myocardial sympathetic nerve damage. In a sample of 37 patients with DLB and 42 patients with AD, Yoshita *et al.* (2006) found that reduced MIBG uptake was 100% specific and 100% sensitive to the diagnosis of DLB, irrespective of the presence of parkinsonism. Additional research has found that MIBG is significantly reduced in DLB relative to both controls and patients with PD (Suzuki *et al.*, 2006; Oka *et al.*, 2007). This research suggests that autonomic postganglionic neurons may be one of the earliest regions of Lewy body pathology in DLB, and it suggests the possibility of using autonomic markers as a measure of preclinical disease.

Overall, autonomic symptoms may be an under-recognized feature of DLB, with severity falling between that of multisystem atrophy and that of PD. The most frequent symptoms are orthostatic hypotension and urinary incontinence, which have a significant negative impact on functional abilities in DLB. Autonomic symptoms tend to occur partway through the disease process, although they have been noted as presenting symptoms in some cases.

Sensitivity to medication and infection

Patients with DLB tend to be particularly "delirium-prone," as they often have disturbances in cognition secondary to even small alterations in neurochemistry. Indeed, the first symptoms of DLB often present in a subacute fashion in the context of a new medication, after surgery with general anesthesia, or during an acute infection. Neuroleptic sensitivity has been found to be a prominent symptom of DLB, occurring in 30–50% of patients (McKeith et al., 1992; Ballard et al., 1998; Sadek and Rockwood, 2003), which places these patients at an increased risk of mortality and morbidity. Specifically, when administered even small doses of neuroleptics, many patients with DLB will show acute sedation, altered mental status and increased parkinsonism (McKeith et al., 1992; Burke et al., 1998; Sechi et al., 2000). In one sample of dementia patients, Aarsland et al. (2005) found high rates of severe neuroleptic reactions following the administration of both typical and atypical antipsychotic drugs in patients with synuclein disorders (53% in DLB, 39% in PDD and 27% in PD) relative to AD (0%). Of note, patients with AD who had pathologically confirmed Lewy body disease in the context of concurrent Alzheimer's pathology were also at increased risk of severe reactions to neuroleptic drugs. This is particularly concerning given the high rate of Lewy body pathology at autopsy in patients with AD who do not meet formal criteria for DLB and thus may not be considered to be at-risk for adverse reactions to neuroleptics.

Additional research suggests that even in the absence of a severe reaction, neuroleptic use may increase levels of tau pathology in DLB. Specifically, a study by Ballard et al. (2005) found that relative to DLB patients who had not received neuroleptic treatment, DLB patients who had received neuroleptic treatment had a 50% increase in tangles within the entorhinal cortex and a 30% increase in plaques in the frontal cortex. The exact mechanisms of neuroleptic sensitivity remain unclear but have been linked to a failure of upregulation of D_2 receptors in the striatum (Piggott et al., 1998) and dopaminergic hypoactivity

(Nishijima and Ishiguro, 1989; Sechi et al., 1996). Overall, these studies clearly highlight the significant risk of neuroleptic medications to individuals with underlying Lewy body pathology and suggest that antipsychotic drugs should be used with caution in individuals with dementia.

Neuropsychiatric findings
Visual hallucinations

Neuropsychiatric symptoms are a core feature of DLB (reviewed by Simard et al., 2000) and have been found to be more prevalent in DLB than in AD (Rockwell et al., 2000). Specifically, recurrent visual hallucinations are one of the core features of DLB and occur in 60–80% of patients with DLB/PDD (Emre, 2003; McKeith et al., 2004b). Typically, these visual hallucinations are complex, well formed and often take the form of people or animals (Ballard et al., 1997) with similar characteristics found across DLB and PDD (Mosimann et al., 2006). Most typically, visual hallucinations in DLB occur daily and consist of complex single objects in the central field of vision lasting minutes at a time (Mosimann et al., 2006). The prevalence of people and animals in the visual hallucinations seen in DLB has suggested underlying dysfunction in the ventral visual stream, although findings suggestive of dorsal stream dysfunction are also seen, albeit less frequently (e.g. palinopsia). Visual hallucinations are also associated with concomitant symptoms of anxiety, apathy and sleep disturbance, which suggests some common underlying mechanisms for all neuropsychiatric symptoms in DLB, perhaps related to cholinergic deficits (Mosimann et al., 2006).

The underlying mechanism for visual hallucinations in DLB is still under debate. However, current theories suggest an interaction between alterations in ACh, brainstem abnormalities and disturbance within the visual system (e.g. Collerton et al., 2005). Specifically, previous research suggests that visual hallucinations can occur secondary to alterations in ACh, as occurs with hallucinogens such as LSD (lysergic acid diethylamide) (Perry and Perry, 1995). In addition, brainstem dysfunction has been known to produce visual hallucinations (e.g. peduncular hallucinosis; see Benke, 2006) via a disturbance of the reticular activating system and associated thalamocortical circuits, which may result in altered sleep–wake cycles and an altered reality monitoring system. In addition, visual hallucinations are also frequently observed in the context of disordered visual input,

11

such as Charles Bonnet syndrome. In this disorder, patients with glaucoma or other eye disorders that result in decreased visual input to the primary visual cortex have been found to have chronic *overactivation* of the bilateral ventral temporal lobes, deemed a *cortical release* phenomenon, which is thought to occur as an attempt to "boost" the decreased visual signal in primary visual cortex (Ffytche *et al.*, 1998; Santhouse *et al.*, 2000). However, one side-effect of this temporal overactivation may be the presence of visual hallucinations.

As discussed throughout this chapter, patients with DLB have significant disturbances in all three factors discussed above. Specifically, they have significant cholinergic deficits, profound brainstem pathology and altered visual processing: a combination of pathologies that likely puts them at very high risk for developing visual hallucinations. As will be discussed below, patients with DLB have been found to have hypoperfusion in the occipital cortex as detected by positron emission tomography (PET) or single-photon emission computed tomography (SPECT), a finding not present in AD. Although this finding occurs in DLB, irrespective of the presence of hallucinations, Imamura *et al.* (1999) found that patients with DLB who had visual hallucinations had relatively *less* hypometabolism in the right temporoparietal region, which the authors hypothesized may lead to the presence of visual hallucinations, perhaps through a cortical release phenomenon similar to that seen in Charles Bonnet syndrome (e.g. Ffytche *et al.*, 1998). The presence of visual hallucinations in DLB has been also linked to increased Lewy body pathology within the temporal lobe (Harding *et al.*, 2002). Additionally, some research has suggested that patients with DLB may have altered visual processing at the level of the retina secondary to synuclein pathology (e.g. Maurage *et al.*, 2003). Consequently, there are potentially many levels at which the visual system in DLB may be impaired. As discussed above, there are multiple factors that may contribute to the presence of visual hallucinations in DLB, which suggests that any model of this complex phenomenon will necessarily be multifactorial.

In addition to complex visual hallucinations, patients with DLB may also experience visual illusions and extracampion hallucinations. Visual illusions occur when a stimuli in the environment is misperceived (e.g. a tree stump looks like an animal), as opposed to a true visual hallucination, which occurs in the absence of visual stimuli. Observations from our clinic suggest that this frequently takes the form of faces "morphing" out of wallpaper or other textured substances. Extracampion hallucinations occur as either dark shadows in the periphery of vision that disappear when looked at, or a false feeling of someone "looking over one's shoulder." Presumably these symptoms reflect similar, but less severe, pathology as that which contributes to the visual hallucinations observed in DLB. Interestingly, the presence of visual hallucinations is associated with a greater response to AChEIs in both DLB and PDD patients (McKeith *et al.*, 2004a; Burn *et al.*, 2006) and visual hallucinations are typically reduced once AChEIs are started (McKeith *et al.*, 2000b; Bullock and Cameron, 2002), suggesting a significant role of acetylcholine in the presence of visual hallucinations in DLB/PDD. Additionally, in one recent study, the administration of donepezil was associated with both a decrease in visual hallucinations and a relative *increase* in occipital perfusion on SPECT, suggesting a potential link between ACh, occipital perfusion and visual hallucinations (Mori *et al.*, 2006).

In summary, recurrent visual hallucinations are a core feature of DLB and often consist of faces, people and/or small animals. The underlying etiology of visual hallucinations in DLB is thought to reflect a complex interaction of deficits in ACh, brainstem function and visual processing. The presence of visual hallucinations is predictive of a good overall response to AChEIs, and treatment with these medications typically leads to a subsequent decrease in visual hallucinations.

Delusions

Delusions are one of the supportive criteria for DLB and in some studies have been found to occur in up to 57% of patients with DLB (e.g. Aarsland *et al.*, 2001). Most frequently, delusions in DLB reflect some type of misperception, resulting in such syndromes as Capgras delusion and reduplicative paramnesia (e.g. Marantz and Verghese, 2002; Hirayama *et al.*, 2003; Ohara and Morita, 2006). Capgras delusions occur when an individual believes that a loved one has been replaced by a nearly identical imposter (e.g. their wife "looks like" their wife but is really an imposter), whereas reduplicative paramnesia is a delusion in which individuals believe that the environment is familiar, but not really the true location (e.g. the house they are in is a duplication of their "real" house). Studies of individuals with Capgras delusions have found that they are able to recognize familiar faces but that they do not demonstrate the appropriate skin conductance responses that are normally associated with the emotional aspects of face recognition (Ellis et al., 1997; Hirstein and Ramachandran, 1997). Thus, Capgras symptoms have been hypothesized to reflect a disconnection of visual information (e.g. occipital lobe) from emotional processing (e.g. amygdala). Given that patients with DLB exhibit both visual deficits and significant Lewy body pathology in the amygdala, it is possible that the combination of these deficits may contribute to the presence of delusions of misperception; however, future studies will be required to explore this hypothesis and its alternatives. Similar to other neuropsychiatric symptoms in DLB, delusions have also been associated with the cholinergic deficits observed in DLB. In one study of patients with pathologically confirmed DLB, delusions were associated with an increase in the upregulation of muscarinic ACh receptors (Ballard et al., 2000). In summary, delusions of misperception are common in DLB and may reflect a disconnection between visual and emotional information and cholinergic deficits; however, additional research is required to fully understand this phenomenon.

Mood symptoms

Historically, research has focused on hallucinations and delusions as the most frequent neuropsychiatric symptoms in DLB. However, it is becoming increasingly recognized that DLB can be a heterogeneous disorder and that additional neuropsychiatric symptoms such as depression and anxiety also frequently occur. Depression is currently listed as a supportive feature for a diagnosis of DLB (McKeith et al., 2005). In addition, a recent study by Borroni et al. (2007) examined behavioral and psychiatric symptoms in patients with DLB and found that anxiety was the most common neuropsychatric symptom, occurring in 65% of patients. In addition, depression (62%), apathy (58%) and agitation and sleep disorders (each 55%) were common features, while psychosis appeared in 50% of patients. These symptoms worsened as the disease progressed and were not associated with the severity of motor symptoms, suggesting a potentially different underlying mechanism.

Overall, current research suggests that visual hallucinations and delusions of misperception are frequently observed in the context of DLB; however, other neuropsychiatric symptoms, such as depression, anxiety, apathy, agitation and sleep disorders, may be just as prevalent and should be taken into consideration when considering a potential diagnosis of DLB.

Of note, many patients with DLB present to clinic having already received a tentative diagnosis of AD and subsequent treatment with an AChEI, which may lessen the likelihood of the presence of hallucination and delusions, as these symptoms typically respond well to AChEIs. Therefore, the absence of these symptoms in the context of treatment with AChEIs should not necessarily dissuade one from a potential diagnosis of DLB provided that other diagnostic criteria are met.

Neuropsychological findings

The classic neuropsychological profile of DLB is prominent deficits in visuospatial, attention and executive abilities, with relatively milder memory difficulties (recall > recognition). Unfortunately, many of the studies that have examined neuropsychological differences between clinically diagnosed DLB and AD are contaminated by the fact that, pathologically, many of these patients likely have both Lewy body and Alzheimer's pathology. The clinical profile of DLB has been known to change depending on the level of concurrent AD pathology (Merdes et al., 2003). Consequently, it is likely that the neuropsychological profile observed in patients with DLB differs depending on the severity and regional distribution of concurrent Alzheimer's pathology, which can make differential diagnosis based on neuropsychological performance alone difficult.

Studies regarding the neuropsychological profiles of patients with clinically diagnosed DLB and AD have found differential patterns of results. Specifically, both groups show impairments in learning and delayed recall; however, patients with DLB demonstrate relatively intact recognition abilities, suggesting a less-severe consolidation deficit relative to AD (Ferman et al., 2006; Crowell et al., 2007). Additionally, both patients with DLB and those with PDD are found to have greater difficulties than those with AD on tasks of attention, inhibition, visuoperceptual skills and constructional praxis (Collerton et al., 2003; Galvin et al., 2006; Guidi et al., 2006). Mori et al. (2000) found that patients with DLB performed worse than those with AD on several visuoperceptual tasks, including object size discrimination, form discrimination, overlapping figure identification and visual counting tasks. In addition, patients with DLB and visual hallucinations and/or misidentification delusions had poorer performance on visual tasks than those without visual neuropsychiatric symptoms, suggesting

13

a potential role for impaired visual function in the presence of visual hallucination and delusions in DLB (Mori *et al.*, 2000).

Consistent with findings suggesting that patients with DLB have difficulty with visuospatial skills, poor pentagon copy performance on the MMSE has been found to be particularly predictive of DLB versus AD (Ala *et al.*, 2001). For example, in their study of patients with MMSE > 25, Ala *et al.* (2001) found that three of four patients with DLB had poor pentagon copy compared with none of the five patients with AD, with a resulting sensitivity and specificity of 88% and 52%, respectively. While impaired pentagon copy in AD has been found to be associated with more globally impaired cognition, impaired pentagon copy in DLB often occurs early in the disorder when other global abilities may be relatively preserved (Ala *et al.*, 2001). Consistent with overlapping clinical profiles in DLB and PDD, similar deficits in pentagon copy have been found across both disorders (Cormack *et al.*, 2004). Overall, these results suggest that poor pentagon copy, particularly in the context of *relatively* intact global abilities, may be particularly predictive of underlying Lewy body pathology and thus this item may be a quick and useful bedside screen.

Data from pathologically confirmed samples of patients with DLB or AD is largely consistent with the neuropsychological profiles observed in clinically diagnosed patients. For example, in a pathologically confirmed sample of 24 patients with DLB and 24 with AD, both groups were found to have impaired total learning and delayed recall scores on the California Verbal Learning Test (CVLT); however, the patients with DLB showed less evidence of rapid forgetting and better recognition scores (Hamilton, 2004). Using groups based on pathological criteria (AD only, DLB only, AD/DLB mixed), Kraybill *et al.* (2005) found that both AD groups (AD and mixed AD/DLB) had poorer memory and naming compared to DLB only, whereas the DLB-only group had more impairment on tasks of executive function (Trails B) and attention (Digit Span) relative to the other two groups. Of note, the mixed AD/DLB group exhibited a more rapid decline in cognition over time than AD or DLB alone, although another group has found similar rates of decline between AD, DLB and mixed AD/DLB (Johnson *et al.*, 2005).

In summary, on neuropsychological testing, DLB is associated with a less-severe consolidation deficit relative to AD, and greater impairment in attention, executive function and visuospatial skills. Poor pentagon copy on the MMSE, particularly in the context of otherwise relatively preserved cognition, is particularly suggestive of DLB. As will be discussed in more detail below, AD and DLB pathology frequently co-occur, which can significantly impact the specific profile observed in DLB patients.

Neuropathology
Pathological criteria

Dementia with Lewy bodies is one of the three disorders termed "synucleinopathies," including PD and multisystem atrophy (MSA). All three have an underlying disorder of α-synuclein, an intracellular protein involved in axonal transport. The most common pathology associated with altered α-synuclein processing is the Lewy body, which is an intracytoplasmic neuronal inclusion that was initially identified as the hallmark pathology found in the brainstem of patients with PD. Although Lewy bodies are typically restricted to the brainstem in PD, in DLB there is profound LB pathology in both the brainstem and neocortical structures. The DLB pathology is thought to start in the brainstem and then progress to the amygdala, limbic cortex and, finally, to neocortex (Marui *et al.*, 2002; McKeith *et al.*, 2005).

Lewy bodies have been thought to reflect an attempt of the neuron to protect itself by collecting the presynaptic α-synuclein aggregates and moving them to the cell body via retrograde axonal transport, where they can be aggregated and deposited in the presumably less-toxic form of a Lewy body (Kopito, 2000; McNaught *et al.*, 2002). However, the severity and location of Lewy body pathology in DLB does not always correlate well with clinical symptoms (Gomez-Tortosa *et al.*, 1999), which has left researchers looking for additional pathological mechanisms that may contribute to clinical symptoms. Interestingly, a recent study suggested that the α-synuclein aggregates themselves might play an important role in the symptoms of DLB. Specifically, Kramer and Schulz-Schaffer (2007) found that DLB is associated with a widespread number of α-synuclein aggregates at the presynaptic terminal, with a concomitant loss of *nearly all* dendritic spines at the adjacent postsynaptic terminal. These findings occurred in the context of relatively few Lewy bodies. Overall, these results suggest that DLB is associated with widespread synaptic dysfunction secondary to presynaptic α-synuclein aggregates and the concomitant loss of postsynaptic dendritic spines. This synaptic dysfunction likely has a huge impact on the clinical symptoms of DLB, exclusive of the number of Lewy bodies. This presynaptic aggregation of α-synuclein necessarily occurs prior to the formation of Lewy bodies, and thus may be an appropriate and important target for future DLB therapies. Chapter 10 has further information on the pathological characteristics of DLB.

Overlap with Alzheimer's disease

In addition to profound Lewy body pathology, patients with DLB also frequently have a significant amount of AD pathology at autopsy. Based on this finding, Marui *et al.* (2004) have proposed an alternative mechanism for classifying DLB pathology: a "pure" form, with significant Lewy body pathology but minimal AD pathology; a "common" form, with significant Lewy body and AD pathology; and an "AD" form, with significant AD pathology but minimal Lewy body pathology (i.e. amygdalar Lewy bodies only). Additionally, using these staging criteria, the three types are further classified by the severity and location of Lewy body pathology (limbic: stage I–II; neocortical: stage III–IV). In their sample, 17/51 individuals with some Lewy body pathology met pathological criteria for the "AD" form. These individuals did not have significant limbic or cortical Lewy body pathology; however, they did have mild amygdala Lewy body pathology. The presence of amygdala Lewy bodies in the absence of other significant Lewy body pathology is frequently seen in AD without obvious clinical correlate (e.g. Hamilton *et al.,* 2000). Of note, amygdalar Lewy bodies tend to co-occur in neurons with neurofibrillary tangles (Schmidt *et al.,* 1996). Marui *et al.* (2004) found that individuals with the "pure" form of DLB had greater pathology in the substantia nigra and locus coeruleus, a younger age of onset and were more likely to have parkinsonism as an early symptom, while those with the "common" form of DLB had greater spongiosis in the transentorhinal cortex, an older age of onset and were more likely to present with dementia as a first symptom (Marui *et al.,* 2004). Overall these results suggest that AD and DLB pathologies frequently overlap and the presence of AD pathology can significantly modify both age of onset and clinical presentation.

The synergistic relationship between α-synuclein and β-amyloid

As discussed above, DLB and AD have frequently been found to be overlapping clinical syndromes. In addition, there is significant pathological evidence suggesting a relationship between α-synuclein and β-amyloid (Aβ) pathology (Saito *et al.,* 2004). Pletnikova *et al.* (2005) found that those with DLB without significant Aβ deposits had significant Lewy neurite pathology in the hippocampus, amygdala, entorhinal cortex and basal forebrain, with relatively little Lewy body or neurite pathology in cingulate cortex and association cortices. However, in those with combined DLB and Aβ pathology, there was an increase in cortical Lewy body pathology, suggesting a potential synergistic effect between α-synuclein and Aβ. In concert with this hypothesis, studies in double-transgenic mice with mutations affecting amyloid precursor protein (APP) and α-synuclein have shown that the presence of Aβ increases α-synuclein aggregation and neuronal degeneration (Masliah *et al.,* 2001). Studies have also found that amyloid plaques in DLB contain an amino acid fragment of α-synuclein, suggesting an interaction of the two pathologies (Yokota *et al.,* 2002; Liu *et al.,* 2005). Recently, a study using nuclear magnetic resonance (NMR) spectroscopy found specific sites of interaction between membrane-bound α-synuclein and Aβ. In particular, they found that the interaction of synaptic membrane-bound α-synuclein with Aβ42 leads to the oligomerization of Aβ42, which is known to be toxic (Mandal *et al.,* 2006). Therefore, much current research suggests a significant interaction between α-synuclein and Aβ pathology and that this relationship is likely synergistic.

In summary, DLB is a disorder of α-synuclein that results in widespread Lewy body pathology which begins in the brainstem and continues out to medial temporal and neocortical regions. Additionally, there are significant synaptic deficits related to a concentration of α-synuclein aggregates in the presynaptic terminal. Concomitant AD pathology frequently occurs in DLB, and there is evidence of a synergisitic relationship between α-synuclein and Aβ pathology. Overall, the significant overlap of the clinical and pathological features of PD, DLB, PDD and AD suggests that these disorders exist on a pathological spectrum, with DLB/PDD representing a midpoint of α-synuclein and Aβ pathology.

Neurotransmitters

Patients with DLB have been found to have profound alterations in cholinergic transmission that are greater than those in AD. Two groups of cholinergic neurons, those in the basal forebrain and the pedunculopontine region, provide cholinergic input to the cerebral cortex and thalamus via their projections. Perry *et al.* (1995) found a 40–50% reduction in nicotinic receptors in the dorsolateral tegmentum of patients with DLB, specifically around the pedunculopontine cholinergic neurons. Additionally, patients with DLB and those with PDD have been found to have a loss of choline acetyltransferase, the enzyme that synthesizes ACh (Perry *et al.*, 1994; Ballard *et al.*, 2000; Tiraboschi *et al.*, 2000).

Patients with DLB also demonstrate significant alterations in dopamine. Indeed, one of the McKeith (2005) diagnostic criteria is decreased dopamine uptake in the basal ganglia on SPECT/PET, which has been shown to be 78% specific for the detection of a clinical diagnosis of DLB and 90% specific for excluding non-DLB dementia (McKeith *et al.*, 2007). Serial SPECT imaging has found significant longitudinal decreases in striatal dopamine binding across PD, DLB, and PDD. Striatal dopamine was found to decrease at similar rates across PD, DLB and PDD and was correlated with both dementia severity and memory impairment (Colloby *et al.*, 2005). In particular, thalamic D_2 receptors have been found to be elevated in patients with DLB and PDD with parkinsonism; however, patients with DLB but *without* parkinsonism show D_2 receptor levels similar to controls, suggesting that upregulated D_2 receptors and parkinsonism are related (Piggott *et al.*, 2007). As noted above, a failure to upregulate D_2 receptors has been linked to the neuroleptic sensitivity observed in DLB (Piggott *et al.*, 1998).

In summary, DLB is associated with significant deficits in both the cholinergic and dopaminergic systems. These alterations in neurotransmitter systems likely contribute significantly to observed deficits in DLB (e.g. decreased arousal, neuropsychiatric symptoms, motor symptoms) that often occur in the absence of significant brain atrophy.

Structural and functional imaging studies

Structural studies

Studies using structural MRI measures have found atrophy in both DLB and AD with similar rates of brain atrophy over 1 year observed in both disorders (O'Brien *et al.*, 2001). Region-of-interest analyses have found relative preservation of medial temporal lobe structures in DLB relative to AD (Hashimoto *et al.*, 1998; Barber *et al.*, 1999). By comparison, there is increased atrophy in DLB relative to AD in subcortical structures such as the putamen (Cousins *et al.*, 2003) and caudate (Almeida *et al.*, 2003; though see Barber *et al.* (2002) for differing results). Although functional imaging research has consistently found occipital lobe abnormalities in DLB (see below), a study using structural MRI methods found no evidence of occipital lobe atrophy in either DLB or AD compared with controls (Middelkoop *et al.*, 2001). Voxel-based morphometry methods have found greater atrophy in bilateral temporal and frontal lobes and insular cortex in DLB relative to controls, but relative preservation of medial temporal lobe regions in comparison with AD (Burton *et al.*, 2002). Another recent study of this type in a large sample of patients (72 DLB, 72 AD, 72 controls) found that, in comparison with patients with AD, patients with DLB showed focused atrophy in the dorsal midbrain, substantia innominata and hypothalamus in the context of relatively preserved temporoparietal association cortex and medial temporal lobe (Whitwell *et al.*, 2007). Of note, the dorsal midbrain, substantia innominata and hypothalamus are all regions containing cholinergic neurons; therefore, atrophy in these regions may directly contribute to the significant cholinergic deficit observed in DLB.

Functional imaging

Multiple studies using SPECT have found that patients with DLB tend to show the same pattern of hypoperfusion as those with AD, namely in bilateral temporoparietal regions and in the posterior cingulate/precuneus (Ishii *et al.*, 1998; Gilman *et al.*, 2005). However, patients with DLB have additional hypoperfusion in the occipital cortex, a finding not observed in AD (Imamura *et al.*, 2001; Lobotesis *et al.*, 2001). Although the cause of occipital hypoperfusion in DLB is still unclear, one study demonstrating an *increase* in focal occipital perfusion following the administration of donepezil is suggestive of a potential cholinergic mechanism (Mori *et al.*, 2006). Consistent with structural imaging studies, patients with DLB show a relative preservation of medial temporal lobe perfusion compared with those with AD (Ishii *et al.*, 1999).

Research using diffusion tensor imaging, which measures the integrity of white matter, found alterations in the frontal, parietal and occipital white matter of patients with DLB relative to controls (Bozzali *et al.*, 2005). In addition, this study found correlations between frontal white matter integrity and verbal fluency, while parietal white matter integrity was correlated with constructional praxis tasks. Interestingly, a previous study of patients with AD found no evidence of involvement of occipital lobe white matter (Bozzali *et al.*, 2002), findings consistent with SPECT research suggesting that occipital lobe dysfunction is a sensitive marker of DLB.

One study to date has used functional MRI to examine regional differences in brain activity in DLB. Sauer *et al.* (2006) examined resting-state and visual cortex activity in nine patients with DLB compared with 10 with AD and 13 age-matched controls. On visuoperceptual tasks, patients with DLB or AD showed equivalent activation in left ventral occipito-temporal regions during a color task; however, those with DLB showed evidence of *less* activity than the AD group during a face processing task (right fusi-form face area) and motion processing task (right V5). Interestingly, resting-state activity was found to be similar in AD and DLB groups, such that both groups demonstrated a relative lack of deactivation in posterior cingulate/precuneus regions compared with controls (Sauer *et al.*, 2006). Although these results are preliminary, they suggest a differential pattern of brain activity between DLB and AD on some visuo-perceptual tasks, and further suggest that functional MRI may be an important tool in the future for clarifying the neuroanatomical correlates of DLB.

Genetics

Research on the genetic epidemiology of DLB is in its relative infancy. However, familial cases of parkin-sonism have been recognized and several published case reports suggest that the clinical and neuropatho-logical profiles of these cases are heterogeneous. Specifically, one study of familial DLB found that all individuals in one kindred developed the "pure" form of DLB with minimal AD pathology, while another kindred developed features consistent with both Lewy body and AD pathology (Galvin *et al.*, 2002). It has also been suggested that the clinical presentation within kindreds may be quite heterogeneous. For example, another study of a DLB kindred found significant variability in the course of the disease, with some individuals presenting with parkinsonism followed by dementia, while others had cognitive decline prior to the onset of their parkinsonism (e.g. Tsuang *et al.*, 2002). Studies examining the family history of dementia and PD in patients with PD, PDD and DLB have found that a positive family

history of PD was equally as frequent across PD, PDD and DLB; however, a positive family history of dementia was four times as likely in the DLB group compared with either PD or PDD (Papapetropoulos *et al.*, 2006).

Similarities of the presentations in families with DLB and PDD suggest similar underlying genetic mechanisms, and, indeed, several mutations have been found that alter α-synuclein and lead to symp-toms of DLB/PDD (review by Gwinn-Hardy, 2002). *PARK1* is a mutation of the α-synuclein gene that has been associated with familial parkinsonism, including DLB and PDD, with specific mutations having been identified at A53T (Polymeropoluos *et al.*, 1997), A30P (Kruger *et al.*, 2001) and E46K (Zarranz *et al.*, 2004). *PARK2* is a mutation in the *parkin* gene, which is most frequently associated with severe degeneration of dopaminergic neurons in the substantia nigia pars compacta and subsequent early-onset parkinsonism (Abbas *et al.*, 1999); however, *PARK2* has also been associated with Lewy body pathology (Farrer *et al.*, 2001), consistent with a potential link between *parkin* and α-synuclein (Schlossmacher *et al.*, 2002). *PARK3* is associated with a course similar to idiopathic PD (Gasser *et al.*, 1994) while *PARK4* causes a more variable phenotype ranging from PD to DLB (Muenter *et al.*, 1998). *PARK6*, *PARK7* and *PARK8* are all muta-tions on chromosome 1. *PARK6*, in particular, is associ-ated with autosomal recessive early-onset parkinsonism (Valente *et al.*, 2001). Recently, a region of *PARK6*, *PINK1* (coding for the PTEN-induced kinase 1) has been linked to α-synuclein disorders. Specifically, an examination of pathologically confirmed patients with PD, DLB and multisystem atrophy found that PINK1, a putative mitochondrial protein, is present in both the glial cytoplasmic inclusions seen in multi-system atrophy and the Lewy bodies of DLB and PD (Murakami *et al.*, 2007). Although the precise mech-anisms by which PINK1 is associated with Lewy bodies and glial cytoplasmic inclusions is unclear, these results do suggest that PINK1 plays a role in the pathology associated with disorders of α-synuclein.

Another set of studies has found that the triplica-tion of a region within the gene for α-synuclein is associated with autosomal dominant Lewy body dis-ease with a heterogeneous clinical phenotype ranging from typical PD to DLB (Farrer *et al.*, 2004; Singleton *et al.*, 2004), These results suggest that the genetic overexpression of wild-type α-synuclein may lead to clinically significant disease. However, in a large study of sporadic DLB and early-onset PD, examination of the α-synuclein gene did not reveal any significant duplications and/or multiplications in this population, which suggests that this phenomenon may not be a common cause of sporadic parkinsonism and related disorders (Hofer *et al.*, 2005).

In addition to genetic factors that affect α-synuclein expression, DLB/PDD is also associated with genes normally associated with AD. The gene *APOE* encodes apolipoprotein E and is polymorphic. There are three alleles: ε2, ε3 and ε4, giving rise to three isoforms APOE2, APOE3 and APOE4. The *APOE* gene, and in particular the ε4 allele, have previously been associated with an increased risk of AD, with the highest risk occurring in homozygous individuals (i.e. ε4/ε4) (Corder *et al.*, 1993). Given the previously described overlap between DLB and AD pathology, it is not surprising that the APOE4 isoform has also been found to contribute to the presentation of DLB. Patients with DLB have been found to have similarly elevated levels of the ε4 allele when compared with AD; however, patients with DLB show normal levels of ε2 allele, which may be neuroprotective, whereas AD patients have reduced ε2 levels (Singleton *et al.*, 2002). One recent study has suggested an increased frequency of the ε3/ε4 genotype in males with DLB (Rosenberg *et al.*, 2001). Status for ε4 may also increase the risk of developing PDD. Specifically, Pankratz *et al.* (2006) found that patients with PD who had at least one ε4 allele were at an increased risk for developing dementia and also had an earlier age of onset. In another study examining the effects of APOE4 on individuals with either AD only or combined AD/DLB, results suggested that, in individuals with at least one ε4 allele, the odds of having combined AD/DLB were increased nine-fold relative to controls (ε2/ε2), while the odds of having AD/DLB relative to AD only were increased two-fold (Tsuang *et al.*, 2005). These results suggest that individuals carrying ε4 are at increased risk for coexistent Lewy body pathology. As seen in other studies, this effect appeared to be somewhat stronger in males, although the effects were not significant. In one study examining 22 famiilies with a history of AD and DLB, four of the families at neuropathological examinination had a demonstrated linkage to chromosome 12p (Trembath *et al.*, 2003), which has previously been found to be associated with late-onset AD and coexistent synuclein pathology. In particular, it has been suggested that chromosome 12p may be a strong predictor of late-onset combined DLB/AD pathology in individuals lacking an ε4 allele (Scott *et al.*, 2002).

Additionally, significant Lewy body pathology in the context of familial AD has been observed in association with the encoding presenilin-1 mutation E184D (Yokota *et al.*, 2002), as well as other mutations affecting both presenilin and APP (Lippa *et al.*, 1998).

In summary, current results suggest that specific mutations of the α-synuclein gene, including *PARK1* and *PARK6*, are associated with familial parkinsonism, with variable clinical phenotypes including PD, PDD and DLB. Replications within the α-synuclein gene itself can also lead to clinically significant Lewy body disease, although this is an unlikely cause of sporadic disease. The presence of an ε4 allele increases the risk of combined AD/DLB pathology, and mutations in genes for presenilin and APP may also increase α-synuclein pathology, again highlighting the link between AD and DLB pathology.

Treatment/management

Data regarding the efficacy of various pharmacological treatments in DLB are relatively sparse; consequently much of the treatment and management strategies for patients with DLB is derived from clinical observation. However, there is significant evidence suggesting the efficacy of AChEIs and the danger of neuroleptic medications in this population.

Anticholinesterase inhibitors

As described above, patients with DLB have more severe deficits in ACh than those with AD. Therefore, it follows that patients with DLB might be expected to benefit significantly from AChEIs such as donepezil, rivastigmine and galantamine, which are medicines typically prescribed for AD. Kaufer *et al.* (1998) initially described two case studies of patients with DLB who showed significant improvements in attention upon the administration of donepezil. More carefully designed clinical trials have also suggested that AChEIs benefit in DLB. A double-blind placebo-controlled study of 20 weeks of rivastigmine in 487 patients with PDD found decreases in apathy, anxiety, delusions and visual hallucinations and increases in attention and memory (McKeith *et al.*, 2000b). An open-label 20 week trial of donepezil in 30 patients with DLB and 40 with PDD found a 12–15 point decrease in neuropsychiatric symptoms on the NPI and a 3–4 point improvement in MMSE scores (Thomas *et al.*, 2005). Rivastigmine has been noted to improve attention in PDD (Wesnes *et al.*, 2005), while donepezil has been found to lead to improvements in continuity of attention and decreased reaction time variability in both DLB and PDD on computerized tasks of attention (Rowan et al., 2007). Overall, studies examining the effects of AChEIs in DLB/PDD have generally found positive benefits, particularly for reducing neuropsychiatric symptoms and fluctuations in attention. Of note, given the severe cholinergic deficits in DLB, all attempts should be made to avoid medications that have anticholinergic properties, as they contribute to a worsening of symptoms.

Dopaminergic agents
Historically, patients with DLB have been found to show variable effects of levodopa on motor function, and in some cases patients have experienced adverse effects on cognition, including increased hallucinations and confusion (Molloy et al., 2005). However, a more recent study examining the effect of levodopa on cognition in DLB and PDD found that after 3 months both groups demonstrated increases in motor function and subjective alertness in the context of stable cognitive abilities, suggesting that levodopa might benefit some patients with DLB/PDD (Molloy et al., 2006). However, patients with DLB are less likely to respond to levodopa than those with PDD or PD (Bonelli et al., 2004). Specifically, one study found that after 6 months of levodopa treatment, followed by an acute levodopa challenge in the "off" state, only 36% of patients with DLB responded, in comparison to 70% in a PDD group and 57% in a PD group, with a positive response more likely in younger patients (Molloy et al., 2005). Overall, these results suggest that treatment with levodopa will produce a significant motor response in some patients with DLB; however, some patients will demonstrate increased neuropsychiatric symptoms and confusion during levodopa treatment. Therefore, the risks and benefits of using levodopa in patients with DLB should be assessed on an individual patient-by-patient basis.

Neuroleptic sensitivity
As noted previously, patients with DLB are at a significantly increased risk of severe reactions to neuroleptic medications, including an increased risk of mortality, suggesting that the use of typical and atypical antipsychotic medications should generally be avoided in these patients. As described above, many neuropsychiatric symptoms in DLB respond well to AChEIs, thus potentially alleviating the need for

antipsychotic treatment. When needed, low doses of quietiapine have been found to benefit neuropsychiatric symptoms in DLB, with minimal motor side-effects (Fernandez et al., 2002). In addition to the effects of neuroleptics, the use of general anesthesia in patients with DLB can cause delirium with significant confusion and neuropsychiatric symptoms. Therefore, minimizing the length of exposure and strength of anesthesia may be particularly beneficial to these patients.

In summary, there is good evidence suggesting that patients with DLB benefit significantly from treatment with AChEI therapies, with improvements in arousal and cognitive function, as well as observed decreases in neuropsychiatric symptoms such as hallucinations, delusions and anxiety. Evidence is mixed regarding the efficacy of levodopa in the treatment of motor symptoms in DLB, with some studies suggesting that approximately one-third of patients show significant benefit; however, in some cases, levodopa treatment is associated with an increase in neuropsychiatric symptoms. Sensitivity to both neuroleptics and general anesthesia is common in DLB and suggests that extreme caution should be used when administering these treatments. Low doses of quetiapine may be a useful treatment for severe neuropsychiatric symptoms; however, AChEI therapies should typically be the first line of treatment in DLB as they may prevent the need for antipsychotic drugs altogether.

Future research
As discussed throughout the chapter, much of the research on DLB is in its relative infancy. Consequently, the next several decades will prove to be particularly enlightening with respect to understanding the genetic and neuropathological mechanisms that contribute to the clinical syndrome of DLB. One area that would benefit from specific attention is the development of criteria for the early diagnosis of DLB (e.g. mild cognitive impairment DLB [MCI-DLB]). Diagnostic criteria for DLB require the presence of dementia as a core feature of the disorder. However, some individuals have clinical symptoms suggestive of underlying Lewy body pathology (e.g. hallucinations and mild parkinsonism) in the absence of dementia, and thus would not meet the criteria set out by McKeith et al. (2005). The criteria of MCI was created to represent a clinical syndrome predictive of those at-risk for developing AD, and has historically

been focused on the early predominance of memory symptoms (e.g. Petersen *et al.*, 1999; Morris *et al.*, 2001; Grundman *et al.*, 2004.) Patients with DLB may not fit into the "standard" amnestic-MRI criteria owing to their lack of substantial memory impairment; however, there are currently no diagnostic criteria to define "MCI-DLB." Current research suggests that dysautonomia, RBD and neuroleptic sensitivity may all be early features of DLB and could potentially be included in research criteria for MCI-DLB for multiple reasons. First, it is possible that there are individuals who do not yet meet DLB research criteria but who are at-risk for potentially life-threatening neuroleptic reactions and would benefit from early identification. Second, the knowledge that patients with DLB benefit significantly from AChEI therapy begs the question of how individuals with MCI-DLB would respond to early intervention. Last, as clinical trials become available for DLB, the identification of individuals at-risk for developing DLB will be of great importance. In summary, future research into the early identification of the individual at-risk for developing DLB/PDD will expand our knowledge regarding this prevalent disorder and assist with providing these patients with better and earlier therapies.

Summary

In summary, DLB is a clinical disorder characterized by dementia, neuropsychiatric symptoms, parkinsonism and fluctuations in attention. Pathologically, DLB is associated with alterations in α-synuclein, with Lewy body pathology that begins in the brainstem, progresses to the amygdala and limbic cortex, and finally extends into neocortex. Patients with DLB exhibit profound cholinergic deficits that likely contribute to the development of visual hallucinations and fluctuations in attention, and accordingly tend to show excellent response to AChEI therapies. Importantly, these patients are at increased risk for mortality secondary to neuroleptic sensitivity; therefore, antipsychotic drugs should be used with extreme caution in this population. There are many significant clinical and pathological features that overlap in DLB and AD, suggesting that these two disorders may exist on a spectrum. Future research regarding the prodrome of DLB (e.g. "MCI-DLB") would be beneficial in clarifying the earliest features of the disorder and allow for the early identification of patients that may benefit from intervention.

References

Aarsland D, Ballard C, Larsen JP, McKeith I. (2001). A comparative study of psychiatric symptoms in dementia with Lewy bodies and Parkinson's disease with and without dementia. *Int J Geriatr Psychiatry* **16**(5): 528–36.

Aarsland D, Perry R, Larsen JP *et al.* (2005). Neuroleptic sensitivity in Parkinson's disease and parkinsonian dementias. *J Clin Psychiatry* **66**(5): 633–7.

Abbas N, Lucking CB, Richard S *et al.* (1999). A wide variety of mutations in the parkin gene are responsible for autosomal recessive parkinsonism in Europe. French Parkinson's Disease Genetics Study Group and the European Consortium on Genetic Susceptibility in Parkinson's Disease. *Hum Mol Genet* **8**(4): 567–74.

Ala TA, Hughes LF, Kyrouac GA *et al.* (2001). Pentagon copying is more impaired in dementia with Lewy bodies than in Alzheimer's disease. *J Neurol Neurosurg Psychiatry* **70**(4): 483–8.

Allan L, McKeith I, Ballard C, Kenny RA. (2005). Prevalence and severity of gait disorders in Alzheimer's and non-Alzheimer's dementias. *J Am Geriatr Soc* **53**(10): 1681–7.

Allan LM, Ballard CG, Burn DJ, Kenny RA. (2006). The prevalence of autonomic symptoms in dementia and their association with physical activity, activities of daily living and quality of life. *Dement Geriatr Cogn Disord* **22**(3): 230–7.

Allan LM, Ballard CG, Allan, J *et al.* (2007). Autonomic dysfunction in dementia. *J Neurol Neurosurg Psychiatry* **78**: 671–7.

Almeida OP, Burton EJ, McKeith I *et al.* (2003). MRI study of caudate nucleus volume in Parkinson's disease with and without dementia with Lewy bodies and Alzheimer's disease. *Dement Geriatr Cogn Disord* **16**(2): 57–63.

Ballard CG, Grace J, McKeith I, Holmes C. (1997). A detailed phenomenological comparison of complex visual hallucinations in dementia with Lewy bodies and Alzheimer's disease. *International Psychogeriatrics* **9**(4): 381–8.

Ballard CG, McKeith I, Harrison R *et al.* (1998). Neuroleptic sensitivity in dementia with Lewy bodies and Alzheimer's disease. *Lancet* **351**(9108): 1032–3.

Ballard CG, Piggott M, Johnson M *et al.* (2000). Delusions associated with elevated muscarinic binding in dementia with Lewy bodies. *Ann Neurol* **48**(6): 868–76.

Ballard CG, Aarsland D, McKeith I *et al.* (2002). Fluctuations in attention: PD dementia vs DLB with parkinsonism. *Neurology* **59**(11): 1714–20.

Ballard CG, Perry RH, McKeith IG, Perry EK. (2005). Neuroleptics are associated with more severe tangle pathology in dementia with Lewy bodies. *Int J Geriatr Psychiatry* **20**(9): 872–5.

Barber R, Gholkar A, Scheltens P et al. (1999). Medial temporal lobe atrophy on MRI in dementia with Lewy bodies. Neurology 52(6): 1153–8.

Barber R, McKeith I, Ballard C, O'Brien J. (2002). Volumetric MRI study of the caudate nucleus in patients with dementia with Lewy bodies, Alzheimer's disease, and vascular dementia. J Neurol Neurosurg Psychiatry 72(3): 406–7.

Benke T. (2006). Peduncular hallucinosis: a syndrome of impaired reality monitoring. J Neurol 253(12): 1561–71.

Boddy F, Rowan EN, Lett D et al. (2007). Subjectively reported sleep quality and excessive daytime somnolence in Parkinson's disease with and without dementia, dementia with Lewy bodies and Alzheimer's disease. Int J Geriatr Psychiatry 22: 529–35.

Boeve BF, Silber MH, Ferman TJ et al. (1998). REM sleep behavior disorder and degenerative dementia: an association likely reflecting Lewy body disease. Neurology 51(2): 363–70.

Boeve BF, Silber MH, Parisi JE et al. (2001). Association of REM sleep behavior disorder and neurodegenerative disease may reflect an underlying synucleinopathy. Mov Disord 16(4): 622–30.

Boeve BF, Silber MH, Ferman TJ. (2003). Synucleinopathy pathology and REM sleep behavior disorder plus dementia or parkinsonism. Neurology 61(1): 40–5.

Boeve BF, Silber MH, Ferman TJ et al. (2004). REM sleep behavior disorder in Parkinson's disease and dementia with Lewy bodies. J Geriatr Psychiatry Neurol 17(3): 146–57.

Boeve BF, Silber MH, Saper CB et al. (2007). Pathophysiology of REM sleep behavior disorder and relevance to neurodegenerative disease. Brain 130: 2770–88.

Bonelli SB, Ransmayr G, Steffelbauer M et al. (2004). L-Dopa responsiveness in dementia with Lewy bodies, Parkinson disease with and without dementia. Neurology 63: 376–8.

Borroni B, Agosti C, Padovani A. (2007). Behavioral and psychological symptoms in dementia with Lewy-bodies (DLB): frequency and relationship with disease severity and motor impairment. Arch Gerontol Geriatr 46: 101–6.

Bostrom F, Jonsson L, Minthon L, Londos E. (2006). Patients with Lewy body dementia use more resources than those with Alzheimer's disease. Int J Geriatr Psychiatry 22: 713–19.

Bozzali M, Falini A, Cercignani M et al. (2002). White matter damage in Alzheimer's disease assessed in vivo using diffusion tensor magnetic resonance imaging. J Neurol Neurosurg Psychiatry 72(6): 742–6.

Bozzali M, Falini A, Franceschi M et al. (2005). Brain tissue damage in dementia with Lewy bodies: an in vivo diffusion tensor MRI study. Brain 128(Pt 7): 1595–604.

Braak H, Del Tredici K, Rub U et al. (2003). Staging of brain pathology related to sporadic Parkinson's disease. Neurobiol Aging 24(2): 197–211.

Bradshaw J, Saling M, Hopwood M et al. (2004). Fluctuating cognition in dementia with Lewy bodies and Alzheimer's disease is qualitatively distinct. J Neurol Neurosurg Psychiatry 75(3): 382–7.

Briel RC, McKeith IG, Barker WA et al. (1999). EEG findings in dementia with Lewy bodies and Alzheimer's disease. J Neurol Neurosurg Psychiatry 66(3): 401–3.

Bullock R, Cameron A. (2002). Rivastigmine for the treatment of dementia and visual hallucinations associated with Parkinson's disease: a case series. Curr Med Res Opin 18(5): 258–64.

Burke WJ, Pfeiffer RF, McComb RD. (1998). Neuroleptic sensitivity to clozapine in dementia with Lewy bodies. J Neuropsychiatry Clin Neurosci 10(2): 227–9.

Burn D, Emre M, McKeith I et al. (2003). Extrapyramidal features in Parkinson's disease with and without dementia and dementia with Lewy bodies: a cross-sectional comparative study. Mov Disord 18(8): 884–9.

Burn DJ, Rowan EN, Minett T et al. (2006). Effects of rivastigmine in patients with and without visual hallucinations in dementia associated with Parkinson's disease. Mov Disord 21(11): 1899–907.

Burton EJ, Karas G, Paling SM et al. (2002). Patterns of cerebral atrophy in dementia with Lewy bodies using voxel-based morphometry. Neuroimage 17(2): 618–30.

Collerton D, Burn D, McKeith I, O'Brien J. (2003). Systematic review and meta-analysis show that dementia with Lewy bodies is a visual-perceptual and attentional-executive dementia. Dement Geriatr Cogn Disord 16(4): 229–37.

Collerton D, Perry E, McKeith I. (2005). Why people see things that are not there: a novel perception and attention deficit model for recurrent complex visual hallucinations. Behav Brain Sci 28(6): 737–57; discussion 757–94.

Colloby SJ, Williams ED, Burn DJ et al. (2005). Progression of dopaminergic degeneration in dementia with Lewy bodies and Parkinson's disease with and without dementia assessed using ^{123}I-FP-CIT SPECT. Eur J Nucl Med Mol Imaging 32(10): 1176–85.

Corder EH, Saunders AM, Strittmatter WJ et al. (1993). Gene dose of apolipoprotein E type 4 allele and the risk of Alzheimer's disease in late onset families. Science 261(5123): 921–3.

Cormack F, Aarsland D, Ballard C, Tovee MJ. (2004). Pentagon drawing and neuropsychological performance in dementia with Lewy bodies, Alzheimer's disease, Parkinson's disease and Parkinson's disease with dementia. Int J Geriatr Psychiatry 19(4): 371–7.

Cousins DA, Burton EJ, Burn D et al. (2003). Atrophy of the putamen in dementia with Lewy bodies but not Alzheimer's disease: an MRI study. Neurology 61(9): 1191–5.

Crowell TA, Luis CA, Cox DE, Mullan M. (2007). Neuropsychological comparison of Alzheimer's disease and dementia with Lewy bodies. *Dement Geriatr Cogn Disord* **23**(2): 120–5.

Del Ser T, McKeith I, Anand R *et al.* (2000). Dementia with Lewy bodies: findings from an international multicentre study. *Int J Geriatr Psychiatry* **15**(11): 1034–45.

Doran M, Larner AJ. (2004). EEG findings in dementia with Lewy bodies causing diagnostic confusion with sporadic Creutzfeldt–Jakob disease. *Eur J Neurol* **11**(12): 838–41.

Ellis HD, Young AW, Quayle AH, De Pauw KW. (1997). Reduced autonomic responses to faces in Capgras delusion. *Proc Biol Sci* **264**(1384): 1085–92.

Emre M. (2003). Dementia associated with Parkinson's disease. *Lancet Neurol* **2**(4): 229–37.

Farrer M, Chan P, Chen R *et al.* (2001). Lewy bodies and parkinsonism in families with parkin mutations. *Ann Neurol* **50**(3): 293–300.

Farrer M, Kachergus J, Forno L *et al.* (2004). Comparison of kindreds with parkinsonism and alpha-synuclein genomic multiplications. *Ann Neurol* **55**(2): 174–9.

Ferman TJ, Boeve BF, Smith GE *et al.* (1999). REM sleep behavior disorder and dementia: cognitive differences when compared with AD. *Neurology* **52**(5): 951–7.

Ferman TJ, Smith GE, Boeve BF *et al.* (2004). DLB fluctuations: specific features that reliably differentiate DLB from AD and normal aging. *Neurology* **62**(2): 181–7.

Ferman TJ, Smith GE, Boeve BF *et al.* (2006). Neuropsychological differentiation of dementia with Lewy bodies from normal aging and Alzheimer's disease. *Clin Neuropsychol* **20**(4): 623–36.

Fernandez HH, Trieschmann ME, Burke MA, Friedman JH. (2002). Quetiapine for psychosis in Parkinson's disease versus dementia with Lewy bodies. *J Clin Psychiatry* **63**(6): 513–5.

Ffytche DH, Howard RJ, Brammer MJ *et al.* (1998). The anatomy of conscious vision: an fMRI study of visual hallucinations. *Nat Neurosci* **1**(8): 738–42.

Galasko D, Saitoh T, Xia Y *et al.* (1994). The apolipoprotein E allele epsilon 4 is overrepresented in patients with the Lewy body variant of Alzheimer's disease. *Neurology* **44**(10): 1950–1.

Galvin JE, Lee SL, Perry A *et al.* (2002). Familial dementia with Lewy bodies: clinicopathologic analysis of two kindreds. *Neurology* **59**(7): 1079–82.

Galvin JE, Pollack J, Morris JC. (2006). Clinical phenotype of Parkinson disease dementia. *Neurology* **67**(9): 1605–11.

Gasser T, Wszolek ZK, Trofatter J *et al.* (1994). Genetic linkage studies in autosomal dominant parkinsonism: evaluation of seven candidate genes. *Ann Neurol* **36**(3): 387–96.

Gilman S, Koeppe RA, Little R *et al.* (2005). Differentiation of Alzheimer's disease from dementia with Lewy bodies utilizing positron emission tomography with [^{18}F] fluorodeoxyglucose and neuropsychological testing. *Exp Neurol* **191**(Suppl 1): S95–103.

Gnanalingham KK, Byrne EJ, Thornton A *et al.* (1997). Motor and cognitive function in Lewy body dementia: comparison with Alzheimer's and Parkinson's diseases. *J Neurol Neurosurg Psychiatry* **62**(3): 243–52.

Gomez-Tortosa E, Newell K, Irizarry MC *et al.* (1999). Clinical and quantitative pathologic correlates of dementia with Lewy bodies. *Neurology* **53**(6): 1284–91.

Grace JB, Walker MP, McKeith IG. (2000). A comparison of sleep profiles in patients with dementia with Lewy bodies and Alzheimer's disease. *Int J Geriatr Psychiatry* **15**(11): 1028–33.

Grundman M, Petersen RC, Ferris SH *et al.* (2004). Mild cognitive impairment can be distinguished from Alzheimer disease and normal aging for clinical trials. *Arch Neurol* **61**(1): 59–66.

Guidi M, Paciaroni L, Paolini S *et al.* (2006). Differences and similarities in the neuropsychological profile of dementia with Lewy bodies and Alzheimer's disease in the early stage. *J Neurol Sci* **248**(1–2): 120–3.

Gwinn-Hardy K. (2002). Genetics of parkinsonism. *Mov Disord* **17**(4): 645–56.

Hamilton JM, Salmon DP, Galasko D *et al.* (2000). Lewy bodies in Alzheimer's disease: a neuropathological review of 145 cases using alpha-synuclein immunohistochemistry. *Brain Pathol* **10**(3): 378–84.

Hamilton RL. (2004). A comparison of episodic memory deficits in neuropathologically confirmed dementia with Lewy bodies and Alzheimer's disease. *J Int Neuropsychol Soc* **10**(5): 689–97.

Harding AJ, Broe GA, Halliday GM. (2002). Visual hallucinations in Lewy body disease relate to Lewy bodies in the temporal lobe. *Brain* **125**(Pt 2): 391–403.

Hashimoto M, Kitagaki H, Imamura T *et al.* (1998). Medial temporal and whole-brain atrophy in dementia with Lewy bodies: a volumetric MRI study. *Neurology* **51**(2): 357–62.

Hirayama K, Meguro K, Shimada M *et al.* (2003). [A case of probable dementia with Lewy bodies presenting with geographic mislocation and nurturing syndrome.] *No To Shinkei* **55**(9): 782–9.

Hirstein W, Ramachandran VS. (1997). Capgras syndrome: a novel probe for understanding the neural representation of the identity and familiarity of persons. *Proc Biol Sci* **264**(1380): 437–44.

Hofer A, Berg D, Asmus F *et al.* (2005). The role of alpha-synuclein gene multiplications in early-onset Parkinson's disease and dementia with Lewy bodies. *J Neural Transm* **112**(9): 1249–54.

Horimoto Y, Matsumoto M, Akatsu H *et al.* (2003). Autonomic dysfunctions in dementia with Lewy bodies. *J Neurol* **250**(5): 530–3.

22

Imamura T, Ishii K, Hirono N et al. (1999). Visual hallucinations and regional cerebral metabolism in dementia with Lewy bodies (DLB). Neuroreport 10(9): 1903–7.

Imamura T, Ishii K, Hirono N et al. (2001). Occipital glucose metabolism in dementia with Lewy bodies with and without Parkinsonism: a study using positron emission tomography. Dement Geriatr Cogn Disord 12(3): 194–7.

Ishii K, Imamura T, Sasaki M et al. (1998). Regional cerebral glucose metabolism in dementia with Lewy bodies and Alzheimer's disease. Neurology 51(1): 125–30.

Ishii K, Yamaji S, Kitagaki H et al. (1999). Regional cerebral blood flow difference between dementia with Lewy bodies and AD. Neurology 53(2): 413–6.

Jankovic J, McDermott M, Carter J et al. (1990). Variable expression of Parkinson's disease: a base-line analysis of the DATATOP cohort. The Parkinson Study Group. Neurology 40(10): 1529–34.

Johnson DK, Morris JC, Galvin JE. (2005). Verbal and visuospatial deficits in dementia with Lewy bodies. Neurology 65(8): 1232–8.

Kaufer DI, Catt KE, Lopez OL, DeKosky ST. (1998). Dementia with Lewy bodies: response of delirium-like features to donepezil. Neurology 51(5): 1512.

Kaufmann H, Nahm K, Purohit D, Wolfe D. (2004). Autonomic failure as the initial presentation of Parkinson disease and dementia with Lewy bodies. Neurology 63(6): 1093–5.

Kopito RR. (2000). Aggresomes, inclusion bodies and protein aggregation. Trends Cell Biol 10(12): 524–30.

Kramer ML, Schulz-Schaeffer WJ. (2007). Presynaptic alpha-synuclein aggregates, not Lewy bodies, cause neurodegeneration in dementia with Lewy bodies. J Neurosci 27(6): 1405–10.

Kraybill ML, Larson EB, Tsuang DW et al. (2005). Cognitive differences in dementia patients with autopsy-verified AD, Lewy body pathology, or both. Neurology 64(12): 2069–73.

Kruger R, Kuhn W, Leenders KL et al. (2001). Familial parkinsonism with synuclein pathology: clinical and PET studies of A30P mutation carriers. Neurology 56(10): 1355–62.

Lippa CF, Smith TW, Saunders AM et al. (1995). Apolipoprotein E genotype and Lewy body disease. Neurology 45: 97–103.

Lippa CF, Fujiwara H, Mann DM et al. (1998). Lewy bodies contain altered alpha-synuclein in brains of many familial Alzheimer's disease patients with mutations in presenilin and amyloid precursor protein genes. Am J Pathol 153(5): 1365–70.

Lippa CF, Duda JE, Grossman M et al. (2007). DLB and PDD boundary issues: diagnosis, treatment, molecular pathology, and biomarkers. Neurology 68(11): 812–9.

Litvan I, MacIntyre A, Goetz CG et al. (1998). Accuracy of the clinical diagnoses of Lewy body disease, Parkinson disease, and dementia with Lewy bodies: a clinicopathologic study. Arch Neurol 55(7): 969–78.

Liu CW, Giasson BI, Lewis KA et al. (2005). A precipitating role for truncated alpha-synuclein and the proteasome in alpha-synuclein aggregation: implications for pathogenesis of Parkinson disease. J Biol Chem 280(24): 22670–8.

Lobotesis K, Fenwick JD, Phipps A et al. (2001). Occipital hypoperfusion on SPECT in dementia with Lewy bodies but not AD. Neurology 56(5): 643–9.

Lopez OL, Becker JT, Kaufer DI et al. (2002). Research evaluation and prospective diagnosis of dementia with Lewy bodies. Arch Neurol 59(1): 43–6.

Mandal PK, Pettegrew JW, Masliah E et al. (2006). Interaction between Abeta peptide and alpha synuclein: molecular mechanisms in overlapping pathology of Alzheimer's and Parkinson's in dementia with Lewy body disease. Neurochem Res 31(9): 1153–62.

Marantz AG, Verghese J. (2002). Capgras' syndrome in dementia with Lewy bodies. J Geriatr Psychiatry Neurol 15(4): 239–41.

Marui W, Iseki E, Kato M et al. (2002). Progression and staging of Lewy pathology in brains from patients with dementia with Lewy bodies. J Neurol Sci 195(2): 153–9.

Marui W, Iseki E, Nakai T et al. (2004). Pathological entity of dementia with Lewy bodies and its differentiation from Alzheimer's disease. Acta Neuropathol (Berl) 108(2): 121–8.

Masliah E, Rockenstein E, Veinbergs I et al. (2001). Beta-amyloid peptides enhance alpha-synuclein accumulation and neuronal deficits in a transgenic mouse model linking Alzheimer's disease and Parkinson's disease. Proc Natl Acad Sci USA 98(21): 12245–50.

Maurage CA, Ruchoux MM, de Vos R et al. (2003). Retinal involvement in dementia with Lewy bodies: a clue to hallucinations? Ann Neurol 54(4): 542–7.

McKeith IG. (2000). Spectrum of Parkinson's disease, Parkinson's dementia, and Lewy body dementia. Neurol Clin 18(4): 865–902.

McKeith IG. (2002). Dementia with Lewy bodies. Br J Psychiatry 180: 144–7.

McKeith IG, Fairbairn A, Perry R et al. (1992). Neuroleptic sensitivity in patients with senile dementia of Lewy body type. BMJ 305(6855): 673–8.

McKeith IG, Galasko D, Kosaka K et al. (1996). Consensus guidelines for the clinical and pathologic diagnosis of dementia with Lewy bodies (DLB): report of the consortium on DLB international workshop. Neurology 47(5): 1113–24.

McKeith IG, Ballard CG, Perry RH et al. (2000a). Prospective validation of consensus criteria for the diagnosis of dementia with Lewy bodies. *Neurology* **54**(5): 1050–8.

McKeith IG, Del Sero T, Spano P *et al.* (2000b). Efficacy of rivastigmine in dementia with Lewy bodies: a randomised, double-blind, placebo-controlled international study. *Lancet* **356**(9247): 2031–6.

McKeith IG, Mintzer J, Aarsland D *et al.* (2004a). Dementia with Lewy bodies. *Lancet Neurol* **3**(1): 19–28.

McKeith IG, Wesnes KA, Perry E, Ferrara R. (2004b). Hallucinations predict attentional improvements with rivastigmine in dementia with Lewy bodies. *Dement Geriatr Cogn Disord* **18**(1): 94–100.

McKeith IG, Dickson DW, Lowe J *et al.* (2005). Diagnosis and management of dementia with Lewy bodies: third report of the DLB Consortium. *Neurology* **65**(12): 1863–72.

McKeith I, O'Brien J, Walker Z *et al.* (2007). Sensitivity and specificity of dopamine transporter imaging with ^{123}I-FP-CIT SPECT in dementia with Lewy bodies: a phase III, multicentre study. *Lancet Neurol* **6**(4): 305–13.

McNaught KS, Shashidharan P, Perl DP *et al.* (2002). Aggresome-related biogenesis of Lewy bodies. *Eur J Neurosci* **16**(11): 2136–48.

Merdes AR, Hansen LA, Jeste DV *et al.* (2003). Influence of Alzheimer pathology on clinical diagnostic accuracy in dementia with Lewy bodies. *Neurology* **60**(10): 1586–90.

Middelkoop HA, van der Flier WM, Burton EJ *et al.* (2001). Dementia with Lewy bodies and AD are not associated with occipital lobe atrophy on MRI. *Neurology* **57**(11): 2117–20.

Molloy S, McKeith IG, O'Brien JT, Burn DJ. (2005). The role of levodopa in the management of dementia with Lewy bodies. *J Neurol Neurosurg Psychiatry* **76**(9): 1200–3.

Molloy SA, Rowan EN, O'Brien JT *et al.* (2006). Effect of levodopa on cognitive function in Parkinson's disease with and without dementia and dementia with Lewy bodies. *J Neurol Neurosurg Psychiatry* **77**(12): 1323–8.

Mori E, Shimomura T, Fujimori M *et al.* (2000). Visuoperceptual impairment in dementia with Lewy bodies. *Arch Neurol* **57**(4): 489–93.

Mori T, Ikeda M, Fukuhara R *et al.* (2006). Correlation of visual hallucinations with occipital rCBF changes by donepezil in DLB. *Neurology* **66**(6): 935–7.

Morris JC, Storandt M, Miller JP *et al.* (2001). Mild cognitive impairment represents early-stage Alzheimer disease. *Arch Neurol* **58**(3): 397–405.

Mosimann UP, Rowan EN, Partington CE *et al.* (2006). Characteristics of visual hallucinations in Parkinson disease dementia and dementia with Lewy bodies. *Am J Geriatr Psychiatry* **14**(2): 153–60.

Muenter MD, Forno LS, Hornykiewicz O *et al.* (1998). Hereditary form of parkinsonism–dementia. *Ann Neurol* **43**(6): 768–81.

Murakami T, Moriwaki Y, Kawarabayashi T *et al.* (2007). PINK1, a gene product of *PARK6*, accumulates in α-synucleinopathy brains. *J Neurol Neurosurg Psychiatry* **78**: 653–4.

Murman DL, Kuo SB, Powell MC, Colenda CC. (2003). The impact of parkinsonism on costs of care in patients with AD and dementia with Lewy bodies. *Neurology* **61**(7): 944–9.

Nishijima K, Ishiguro T. (1989). [Clinical course and CSF monoamine metabolism in neuroleptic malignant syndrome: a study of nine typical cases and five mild cases.] *Seishin Shinkeigaku Zasshi [Psychiatr Neurol Jpn]* **91**(6): 429–56.

O'Brien JT, Paling S, Barber R *et al.* (2001). Progressive brain atrophy on serial MRI in dementia with Lewy bodies, AD, and vascular dementia. *Neurology* **56**(10): 1386–8.

Ohara K, Morita Y. (2006). [Case with probable dementia with Lewy bodies, who shows reduplicative paramnesia and Capgras syndrome.] *Seishin Shinkeigaku Zasshi [Psychiatr Neurol Jpn]* **108**(7): 705–14.

Oka H, Morita M, Onouchi K *et al.* (2007). Cardiovascular autonomic dysfunction in dementia with Lewy bodies and Parkinson's disease. *J Neurol Sci* **254**(1–2): 72–7.

Olson EJ, Boeve BF, Silber MH. (2000). Rapid eye movement sleep behavior disorder: demographic, clinical and laboratory findings in 93 cases. *Brain* **123** (Pt 2): 331–9.

Pankratz N, Byder L, Halter C *et al.* (2006). Presence of an *APOE4* allele results in significantly earlier onset of Parkinson's disease and a higher risk with dementia. *Mov Disord* **21**(1): 45–9.

Papapetropoulos S, Lieberman A, Gonzalez J *et al.* (2006). Family history of dementia: dementia with Lewy bodies and dementia in Parkinson's disease. *J Neuropsychiatry Clin Neurosci* **18**(1): 113–6.

Perriol MP, Dujardin K, Derambure P *et al.* (2005). Disturbance of sensory filtering in dementia with Lewy bodies: comparison with Parkinson's disease dementia and Alzheimer's disease. *J Neurol Neurosurg Psychiatry* **76**(1): 106–8.

Perry EK, Haroutunian V, Davis KL *et al.* (1994). Neocortical cholinergic activities differentiate Lewy body dementia from classical Alzheimer's disease. *Neuroreport* **5**(7): 747–9.

Perry EK, Morris CM, Court JA *et al.* (1995). Acetylcholine and hallucinations: disease-related compared to drug-induced alterations in human consciousness. *Brain Cogn* **28**(3): 240–58.

Perry EK, Perry RH. (1995). Alteration in nicotine binding sites in Parkinson's disease, Lewy body dementia and Alzheimer's disease: possible index of early neuropathology. *Neuroscience* **64**(2): 385–95.

Petersen RC, Smith GE, Waring SC et al. (1999). Mild cognitive impairment: clinical characterization and outcome. Arch Neurol 56(3): 303–8.

Piggott MA, Perry EK, Marshall EF et al. (1998). Nigrostriatal dopaminergic activities in dementia with Lewy bodies in relation to neuroleptic sensitivity: comparisons with Parkinson's disease. Biol Psychiatry 44(8): 765–74.

Piggott MA, Ballard CG, Dickinson HO et al. (2007). Thalamic D_2 receptors in dementia with Lewy bodies, Parkinson's disease, and Parkinson's disease dementia. Int J Neuropsychopharmacol 10(2): 231–44.

Pletnikova O, West N, Lee MK et al. (2005). Abeta deposition is associated with enhanced cortical alpha-synuclein lesions in Lewy body diseases. Neurobiol Aging 26(8): 1183–92.

Polymeropoulos MH, Lavedan C, Leroy E et al. (1997). Mutation in the alpha-synuclein gene identified in families with Parkinson's disease. Science 276(5321): 2045–7.

Rahkonen T, Eloniemi-Sulkava U, Rissanen S et al. (2003). Dementia with Lewy bodies according to the consensus criteria in a general population aged 75 years or older. J Neurol Neurosurg Psychiatry 74(6): 720–4.

Rockwell E, Choure J, Galasko D et al. (2000). Psychopathology at initial diagnosis in dementia with Lewy bodies versus Alzheimer disease: comparison of matched groups with autopsy-confirmed diagnoses. Int J Geriatr Psychiatry 15(9): 819–23.

Rosenberg CK, Cummings TJ, Saunders AM et al. (2001). Dementia with Lewy bodies and Alzheimer's disease. Acta Neuropathol (Berl) 102(6): 621–6.

Rowan E, McKeith IG, Saxby BK et al. (2007). Effects of donepezil on central processing speed and attentional measures in Parkinson's disease with dementia and dementia with Lewy bodies. Dement Geriatr Cogn Disord 23(3): 161–7.

Sadek J, Rockwood K. (2003). Coma with accidental single dose of an atypical neuroleptic in a patient with Lewy body dementia. Am J Geriatr Psychiatry 11(1): 112–3.

Saito Y, Ruberu NN, Sawabe M et al. (2004). Lewy body-related alpha-synucleinopathy in aging. J Neuropathol Exp Neurol 63(7): 742–9.

Sakakibara R, Ito T, Uchiyama T et al. (2005). Lower urinary tract function in dementia of Lewy body type. J Neurol Neurosurg Psychiatry 76(5): 729–32.

Santhouse AM, Howard RJ, ffytche DH (2000). Visual hallucinatory syndromes and the anatomy of the visual brain. Brain 123(Pt 10): 2055–64.

Sauer J, ffytche DH, Ballard C et al. (2006). Differences between Alzheimer's disease and dementia with Lewy bodies: an fMRI study of task-related brain activity. Brain 129(Pt 7): 1780–8.

Schenck CH, Bundlie SR Ettinger MG, Mahowald MW. (2002). REM sleep behavior disorder: clinical, developmental, and neuroscience perspectives 16 years after its formal identification in SLEEP. Sleep 25(2): 120–38.

Schenck CH, Mahowald MW (2002). Chronic behavioral disorders of human REM sleep: a new category of parasomnia. 1986 [classical article]. Sleep 25(2): 293–308.

Schlossmacher MG, Frosch MP, Gai WP et al. (2002). Parkin localizes to the Lewy bodies of Parkinson disease and dementia with Lewy bodies. Am J Pathol 160(5): 1655–67.

Schmidt ML, Martin JA, Lee VM, Trojanowski JQ. (1996). Convergence of Lewy bodies and neurofibrillary tangles in amygdala neurons of Alzheimer's disease and Lewy body disorders. Acta Neuropathol (Berl) 91(5): 475–81.

Scott WK, Vance JM, Haines JL, Pericak-Vance MA. (2002). Linkage of parkinsonism and Alzheimer's disease with Lewy body pathology to chromosome 12. Ann Neurol 52(4): 524; author reply 524.

Sechi G, Agnetti V, Masuri R et al. (1996). Acute hyponatremia and neuroleptic malignant syndrome in Parkinson's disease. Prog Neuropsychopharmacol Biol Psychiatry 20(3): 533–42.

Sechi G, Manca S, Deiana GA et al. (2000). Risperidone, neuroleptic malignant syndrome and probable dementia with Lewy bodies. Prog Neuropsychopharmacol Biol Psychiatry 24(6): 1043–51.

Simard M, van Reekum R, Cohen T. (2000). A review of the cognitive and behavioral symptoms in dementia with Lewy bodies. J Neuropsychiatry Clin Neurosci 12(4): 425–50.

Singleton A, Gwinn-Hardy K, Sharabi Y et al. (2002). Clinical and neuropathological correlates of apolipoprotein E genotype in dementia with Lewy bodies. Dement Geriatr Cogn Disord 14(4): 167–75.

Singleton AB, Wharton A, O'Brien KK et al. (2004). Association between cardiac denervation and parkinsonism caused by alpha-synuclein gene triplication. Brain 127(Pt 4): 768–72.

Stavitsky K, Brickman AM, Scarmeas N et al. (2006). The progression of cognition, psychiatric symptoms, and functional abilities in dementia with Lewy bodies and Alzheimer disease. Arch Neurol 63(10): 1450–6.

Suzuki M, Kurita A, Hashimoto M et al. (2006). Impaired myocardial ^{123}I-metaiodobenzylguanidine uptake in Lewy body disease: comparison between dementia with Lewy bodies and Parkinson's disease. J Neurol Sci 240(1–2): 15–19.

Tan A, Salgado M, Fahn S. (1996). Rapid eye movement sleep behavior disorder preceding Parkinson's disease with therapeutic response to levodopa. Mov Disord 11(2): 214–6.

Thaisetthawatkul P, Boeve BF, Benarroch EE *et al.* (2004). Autonomic dysfunction in dementia with Lewy bodies. *Neurology* **62**(10): 1804–9.

Thomas DA, Libon DJ, Ledakis GE. (2005). Treating dementia patients with vascular lesions with donepezil: a preliminary analysis. *Appl Neuropsychol* **12**(1): 12–18.

Tiraboschi P, Hansen LA, Alford M *et al.* (2000). Cholinergic dysfunction in diseases with Lewy bodies. *Neurology* **54**(2): 407–11.

Trembath Y, Rosenberg C, Ervin JF *et al.* (2003). Lewy body pathology is a frequent co-pathology in familial Alzheimer's disease. *Acta Neuropathol (Berl)* **105**(5): 484–8.

Tsuang DW, Dalan AM, Eugenio CJ *et al.* (2002). Familial dementia with Lewy bodies: a clinical and neuropathological study of 2 families. *Arch Neurol* **59**(10): 1622–30.

Tsuang DW, Wilson RK, Lopez OL *et al.* (2005). Genetic association between the *APOE*4* allele and Lewy bodies in Alzheimer disease. *Neurology* **64**(3): 509–13.

Valente EM, Bentivoglio AR, Dixon PH *et al.* (2001). Localization of a novel locus for autosomal recessive early-onset parkinsonism, *PARK6*, on human chromosome 1p35–p36. *Am J Hum Genet* **68**(4): 895–900.

Walker MP, Ayre GA, Cummings JL *et al.* (2000a). The Clinician Assessment of Fluctuation and the One Day Fluctuation Assessment Scale. Two methods to assess fluctuating confusion in dementia. *Br J Psychiatry* **177**: 252–6.

Walker MP, Ayre GA, Cummings JL *et al.* (2000b). Quantifying fluctuation in dementia with Lewy bodies, Alzheimer's disease, and vascular dementia. *Neurology* **54**(8): 1616–25.

Wenning GK, Scherfler C, Granata R *et al.* (1999). Time course of symptomatic orthostatic hypotension and urinary incontinence in patients with postmortem confirmed parkinsonian syndromes: a clinicopathological study. *J Neurol Neurosurg Psychiatry* **67**(5): 620–3.

Wesnes KA, McKeith I, Edgar C *et al.* (2005). Benefits of rivastigmine on attention in dementia associated with Parkinson disease. *Neurology* **65**(10): 1654–6.

Whitwell JL, Weigand SD, Shiung MM *et al.* (2007). Focal atrophy in dementia with Lewy bodies on MRI: a distinct pattern from Alzheimer's disease. *Brain* **130**(Pt 3): 708–19.

Williams MM, Xiong C, Morris JC, Galvin JE. (2006). Survival and mortality differences between dementia with Lewy bodies vs Alzheimer disease. *Neurology* **67**(11): 1935–41.

Yamamoto T, Imai T. (1988). A case of diffuse Lewy body and Alzheimer's diseases with periodic synchronous discharges. *J Neuropathol Exp Neurol* **47**(5): 536–48.

Yokota O, Terada S, Ishizu H *et al.* (2002). NACP/alpha-synuclein immunoreactivity in diffuse neurofibrillary tangles with calcification (DNTC). *Acta Neuropathol (Berl)* **104**(4): 333–41.

Yoshita M, Taki J, Yokoyama K *et al.* (2006). Value of ^{123}I-MIBG radioactivity in the differential diagnosis of DLB from AD. *Neurology* **66**(12): 1850–4.

Zaccai J, McCracken C, Brayne C. (2005). A systematic review of prevalence and incidence studies of dementia with Lewy bodies. *Age Ageing* **34**(6): 561–6.

Zarranz JJ, Alegre J, Gomez-Esteban JC *et al.* (2004). The new mutation, E46K, of alpha-synuclein causes Parkinson and Lewy body dementia. *Ann Neurol* **55**(2): 164–73.

Chapter 3

Neurogenetics of dementia

Huidy Shu

The molecular era of human genetics began in 1983 when an intrepid group of clinicians and scientists led by James Gusella and Nancy Wexler mapped the gene mutation that causes Huntington's disease (HD) to the short arm of human chromosome 4.[1] In the 25 years since this discovery, the new field of human neurogenetics has provided an unprecedented explosion in our molecular understanding of dementia. Aided by the "completion" of the Human Genome Project, scientists continue to discover new gene mutations that cause rare but highly penetrant familial dementia syndromes. The study of these genes and the proteins they encode have provided us with plausible hypotheses for the biochemical underpinnings of these rare diseases as well as the more common syndromes to which they are related.

Traditional disease gene discovery has been performed through the processes of "linkage analysis" and "positional cloning."[2,3] These methods make no a priori assumptions about the biochemical function of the protein corresponding to the mutant gene but instead rely upon the discovery of the physical location of the mutation on one of the chromosomes. They require the phenotypic characterization of one or more large families through which the disease phenotype segregates. In general, larger families provide more genetic information through the number of meiotic recombination events. Genetic material from each available member of the family is scored for a panel of DNA polymorphisms, or "markers", spanning each human chromosome. The goal is to find a statistical linkage between the disease phenotype and individual marker alleles, which is represented statistically as a "logarithm of the odds" or LOD score. A value of $+3$, in general, represents a significant genetic linkage, corresponding to the conventional $p < 0.05$ threshold for statistical significance. Once

linkage is established with one "marker", more precise mapping can be performed with even more closely spaced DNA polymorphisms in the local chromosomal region. The most optimistic scenario for this type of analysis is linkage to a chromosomal region approximately 1 million base pairs of DNA in length. In analyses with no linkage, confounding factors can include phenotypic uncertainty caused by incomplete penetrance, variable expressivity, complex inheritance, non-paternity or just plain misdiagnosis.

Once the candidate region has been narrowed to the limit of resolution made possible by the number of meiotic events within the affected family, a search for the causative mutation can begin.[3] A map of every gene within nearly every chromosomal region is available online now through the Human Genome Project.[4,5] Large-scale sequencing of the coding regions of these candidate genes in DNA samples from family members is then usually necessary to find the specific mutation that is associated with the disease phenotype. Both the severity of the amino acid change caused by mutation as well as the importance of the amino acid to the overall function of the protein (determined by evaluation for evolutionary conservation) influence the likelihood that discovered mutations are disease-causing rather than benign polymorphisms. Confirmation that the discovered mutation causes the disease can sometimes be difficult and may entail experiments such as mutation screening in other individuals or families with the same disease, development of a transgenic or knockout mouse model of the disease or by "rescue" of the disease phenotype in cell culture by gene replacement.

The vast majority of human neurogenetics research over the past 20 years has followed this outline of linkage analysis and positional cloning. In this chapter, I hope to summarize the major discoveries in the neurogenetics of the major dementia syndromes. I hope also to convey how these genetic findings have shaped our understanding of the molecular and cellular pathogenesis of dementia and how our increased

The Behavioral Neurology of Dementia, eds. Bruce L. Miller and Bradley F. Boeve. Published by Cambridge University Press.
© Cambridge University Press 2009.

understanding of disease pathogenesis is bringing us closer to effective therapies for dementia.

Alzheimer's disease

Alzheimer's disease (AD) is the most common cause of dementia.[6] There are at least an estimated 15 million people worldwide with AD. Because age is the strongest risk factor for the development of AD, improvements in public health and medical treatment during the twentieth century have extended the average lifespan worldwide but have also contributed to epidemic numbers of AD cases. Chapter 5 has a more extensive discussion of the clinical presentation, diagnosis and treatment of AD.

Family history is a strong risk-factor for the development of AD.[7] Three factors argue for the link between genes and AD. First, there are very rare families (< 5% of cases) where early-onset AD (before age 60) is inherited in an autosomal dominant fashion (Familial AD [FAD]). The study of these families has led to extensive molecular genetic analysis of this disease since the early 1990s and is reviewed within this chapter. Second, late-onset AD (after age 65) carries a cumulative risk of approximately 25% in first-degree relatives of patients with AD.[8–10] Finally, the vast majority of individuals with Down syndrome will develop AD neuropathology if they survive to 40 years of age.[11,12] Because Down syndrome is caused by trisomy of chromosome 21, this suggests that changes in expression of one or more genes on this chromosome may predispose individuals to AD.

The amyloid hypothesis

The central role of the β-amyloid peptide in the pathogenesis of AD has been established through a combination of genetic and biochemical analysis since the mid 1980s. Biochemical analysis first identified β-amyloid as the major component of senile plaques, the distinguishing neuropathological signature of AD. The gene that encodes the precursor to β-amyloid, or amyloid precursor protein (APP), was then found mutated in certain families with autosomal dominant AD. Two other genes have been isolated that also segregate with early-onset FAD in an autosomal dominant fashion. Amazingly, these other two genes produce proteins that are critical for the protease-dependent processing of APP into β-amyloid. These data taken together provide overwhelming evidence that the proteolytic formation of the β-amyloid peptide from APP is a key step in the pathogenesis of AD.

In 1984, Glenner and Wong purified the protein component of the cerebrovascular amyloid found in AD brains.[13] This 4.2 kDa protein consisted of 24 amino acid residues and was named β-amyloid protein. A second group led by Masters confirmed this finding in 1985 with the discovery of an identical 40 amino acid residue protein in both AD and Down syndrome brains.[14,15] When the gene encoding this protein was cloned in 1987, it was found that β-amyloid protein, also called Aβ40, was a proteolytic fragment of the large transmembrane domain protein APP.[16–19]

The gene for APP includes 19 exons and its mRNA is extensively alternatively spliced.[20] The three major APP isoforms consist of 695 (APP695), 751 (APP751) and 770 (APP770) amino acid residues, but APP695 is the predominant isoform expressed in the brain.[21] Extensive post-translational modification also occurs with APP; it can be processed by three different proteolytic enzymes: α-, β- and γ-secretases (reviewed by Blennow et al. [6]). Alpha-secretase cleaves APP within the amyloid domain and so is not involved in β-amyloid peptide formation. Beta-secretase releases the N-terminal end of β-amyloid peptide from APP, and γ-secretase cleavage releases the C-terminal end within the transmembrane domain of APP. The resulting proteolytic fragments from β- and γ-secretase cleavage include Aβ40 and Aβ42, both amyloidogenic peptides that differ only by two amino acid residues at their C-terminus.

The initial genetic linkage between the familial AD phenotype and the APP locus on chromosome 21 was difficult to prove. Only after a mutation in *APP* (G693Q) was found to cause a rare syndrome of hereditary cerebral hemorrhage with amyloidosis did direct sequencing of *APP* in samples from patients with FAD commence in earnest.[22] In 1991, John Hardy and colleagues found that rare cases of FAD are caused by a missense mutation (leading to V717I) within the APP gene.[23] A number of other APP mutations have subsequently been found within other AD families (over 30) but this first mutation (V717I) remains the most common. These mutations can be divided into two groups: those that cause early-onset AD and those that cause cerebral amyloidosis with or without AD. Interestingly, mutations that cause cerebral amyloidosis (causing changes E693Q, E693K, N694D) cluster within the β-amyloid domain of APP, while the majority of those that cause early-onset AD cluster near the γ-secretase cleavage site within the transmembrane domain.

Shortly after these mutations in APP were described, genetic linkage was found with other early-onset AD families and two other genetic loci on chromosomes 1 and 14. In 1995, a group led by Peter St. George-Hyslop cloned the gene for presenilin 1 (*PS1*) on chromosome 14.[24] This gene consists of 13 exons encoding multiple protein isoforms through alternative mRNA splicing. The full-length protein has 467 amino acid residues and has a complex structural topology with nine transmembrane domains. Two months later, a group led by Gerald Schellenberg published details of a *PS2* gene with linkage to early-onset familial AD on chromosome 1.[25] The amino acid sequence from *PS2* is nearly identical to that from *PS1* with 80% sequence similarity. The *PS2* gene comprises 12 exons whose organization is again remarkably similar to *PS1*, implying that these genes arose through evolution by duplication. Genetic studies in mice have confirmed that *PS1* and *PS2* are in part genetically redundant, suggesting that their biochemical functions are quite similar.[26]

The majority of families segregating early-onset AD harbor mutations in *PS1* while *APP* and *PS2* mutations are much rarer.[27] More than 160 different mutations in *PS1* have been described and they are associated with the most aggressive forms of FAD. [28–32] Mean age of disease onset is very early (usually under age 50), and the duration of disease is rather short (usually less than 8 years). Phenotypically, those with *PS1* exhibit severe dementia with more prominent aphasia, myoclonus, seizures and parkinsonism compared with those with *APP* mutations.[28] Pathologically, senile amyloid plaques, neurofibrillary tangles, and amyloid angiopathy have all been commonly found in those with *PS1* mutations. Mutations in *PS2* are very rarely found as a cause of FAD, with only 12 pathogenic mutations described to date. The most-extensively studied family has an average age of onset of 54.9 years and the penetrance of *PS2*-mediated disease is far from 100%.[33] In fact, there is significant variability in the age of onset within the same family, extending from the forties to the seventies, and this variability may be influenced by allele status in the gene for apolipoprotein E (*APOE*). The disease phenotype is otherwise indistinguishable from sporadic AD, both clinically and pathologically.

Presenilin 1 protein (and possibly presenilin 2 as well) has been shown to be an important contributor to the γ-secretase cleavage activity required for β-amyloid formation from APP (reviewed by de Strooper [34]). Presenilin forms a protein complex with three other proteins within neuronal membranes: nicastrin, anterior pharynx-defective 1 (Aph1) and presenilin enhancer 2 (Pen2). Each of these proteins contributes to the complex's aspartyl protease activity, which cleaves APP within the transmembrane domain liberating the C-terminal fragment of APP. This activity, often called γ-secretase, is the final enzymatic step in the production of Aβ40 and Aβ42. In vitro studies have shown that pathogenic mutations within PS1 and PS2 decrease the production of Aβ40 in favor of the more amyloidogenic Aβ42.[35,36] These data, taken together, suggest a molecular mechanism for amyloid deposition in AD and they have highlighted the γ-secretase as an attractive target for rational drug design. Unfortunately, γ-secretase activity is required in a number of other essential biochemical pathways, most notably the Notch signaling pathway during embryogenesis. [37,38] The broad range of essential γ-secretase activities has been a formidable barrier to the development of specific inhibitors of APP processing for the treatment of AD.

Apolipoprotein E

While causative mutations in the genes for APP and presenilin have been found in cases of early-onset AD, these genes play a much smaller role in the development of late-onset AD. Instead, polymorphisms within the gene encoding APOE are the most important genetic determinants of late-onset AD risk. The *ApoE* gene maps to the long arm of chromosome 19 and it encodes a polypeptide of 299 residues. There are three common isoforms of ApoE resulting from polymorphisms at two amino acids within the protein, residues 112 and 158. The most common allele, *ApoE3* (ε3) (70–80%), gives rise to an isoform with cysteine at residue 112 and arginine at 158. The less common isoforms ApoE2 (5–10%) and ApoE4 (10–20%) contain cysteines or arginines at both sites, respectively. Apolipoprotein E is a component of both chylomicrons and very low density lipoproteins (VLDL) and these small variations in ApoE sequence cause significant differences in the risk of type III hyperlipoproteinemia and atherosclerotic disease.

In 1991, a group led by M. Pericak-Vance established genetic linkage to chromosome 19 in families with late-onset AD.[39] Shortly thereafter, they found that the *ApoE4* allele was highly associated with the development of sporadic and familial late-onset AD. [40,41] In their initial study, the ApoE4 allele frequency was 0.50 in patients with AD versus 0.16 in controls.[42] This association has been replicated by a large number of other groups in a variety of clinical settings and the effect has remained consistent. A recent meta-analysis of all published *ApoE* allele case–control and family-based studies provides an odds ratio of 2.8 to 4.3 for the development of AD with one *ApoE4* allele.[43] The effect seems to be dosage dependent because *ApoE4* homozygotes have an odds ratio of 11.8 to 21.8. Other studies have shown that *ApoE4* alleles are associated with an earlier onset of AD.[40,44] The *ApoE4* allele is not necessary for the development of AD, as nearly half of all patients with AD do not have an *ApoE4* allele, but it could be considered sufficient because more than 90% of all *ApoE4* homozygotes develop disease.[40]

In 1994, three different groups found a different relationship between APOE and AD.[45–47] In similar association studies, they found that the rare *ApoE2* allele was associated with a lower risk of AD when compared with patients homozygous for *ApoE3*. This has been confirmed by a number of other studies, including the same recent meta-analysis, which provided an odds ratio of 0.3 to 0.7 for the development of AD with one *ApoE2* allele.[43] This is consistent with a model where *ApoE2* confers protection from AD where *ApoE4* confers additional risk of the disease.

That different alleles of *ApoE* impart opposite tendencies for the development of sporadic AD implies that ApoE is important for the AD pathogenesis. Unfortunately, the mechanism of ApoE's effects on AD risk remains obscure. Some studies have suggested that ApoE is necessary for β-amyloid deposition in a mouse model of AD.[48] In vitro studies have revealed that ApoE3 interacts with β-amyloid with extremely high affinity, whereas ApoE4 binds 20 times less tightly.[49] This suggests that ApoE may be part of a β-amyloid clearance mechanism where ApoE4 is less efficient than ApoE3. Still other studies have implicated ApoE's inhibitory effects on neurite extension and branching as the culprit.[50]

Other genetic risk factors

Mutations in the genes for APP and presenilin cause rare but highly penetrant early-onset AD phenotypes, but they only account for less than 5% of all AD cases: 95% of AD cases are typically of the late-onset variety and more than half of the patients have risk conferred by the *ApoE4* allele described above. This leaves nearly half of all AD cases with unknown genetic risk factors. Owing to the explosion of genetic sequence

data collection since the late 1980s, there has been a flood of small studies either suggesting or refuting newly discovered small genetic risk factors for AD, but the complete collection of these papers has been nearly impossible to digest for individual investigators simply because of the sheer volume.

A catalogue of all of the published genetic association studies has now been compiled and is available to the public through the Alzgene website (http://www.alzforum.org/res/com/gen/alzgene/default.asp). In addition, a meta-analysis has been performed for each gene for which there are at least two independent association studies and these data are also available online. The result of this undertaking is a continually compiled and updated database of all gene association studies for AD with an up-to-date rank list of significant odds ratios for each genetic risk factor in question. This database will certainly be an invaluable resource for the research community as their collective focus shifts from rare but highly penetrant genetic causes of early-onset AD to common, but poorly penetrant genetic risk factors of late-onset AD.

Frontotemporal dementias

Frontotemporal dementia (FTD) is the most common member of a group of dementia syndromes characterized by focal degeneration of the frontal and anterior temporal lobes of the brain. Those patients with frontotemporal lobar degeneration (FTLD) differ from patients with AD in that they present with behavioral symptoms (FTD), non-fluent aphasia (progressive non-fluent aphasia [PNFA]) or loss of semantic knowledge (semantic dementia [SD]) rather than with memory loss. For an extensive discussion of the clinical features of these syndromes, see Ch. 4, 18 and 19.

A recent study of pedigrees in a large clinical cohort has revealed a strong genetic influence on the development of FTLD.[51] Nearly 38% of those with FTLD have a family history of dementia and in 13% there is evidence for autosomal dominant inheritance. In addition, individual clinical syndromes have differences in heritability: 59% of those with FTD/amyotrophic lateral sclerosis (ALS) have a family history of dementia or ALS while only 17% of patients with SD have such a family history.

The study of FTLD neuropathology has revealed a great deal of confusing heterogeneity within clinical syndromes and clinical overlap between these same syndromes. Over the last several years, it has become clear that most cases of FTLD are pathologically associated with neuronal inclusions filled with either filamentous phosphorylated microtubule-associated protein tau (MAP-τ) or ubiquitinated TAR DNA-binding protein (TDP-43). This dichotomy has suggested for many years that the pathogenetic mechanisms underlying FTLD may be heterogeneous as well; an idea supported by genetic data collected since the mid 1990s.

In 1998, Michael Hutton and colleagues isolated causative mutations for autosomal dominant FTD with parkinsonism (FTDP-17) in the gene encoding MAP-τ on human chromosome 17.[52] Tau is a 352 to 441 amino acid residue protein that functions to promote microtubule polymerization through an interaction with four microtubule binding repeats at the protein's C-terminus. The gene *MAPT* has 14 exons whose splicing is regulated in a complex fashion.[53] Alternative splicing occurs at exons 2, 3 and 10 and each of the six possible splice variants is expressed in the human brain. Three of the resulting isoforms contain four microtubule binding repeats (4R) while the others contain three (3R).

More than 30 pathogenic mutations have been isolated in the *MAPT* gene. Most are missense mutations affecting the C-terminal microtubule repeat domains (G272V and R406W), most prominently the variable repeat encoded by exon 10 (R301L). In addition, another set of mutations lie within the intron preceding exon 10, and molecular analysis has shown that these mutations increase the inclusion of exon 10 within the spliced mRNA.[52] These mutations, therefore, pathogenically increase the proportion of 4R MAP-τ compared with 3R MAP-τ within the brain. In vitro studies have shown that many of these mutations disrupt MAP-τ interactions with microtubules and cause accumulation of MAP-τ within neurons.[54,55] Despite these discoveries, however, it remains unclear which of these mechanisms are causative rather than just associated with the disease phenotype.

Most of these patients with *MAPT* mutations present with clinical early-onset FTD (age 30–60) with or without parkinsonism.[56] There are, however, exceptions, including those that present primarily with parkinsonism,[57] memory loss,[58,59] aphasia,[60] corticobasal syndrome [61] and even a clinical syndrome consistent with progressive supranuclear palsy (PSP).[62,63] Pathologically, these brains have atrophy, neuronal loss and some combination of neurofibrillary tangles, Pick bodies, and other MAP-τ-positive staining cytoplasmic neuronal inclusions.

Genetic studies in both mice and fruit flies have shown that MAP-τ is not essential for animal viability. [64,65] Homozygous loss-of-function mutations in *MAPT*, however, can enhance the neuronal migration and axon outgrowth defects exhibited by mutants for the other major microtubule-associated protein in mammals, MAP1B, suggesting that there is functional redundancy between these related genes.[66] Overproduction of mutant MAP-τ within the *Drosophila* nervous system induces cell death, and genetic screens for interacting genes have isolated the gene for glycogen synthase kinase 3β (*GSK3β*) as a critical partner for the cell death phenotype through its ability to phosphorylate MAP-τ.[67] Transgenic mice overproducing mutant MAP-τ species within the brain have recapitulated cognitive deficits, neurodegeneration and neurofibrillary tangles seen in human tauopathies as hypothesized.[68] One recent study however has dissociated MAP-τ accumulation in neurofibrillary tangles from cognitive decline and neuronal death in a specific mouse model, suggesting that neurofibrillary tangles are not the proximal cause of FTLD or AD.[69]

The second gene associated with FTD was mapped to chromosome 9p13 and isolated by Virginia Kimonis and colleagues in 2004.[70] They studied 13 families through which segregated a rare syndrome involving inclusion body myopathy associated with Paget's disease of the bone and FTD (IBMPFD). Individual patients with this syndrome may not manifest each of these component symptoms. For instance, in the largest series of patients reported, myopathy is the most common phenotype, but only 30% of the patients exhibited FTD.[70] A more recent description of two French families with confirmed mutations revealed an FTD penetrance of 70–100%, with a lower rate of myopathy.[71] Initial neuropathological studies have revealed the presence of ubiquitin-containing inclusions uniquely within neuronal nuclei within neocortex.[72,73]

Causative mutations in the gene encoding valosin-containing protein (VCP) were found by sequencing through candidate genes residing at 9p13.[70] This protein is a 97 kDa protein in the type II AAA-ATPase family. It is ubiquitously expressed and highly conserved from yeast to humans. Evidence suggests that VCP may act as a molecular chaperone, shuttling ubiquitinated proteins to the proteasome complex to initiate degradation and thus regulating a host of cellular processes. All of the published mutations in IBMPFD families affect the N-terminal domain, which

31

is thought to interact with ubiquitinated proteins. In fact, 11 of 16 affected families in the literature harbor mutations affecting a highly conserved arginine at position 155 within this CDC48-homologous domain of VCP. These data suggest that impaired targeting of misfolded proteins to the proteasome may be relevant in the study of neurodegenerative diseases, many of which involve the abnormal accumulation of specific proteins within the brain.

Valosin-containing protein is highly conserved through evolution and has been studied most extensively in yeast, flies and in mammalian cell culture. [74] The yeast and mammalian versions of VCP have been implicated in membrane fusion, cell cycle control, transcriptional regulation, apoptosis and endoplasmic reticulum-associated degradation of misfolded proteins. Homozygous mutations within *ter94*, the *Drosophila* orthologue of VCP, are lethal but heterozygous loss-of-function mutants have no obvious phenotype.[75] It was also isolated in a genetic screen for dosage-dependent modifiers of polyglutamine-induced neurodegeneration.[76] More recently, overexpression of human VCP has been shown to genetically suppress neurodegeneration induced by overproduction of *Drosophila* ataxin-3, a polyglutamine-containing protein.[77] These studies, along with the finding that *VCP* mutations cause IBMPFD, suggest that VCP may be part of a common mechanism of neurodegeneration caused by a number of molecular etiologies.

The third gene associated with FTD was isolated by Elizabeth Fisher and colleagues in 2005.[78] They studied 11 affected members of a large Danish family from Jutland segregating an autosomal dominant dementia syndrome. The causative mutation on chromosome 3 was found in the gene encoding the charged multivesicular body protein 2B (CHMP2B). [78] This is a 213 amino acid residue protein conserved throughout species and contains coiled coil, SNF-7 and C-terminal acidic domains. It is a known component of the endosomal secretory complex required for transport III (ESCRTIII) that regulates trafficking of specific vesicular compartments within cells.

Affected individuals from this Danish family have been extensively studied over the last 30 years.[79] The average age of onset for this syndrome is 57 years and the onset is insidious. It presents with subtle personality change, disinhibition, apathy, dyscalculia and hyperorality. Late in the disease course, motoric abnormalities are prominent, with parkinsonism, dystonia, pyramidal signs and myoclonus. The average disease course is 8 years. Recent neuropathologic

analysis was performed in two patients and signs of Alzheimer's pathology, MAP-τ inclusions and ubiquitin-containing inclusions were not seen.[79]

The Jutland mutation within *CHMP2B* lies in the splice acceptor site of exon 6.[78] Molecular analysis of amplification products of CHMP2B by reverse transcriptase polymerase chain reaction in these affected individuals revealed two aberrant mRNAs not seen in unaffected family members. One product contained 201 base pairs of intronic sequence between exon 5 and exon 6. The other product utilized a cryptic splice acceptor site within exon 6. Both predicted protein translations have different (or missing) amino acid sequences for the final 30 or so residues of the protein. Further screening of 400 unrelated Europeans with FTD for mutations within *CHMP2B* revealed only one change affecting a conserved residue (G442T).[78] Extensive genetic analysis in hundreds of other American FTD families has shown that *CHMP2B* mutations are an extremely rare cause of disease.[80] In fact, a nonsense mutation was recently found in an Afrikaner non-demented control that causes a similar effect upon the CHMP2B C-terminus as seen in the Danish mutation. More recent analyses in a Belgian FTD cohort have revealed one family with a nonsense mutation that also causes a truncation of the protein's C-terminus.[81] Overproduction of these truncated proteins has been shown to cause endosomal accumulation in cell culture as well as autophagy and neurodegeneration in the *Drosophila* nervous system. [81,82] These findings suggest that there may be incomplete penetrance of the CHMP2B FTD phenotype, but that C-terminal truncation of CHMP2B is likely to be a rare, bonafide cause of genetic FTD.

A much more common genetic cause of FTD was found independently by groups led by Christina van Broeckhoven and Michael Hutton in 2006.[83,84] This work arose from the discovery of mutations within the gene encoding MAP-τ that cause FTDP-17.[52] Over the years since this discovery, a number of other families have been described that segregated the FTD phenotype with strong linkage to the chromosomal region of *MAPT*, but they did not harbor mutations within *MAPT*.[85,86] Moreover, postmortem analysis of these brains revealed ubiquitin-positive neuronal inclusions, rather than the MAP-τ-positive neuronal inclusions seen in those with *MAPT* mutations.[85–89] These data suggested the presence of another FTD-associated gene in the vicinity of *MAPT*, and subsequent positional cloning led to the discovery of pathogenic mutations within the progranulin gene.

The gene *PGRN* encodes progranulin a 593 amino acid residue protein that is, cysteine rich and secreted by cells (reviewed by He and Bateman [90]). The sequence contains 7.5 "granulin" repeats each forming a stacked β-hairpin structure reminiscent of epidermal growth factor.[91] Proteolytic fragments of the full-length progranulin protein, called "granulins," were first purified from inflammatory exudates, and, therefore, progranulin has been implicated in wound repair as well as in angiogenesis and cancer.[92] Progranulin is produced throughout the developing brain, among other tissues, but little is known about the function of the protein.[93] One study showed that progranulin is upregulated in the hypothalamus of rats as a result of androgen exposure during the perinatal period, and that this expression may be important for the development of male mating behavior.[94,95]

Researchers at the Mayo Clinic have sequenced *PGRN* in all 378 cases of FTLD in their cohort.[96] This analysis has revealed that 10% have mutations affecting progranulin, including 23% of those with positive family histories for dementia. The average age of onset was 59 years and the average age of death was 65 years; however, there is significant variability in both. Presentation was with primary language dysfunction in 24%, a number that is twice that of all other FTLD cases within their cohort.[96]

Further clinical descriptions of these patients with *PGRN* mutations have been sparse, although they have presented with the clinical syndromes of FTD, PNFA [97] and corticobasal syndrome.[98] A number of cases independently described by groups led by Mesulam and Neary have qualified for diagnoses of primary progressive aphasia.[97,99,100] Many of these cases do not meet criteria for PNFA or SD and may represent overlap between the two or a new clinical syndrome altogether. Pathologic studies have shown that patients with FTLD with mutations affecting progranulin harbor ubiquitin-containing neuronal intranuclear inclusions within the cortex that are not found in sporadic cases of FTLD.[101] Lee and colleagues have since found that these neuronal inclusions in both progranulin-mediated and sporadic FTD are filled with TDP-43.[102] Chapter 4 has a more extensive discussion of TDP-43 in the pathogenesis of FTLD.

More than 30 different mutations have now been described within *PGRN*. Most of them insert a premature stop codon within the message, forming a so-called "nonsense" mutation. Interestingly, these mRNAs with premature stop codons are degraded very shortly after transcription through the process of nonsense-mediated decay, and, therefore, these mutations behave genetically as null alleles. Because of this, the autosomal dominant inheritance pattern seen in these families is mediated through the unusual mechanism of "haplo-insufficiency," or the inability of a carrier to avoid the FTD phenotype with 50% of normal progranulin activity. This unusual mechanism of inheritance offers the tantalizing prospect that exogenous replacement of progranulin activity in gene carriers or those with FTD may be an effective preventative measure or treatment. More recently, missense progranulin variants have also been described within patients with FTD, but the molecular mechanism of their disease pathogenesis awaits further research.[103]

Parkinsonian syndromes
Synucleinopathies

Dementia with Lewy bodies (DLB) is a common and important cause of cognitive impairment. Unfortunately, because of substantial clinical and pathological overlap with AD and Parkinson's disease (PD) with dementia, genetic studies of DLB have not been plentiful. Many families harbor a genetic syndrome that may express itself as dementia in one member and a movement disorder in another. This phenotypic heterogeneity, along with the pathological similarity between DLB and PD, suggests that these entities have related molecular and genetic risk factors. Chapter 2 has an extensive discussion of the clinical features of DLB.

The genetic analysis of these diseases began in the 1990s with the discovery of the large Italian and American "Contursi" kindred and three ancestral Greek families that harbored an autosomal dominant form of early-onset PD. In 1996, Robert Nussbaum and colleagues mapped a mutation in these families to chromosome 4q21–23 [104] and in 1997, a causative mutation was found in the gene encoding α-synuclein (*SNCA*).[105] Alpha-synuclein is a 140 amino acid residue protein localized to the synapse but of unknown function.[106] The causative mutation in the Contursi kindred (A53T) initiates a disease with an early average age of onset at 46 years and an estimated phenotypic penetrance of 85%.[105] The clinical phenotype is variable. Patients often present with a typical parkinsonian movement disorder, an early-onset dementia or a mixture of the two. More recently, two other mutations (leading to A30P and

E46K) have been found in a German and a Spanish family, respectively.[107,108] Finally, α-synuclein was subsequently found to be the major component of the characteristic pathological signature of PD and DLB, the Lewy body, cementing its importance in the pathogenesis of both syndromes.[109]

Mutations in *SNCA* do not cause disease by disrupting the normal function of the protein. It is not required for animal viability, as mice engineered to have no *SNCA* gene activity develop normally despite mild neurotransmission deficits.[110] Instead, two lines of evidence suggest that *SNCA* gain-of-function may be more important for disease pathogenesis. First, increasing *SNCA* gene dosage can cause PD/DLB. The Iowa kindred, where members are affected in their thirties with either parkinsonism or DLB, was found in 2003 to harbor a triplication of the *SNCA* locus.[111] Since this discovery, other families have been found to harbor duplications of this locus, [112,113] and increasing copy number of the *SNCA* has been found to be associated with decreasing age of onset of disease. Second, polymorphisms in dinucleotide repeats within upstream transcriptional enhancer elements affect the efficiency of *SNCA* expression. [114] A case–control study of over 2000 patients with idiopathic PD and controls demonstrated that one particular allele (263 base pairs) of the REP1 dinucleotide repeat was associated with the PD phenotype with an odds ratio of 1.43.[115]

The initial work on α-synuclein has led to the discovery of a number of other genes that cause autosomal dominant and recessive PD. Most of these gene mutations are rare causes of PD: *parkin, PINK1, UCHL-1* and *DJ-1*.[116–119] The discovery of these genes has highlighted the profound importance of the ubiquitin–proteasome system as well as mitochondrial function in the pathogenesis of PD. A sixth gene, which encodes leucine-rich repeat kinase 2 (*LRRK2*) or "dardarin," is the most common genetic cause of PD yet identified.

In 2004, two groups isolated causative mutations in the gene *LRRK2* through work with a number of British, American, German–Canadian and Basque families.[120,121] Pathological studies on these families have shown striking neuropathological heterogeneity, with some cases harboring classic Lewy bodies, others with MAP-τ-positive neurofibrillary tangles, and others with neither of these distinctive lesions.[121–123] A recent worldwide study has shown that six specific autosomal dominant missense mutations in *LRRK2* are robustly associated with disease:

giving changes G2019S, R1441G, R1441C, R1441H, I2020T and Y1699C.[124] The single most common mutant, G2019S, accounts for 1% of all sporadic PD and 4% of all hereditary cases.[124] Clinically, age of onset is variable with an average of 58.1 years and a distribution very similar to idiopathic PD.[124] Mutations are seen only rarely in unaffected individuals, although they are quite common in affected individuals with Ashkenazi Jewish, North African Arab or Portuguese heritage.[124]

The gene *LRRK2* encodes a large multidomain protein with 2482–2527 residues. Its domains include a leucine-rich repeat, a small GTPase, a kinase and a WD-40 domain, all of which are common modular domains in known signal transduction cascades. Mutations have been found causing changes scattered throughout the LRRK2 protein and associated with the PD phenotype; however, there is some evidence to suggest that both GTPase and kinase activities are important for disease pathogenesis. The most common mutation worldwide is a missense mutation affecting the LRRK2's kinase domain (G2019S) that significantly increases the kinase activity.[125] Another common mutation has recently been found to decrease LRRK2's GTPase activity as well as increase the kinase activity (R1441C).[125,126] The mechanism by which these biochemical perturbations cause striatonigral degeneration and Lewy body formation may be important for the development of effective pharmacologic interventions over the next several years.

Tauopathies

The clinical entities of PSP and corticobasal degeneration (CBD) are parkinsonian syndromes that are often confused with idiopathic PD as well as each other. The clinical presentation of PSP remains relatively specific for PSP neuropathology, but the clinical "corticobasal syndrome" can be caused by underlying CBD, PSP, TDP-43, AD and Creutzfeldt–Jakob disease (CJD) pathologies among others. This pathologic heterogeneity has hampered genetic studies of both of these diseases, but it may not reflect molecular heterogeneity as both PSP and CBD pathologies involve abnormal accumulation of MAP-τ. In fact, an informative family has been described where a corticobasal syndrome is inherited in an autosomal dominant fashion, but where two siblings at autopsy had either PSP or CBD pathology.[127] The underlying mutation in this family has not yet been described. Chapter 20 has an extensive discussion of these clinical and pathological entities.

In 1999, Michael Hutton and colleagues described two extended haplotypes (H1 and H2) of linked polymorphisms that cover over 100 kilobases of the *MAPT*.[128] The H1 homozygotes account for 63% of Caucasian-Americans, while heterozygotes account for 31% and H2 homozygotes account for 6%. They proposed that either recombination was suppressed across this gene, or that recombinant genes have an evolutionary selective disadvantage. Interestingly, in a genetic study of 64 unrelated patients with PSP, they found that H1 homozygotes accounted for 87.5% and heterozygotes were found in 12.5%. That no patients with PSP in their cohort carried two H2 haplotypes solidified the association between PSP and the H1 haplotype. This suggests that the H1 haplotype may be necessary for the development of PSP, but that it is not sufficient as the vast majority of H1 homozygotes in the population never develop disease.

More recently, a small number of individuals with PSP and CBD have been found to harbor missense mutations within *MAPT*. The first mutation affects a functionally important and conserved residue near the N-terminus of the protein (R5L), but it has not been shown to segregate with the disease in familial cases.[62] The second (G303V) segregates with disease in one family, and it alters the splicing of *MAPT* exon 10, leading to the overproduction of 4R MAP-τ compared with 3R.[63] A clinical syndrome most consistent with FTD but pathologically consistent with CBD was found to harbor a seemingly silent N296N mutation that also causes disease by increasing the production of 4R MAP-τ in the brain.[129] Finally, a sporadic case of corticobasal syndrome was recently found to harbor a G389R change with MAP-τ. [61] These data taken together suggest that increased ratios of 4R/3R MAP-τ may be sufficient to cause abnormal MAP-τ accumulation as well as clinical neurodegenerative disease.

Prion diseases

Creutzfeldt–Jakob disease is the prototypic human prion disease, first described by Jakob in 1921. Although it is extremely rare, it is notable for its rapidity of progression, usually over a few months, and its unusual pathogenesis, which has been eloquently described in efforts led by Stanley Prusiner. Definitive diagnosis can only be made by neuropathology, but a probable diagnosis currently depends on satisfaction of World Health Organization criteria including dementia, myoclonus, electroencephalographic findings and 14-3-3 protein. Chapter 23 has an extensive clinical description of CJD and related disorders.

Many early cases of CJD were known to be familial, some in an autosomal dominant mode of inheritance, but this did not aid in the understanding of CJD pathogenesis until relatively recently. A Herculean research effort on CJD and a related prion disease of the Fore people from Papua-New Guinea led by Carleton Gajdusek showed that these "spongiform encephalopathies" were transmissible to laboratory animals through inoculation and to other people through cannibalism.[130,131] Gajdusek and colleagues later went on to show that even familial cases of CJD were transmissible to non-human primates, [132] marking the first example of a disease that is simultaneously inherited and infectious. The pathogenesis of familial and transmissible spongiform encephalopathies (TSEs) was presumed to be caused by a "slow virus" by Gajdusek and others for many years. However in 1982, Stanley Prusiner and colleagues isolated a protein that accumulates in hamster brains infected with scrapie, a TSE found in sheep that is pathologically similar to CJD.[133] The identification of the prion protein (PrP) as the infectious agent in all TSEs including CJD has provided a unique but controversial molecular basis for the pathogenesis of these slow and non-inflammatory infections.[134] Molecular genetic studies confirmed the importance of PrP in the pathogenesis of the TSEs through the isolation of mutations in the human gene for PrP (*PRNP*) in families with CJD, the related Gerstmann–Straussler–Scheinker disease (GSS) and fatal familial insomnia (FFI).[135–138] Chapter 22 has an extensive discussion of these different prion disease phenotypes.

The *PRNP* gene is located on human chromosome 20p12. It comprises two exons with the entire open reading frame within exon 2. The protein product consists of 253 amino acid residues and is widely expressed in the nervous system, but its normal function is unknown. The protein's N-terminal domain centers around a repeated sequence consisting of a nine-mer peptide immediately followed by four identical octapeptide repeats. The C-terminal domain contains two glycosylation sites and is relatively unstructured. It has been reasonably postulated that pathogenic mutations in *PRNP* promote disease by destabilizing the native PrP^c (cellular) conformer in favor of the disease-causing PrP^{Sc} (scrapie) version. While this may be the case for some mutations,[139] other mutations may promote PrP^{Sc} formation by

35

perturbing molecular interactions between PrP and other proteins.[140,141]

There are a handful of common polymorphisms that have been found throughout *PRNP*, and two of these polymorphisms have been proposed to influence disease phenotype in all categories of prion disease. In the Caucasian population of North America and Europe, most people carry at least one allele of *PRNP*, coding for methionine at codon 129 (129M): 43% MM homozygotes and 49% MV heterozygotes. Homozygotes for valine at codon 129 (129V) are rare (8%).[142] These ratios vary from population to population, with much lower frequencies of 129V in China and Japan and much higher frequencies in Papua-New Guinea and in some Native American groups. A second polymorphism involves either a common glutamine or a rare lysine at codon 219 (E219K) in Japanese populations.[143]

More than 50 unique *PRNP* mutations have been described in families harboring autosomal dominant prion disease. These mutations fall into four major categories: missense point mutations that cause amino acid substitutions; nonsense point mutations that cause premature protein termination; insertion of additional octapeptide repeats; and, most rarely, deletion of octapeptide repeats. The first mutation reported by Prusiner and colleagues in 1989 produces P102L and causes the GSS phenotype with a median age of onset of 50 and disease duration of approximately 4 years.[135] The most common mutation (causing E200K) was first described in a large cluster of Libyan and Tunisian Jews where the incidence of CJD is 100 times higher than the worldwide baseline. The disease phenotype resembles sporadic CJD, with a mean age of onset of 58 years and a mean duration of disease of 6 months.[144,145] The D178N change causes disease with either CJD or FFI phenotypes beginning at an average age of 50 with disease lasting an average duration of 11 months.[146] Finally, insertional mutations within the octapeptide repeat domain of PrP with at least four additional repeats can also cause clinical CJD.[147]

There is significant variability in the phenotypic expression of all *PRNP* mutations, but the mechanism of this variability remains unclear. For instance, patients with the mutation leading to E200K can have extremely atypical presentations, with peripheral neuropathy or PSP.[148] The age of disease onset with any of these mutations can span from the third decade to the eighth decade of life, and even some asymptomatic carriers have been found as well.[146]

The duration of disease can be as short as a few months but as long as 17 years with the same *PRNP* mutations. However, some of the phenotypic variability has been found to be associated with certain molecular changes in the PrP protein. Subjects with less than four octapeptide insertions tend to have a CJD phenotype and a low penetrance of disease, whereas subjects with greater than four tend to have a GSS phenotype with high penetrance.[149]

Perhaps the greatest known influence on the variable expressivity of all prion disease is a polymorphism at codon 129 (M129V). Because of this influence, genetic prion disorders are often categorized by the molecular haplotype, which includes both the primary mutation (i.e. D178N) as well as any modifying polymorphisms (i.e. 129M versus 129V). For instance, patients carrying D178N can present with either CJD or FFI phenotypes. The particular phenotype is strongly associated with a particular allelic variation in codon 129 acting genetically in *cis* to the D178N mutation. D178N coupled with 129V is associated with the CJD phenotype while D178N coupled with 129M is associated with the FFI phenotype.[137] In other instances, this polymorphism may have an effect on the age of onset of prion disease. Kuru, the acquired form of prion disease of the Fore people of Papua-New Guinea, has an earlier and more aggressive course in the context of MM and VV homozygosity.[150,151] Sporadic CJD is also affected by the M129V polymorphism, where disease is also associated with MM and VV homozygosity.[152] The most striking effect of this polymorphism, however, occurs in patients with variant CJD, where every case of variant CJD that has been tested has been MM homozygous at codon 129.[153] Unfortunately, the mechanism by which these subtle amino acid substitutions affect prion disease pathogenesis remains to be determined.

Huntington's disease

It was clear from George Huntington's initial description in 1872 that HD was hereditary. In retrospect, his presentation perfectly described an autosomal dominant inheritance pattern, decades before the scientific community's "rediscovery" of Gregor Mendel's original research on genetics: "When either or both the parents have shown manifestation of the disease . . . one or more of the offspring almost invariably suffer from the disease, if they live to adult age. But if by any chance these children go through life without it, the thread is broken and the grandchildren and great-grandchildren of the original shakers may rest assured that they are free from the disease." Work by a number of physicians over the next several decades firmly established Huntington's disease as a Mendelian disorder.

Because HD was so obviously genetic in origin, it was an early target for disease gene hunters in the 1970s and 1980s. James Gusella and colleagues established genetic linkage between the HD phenotype and a marker called G8 on the short arm of chromosome 4 in 1983.[1] But despite this early triumph and the collaborative efforts of six laboratories in the USA and UK (called the Huntington's Disease Collaborative Research Group), 10 more years elapsed before the discovery of the specific gene mutation.[154] The *IT15* gene contains 67 exons and encodes a protein with a predicted weight of 348 kDa named huntingtin. The causative mutation is trinucleotide repeat expansion (CAG) within exon 1 of *IT15*. These CAG repeats are transcribed and translated into a long run of tandem glutamine residues within the protein, termed "polyglutamine repeats." Normal alleles usually give rise to 16 repeats, but they fall along a Gaussian distribution with an upper limit of 35 repeats. Pathogenic, or "expanded" alleles give rise to a range from 36 repeats to over 100, with most alleles producing between 40 and 50 CAGs. [155] There is a small range where the disease is possible but phenotypic penetrance is less than 100% (36–39 repeats).[156]

The discovery of a trinucleotide repeat expansion as the molecular cause of HD has provided new insights into certain peculiarities of HD genetics from the pre-molecular era. Nearly 40 years ago, it was found that the vast majority of those with juvenile HD inherited it from a father and not a mother.[157] Researchers also established that this disease, like myotonic dystrophy, develops earlier and more severely in successive generations, a genetic phenomenon called "anticipation".[158] These unusual genetic features now have a clear molecular basis determined by the size of pathogenic trinucleotide repeat. First, there is a strong inverse correlation between the number of CAG repeats and the age of disease onset. [159–161] In other words, higher repeat numbers are associated with younger age of onset. Families with HD that clinically exhibited anticipation were found to have increasing numbers of CAG repeats in successive generations.[159,160,162] Finally, while both male and female meioses are associated with repeat-length

instability, only paternal transmission tends to cause net repeat expansion in the next generation.[162] In other words, male, but not female, gametogenesis tends to cause expansion of the repeats, thus increasing the likelihood of intergenerational worsening of disease severity.

Huntingtin is a ubiquitously expressed protein found with high levels in the brain.[163,164] Mouse studies have shown that it is essential for organismal survival, but loss-of-function mutations cause an embryonic developmental phenotype that does not resemble HD.[165–167] Instead, because overexpression of mutant huntingtin in mice causes motor dysfunction, behavioral abnormalities and neurodegeneration, it is generally accepted that the pathogenically expanded polyglutamine tract in the context of the huntingtin protein causes a toxic gain of function.[168–171]

The biochemical and cellular mechanisms by which mutant huntingtin causes neurodegeneration, however, continues to be hotly debated. The polyglutamine tract clearly is a critical factor in the neurodegeneration seen in HD brains, but the protein context for the polyglutamine tract is also likely to be important for disease pathogenesis. This is because the different polyglutamine diseases (HD, spinobulbar muscular atrophy, dentatorubropallidoluysian atrophy, etc.) are all neurodegenerative, but in distinctively different patterns within the nervous system. The most influential theory of molecular pathogenesis over the last decade invokes the tendency of mutant huntingtin to form insoluble protein aggregates within neurons, often seen pathologically as nuclear inclusions, as the "toxic" form of the mutant protein. The extensive evidence in favor of this theory is beyond the scope of this chapter, but most of this evidence is circumstantial. A smaller number of studies have argued that these inclusions may, instead, be protective. More recent automated microscopy studies have shown that inclusion body formation within cultured neurons predicts cell survival, while intracellular mutant huntingtin levels predict cell death.[172] This is instead consistent with a model where mutant huntingtin aggregates are part of a cellular coping mechanism operating against huntingtin toxicity.[172,173]

Future of neurogenetics

There is no argument over the profound impact that traditional Mendelian genetic analysis has had on our understanding of the dementia syndromes. Unbiased genetic analyses of familial FAD, FTD, PD, CJD and

HD have confirmed the biological importance of the abnormally accumulated proteins found in the brains of patients with these diseases (APP, MAP-τ, α-synuclein, PrP, and huntingtin, respectively). Despite these amazing achievements, however, the question always remains whether the study of rare, early-onset, genetic forms of dementia is truly informative about the pathogenesis of common, late-onset, sporadic forms of dementia. In a nutshell, is the knowledge we are gaining about genetic dementia relevant to the study of sporadic dementia? Are these really the same diseases?

Sporadic dementia is, in fact, not completely sporadic. As we discussed earlier, *ApoE4* is an important genetic risk factor for late-onset AD. Therefore, sporadic dementia must result from a combination of genetic risk and protective factors interacting with environment, a non-Mendelian form of inheritance termed "complex genetics." The molecular dissection of complex genetic disorders has been beyond the scope of neurogenetics research until the completion of the Human Genome Project in 2004.[174] Data from this project as well as the more recent International Hap Map Project have provided the scientific community with a map of the millions of molecular genetic "markers" that span the human genome in the form of single nucleotide polymorphisms (SNPs). [175] These "common" genetic variants represent the small genetic differences between individuals of our species, including perhaps our individual susceptibilities to complex genetic diseases. This idea that common diseases are in part caused by common genetic variants is termed the "common disease common variant (CDCV) hypothesis".[2]

The availability of millions of informative SNPs along with automated DNA microarray technology, has presented the scientific community with the opportunity to test this CDCV hypothesis. Whole genome association studies have now been initiated to search for genetic risk and protective factors for a number of sporadic dementias. These studies compare allelic frequencies in 10^5–10^6 SNPs between patients with dementia and age-matched controls. One recent study used this method to confirm the status of the *ApoE4* allele as the most powerful genetic risk factor for late-onset AD,[176] but few other studies have yet provided us with any reproducible new risk factors. The reasons are still unclear but may include the statistical problem of multiple comparisons, genetic interactions between multiple risk factors, genetic heterogeneity, gene–environment interactions, and, of course, the possibility that the

CDCV hypothesis is incorrect. What is clear is that the "old, reliable" Mendelian approach to genetic disease continues to provide us with new theories on the biological basis of dementia while the kinks are being worked out on the "new fangled" whole genome approach.

References

1. Gusella, J. F., N. S. Wexler, P. M. Conneally *et al.* A polymorphic DNA marker genetically linked to Huntington's disease. *Nature*, 1983; **306**(5940): 234–8.

2. Botstein, D. and N. Risch. Discovering genotypes underlying human phenotypes: past successes for mendelian disease, future approaches for complex disease. *Nat Genet*, 2003; **33**(Suppl): 228–37.

3. Strachan, T. and A. P. Read. *Human Molecular Genetics 3*, 3rd edn. London: Garland Press, 2004.

4. Lander, E. S., L. M. Linton, B. Birren *et al.* Initial sequencing and analysis of the human genome. *Nature*, 2001; **409**(6822): 860–921.

5. Venter, J. C., M. D. Adams, E. W. Myers *et al.* The sequence of the human genome. *Science*, 2001; **291** (5507): 1304–51.

6. Blennow, K., M. J. de Leon and H. Zetterberg. Alzheimer's disease. *Lancet*, 2006; **368**(9533): 387–403.

7. Pulst, S.-M. *Contemporary Neurology Series: Neurogenetics*. New York: Oxford University Press, 2000.

8. Hirst, C., I. M. Yee and A. D. Sadovnick. Familial risks for Alzheimer disease from a population-based series. *Genet Epidemiol*, 1994; **11**(4): 365–74.

9. Hocking, L. B. and J. C. Breitner. Cumulative risk of Alzheimer-like dementia in relatives of autopsy-confirmed cases of Alzheimer's disease. *Dementia*, 1995; **6**(6): 355–6.

10. Farrer, L. A., D. M. O'Sullivan, L. A. Cupples, J. H. Growdon and R. H. Myers. Assessment of genetic risk for Alzheimer's disease among first-degree relatives. *Ann Neurol*, 1989; **25**(5): 485–93.

11. Lai, F. and R. S. Williams. A prospective study of Alzheimer disease in Down syndrome. *Arch Neurol*, 1989; **46**(8): 849–53.

12. Burger, P. C. and F. S. Vogel. The development of the pathologic changes of Alzheimer's disease and senile dementia in patients with Down's syndrome. *Am J Pathol*, 1973; **73**(2): 457–76.

13. Glenner, G. G. and C. W. Wong. Alzheimer's disease: initial report of the purification and characterization of a novel cerebrovascular amyloid protein. *Biochem Biophys Res Commun*, 1984; **120**(3): 885–90.

14. Masters, C. L., G. Multhaup, G. Simms *et al.* Neuronal origin of a cerebral amyloid: neurofibrillary tangles of Alzheimer's disease contain the same protein as the

amyloid of plaque cores and blood vessels. *Embo J*, 1985; **4**(11): 2757–63.

15. Masters, C. L., G. Simms, N. A. Weinman *et al.* Amyloid plaque core protein in Alzheimer disease and Down syndrome. *Proc Natl Acad Sci USA*, 1985; **82**(12): 4245–9.

16. Robakis, N. K., N. Ramakrishna, G. Wolfe, and H. M. Wisniewski. Molecular cloning and characterization of a cDNA encoding the cerebrovascular and the neuritic plaque amyloid peptides. *Proc Natl Acad Sci USA*, 1987; **84**(12): 4190–4.

17. Tanzi, R. E., J. F. Gusella, P. C. Watkins *et al.* Amyloid beta protein gene: cDNA, mRNA distribution, and genetic linkage near the Alzheimer locus. *Science*, 1987; **235**(4791): 880–4.

18. Kang, J., H. G. Lemaire, A. Unterbeck *et al.* The precursor of Alzheimer's disease amyloid A4 protein resembles a cell-surface receptor. *Nature*, 1987; **325**(6106): 733–6.

19. Goldgaber, D., M. I. Lerman, O. W. McBride, U. Saffiotti and D. C. Gajdusek. Characterization and chromosomal localization of a cDNA encoding brain amyloid of Alzheimer's disease. *Science*, 1987; **235**(4791): 877–80.

20. Yoshikai, S., H. Sasaki, K. Doh-ura, H. Furuya and Y. Sakaki. Genomic organization of the human amyloid beta-protein precursor gene. *Gene*, 1990; **87**(2): 257–63.

21. Tanaka, S., S. Nakamura, K. Ueda *et al.* Three types of amyloid protein precursor mRNA in human brain: their differential expression in Alzheimer's disease. *Biochem Biophys Res Commun*, 1988; **157**(2): 472–9.

22. Levy, E., M. D. Carman, I. J. Fernandez-Madrid *et al.* Mutation of the Alzheimer's disease amyloid gene in hereditary cerebral hemorrhage, Dutch type. *Science*, 1990; **248**(4959): 1124–6.

23. Goate, A., M. C. Chartier-Harlin, M. Mullan *et al.* Segregation of a missense mutation in the amyloid precursor protein gene with familial Alzheimer's disease. *Nature*, 1991; **349**(6311): 704–6.

24. Sherrington, R., E. I. Rogaev, Y. Liang *et al.* Cloning of a gene bearing missense mutations in early-onset familial Alzheimer's disease. *Nature*, 1995; **375**(6534): 754–60.

25. Levy-Lahad, E., E. M. Wijsman, E. Nemens *et al.* A familial Alzheimer's disease locus on chromosome 1. *Science*, 1995; **269**(5226): 970–3.

26. Herreman, A., D. Hartmann, W. Annaert *et al.* Presenilin 2 deficiency causes a mild pulmonary phenotype and no changes in amyloid precursor protein processing but enhances the embryonic lethal phenotype of presenilin 1 deficiency. *Proc Natl Acad Sci USA*, 1999; **96**(21): 11872–7.

27. Janssen, J. C., J. A. Beck, T. A. Campbell *et al.* Early onset familial Alzheimer's disease: Mutation frequency in 31 families. *Neurology*, 2003; **60**(2): 235–9.

28. Lampe, T. H., T. D. Bird, D. Nochlin *et al.* Phenotype of chromosome 14-linked familial Alzheimer's disease in a large kindred. *Ann Neurol*, 1994; **36**(3): 368–78.

29. Lippa, C. F., J. M. Swearer, K. J. Kane *et al.* Familial Alzheimer's disease: site of mutation influences clinical phenotype. *Ann Neurol*, 2000; **48**(3): 376–9.

30. Lopera, F., A. Ardilla, A. Martinez *et al.* Clinical features of early-onset Alzheimer disease in a large kindred with an E280A presenilin-1 mutation. *JAMA* 1997; **277**(10): 793–9.

31. Ikeda, M., V. Sharma, S. M. Sumi *et al.* The clinical phenotype of two missense mutations in the presenilin I gene in Japanese patients. *Ann Neurol*, 1996; **40**(6): 912–7.

32. Axelman, K., H. Basun, and L. Lannfelt. Wide range of disease onset in a family with Alzheimer disease and a His163Tyr mutation in the presenilin-1 gene. *Arch Neurol*, 1998; **55**(5): 698–702.

33. Bird, T. D., E. Levy-Lahad, P. Poorkaj *et al.* Wide range in age of onset for chromosome 1-related familial Alzheimer's disease. *Ann Neurol*, 1996; **40**(6): 932–6.

34. de Strooper, B. Aph-1, Pen-2, and nicastrin with presenilin generate an active gamma-secretase complex. *Neuron*, 2003; **38**(1): 9–12.

35. Duff, K., C. Eckman, C. Zehr *et al.* Increased amyloid-beta42(43) in brains of mice expressing mutant presenilin 1. *Nature*, 1996; **383**(6602): 710–3.

36. Scheuner, D., C. Eckman, M. Jensen *et al.* Secreted amyloid beta-protein similar to that in the senile plaques of Alzheimer's disease is increased in vivo by the presenilin 1 and 2 and APP mutations linked to familial Alzheimer's disease. *Nat Med*, 1996; **2**(8): 864–70.

37. Donoviel, D. B., A. K. Hadjantonakis, M. Ikeda *et al.* Mice lacking both presenilin genes exhibit early embryonic patterning defects. *Genes Dev*, 1999; **13**(21): 2801–10.

38. Shen, J., R. T. Bronson, D. F. Chen *et al.* Skeletal and CNS defects in presenilin-1-deficient mice. *Cell*, 1997; **89**(4): 629–39.

39. Pericak-Vance, M. A., J. L. Bebout, P. C. Gaskell, Jr. *et al.* Linkage studies in familial Alzheimer disease: evidence for chromosome 19 linkage. *Am J Hum Genet*, 1991; **48**(6): 1034–50.

40. Corder, E. H., A. M. Saunders, W. J. Strittmatter *et al.* Gene dose of apolipoprotein E type 4 allele and the risk of Alzheimer's disease in late onset families. *Science*, 1993; **261**(5123): 921–3.

41. Saunders, A. M., W. J. Strittmatter, D. Schmechel *et al.* Association of apolipoprotein E allele epsilon 4 with late-onset familial and sporadic Alzheimer's disease. *Neurology*, 1993; **43**(8): 1467–72.

42. Strittmatter, W. J., A. M. Saunders, D. Schmechel *et al.* Apolipoprotein E: high-avidity binding to beta-amyloid and increased frequency of type 4 allele in

late-onset familial Alzheimer disease. *Proc Natl Acad Sci USA*, 1993; **90**(5): 1977–81.

43. Bertram, L., M. B. McQueen, K. Mullin, D. Blacker and R. E. Tanzi. Systematic meta-analyses of Alzheimer disease genetic association studies: the AlzGene database. *Nat Genet*, 2007; **39**(1): 17–23.

44. Blacker, D., J. L. Haines, L. Rodes *et al.* ApoE-4 and age at onset of Alzheimer's disease: the NIMH genetics initiative. *Neurology*, 1997; **48**(1): 139–47.

45. Corder, E. H., A. M. Saunders, N. J. Risch *et al.* Protective effect of apolipoprotein E type 2 allele for late onset Alzheimer disease. *Nat Genet*, 1994; **7**(2): 180–4.

46. Talbot, C., C. Lendon, N. Craddock *et al.* Protection against Alzheimer's disease with apoE epsilon 2. *Lancet*, 1994; **343**(8910): 1432–3.

47. West, H. L., G. W. Rebeck and B. T. Hyman. Frequency of the apolipoprotein E epsilon 2 allele is diminished in sporadic Alzheimer disease. *Neurosci Lett*, 1994; **175**(1–2): 46–8.

48. Bales, K. R., T. Verina, D. J. Cummins *et al.* Apolipoprotein E is essential for amyloid deposition in the APP(V717F) transgenic mouse model of Alzheimer's disease. *Proc Natl Acad Sci USA*, 1999; **96**(26): 15233–8.

49. LaDu, M. J., M. T. Falduto, A. M. Manelli *et al.* Isoform-specific binding of apolipoprotein E to beta-amyloid. *J Biol Chem*, 1994; **269**(38): 23403–6.

50. Nathan, B. P., S. Bellosta, D. A. Sanan *et al.* Differential effects of apolipoproteins E3 and E4 on neuronal growth in vitro. *Science*, 1994; **264**(5160): 850–2.

51. Goldman, J. S., J. M. Farmer, E. M. Wood *et al.* Comparison of family histories in FTLD subtypes and related tauopathies. *Neurology*, 2005; **65**(11): 1817–9.

52. Hutton, M., C. L. Lendon, P. Rizzu *et al.* Association of missense and 5′-splice-site mutations in tau with the inherited dementia FTDP-17. *Nature*, 1998; **393**(6686): 702–5.

53. Goedert, M., M. G. Spillantini, R. Jakes, D. Rutherford and R. A. Crowther. Multiple isoforms of human microtubule-associated protein tau: sequences and localization in neurofibrillary tangles of Alzheimer's disease. *Neuron*, 1989; **3**(4): 519–26.

54. Hasegawa, M., M. J. Smith and M. Goedert. Tau proteins with FTDP-17 mutations have a reduced ability to promote microtubule assembly. *FEBS Lett*, 1998; **437**(3): 207–10.

55. Hong, M., V. Zhukareva, V. Vogelsberg-Ragaglia *et al.* Mutation-specific functional impairments in distinct tau isoforms of hereditary FTDP-17. *Science*, 1998; **282**(5395): 1914–17.

56. Heutink, P., M. Stevens, P. Rizzu *et al.* Hereditary frontotemporal dementia is linked to chromosome 17q21–q22: a genetic and clinicopathological study of three Dutch families. *Ann Neurol*, 1997; **41**(2): 150–9.

57. Wszolek, Z. K., R. F. Pfeiffer, M. H. Bhatt *et al.* Rapidly progressive autosomal dominant parkinsonism and dementia with pallido-ponto-nigral degeneration. *Ann Neurol*, 1992; **32**(3): 312–20.

58. Lindquist, S. G., I. E. Holm, M. Schwartz *et al.* Alzheimer disease-like clinical phenotype in a family with FTDP-17 caused by a MAPT R406W mutation. *Eur J Neurol*, 2008; **15**(4): 377–85.

59. Ostojic, J., C. Elfgren, U. Passant *et al.* The tau R406W mutation causes progressive presenile dementia with bitemporal atrophy. *Dement Geriatr Cogn Disord*, 2004; **17**(4): 298–301.

60. Ghetti, B., J. R. Murrell, P. Zolo, M. G. Spillantini and M. Goedert. Progress in hereditary tauopathies: a mutation in the tau gene (G389R) causes a Pick disease-like syndrome. *Ann N Y Acad Sci*, 2000; **920**: 52–62.

61. Rossi, G., C. Marelli, L. Farina *et al.* The G389R mutation in the MAPT gene presenting as sporadic corticobasal syndrome. *Mov Disord*, 2008; **23**(6): 892–5.

62. Poorkaj, P., N. A. Muma, V. Zhukareva *et al.* An R5L tau mutation in a subject with a progressive supranuclear palsy phenotype. *Ann Neurol*, 2002; **52**(4): 511–16.

63. Ros, R., S. Thobois, N. Streichenberger *et al.* A new mutation of the tau gene, G303V, in early-onset familial progressive supranuclear palsy. *Arch Neurol*, 2005; **62**(9): 1444–50.

64. Doerflinger, H., R. Benton, J. M. Shulman and D. St Johnston. The role of PAR-1 in regulating the polarised microtubule cytoskeleton in the *Drosophila* follicular epithelium. *Development*, 2003; **130**(17): 3965–75.

65. Harada, A., K. Oguchi, S. Okabe *et al.* Altered microtubule organization in small-calibre axons of mice lacking tau protein. *Nature*, 1994; **369**(6480): 488–91.

66. Takei, Y., J. Teng, A. Harada and N. Hirokawa. Defects in axonal elongation and neuronal migration in mice with disrupted tau and map1b genes. *J Cell Biol*, 2000; **150**(5): 989–1000.

67. Jackson, G. R., M. Wiedau-Pazos, T. K. Sang *et al.* Human wild-type tau interacts with wingless pathway components and produces neurofibrillary pathology in *Drosophila*. *Neuron*, 2002; **34**(4): 509–19.

68. Ramsden, M., L. Kotilinek, C. Forster *et al.* Age-dependent neurofibrillary tangle formation, neuron loss, and memory impairment in a mouse model of human tauopathy (P301L). *J Neurosci*, 2005; **25**(46): 10637–47.

69. Santacruz, K., J. Lewis, T. Spires *et al.* Tau suppression in a neurodegenerative mouse model improves memory function. *Science*, 2005; **309**(5733): 476–81.

70. Watts, G. D., J. Wymer, M. J. Kovach *et al.* Inclusion body myopathy associated with Paget disease of bone and frontotemporal dementia is caused by mutant valosin-containing protein. *Nat Genet*, 2004; **36**(4): 377–81.

71. Guyant-Marechal, L., A. Laquerriere, C. Duyckaerts *et al.* Valosin-containing protein gene mutations: clinical and neuropathologic features. *Neurology*, 2006; **67**(4): 644–51.

72. Forman, M. S., I. R. Mackenzie, N. J. Cairns *et al.* Novel ubiquitin neuropathology in frontotemporal dementia with valosin-containing protein gene mutations. *J Neuropathol Exp Neurol*, 2006; **65**(6): 571–81.

73. Neumann, M., I. R. Mackenzie, N. J. Cairns *et al.* TDP-43 in the ubiquitin pathology of frontotemporal dementia with VCP gene mutations. *J Neuropathol Exp Neurol*, 2007; **66**(2): 152–7.

74. Wang, Q., C. Song and C. C. Li. Molecular perspectives on p97-VCP: progress in understanding its structure and diverse biological functions. *J Struct Biol*, 2004; **146**(1–2): 44–57.

75. Ruden, D. M., V. Sollars, X. Wang *et al.* Membrane fusion proteins are required for oskar mRNA localization in the Drosophila egg chamber. *Dev Biol*, 2000; **218**(2): 314–25.

76. Higashiyama, H., F. Hirose, M. Yamaguchi *et al.* Identification of ter94, Drosophila VCP, as a modulator of polyglutamine-induced neurodegeneration. *Cell Death Differ*, 2002; **9**(3): 264–73.

77. Boeddrich, A., S. Gaumer, A. Haacke *et al.* An arginine/lysine-rich motif is crucial for VCP/p97-mediated modulation of ataxin-3 fibrillogenesis. *Embo J*, 2006; **25**(7): 1547–58.

78. Skibinski, G., N. J. Parkinson, J. M. Brown *et al.* Mutations in the endosomal ESCRTIII-complex subunit CHMP2B in frontotemporal dementia. *Nat Genet*, 2005; **37**(8): 806–8.

79. Gydesen, S., J. M. Brown, A. Brun *et al.* Chromosome 3 linked frontotemporal dementia (FTD-3). *Neurology*, 2002; **59**(10): 1585–94.

80. Momeni, P., E. Rogaeva, V. van Deerlin *et al.* Genetic variability in CHMP2B and frontotemporal dementia. *Neurodegener Dis*, 2006; **3**(3): 129–33.

81. van der Zee, J., H. Urwin, S. Engelborghs *et al.* CHMP2B C-truncating mutations in frontotemporal lobar degeneration are associated with an aberrant endosomal phenotype in vitro. *Hum Mol Genet*, 2008; **17**(2): 313–22.

82. Lee, J. A., A. Beigneux, S. T. Ahmad, S. G. Young and F. B. Gao. ESCRT-III dysfunction causes autophagosome accumulation and neurodegeneration. *Curr Biol*, 2007; **17**(18): 1561–7.

83. Cruts, M., I. Gijselinck, J. van der Zee *et al.* Null mutations in progranulin cause ubiquitin-positive frontotemporal dementia linked to chromosome 17q21. *Nature*, 2006; **442**(7105): 920–4.

84. Baker, M., I. R. Mackenzie, S. M. Pickering-Brown *et al.* Mutations in progranulin cause tau-negative frontotemporal dementia linked to chromosome 17. *Nature*, 2006; **442**(7105): 916–19.

85. Rademakers, R., M. Cruts, B. Dermaut *et al.* Tau negative frontal lobe dementia at 17q21: significant finemapping of the candidate region to a 4.8 cM interval. *Mol Psychiatry*, 2002; **7**(10): 1064–74.

86. Mackenzie, I. R., M. Baker, G. West *et al.* A family with tau-negative frontotemporal dementia and neuronal intranuclear inclusions linked to chromosome 17. *Brain*, 2006; **129**(Pt 4): 853–67.

87. Rosso, S. M., W. Kamphorst, B. de Graaf *et al.* Familial frontotemporal dementia with ubiquitin-positive inclusions is linked to chromosome 17q21–22. *Brain*, 2001; **124**(Pt 10): 1948–57.

88. Kertesz, A., T. Kawarai, E. Rogaeva *et al.* Familial frontotemporal dementia with ubiquitin-positive, tau-negative inclusions. *Neurology*, 2000; **54**(4): 818–27.

89. Lendon, C. L., T. Lynch, J. Norton *et al.* Hereditary dysphasic disinhibition dementia: a frontotemporal dementia linked to 17q21–22. *Neurology*, 1998; **50**(6): 1546–55.

90. He, Z. and A. Bateman. Progranulin (granulin-epithelin precursor, PC-cell-derived growth factor, acrogranin) mediates tissue repair and tumorigenesis. *J Mol Med*, 2003; **81**(10): 600–12.

91. Hrabal, R., Z. Chen, S. James, H. P. Bennett and F. Ni. The hairpin stack fold, a novel protein architecture for a new family of protein growth factors. *Nat Struct Biol*, 1996; **3**(9): 747–52.

92. Bateman, A., D. Belcourt, H. Bennett, C. Lazure and S. Solomon. Granulins, a novel class of peptide from leukocytes. *Biochem Biophys Res Commun*, 1990; **173**(3): 1161–8.

93. Daniel, R., E. Daniels, Z. He and A. Bateman. Progranulin (acrogranin/PC cell-derived growth factor/granulin-epithelin precursor) is expressed in the placenta, epidermis, microvasculature, and brain during murine development. *Dev Dyn*, 2003; **227**(4): 593–9.

94. Suzuki, M. and M. Nishiahara. Granulin precursor gene: a sex steroid-inducible gene involved in sexual differentiation of the rat brain. *Mol Genet Metab*, 2002; **75**(1): 31–7.

95. Suzuki, M., S. Yoshida, M. Nishihara and M. Takahashi. Identification of a sex steroid-inducible gene in the neonatal rat hypothalamus. *Neurosci Lett*, 1998; **242**(3): 127–30.

96. Gass, J., A. Cannon, I. R. Mackenzie *et al.* Mutations in progranulin are a major cause of ubiquitin-positive frontotemporal lobar degeneration. *Hum Mol Genet*, 2006; **15**(20): 2988–3001.

97. Snowden, J. S., S. M. Pickering-Brown, I. R. Mackenzie *et al.* Progranulin gene mutations associated with frontotemporal dementia and progressive non-fluent aphasia. *Brain*, 2006; **129**(Pt 11): 3091–102.

98. Masellis, M., P. Momeni, W. Meschino *et al.* Novel splicing mutation in the progranulin gene causing familial corticobasal syndrome. *Brain*, 2006; **129**(Pt 11): 3115–23.

99. Mesulam, M., N. Johnson, T. A. Krefft *et al.* Progranulin mutations in primary progressive aphasia: the PPA1 and PPA3 families. *Arch Neurol*, 2007; **64**(1): 43–7.

100. Davion, S., N. Johnson, S. Weintraub *et al.* Clinicopathologic correlation in PGRN mutations. *Neurology*, 2007; **69**(11): 1113–21.

101. Mackenzie, I. R., M. Baker, S. Pickering-Brown *et al.* The neuropathology of frontotemporal lobar degeneration caused by mutations in the progranulin gene. *Brain*, 2006; **129**(Pt 11): 3081–90.

102. Neumann, M., D. M. Sampathu, L. K. Kwong *et al.* Ubiquitinated TDP-43 in frontotemporal lobar degeneration and amyotrophic lateral sclerosis. *Science*, 2006; **314**(5796): 130–3.

103. van der Zee, J., I. Le Ber, S. Maurer-Stroh *et al.* Mutations other than null mutations producing a pathogenic loss of progranulin in frontotemporal dementia. *Hum Mutat*, 2007; **28**(4): 416.

104. Polymeropoulos, M. H., J. J. Higgins, L. I. Golbe *et al.* Mapping of a gene for Parkinson's disease to chromosome 4q21–q23. *Science*, 1996; **274**(5290): 1197–9.

105. Polymeropoulos, M. H., C. Lavedan, E. Leroy *et al.* Mutation in the alpha-synuclein gene identified in families with Parkinson's disease. *Science*, 1997; **276**(5321): 2045–7.

106. Kahle, P. J., M. Neumann, L. Ozmen *et al.* Subcellular localization of wild-type and Parkinson's disease-associated mutant alpha-synuclein in human and transgenic mouse brain. *J Neurosci*, 2000; **20**(17): 6365–73.

107. Zarranz, J. J., J. Alegre, J. C. Gomez-Esteban *et al.* The new mutation, E46K, of alpha-synuclein causes Parkinson and Lewy body dementia. *Ann Neurol*, 2004; **55**(2): 164–73.

108. Kruger, R., W. Kuhn, T. Muller *et al.* Ala30Pro mutation in the gene encoding alpha-synuclein in Parkinson's disease. *Nat Genet*, 1998; **18**(2): 106–8.

109. Spillantini, M. G., M. L. Schmidt, V. M. Lee *et al.* Alpha-synuclein in Lewy bodies. *Nature*, 1997; **388**(6645): 839–40.

110. Abeliovich, A., Y. Schmitz, I. Farinas *et al.* Mice lacking alpha-synuclein display functional deficits in the nigrostriatal dopamine system. *Neuron*, 2000; **25**(1): 239–52.

111. Singleton, A. B., M. Farrer, J. Johnson *et al.* Alpha-synuclein locus triplication causes Parkinson's disease. *Science*, 2003; **302**(5646): 841.

112. Ibanez, P., A. M. Bonnet, B. Debarges *et al.* Causal relation between alpha-synuclein gene duplication and familial Parkinson's disease. *Lancet*, 2004; **364**(9440): 1169–71.

113. Chartier-Harlin, M. C., J. Kachergus, C. Roumier *et al.* Alpha-synuclein locus duplication as a cause of familial Parkinson's disease. *Lancet*, 2004; **364**(9440): 1167–9.

114. Chiba-Falek, O. and R. L. Nussbaum. Effect of allelic variation at the NACP-Rep1 repeat upstream of the alpha-synuclein gene (SNCA) on transcription in a cell culture luciferase reporter system. *Hum Mol Genet*, 2001; **10**(26): 3101–9.

115. Maraganore, D. M., M. de Andrade, A. Elbaz *et al.* Collaborative analysis of alpha-synuclein gene promoter variability and Parkinson disease. *JAMA* 2006; **296**(6): 661–70.

116. Kitada, T., S. Asakawa, N. Hattori *et al.* Mutations in the *parkin* gene cause autosomal recessive juvenile parkinsonism. *Nature*, 1998; **392**(6676): 605–8.

117. Valente, E. M., P. M. Abou-Sleiman, V. Caputo *et al.* Hereditary early-onset Parkinson's disease caused by mutations in *PINK1*. *Science*, 2004; **304**(5674): 1158–60.

118. Leroy, E., R. Boyer, G. Auburger *et al.* The ubiquitin pathway in Parkinson's disease. *Nature*, 1998; **395** (6701): 451–2.

119. Bonifati, V., P. Rizzu, M. J. van Baren *et al.* Mutations in the *DJ-1* gene associated with autosomal recessive early-onset parkinsonism. *Science*, 2003; **299**(5604): 256–9.

120. Paisan-Ruiz, C., S. Jain, E. W. Evans *et al.* Cloning of the gene containing mutations that cause PARK8-linked Parkinson's disease. *Neuron*, 2004; **44**(4): 595–600.

121. Zimprich, A., S. Biskup, P. Leitner *et al.* Mutations in LRRK2 cause autosomal-dominant parkinsonism with pleomorphic pathology. *Neuron*, 2004; **44**(4): 601–7.

122. Giasson, B. I., J. P. Covy, N. M. Bonini *et al.* Biochemical and pathological characterization of Lrrk2. *Ann Neurol*, 2006; **59**(2): 315–22.

123. Ross, O. A., M. Toft, A. J. Whittle *et al.* Lrrk2 and Lewy body disease. *Ann Neurol*, 2006; **59**(2): 388–93.

124. Healy, D. G., M. Falchi, S. S. O'Sullivan *et al.* Phenotype, genotype, and worldwide genetic penetrance of LRRK2-associated Parkinson's disease: a case–control study. *Lancet Neurol*, 2008; **7**(7): 583–90.

125. West, A. B., D. J. Moore, S. Biskup *et al.* Parkinson's disease-associated mutations in leucine-rich repeat kinase 2 augment kinase activity. *Proc Natl Acad Sci USA*, 2005; **102**(46): 16842–7.

126. Lewis, P. A., E. Greggio, A. Beilina *et al.* The R1441C mutation of LRRK2 disrupts GTP hydrolysis. *Biochem Biophys Res Commun*, 2007; **357**(3): 668–71.

127. Tuite, P. J., H. B. Clark, C. Bergeron *et al.* Clinical and pathologic evidence of corticobasal degeneration and progressive supranuclear palsy in familial tauopathy. *Arch Neurol*, 2005; 62(9): 1453–7.

128. Baker, M., I. Litvan, H. Houlden *et al.* Association of an extended haplotype in the tau gene with progressive supranuclear palsy. *Hum Mol Genet*, 1999; 8(4): 711–15.

129. Spillantini, M. G., H. Yoshida, C. Rizzini *et al.* A novel tau mutation (N296N) in familial dementia with swollen achromatic neurons and corticobasal inclusion bodies. *Ann Neurol*, 2000; 48(6): 939–43.

130. Gajdusek, D. C., C. J. Gibbs and M. Alpers. Experimental transmission of a Kuru-like syndrome to chimpanzees. *Nature*, 1966; 209(5025): 794–6.

131. Gibbs, C. J., Jr., D. C. Gajdusek, D. M. Asher *et al.* Creutzfeldt–Jakob disease (spongiform encephalopathy): transmission to the chimpanzee. *Science*, 1968; 161(839): 388–9.

132. Roos, R., D. C. Gajdusek and C. J. Gibbs, Jr. The clinical characteristics of transmissible Creutzfeldt–Jakob disease. *Brain*, 1973; 96(1): 1–20.

133. Prusiner, S. B. Novel proteinaceous infectious particles cause scrapie. *Science*, 1982; 216(4542): 136–44.

134. Bendheim, P. E., J. M. Bockman, M. P. McKinley, D. T. Kingsbury and S. B. Prusiner. Scrapie and Creutzfeldt–Jakob disease prion proteins share physical properties and antigenic determinants. *Proc Natl Acad Sci USA*, 1985; 82(4): 997–1001.

135. Hsiao, K., H. F. Baker, T. J. Crow *et al.* Linkage of a prion protein missense variant to Gerstmann–Straussler syndrome. *Nature*, 1989; 338(6213): 342–5.

136. Owen, F., M. Poulter, R. Lofthouse *et al.* Insertion in prion protein gene in familial Creutzfeldt–Jakob disease. *Lancet*, 1989; 1(8628): 51–2.

137. Goldfarb, L. G., R. B. Petersen, M. Tabaton *et al.* Fatal familial insomnia and familial Creutzfeldt–Jakob disease: disease phenotype determined by a DNA polymorphism. *Science*, 1992; 258(5083): 806–8.

138. Medori, R., H. J. Tritschler, A. LeBlanc *et al.* Fatal familial insomnia, a prion disease with a mutation at codon 178 of the prion protein gene. *N Engl J Med*, 1992; 326(7): 444–9.

139. Vanik, D. L. and W. K. Surewicz. Disease-associated F198S mutation increases the propensity of the recombinant prion protein for conformational conversion to scrapie-like form. *J Biol Chem*, 2002; 277(50): 49065–70.

140. Zahn, R., A. Liu, T. Luhrs *et al.* NMR solution structure of the human prion protein. *Proc Natl Acad Sci USA*, 2000; 97(1): 145–50.

141. Zhang, Y., W. Swietnicki, M. G. Zagorski, W. K. Surewicz and F. D. Sonnichsen. Solution structure of the E200K variant of human prion protein. Implications for the mechanism of pathogenesis in familial prion diseases. *J Biol Chem*, 2000; 275(43): 33650–4.

142. Zimmermann, K., P. L. Turecek and H. P. Schwarz. Genotyping of the prion protein gene at codon 129. *Acta Neuropathol*, 1999; 97(4): 355–8.

143. Tanaka, Y., K. Minematsu, H. Moriyasu *et al.* A Japanese family with a variant of Gerstmann–Straussler–Scheinker disease. *J Neurol Neurosurg Psychiatry*, 1997; 62(5): 454–7.

144. Hsiao, K., M. Scott, D. Foster *et al.* Spontaneous neurodegeneration in transgenic mice with prion protein codon 101 proline–leucine substitution. *Ann N Y Acad Sci*, 1991; 640: 166–70.

145. Kahana, E., N. Zilber and M. Abraham. Do Creutzfeldt–Jakob disease patients of Jewish Libyan origin have unique clinical features? *Neurology*, 1991; 41(9): 1390–2.

146. Mead, S. Prion disease genetics. *Eur J Hum Genet*, 2006; 14(3): 273–81.

147. Owen, F., M. Poulter, T. Shah *et al.* An in-frame insertion in the prion protein gene in familial Creutzfeldt–Jakob disease. *Brain Res Mol Brain Res*, 1990; 7(3): 273–6.

148. Rowe, D. B., V. Lewis, M. Needham *et al.* Novel prion protein gene mutation presenting with subacute PSP-like syndrome. *Neurology*, 2007; 68(11): 868–70.

149. Croes, E. A., J. Theuns, J. J. Houwing-Duistermaat *et al.* Octapeptide repeat insertions in the prion protein gene and early onset dementia. *J Neurol Neurosurg Psychiatry*, 2004; 75(8): 1166–70.

150. Lee, H. S., P. Brown, L. Cervenakova *et al.* Increased susceptibility to kuru of carriers of the PRNP 129 methionine/methionine genotype. *J Infect Dis*, 2001; 183(2): 192–6.

151. Cervenakova, L., L. G. Goldfarb, R. Garruto *et al.* Phenotype–genotype studies in kuru: implications for new variant Creutzfeldt–Jakob disease. *Proc Natl Acad Sci USA*, 1998; 95(22): 13239–41.

152. Palmer, M. S., A. J. Dryden, J. T. Hughes and J. Collinge. Homozygous prion protein genotype predisposes to sporadic Creutzfeldt–Jakob disease. *Nature*, 1991; 352(6333): 340–2.

153. Zeidler, M., G. Stewart, S. N. Cousens, K. Estibeiro and R. G. Will. Codon 129 genotype and new variant CJD. *Lancet*, 1997; 350(9078): 668.

154. The Huntington's Disease Collaborative Research Group. A novel gene containing a trinucleotide repeat that is expanded and unstable on Huntington's disease chromosomes. *Cell*, 1993; 72(6): 971–83.

155. Kremer, B., P. Goldberg, S. E. Andrew *et al.* A worldwide study of the Huntington's disease mutation. The sensitivity and specificity of measuring CAG repeats. *N Engl J Med*, 1994; 330(20): 1401–6.

156. Rubinsztein, D. C., J. Leggo, R. Coles *et al.* Phenotypic characterization of individuals with 30–40 CAG repeats in the Huntington disease (HD) gene reveals HD cases with 36 repeats and apparently normal elderly individuals with 36–39 repeats. *Am J Hum Genet*, 1996; **59**(1): 16–22.

157. Merrit, A. D., P. M. Conneally, N. F. Rahman and A. L. Drew. Juvenile Huntington's chorea. In *Progress in Neurogenetics*, A. Barbeau and J. R. Brunnette. (eds.). Amsterdam: Excerpta Medica Foundation, 1969: 645–650.

158. Ridley, R. M., C. D. Frith, T. J. Crow and P. M. Conneally. Anticipation in Huntington's disease is inherited through the male line but may originate in the female. *J Med Genet*, 1988; **25**(9): 589–95.

159. Andrew, S. E., Y. P. Goldberg, B. Kremer *et al.* The relationship between trinucleotide (CAG) repeat length and clinical features of Huntington's disease. *Nat Genet*, 1993; **4**(4): 398–403.

160. Duyao, M., C. Ambrose, R. Myers *et al.* Trinucleotide repeat length instability and age of onset in Huntington's disease. *Nat Genet*, 1993; **4**(4): 387–92.

161. Snell, R. G., J. C. MacMillan, J. P. Cheadle *et al.* Relationship between trinucleotide repeat expansion and phenotypic variation in Huntington's disease. *Nat Genet*, 1993; **4**(4): 393–7.

162. Kremer, B., E. Almqvist, J. Theilmann *et al.* Sex-dependent mechanisms for expansions and contractions of the CAG repeat on affected Huntington disease chromosomes. *Am J Hum Genet*, 1995; **57**(2): 343–50.

163. Strong, T. V., D. A. Tagle, J. M. Valdes *et al.* Widespread expression of the human and rat Huntington's disease gene in brain and nonneural tissues. *Nat Genet*, 1993; **5**(3): 259–65.

164. Sharp, A. H., S. J. Loev, G. Schilling *et al.* Widespread expression of Huntington's disease gene (IT15) protein product. *Neuron*, 1995; **14**(5): 1065–74.

165. Duyao, M. P., A. B. Auerbach, A. Ryan *et al.* Inactivation of the mouse Huntington's disease gene homolog *Hdh*. *Science*, 1995; **269**(5222): 407–10.

166. Nasir, J., S. B. Floresco, J. R. O'Kusky *et al.* Targeted disruption of the Huntington's disease gene results in embryonic lethality and behavioral and morphological changes in heterozygotes. *Cell*, 1995; **81**(5): 811–23.

167. Zeitlin, S., J. P. Liu, D. L. Chapman, V. E. Papaioannou and A. Efstratiadis. Increased apoptosis and early embryonic lethality in mice nullizygous for the Huntington's disease gene homologue. *Nat Genet*, 1995; **11**(2): 155–63.

168. Mangiarini, L., K. Sathasivam, M. Seller *et al.* Exon 1 of the HD gene with an expanded CAG repeat is sufficient to cause a progressive neurological phenotype in transgenic mice. *Cell*, 1996; **87**(3): 493–506.

169. Reddy, P. H., M. Williams, V. Charles *et al.* Behavioural abnormalities and selective neuronal loss in HD transgenic mice expressing mutated full-length HD cDNA. *Nat Genet*, 1998; **20**(2): 198–202.

170. Shelbourne, P. F., N. Killeen, R. F. Hevner *et al.* A Huntington's disease CAG expansion at the murine *Hdh* locus is unstable and associated with behavioural abnormalities in mice. *Hum Mol Genet*, 1999; **8**(5): 763–74.

171. Lin, C. H., S. Tallaksen-Greene, W. M. Chien *et al.* Neurological abnormalities in a knock-in mouse model of Huntington's disease. *Hum Mol Genet*, 2001; **10**(2): 137–44.

172. Arrasate, M., S. Mitra, E. S. Schweitzer, M. R. Segal and S. Finkbeiner. Inclusion body formation reduces levels of mutant huntingtin and the risk of neuronal death. *Nature*, 2004; **431**(7010): 805–10.

173. Saudou, F., S. Finkbeiner, D. Devys and M. E. Greenberg. Huntingtin acts in the nucleus to induce apoptosis but death does not correlate with the formation of intranuclear inclusions. *Cell*, 1998; **95**(1): 55–66.

174. Finishing the euchromatic sequence of the human genome. *Nature*, 2004; **431**(7011): 931–45.

175. International HapMap Consortium. A haplotype map of the human genome. *Nature*, 2005; **437**(7063): 1299–320.

176. Coon, K. D., A. J. Myers, D. W. Craig *et al.* A high-density whole-genome association study reveals that APOE is the major susceptibility gene for sporadic late-onset Alzheimer's disease. *J Clin Psychiatry*, 2007; **68**(4): 613–18.

Chapter 4

Frontotemporal dementia

Indre V. Viskontas and Bruce L. Miller

Introduction

With "baby boomers" now reaching late middle age, degenerative diseases are becoming an increasingly important national health issue. One such disorder, frontotemporal lobar degeneration (FTLD), is particularly devastating to patients and their families, as symptoms include changes in behavior and the erosion of personal relationships, often during the earliest stages. These disease features place great demands on caregivers and the society at large. Understanding the disease and its complexities, and educating the general public with respect to the course and causes of FTLD, is, therefore, acutely important.

The condition typically presents in patients who are between 45 and 65 years of age, and is at least as likely as early-onset Alzheimer's disease (AD) with a prevalence of approximately 15 per 100 000 population between 45 and 64 years of age.[1] Knopman and colleagues[2] have shown that FTLD is more common than AD in patients under the age of 60 years, while other authors suggest that FTLD-spectrum disorders account for up to 20% of all patients with degenerative dementias.[3,4] Genetics remain the only known etiology for FTLD, accounting for up to 40% of all cases, although large epidemiology studies investigating other risk factors have yet to be undertaken.

Frontotemporal lobar degeneration encapsulates a heterogeneous group of clinical and pathological syndromes and can begin with behavioral, cognitive, language or motor signs and symptoms. Although both the frontal and temporal brain regions are involved in nearly all cases, there is significant variability as to whether the left or right frontal or temporal lobe is the most severe and earliest site of involvement. Perhaps the most widely accepted classification system divides FTLD into three (or four) subtypes: behavioral

or frontal-variant frontotemporal dementia (bv-FTD; sometimes simply called FTD); the temporal variant (tv-FTD), or semantic dementia (SD); and a left frontal and insular predominant degeneration called progressive non-fluent aphasia (PNFA). The temporal variant can begin on the right side and when it does deficits in emotion predominate. In contrast, when the disease begins on the left side, patients show a loss of word meaning and conceptual knowledge. The main symptoms of each of these subtypes are listed in Table 4.1. While the subtype classification is based primarily on presenting symptoms, recent findings suggest that bv-FTD, tv-FTD (right and left) and PNFA differ in prevalence, age of onset, sex distributions, genetic susceptibilities, co-associations with other degenerative conditions and neuropathological features. Therefore, we continue to use this somewhat bulky and imperfect nomenclature system, until a more effective and accurate classification system can be devised.

A brief history of frontotemporal lobar degeneration

Arnold Pick first described a set of symptoms resulting from focal temporal atrophy that are now ascribed to FTLD.[5] While most of Pick's original cases had focal temporal atrophy and would now be classified as having SD, he also described patients with focal frontal disease. His early work was supplemented by Alois Alzheimer, who noted that intraneuronal inclusions were seen upon pathological investigation of such patients.[6] Pick emphasized that language loss was typical of his temporal lobe cases and he was particularly interested in showing that degenerative disorders could be associated with highly focal clinical syndromes. Even though cases of FTLD were described early in the twentieth century, patients with FTLD were largely ignored in the literature throughout most of the century, with the exception

The Behavioral Neurology of Dementia, eds. Bruce L. Miller and Bradley F. Boeve. Published by Cambridge University Press.
© Cambridge University Press 2009.

Table 4.1. Variants of frontotemporal lobar degeneration and their affected brain regions

Subtype and anatomy	Behavioral features	Cognitive features	Motor features	Neuropathology and genetics
Progressive non-fluent aphasia (PNFA): left frontoinsular, basal ganglia	Later in the course, apathy and sometimes disinhibition	Non-fluent, apraxia of speech, frontal executive; episodic memory, drawing relatively spared	Overlap with PSP, CBD; asymmetric PD, alien hand, supranuclear gaze disturbance	Tau with CBD or PSP the expected pathology subtypes; some *PGRN* mutations present as PNFA, but most cases of PNFA are not familial
Frontotemporal dementia: right > left frontoinsular, anterior temporal	Disinhibition, lost sympathy/empathy, compulsions, apathy, poor judgement	Poor generation, inhibition and set-shifting; episodic memory, drawing relatively spared	ALS or parkinsonism are very common	Equally divided between tau and TDP-43; when ALS emerges almost always TDP-43; consider mutations affecting tau or *PGRN*
Left temporal variant: left > right anterior temporal, insula, amygdala	Semantic dementia; poor word finding, depression	Semantic anomia/paraphasias; verbal episodic memory problems; visual skills spared, can be enhanced	Usually spared till later; ALS uncommon	Usually TDP-43; also, Pick bodies seen; can be associated with *PGRN* mutations; Alzheimer pathology in 20%
Right temporal variant: right > left anterior temporal, insula, amygdala	Loss of empathy, depression, poor facial recognition, atypical depressive features	Poor recognition of familiar faces and facial emotions; some obsessed with words	Usually spared till later. ALS uncommon	Usually TDP-43 but Pick pathology can occur; Alzheimer pathology in 20%; consider *PGRN* mutations

Notes:
ALS, amyotrophic lateral sclerosis; CBD, corticobasal degeneration; PD, Parkinson's disease; *PGRN*, gene for progranulin; PSP, progressive supranuclear palsy; TDP, TAR DNA-binding protein.

of studies from Constantinidis and Sjögren. In the 1980s, investigators in Manchester, England, and Lund, Sweden, rekindled studies into Pick's disease and began to carefully study non-Alzheimer patients who suffered from focal degenerative disorders of the frontal and anterior temporal lobes.[7,8] At the same time, patients with asymmetrical degeneration of the left hemisphere were described as having a syndrome for which the term "primary progressive aphasia" was coined. In both the symmetrical cases described as "FTD" and the asymmetrical left-sided cases characterized as primary progressive aphasia, non-AD, Pick-like pathology was often found.

With the technical advances in neuroimaging in the late 1980s and early 1990s, patients with atrophy of the frontal and anterior temporal lobes, in conjunction with non-Alzheimer pathology, were found more easily; in approximately 80% of these cases, classical Pick bodies were not found,[4,9,10] leading Arne Brun to coin the term "frontal lobe dementia of the non-Alzheimer-type," emphasizing that Pick's disease was not an invariable feature. By the early 1990s, many cases were reported in the USA.[11,12] As similarities between the language and behavioral syndromes were observed at a pathological level, FTLD was used to capture this constellation of patients with focal frontotemporal clinical syndromes that were thought to be associated with non-Alzheimer pathology.

Further complicating efforts for a streamlined nomenclature syndrome, the overlap between FTLD and motor disorders became apparent. Approximately 15% of all those with FTD show concurrent or developed motor neuron disease (FTD-MND). Conversely, many, if not the majority of patients with amyotrophic lateral sclerosis (ALS), show frontal-executive or behavioral disorders and approximately one-half of patients with FTLD and nearly all with ALS show inclusions with ubiquitinated TAR DNA-binding protein (TDP-43). In addition, linking FTLD to atypical parkinsonian syndromes, there is significant and simultaneous degeneration of basal ganglia structures in FTLD populations, which often leads to the co-expression of parkinsonian features within all of the FTLD subtypes. In the case of PNFA, most patients demonstrate corticobasal degeneration (CBD) or progressive supranuclear palsy (PSP) at autopsy.

Diagnosing frontotemporal lobar degeneration dementia

It can be problematic to diagnose FTLD with clinical accuracy, and in some instances FTLD is difficult to distinguish from AD. Both AD and FTLD have insidious onset, produce a progressive dementia syndrome that can include memory deficits, executive dysfunction and language impairment, and cause alterations in behavior that can make the two disorders difficult to differentiate antemortem.[13]

While definitive differential diagnosis of FTLD and AD can only be made with pathology, great strides in accuracy of antemortem diagnosis have been made. For instance, in patients with early AD, atrophy and dysfunction is most commonly seen in the medial temporal lobes, leading to episodic memory deficits, and an inability to learn new information.[14] As the disease progresses and the atrophy spreads to the frontal, parietal and even occipital lobes, other cognitive, social, emotional and even perceptual impairments are observed.[15]

By contrast, in FTLD, neural degeneration starts in the frontal and anterior temporal lobes, and early symptoms include deficits in behavior, executive control or language function, often coupled with relatively intact episodic memory.[16] Several clinical studies have now shown that FTLD can be reliably differentiated from AD during life based upon the characteristic patterns of decline with these two disorders,[17,18] although, even in specialized clinical centers, approximately 15% of patients diagnosed with FTLD show AD pathology.

Patients with FTLD show remarkable heterogeneity of clinical syndromes and cerebral atrophy patterns within the disease. As discussed above, Neary et al.[19] delineated research criteria to take this heterogeneity into account by dividing the disorder into the three different subtypes: FTD, PNFA and SD. These three clinical syndromes were differentiated primarily on the relative degeneration seen in the frontal and temporal lobes, and the right and left hemispheres.

The FTD subtype presents with asymmetric right but bilateral frontal involvement. Typically, the disease begins in the anterior cingulate, orbitofrontal and anterior insular regions of the frontal lobes, areas that modulate emotion and behavior. This degeneration leads to behavioral abnormalities, including disinhibition, apathy, loss of sympathy or empathy for others, overeating, and repetitive motor behaviors. As FTD progresses, dorsolateral prefrontal cortical involvement becomes apparent and patients begin to exhibit abnormalities in executive control. We have suggested research criteria for FTLD subtypes that classify patients into possible or probable based upon these findings.

Patients with PNFA have selective left frontoinsular degeneration, and present with agrammatism, hesitant, non-fluent speech output and speech apraxia. In some instances, the disorder begins with abnormalities in speech but not language. When supranuclear gaze palsy, frequent falls, dysphagia or asymmetric parkinsonian signs such as focal dystonia or alien hand are seen, the association between the PNFA syndrome and CBD or PSP becomes apparent. However, PSP or CBD are the expected pathological outcomes for PNFA, and the presence of parkinsonian features of both should always be investigated.

In SD, two syndromes emerge: patients with predominantly left temporal degeneration show a profound anomia associated with progressive loss of conceptual knowledge of words, while patients with predominantly right temporal atrophy show deficits in empathy and knowledge about the emotions of others.[20]

As has been discussed, FTLD subtypes overlap with three other disorders: CBD, PSP and FTD-MND.[21] Corticobasal degeneration is characterized by the presence of asymmetric parkinsonism with dystonia, rigidity, limb apraxia and a "useless or alien" limb.[22] At pathology, there are neuronal inclusions with tau present in astrocytes and neurons.[23] More than one-half of the patients diagnosed with CBD pathologically, however, do not show antemortem rigidity or apraxia.[24] Traditionally, PSP has been described as a movement disorder associated with falls, ophthalmoplegia, axial rigidity and a frontal dementia. Like CBD, tau inclusions are seen postmortem.[25] Recent studies suggest that most patients with PNFA show PSP or CBD at postmortem.[21] Some patients with FTD also show PSP or CBD, but patients with SD are only rarely shown to have characteristics of PSP or CBD as well.[26,27]

Even in the 1920s, dementia and MND were observed to be related.[28] Several more reports were published in the 1980s[29–33] and a link with FTD was formally suggested by Neary and colleagues.[34] Generally, patients with FTD-MND show dementia symptoms early in the disease, primarily behavioral changes such as disinhibition. Following the onset of dementia, these patients begin to show muscular weakness and wasting of limb muscles. Typically, patients live approximately 1.4 years from the time of diagnosis, with the respiratory complications of bulbar palsy as the cause of death.[35,36]

Behavioral frontotemporal dementia

The behavioral subtype, also called simply FTD, is the prototypical FTLD syndrome and accounts for approximately 56% of all FTLD.[36,37] This subtype is male predominant by two to one, has the earliest age of onset (around 58 years at diagnosis), progresses most rapidly from time of diagnosis (3.4 years from diagnosis to death), has the highest genetic susceptibility (up to 20% show an autosomal dominant pattern of inheritance) and has a strong association with ALS. At our University of California at San Francisco clinic, patients with FTD are equally divided between those with ubiquitin–TDP-43 and those with tau inclusions postmortem.

The first symptoms of bv-FTD are generally behavioral. These include alterations in social decorum and personal regulation, including disinhibition, apathy, overeating, emotional blunting, personality changes toward coldness and submissiveness, repetitive motor behaviors and impairment in judgement and insight. Along with these behavioral changes, deficits in executive functioning are seen and patients show perseverative behaviors and difficulties with planning, organizing, task switching and generating ideas. Often, patients do not reach the neurologist even after they have exhibited profound lapses in financial or interpersonal judgement, since these behavioral changes are misconstrued as mid-life issues or psychiatric problems. Sadly, unlike in AD, where social decorum is spared and family and acquaintances remain sympathetic, in FTD, patients may be resented by colleagues and family because of their rudeness, coldness and deficits in social modulation.

Approximately 15% of patients develop ALS, and extrapyramidal symptoms are also common. Structural and functional imaging studies typically show greater abnormalities in the right than the left frontal regions. The ventral and medial frontal and insular regions – all paralimbic structures – are affected early in FTD. Often the atrophy here is evident on the first visit to the neurologist, and dysfunction in these critical frontal and anterior temporal regions seems to be driving the disinhibition, apathy and eating disorder.

Semantic dementia

The SD subtype is a temporally predominant syndrome that attacks asymmetrically either the left or the right temporal lobe and accounts for around 20% of all patients with FTLD. Patients with SD have a slightly older age of onset (around 59 years), show the slowest rate of progression (5.2 years from diagnosis to death) and are less likely to have an autosomal dominant pattern of inheritance. Recently, it has been demonstrated that these patients usually show ubiquitin–TDP-43 inclusions postmortem.[36,37]

In our experience, left-sided SD is more commonly recognized than right-sided SD. These patients with left-sided SD begin with word-finding difficulty, often with nouns more than verbs. Category specificity for these naming deficits is common, with knowledge regarding animals lost before tool knowledge. With SD, the specific layering of meaning that surrounds a given word is lost and patients substitute specific words for superordinate categories. For example, an "osprey" may become an "eagle", then a "bird", next an "animal" and finally a "thing" before the word and concept are lost entirely. As SD progresses, speech remains fluent but anomia worsens and patients show trouble not only in naming words but also in recognizing them. Compulsive interests in visually appealing objects emerge, sometimes leading to compulsive card-game playing, coin collecting or even stealing. As the disease spreads to the right side, patients begin to have problems recognizing emotions in others and lose the ability to recognize faces or people or buildings that they once knew. Eventually prosopagnosia and multimodality agnosia for objects develop; even though a patient can see, feel and touch an item, he/she is unable to conjure up its name or recognize its function.

Patients with left-sided SD seem to outnumber those whose SD begins on the right side by approximately two to one. When the disorder begins on the right side, psychiatric features predominate, with loss of empathy for others, atypical depressive features and inability to recognize emotions in faces being common features of the disease. While words are lost first with left-sided SD, familiar face recognition is lost first when the right side is involved. Left-sided SD moves to the right temporal lobe followed by involvement of orbital-frontal cortex and finally spreads throughout the frontotemporal cortex and basal ganglia.

Progressive non-fluent aphasia

The PNFA subtype accounts for approximately 25% of all FTLD, is intermediate in rates of progression (4.3 years from diagnosis) and genetic propensity, has a high association with CBD and PSP and most patients shows tau inclusions postmortem.[21]

Progressive non-fluent aphasia generally presents as a disorder with deficits in language or speech. First symptoms include decreased output for words, shortened phrase length and deficits in articulation. The disease is insidious in onset and the patient often becomes aware of his or her deficits before others have noticed any changes. Unlike in SD, the use of nouns remains intact but deficits in the understanding of grammar are common. Many patients exhibit speech apraxia: a deficit in articulatory planning in which the patients are unable to direct speech musculature to produce sounds in a proper sequence. Patients are usually able to maintain social decorum throughout most of the illness, although some patients do evolve to an FTD syndrome. Motor disorders characteristic of CBD or PSP become common several years after the onset of PNFA. Some patients evolve from PNFA to classical CBD or PSP over a fairly short period of time.

Genetic findings in frontotemporal lobar degeneration

Estimates of the proportion of FTLD patients with a family history have ranged from 10% to 50%.[3,9,13] Part of this variability results from regional differences in the prevalence of genetic mutations, but there is also ample evidence that different FTLD subtypes show different patterns of inheritance: FTD-MND and FTD are perhaps the most likely subtypes to show genetic links suggesting an autosomal dominant pattern, while PNFA and SD are the least likely subtypes to show dominant patterns of inheritance.[39] Yet, recent studies show that both PNFA and SD can be caused by mutations in *PGRN*, which encodes progranulin.

The first genetic discovery related to the FTLD syndrome was the finding that mutations of the gene for the microtubule-associated protein tau (*MAPT*) could cause an autosomal dominant FTD syndrome. The familial forms of FTD that are linked to this gene are grouped under the classification "frontotemporal dementia with parkinsonism linked to chromosome 17" (FTDP-17). This form results from mutations in the exon or intron regions of the tau gene localized to 17q21–22.[40,41] Over 40 distinct pathogenic mutations associated with "toxic gain of function" of the tau protein have been identified in a large number of families with FTDP-17.[42] The proportion of patients with specific mutations is highly skewed: three of the mutations account for more than half of the genetically characterized cases currently reported in the literature. These three mutations are the P301L, associated with the classic FTD phenotype; exon 10 5' splice site +16, associated with a syndrome that includes memory or language impairment and parkinsonism; and N279K, with features of parkinsonism

and PSP, also called pallidopontonigral degeneration.[43] Thus far, those patients with FTDP-17 have shown a filamentous pathology associated with hyperphosphorylation of the tau protein.

Identical genetic mutations may result in different phenotypes, and different genetic mutations may show similar phenotypes. For example, in one family, a tau mutation resulted in a syndrome diagnosed as CBD in the father, and as FTD in the son.[44] In addition to mutations on chromosome 17q21–22, Bird and colleagues[45] found that FTD may also be linked to chromosome 9q21–q22.

Tau mutations

Tau is a protein that binds to and promotes microtubule assembly. In a healthy brain, tau is soluble and expressed as six major protein isoforms that are generated by alternative splicing of a single gene on chromosome 17q21. Inclusion of a 31 amino acid repeat encoded by exon 10 in the mRNA produces three isoforms with four microtubule-binding repeats each (4R tau).[46] If the repeat is excluded (exon 10−), the resulting protein will have only three domains (3R tau). In healthy brains, the ratio of 3R to 4R is 1:1. Many of the tau mutations that are involved in FTLD are clustered around exon 10, with the ultimate result of altering the ratio of 3R to 4R in the brain, or altering the binding affinity of the protein.[47] Tau mutations may be missense, deletion or silent mutations in the coding region, or intronic mutations.[48–50] Generally, these mutations reduce the ability of tau to interact with microtubules or lead to the abnormal accumulation of 4R tau, resulting in a build-up of toxic filaments in the cell body and dendrites, eventually leading to the death of the cell.[43]

Most of the genetic mutations in tau are associated with overproduction of the 4R (longer) form of tau. Additionally, the H1 haplotype, which is overrepresented in both CBD and PSP, is associated with overproduction of 4R tau. This finding has led Hutton and colleagues to suggest that it is the 4R, not the 3R, form of tau that is pathogenetically linked to FTLD spectrum disorders where tau is found.[49] This mechanism appears to be a classical "toxic gain of function" where the production of an abnormal protein or the overproduction of a normal protein is toxic.

Ubiquitin–TDP-43 genetic findings

The study of tau mutations has dominated genetic research into FTLD until recently, even though many

FTD families do not show tau pathology postmortem. Instead, these patients show ubiquitin-immunoreactive neuronal cytoplasmic inclusions and lentiform ubiquitin-immunoreactive neuronal intranuclear inclusions that also stain for TDP-43.[51,52] These inclusions are generally found in layer II of frontal and temporal neocortex and in the dentate gyrus of the hippocampus.[53] Recent reports by Radeamakers and colleagues and Baker and colleagues[54] in families with FTD conclusively linked to chromosome 17q21, with tau-negative but ubiquitin-positive inclusions, missense mutations in the gene for progranulin (*PGRN*) were found to be the cause of the disease. Many of the carriers of *PGRN* mutations present between the ages of 40 to 70, although 10% of carriers remain asymptomatic at the age of 70. Therefore, unlike tau mutations, with *PGRN* the clinical expression is incomplete. Although FTD is the most common type of presentation, PNFA, SD, CBD and AD presentations have been seen.

The exact function of progranulin in neurons remains unknown, although outside of the nervous system it is involved in wound repair and mediates inflammation, influencing cell-cycle progression and cell motility.[55] One hypothesis currently gaining popularity is the possibility that this protein has growth factor activity even in the brain: high levels may be tumorigenic while low levels appear to cause FTD.

Baker and colleagues[56] showed that the mutations in FTD cause a loss in functional progranulin (haplo-insufficiency) by creating a null allele. Hence, ubiquitin inclusions show insufficient levels of progranulin. In contrast to tau mutations where there is toxic gain of function, with *PGRN* mutations the abnormality is caused by a deficiency in the production of sufficient levels of the protein. Strategies for replacing progranulin or its metabolites are being investigated. Shortly after the discovery of *PGRN* mutations, it was found that the protein TDP-43 was nearly universally bound to ubiquitin in those with *PRGN* mutations, in FTD and SD with ubiquitin inclusions and in the inclusions found in ALS. Hence, these inclusions are now called TDP-43 positive. To date, there have been no definitive FTD syndromes associated with TDP-43 mutations although one patient with a polymorphism affecting TDP-43 associated with FTD-ALS has been described.

A less common autosomal dominant FTD has also been observed in association with a mutation in the valosin-containing protein. In these families the FTD syndrome is seen in association with inclusion body myositis, Paget's disease and diabetes. In at least one family, an autosomal form of FTD has been associated with mutations in the gene encoding the charged multivesicular body protein 2B (*CHMP2B*), which is involved in endosomal processing of proteins. Still unaccounted for are the large numbers of patients in whom familial FTD-MND occurs. As this chapter was going to press, several groups were close to mapping a gene on chromosome 9 in FTD-MND.

Pathological findings in frontotemporal lobar degeneration

Two major types of pathological changes are observed in FTLD: gross morphological atrophy in the frontal and anterior temporal lobes, and microscopic changes, including any or all of the following: gliosis, inclusion bodies, swollen neurons and microvacuolation. Increasingly, as our understanding of genetic mutations in FTLD grows, an important distinction is made upon pathology between tau and ubiquitin inclusions within neurons or glia.

Gross anatomical changes

In FTLD, gross anatomical changes range from a mild to a severe decrease in overall brain weight, associated with focal atrophy of the frontal and temporal lobes. Symmetric atrophy of the frontal lobes is characteristic of bv-FTD, while asymmetric atrophy (left > right) is consistent with PNFA (frontal lobes) and SD (temporal lobes). Thinning of the cortical ribbon and discoloration of white matter may also be observed. In rarer cases, atrophy may extend into the parietal lobes, amygdala, hippocampus, insula, thalamus and basal ganglia (head of the caudate nucleus).[57] Ventricular enlargement is often present, as well as pallor of the substantia nigra, atrophy of the anterior nerve roots and discoloration of the lateral funiculus in the spinal cord.

Microscopic findings

Despite the origins of the FTLD classification, only a minority of patients diagnosed with FTLD will show the classical Pick pattern at autopsy. In classical Pick's disease, much of the gross atrophy seen at pathology is a result of a severe and often complete loss of large pyramidal cells in cortical layer III, and the small pyramidal and non-pyramidal cells of layer II.[9] Pyramidal cells in layer V may also be shrunken. The most severe loss of synaptic density is found in the superficial frontal layers. White matter changes include loss of myelin and axons. Recently, Seeley and colleagues[58] have suggested that large neurons found in layer 5b of frontoinsular and anterior cingulate cortex, neurons most extensively described by von Economo, may be the first cells to degenerate in FTD. The von Economo neurons are found in the greatest concentration in humans compared with other great apes and are absent in most other species with the exception of certain cetaceans. Their large size and small dendritic tree suggest that they may be responsible for the quick transmission of signals from paralimbic into adjacent frontal regions involved with higher order cognitive processes. More work is needed to elucidate the role of these neurons in cognition and to understand why they are selectively vulnerable in FTD.

Remaining neurons also show one of two possible distinctive histological features: swelling (called "ballooned" or Pick cell) and an inclusion within the perikaryon, most often in layer II (Pick body). Pick bodies are usually found in limbic (with the greatest concentration in the amygdala and hippocampus, including the dentate gyrus), paralimbic and ventral temporal lobe cortex, but they may also be seen in anterior frontal and dorsal temporal lobes. Pick bodies are composed of randomly arranged filaments of tau.

In patients with FTD-MND, a second histological pattern is observed. Generally, these patients show loss of large pyramidal cells, microvacuolation and mild gliosis.[53] Substantia nigra is pale, with intense reactive fibrous astrocytosis. Inclusions are tau negative but ubiquitin positive and found throughout the frontal cortex and hippocampus (dentate gyrus). The hypoglossus nucleus in the brainstem also shows atrophy. Similarly, in those with ubiquitin-only (tau and α-synuclein negative) immunoreactive neuronal changes (ubiquitin inclusion FTD or FTLD-U), TDP-43, which is normally contained within the nucleus, seems to leave the nucleus and accumulates in the cell bodies and neuronal processes.[59] TDP-43 has been identified in sporadic and familial FTLD-U and ALS, though subtle differences in the TDP-43 variants may reflect different pathogenic mechanisms in the different disease subtypes.

In CBD, the brain has ballooned or swollen neurons similar to those seen in Pick's disease, but the neurons do not contain Pick bodies. These ballooned neurons may be found throughout the neocortex, but mostly in the superior frontal and parietal lobes, including primary motor or sensory cortex. There is also neuronal loss and gliosis in affected regions, often in the basal ganglia. Finally, astrocytic plaques that stain with anti-tau antibodies are found

in CBD.[60] Tau inclusions in neurons and glia is also seen in PSP. Neurofibrillary tangles are evident in cortex and midbrain. Cortical atrophy is relatively mild while midbrain and brainstem atrophy is evident.[61]

Diagnosing frontotemporal lobar degeneration using neuroimaging

With advances in neuroimaging techniques, several tools have emerged that are fairly effective in differentiating FTLD subtypes from each other and from other disorders. Bilateral frontal hypoperfusion is observed in patients with bv-FTD using ^{99}Tc-hexamethylylpropyleneamine (HMPAO) single-photon emission computed tomography (SPECT)[12] and ^{18}F-fluorodeoxyglucose positron emission tomography (FDG-PET).[62] Furthermore, cortical atrophy in the ventromedial frontal cortex, posterior orbitofrontal cortex, insula, anterior cingulate cortex, right dorsolateral frontal cortex and left premotor cortex, as seen in T_1-weighted structural magnetic resonance imaging (MRI) scans, also marks bv-FTD.[63] Distinguishing FTLD from AD, patients with FTLD show faster rates of frontal atrophy (4.1–4.5% per year) as seen on longitudinal MRI scans but similar rates of parieto-occipital atrophy (2.2–2.4% per year) when compared with patients with AD.[64] A promising new approach for differentiating FTD from AD involves the new amyloid agent Pittsburgh compound B (PIB). This compound binds to β-amyloid proteins in living tissue and may be detected using PET. Since accumulation of β-amyloid is not a marker of FTLD, PIB imaging may be useful in excluding FTLD from AD.[65]

Patients with SD, in contrast, show severe, bilateral, but still asymmetric, hypoperfusion in the anterior temporal lobes on HMPAO-SPECT.[66] Temporal lobe atrophy is also clearly seen on structural MRI scans and SD may be differentiated from AD even by simple visual inspection.[67] Detailed volumetric measures show that hippocampal atrophy is more severe in SD than in AD, particularly in the anterior hippocampus. Usually the degeneration in SD is asymmetric, accompanied by more severe atrophy of the amygdalae, temporal pole, fusiform and inferolateral temporal gyri.[68] Mummery et al.[69] have also shown that FDG-PET reveals brain activation changes in regions outside of the temporal lobes, reflecting the disruption that semantic memory impairments cause in other brain regions. There have been few efforts to distinguish PNFA from other subtypes with neuroimaging, but structural MRI has shown left perisylvian atrophy.[70,71]

51

Treatment and therapy

Unfortunately, as of yet, there are no effective pharmacological treatments to reverse or halt the progression of FTLD. Current treatment of patients with FTLD involves treating specific symptoms and improving quality of life. Acetylcholinesterase inhibitors developed to improve symptoms of AD do not seem to be effective in managing symptoms of FTD, perhaps because the cholinergic neurons in the nucleus basalis of Meynert are relatively spared in FTLD. Furthermore, acetylcholinesterase inhibitors may cause agitation in patients with FTLD and are particularly dangerous for patients with FTD-MND, since they may cause increased production of oral secretions.

Selective serotonin reuptake inhibitors (SSRIs), in contrast, have shown some success in treating compulsions and carbohydrate cravings in patients with FTLD.[72] Generally, SSRIs are well tolerated by patients. Patients who do not respond to SSRIs, and who show aggressive or delusional behaviors may benefit from low doses of atypical antipsychotic drugs such as olanzepine, quetiapine or risperidone. Typical antipsychotic drugs known to result in extrapyramidal side-effects should be avoided, since those with FTLD are likely to show parkinsonism. In the only placebo-controlled study of FTLD, the antidepressant trazodone was shown to be effective compared with placebo in controlling behavior.[73]

Since behavioral changes figure prominently in the disease, the safety of the patient and those with whom he/she interacts must be a primary concern. Removing dangerous items from the home, eliminating driving later in the disease and educating caregivers are all methods of preventing injury and distress. In addition to education, caregivers should also be provided with support and respite. Depression in caregivers is common and leads to earlier placement in nursing homes for the patients.[74] Speech therapy for patients with PNFA is often appreciated by the patient and offers temporary gains that are eventually overwhelmed by the illness.

Future directions

There remain many challenges in the treatment and diagnosis of FTLD and related disorders. As FTLD has finally been recognized as important, relatively common and distinctive from AD, research into its causes and treatment has accelerated in recent years.

Furthermore, it is becoming evident that the three major FTLD subtypes have distinctive demographics, rates of progression and possibly even etiologies. As diagnosis has improved, new challenges have emerged. Even at research centers, many patients diagnosed with FTLD turn out to have AD upon pathology, and close to perfect separation of these two disorders remains a goal of the coming decade. A further challenge for clinicians, we suspect, is that in the future diagnoses will separate tau-related FTLD from ubiquitin-related FTLD, as distinctive therapies for these subtypes are developed. Whenever therapies become available, more accurate and earlier diagnosis of FTLD will be needed.

The recent discovery of the *PGRN* mutations and progranulin changes as a cause for FTD has greatly excited the field. Unlike tau mutations, the progranulin changes may be relatively common, which may require more widespread screening for these mutations in patients with FTD. Importantly, the potential for therapy has been stimulated by this finding since progranulin appears to have growth factor activity. Other therapeutic approaches are under active study in animal models of FTLD associated with tau and valosin mutations. Finally, genes linked to FTD-ALS will soon be discovered, offering still more hopes and challenges.

References

1. Ratnavalli, E., C. Brayne, K. Dawson *et al.* The prevalence of frontotemporal dementia. *Neurology*, 2002; **58**(11): 1615–21.

2. Knopman, D. S., R. C. Petersen, S. D. Edland *et al.* The incidence of frontotemporal lobar degeneration in Rochester, Minnesota, 1990 through 1994. *Neurology*, 2004; **62**(3): 506–8.

3. Neary, D., J. S. Snowden, B. Northen *et al.* Dementia of frontal lobe type. *J Neurol Neurosurg Psychiatry*, 1988; **51**(3): 353–61.

4. Brun, A. Frontal lobe degeneration of non-Alzheimer type. I. *Neuropathol Arch Gerontol Geriatr*, 1987; **6**(3): 193–208.

5. Pick, A. Uber die Beziehungen der senilen Hirnatrophie zur Aphasie. *Prager Med Wochensch*, 1892; **17**: 165–7.

6. Alzheimer, A. Uber eigenartige Krankheitsfalle des spateren Alters. *Z Ges Neurol Psychiatr*, 1911; **4**: 356–85.

7. Neary, D., J. S. Snowden, D. M. Bowen *et al.* Neuropsychological syndromes in presenile dementia due to cerebral atrophy. *J Neurol Neurosurg Psychiatry*, 1986; **49**(2): 163–74.

8. Gustafson, L. Frontal lobe degeneration of non-Alzheimer type. II. Clinical picture and differential diagnosis. *Arch Gerontol Geriatr*, 1987; **6**(3): 209–23.

9. Mann, D. M. A., P. W. South, J. S. Snowden *et al.* Dementia of frontal lobe type: neuropathology and immunohistochemistry. *J Neurol Neurosurg Psychiatry*, 1993; **56**: 605–14.

10. Knopman, D. S., A. R. Mastri, W. H. D. Frey *et al.* Dementia lacking distinctive histologic features: a common non-Alzheimer degenerative dementia. *Neurology*, 1990; **40**(2): 251–6.

11. Jagust, W. J., B. R. Reed, J. P. Seab *et al.* Clinical-physiologic correlates of Alzheimer's disease and frontal lobe dementia. *Am J Physiol Imaging*, 1989; **4**: 89–96.

12. Miller, B. L., J. L. Cummings, J. Villanueva-Meyer *et al.* Frontal lobe degeneration: clinical, neuropsychological, and SPECT characteristics. *Neurology*, 1991; **41**(9): 1374–82.

13. Varma, A. R., J. S. Snowden, J. J. Lloyd *et al.* Evaluation of the NINCDS–ADRDA criteria in the differentiation of Alzheimer's disease and frontotemporal dementia. *J Neurol Neurosurg Psychiatry*, 1999; **66**(2): 184–8.

14. de Leon, M. J., A. Convit, S. DeSanti *et al.* Contribution of structural neuroimaging to the early diagnosis of Alzheimer's disease. *Int Psychogeriatr*, 1997; **9**(Suppl 1): 183–90; discussion 247–52.

15. Thompson, P. M., K. M. Hayashi, G. de Zubicaray *et al.* Dynamics of gray matter loss in Alzheimer's disease. *J Neurosci*, 2003; **23**(3): 994–1005.

16. Kitagaki, H., E. Mori, S. Yamaji *et al.* Frontotemporal dementia and Alzheimer disease: evaluation of cortical atrophy with automated hemispheric surface display generated with MR images. *Radiology*, 1998; **208**(2): 431–9.

17. Read, S. L., B. L. Miller, I. Mena *et al.* SPECT in dementia: clinical and pathological correlation. *J Am Geriatr Soc*, 1995; **43**(11): 1243–7.

18. Miller, B. L. Clinical advances in degenerative dementias. [See comments.] *Br J Psychiatry*, 1997; **171**(18): 1–3.

19. Neary, D., J. S. Snowden, L. Gustafson *et al.* Frontotemporal lobar degeneration: a consensus on clinical diagnostic criteria. *Neurology*, 1998; **51**(6): 1546–54.

20. Boxer, A. L. and B. L. Miller Clinical features of frontotemporal dementia. *Alzheimer Dis Assoc Disord*, 2005; **19**(Suppl 1): S3–6.

21. Josephs, K. A., R. C. Petersen, D. S. Knopman *et al.* Clinicopathologic analysis of frontotemporal and corticobasal degenerations and PSP. *Neurology*, 2006; **66**(1): 41–8.

22. Litvan, I., Y. Agid, C. Goetz *et al.* Accuracy of the clinical diagnosis of corticobasal degeneration: a clinicopathologic study. *Neurology*, 1997; **48**(1): 119–25.

23. Schneider, J. A., R. L. Watts, M. Gearing *et al.* Corticobasal degeneration: neuropathologic and clinical heterogeneity. *Neurology*, 1997; **48**(4): 959–69.

24. Boeve, B. F., D. M. Maraganore, J. E. Parisi *et al.* Pathologic heterogeneity in clinically diagnosed corticobasal degeneration. *Neurology*, 1999; **53**(4): 795–800.

25. Verny, M., K. A. Jellinger, J. J. Hauw *et al.* Progressive supranuclear palsy: a clinicopathological study of 21 cases. *Acta Neuropathol*, 1996; **91**(4): 427–31.

26. Mathuranath, P. S., J. H. Xuereb, T. Bak *et al.* Corticobasal ganglionic degeneration and/or frontotemporal dementia? A report of two overlap cases and review of literature. *J Neurol Neurosurg Psychiatry*, 2000; **68**(3): 304–12.

27. Kertesz, A. and D. G. Munoz. Diagnostic controversies: is CBD part of the "pick complex". *Adv Neurol*, 2000; **82**: 223–31.

28. Meyer, A. Uber eine der amyotrophischen Lateralsklerose nahestehende Erkrankung mit psychischen Storungen. *Zeitschrift Ges Neurol Psychiatr*, 1929; **121**: 107–138.

29. Hudson, A. J. Amyotrophic lateral sclerosis and its association with dementia, parkinsonism and other neurological disorders: a review. *Brain*, 1981; **104**(2): 217–47.

30. Mitsuyama, Y., H. Fukunaga and M. Yamashita. Alzheimer's disease with widespread presence of Lewy bodies. *Folia Psychiatr Neurol Jpn*, 1984; **38**(1): 81–8.

31. Morita, K., H. Kaiya, T. Ikeda *et al.* Presenile dementia combined with amyotrophy: a review of 34 Japanese cases. *Arch Gerontol Geriatr*, 1987; **6**(3): 263–77.

32. Salazar, A. M., C. L. Masters, D. C. Gajdusek *et al.* Syndromes of amyotrophic lateral sclerosis and dementia: relation to transmissible Creutzfeldt–Jakob disease. *Ann Neurol*, 1983; **14**(1): 17–26.

33. Clark, A. W., H. J. Manz, C. L. White III *et al.* Cortical degeneration with swollen chromatolytic neurons: its relationship to Pick's disease. *J Neuropathol Exp Neurol*, 1986; **45**(3): 268–84.

34. Neary, D., J. S. Snowden, D. M. Mann *et al.* Frontal lobe dementia and motor neuron disease. *J Neurol Neurosurg Psychiatry*, 1990; **53**(1): 23–32.

35. Snowden, J. S., D. Neary and D. M. A. Mann. *Fronto-temporal Lobar Degeneration: Fronto-temporal Dementia, Progressive Aphasia, Semantic Dementia.* New York: Churchill Livingstone, 1996.

36. Roberson, E. D., J. H. Hesse, K. D. Rose *et al.* Frontotemporal dementia progresses to death faster than Alzheimer disease. *Neurology*, 2005; **65**(5): 719–25.

37. Johnson, J. K., J. Diehl, M. F. Mendez *et al.* Frontotemporal lobar degeneration: demographic

53

characteristics of 353 patients. *Arch Neurol*, 2005; **62**(6): 925–30.

38. Chow, T. W., B. L. Miller, V. N. Hayashi *et al.* Inheritance of frontotemporal dementia. *Arch Neurol*, 1999; **56**(7): 817–22.

39. Goldman, J. S., J. M. Farmer, E. M. Wood *et al.* Comparison of family histories in FTLD subtypes and related tauopathies. *Neurology*, 2005; **65**(11): 1817–19.

40. van Swieten, J. C., M. Stevens, S. M. Rosso *et al.* Phenotypic variation in hereditary frontotemporal dementia with tau mutations. *Ann Neurol*, 1999; **46**(4): 617–26.

41. Wilhelmsen, K. C., T. Lynch, E. Pavlou *et al.* Localization of disinhibition–dementia–parkinsonism–amyotrophy complex to 17q21–22. *Am J Hum Genetics*, 1994; **55**: 1159–65.

42. Tsuboi, Y. Neuropathology of familial tauopathy. *Neuropathology*, 2006; **26**(5): 471–4.

43. Spillantini, M. G., J. C. van Swieten and M. Goedert. Tau gene mutations in frontotemporal dementia and parkinsonism linked to chromosome 17 (FTDP-17). *Neurogenetics*, 2000; **2**(4): 193–205.

44. Bugiani, O., J. R. Murrell, G. Giaccone *et al.* Frontotemporal dementia and corticobasal degeneration in a family with a P301S mutation in tau. *J Neuropathol Exp Neurol*, 1999; **58**(6): 667–77.

45. Bird, T., D. Knopman, J. van Swieten *et al.* Epidemiology and genetics of frontotemporal dementia/ Pick's disease. *Ann Neurol*, 2003; **54**(Suppl 5): S29–31.

46. Goedert, M. and R. Jakes. Expression of separate isoforms of human tau protein: correlation with the tau pattern in brain and effects on tubulin polymerization. *Embo J*, 1990; **9**(13): 4225–30.

47. Hong, M., V. Zhukareva, V. Vogelsberg-Ragaglia *et al.* Mutation-specific functional impairments in distinct tau isoforms of hereditary FTDP-17. *Science*, 1998; **282**(5395): 1914–17.

48. Poorkaj, P., T. D. Bird, E. Wijsman *et al.* Tau is a candidate gene for chromosome 17 frontotemporal dementia. *Ann Neurol*, 1998; **43**(6): 815–25. [Published erratum appears in *Ann Neurol* 1998; 44(3): 428.]

49. Hutton, M., C. L. Lendon, P. Rizzu *et al.* Association of missense and 5'-splice-site mutations in tau with the inherited dementia FTDP-17. *Nature*, 1998; **393**(6686): 702–5.

50. Spillantini, M. G., J. R. Murrell, M. Goedert *et al.* Mutation in the tau gene in familial multiple system tauopathy with presenile dementia. *Proc Natl Acad Sci USA*, 1998; **95**(13): 7737–41.

51. van der Zee, J., R. Rademakers, S. Engelborghs *et al.* A Belgian ancestral haplotype harbours a highly prevalent mutation for 17q21-linked tau-negative FTLD. *Brain*, 2006; **129**(Pt 4): 841–52.

52. Mackenzie, I. R., M. Baker, G. West *et al.* A family with tau-negative frontotemporal dementia and neuronal intranuclear inclusions linked to chromosome 17. *Brain*, 2006; **129**(Pt 4): 853–67.

53. Neary, D., J. S. Snowden and D. M. Mann. Classification and description of frontotemporal dementias. *Ann N Y Acad Sci*, 2000; **920**(51–52): 46–51.

54. Baker, M., I. R. Mackenzie, S. M. Pickering-Brown *et al.* Mutations in progranulin cause tau-negative frontotemporal dementia linked to chromosome 17. *Nature*, 2006; **442**(7105): 916–19.

55. He, Z., C. H. Ong, J. Halper *et al.* Progranulin is a mediator of the wound response. *Nat Med*, 2003; **9**(2): 225–9.

56. Baker, M., I. R. Mackenzie, S. M. Pickering-Brown *et al.* Mutations in progranulin cause tau-negative frontotemporal dementia linked to chromosome 17. *Nature*, 2006; **442**(7105): 916–19.

57. Mann, D. M. and P. W. South. The topographic distribution of brain atrophy in frontal lobe dementia. *Acta Neuropathol*, 1993; **85**(3): 334–40.

58. Seeley, W. W., D. A. Carlin, J. M. Allman *et al.* Early frontotemporal dementia targets neurons unique to apes and humans. *Ann Neurol*, 2006; **60**(6): 660–7.

59. Neumann, M., D. M. Sampathu, L. K. Kwong *et al.* Ubiquitinated TDP-43 in frontotemporal lobar degeneration and amyotrophic lateral sclerosis. *Science*, 2006; **314**(5796): 130–3.

60. Dickson, D. W., C. Bergeron, S. S. Chin *et al.* Office of Rare Diseases neuropathologic criteria for corticobasal degeneration. *J Neuropathol Exp Neurol*, 2002; **61**(11): 935–46.

61. Boxer, A. L., M. D. Geschwind, N. Belfor *et al.* Patterns of brain atrophy that differentiate corticobasal degeneration syndrome from progressive supranuclear palsy. *Arch Neurol*, 2006; **63**(1): 81–6.

62. Hoffman, J. M., K. A. Welsh-Bohmer, M. Hanson *et al.* FDG PET imaging in patients with pathologically verified dementia. *J Nucl Med*, 2000; **41**(11): 1920–8.

63. Rosen, H. J., M. L. Gorno-Tempini, W. P. Goldman *et al.* Patterns of brain atrophy in frontotemporal dementia and semantic dementia. *Neurology*, 2002; **58**(2): 198–208.

64. Chan, D., N. C. Fox, R. Jenkins *et al.* Rates of global and regional cerebral atrophy in AD and frontotemporal dementia. *Neurology*, 2001; **57**(10): 1756–63.

65. Rabinovici, G. D., A. J. Furst, J. P. O'Neil *et al.* ^{11}C-PIB PET imaging in Alzheimer disease and frontotemporal lobar degeneration. *Neurology*, 2007; **68**(15): 1205–12.

66. Edwards-Lee, T., B. L. Miller, D. F. Benson *et al.* The temporal variant of frontotemporal dementia. *Brain*, 1997; **120**(Pt 6): 1027–40.

67. Galton, C. J., K. Patterson, K. Graham *et al.* Differing patterns of temporal atrophy in Alzheimer's disease

and semantic dementia. *Neurology*, 2001; **57**(2): 216–25.

68. Chan, D., N. C. Fox, R. I. Scahill *et al.* Patterns of temporal lobe atrophy in semantic dementia and Alzheimer's disease. *Ann Neurol*, 2001; **49**(4): 433–42.

69. Mummery, C. J., K. Patterson, R. J. Wise *et al.* Disrupted temporal lobe connections in semantic dementia. *Brain*, 1999; **122**(Pt 1): 61–73.

70. Hodges, J. R. and K. Patterson. Nonfluent progressive aphasia and semantic dementia: a comparative neuropsychological study. *J Int Neuropsychol Soc*, 1996; **2**(6): 511–24.

71. Rosen, H. J., J. H. Kramer, M. L. Gorno-Tempini *et al.* Patterns of cerebral atrophy in primary progressive aphasia. *Am J Geriatr Psychiatry*, 2002; **10**(1): 89–97.

72. Swartz, J. R., B. L. Miller, I. M. Lesser and A. L. Darby. Frontotemporal dementia: treatment response to serotonin selective reuptake inhibitors. *J Clin Psychiatry*, 1997; **58**(5): 212–16.

73. Pasquier, F., T. Fukui, M. Sarazin *et al.* Laboratory investigations and treatment in frontotemporal dementia. *Ann Neurol*, 2003; **54**(Suppl 5): S32–5.

74. Litvan, I. Therapy and management of frontal lobe dementia patients. *Neurology*, 2001; **56**(Suppl 4): S41–5.

Chapter 5

Alzheimer's disease

Brandy R. Matthews and Bruce L. Miller

Introduction

While dementia is characterized by a change in cognition that is sufficient to adversely affect a person's daily function in the absence of an acute confusional state or delirium, Alzheimer's disease (AD) more specifically refers to dementia that is slowly progressive with prominent memory dysfunction occurring early in the clinical course.[1] Alois Alzheimer initially described the illness in 1901 with the clinical case of Auguste D., a 51-year-old woman with cognitive disturbance, disorientation, delusions, aphasia and behavioral dyscontrol. A postmortem presentation followed in 1906 and revealed the presenile dementia to be associated with striking generalized cortical atrophy and unique neuropathological changes. In a subsequent 1911 publication, Dr. Alzheimer described in histological detail the now disease-defining neurofibrillary tangles (NFT) and neuritic plaques observed at autopsy, with apparent surprise that the eponymous "Alzheimer's disease" had already been suggested in a textbook by Kraepelin in 1910.[2] Alzheimer's disease now represents the leading cause of dementia worldwide and is a well-known cause of death, disability, and financial burden across cultures.[3–5]

Epidemiology

In 1990, 4 million people in the USA were estimated to have AD, with an associated projection that this number would escalate to 14 million by 2050.[6] The incidence of AD is age related, doubling every 5 years after the age of 65 years. The prevalence doubles with the same pattern, rendering the illness relatively common in the seventh and eighth decades of life. [7–9] Beyond the age of 85, the annual incidence of AD is 6–8%,[5] with an associated prevalence in

Western countries of 24–33%. The incidence and prevalence in developing nations is less well defined, but it is estimated that 60–70% of people with dementia live in developing countries, with a disproportionate number in India, China and other Asian-Pacific nations.[4] A slightly higher prevalence in women may reflect gender-specific longevity.[10,11] However, the source of higher incidence rates in African-Americans and Hispanics remains to be determined.[12,13] Disease duration from onset varies widely from 2 to 20 years and influences prevalence rates, with population-based studies suggesting a median survival of 4–6 years from diagnosis.[14–16]

Risk modifiers

As clearly demonstrated by epidemiological data, advancing age is the primary risk factor for the development of AD. However, many other environmental and genetic risk factors have been described and are considered potential routes for modification of disease development and course. While AD is considered an illness of the elderly, recent evidence suggests that early-life exposures may influence the clinical expression of the illness.[17] The earliest of these exposures are genetic influences, which may begin in utero, with identified mutations and genetic predispositions for disease development to be considered in a subsequent section of this chapter. Other early-life contributions to AD neuropathological changes include head injury, [18–21] obesity and insulin resistance,[22,23] and other identified vascular risk factors.[24–27] Risk modifiers for clinical expression of the disease from early life also include head circumference and brain weight as determined through the first decade of life,[28] general body growth continuing through the second decade of life,[29,30] and socioeconomic status, known to be associated with nutritional status and environmental enrichment.[31–35]

When considering risk factors for AD, it may be prudent to consider separately risk factors that predict

The Behavioral Neurology of Dementia, eds. Bruce L. Miller and Bradley F. Boeve. Published by Cambridge University Press. © Cambridge University Press 2009.

pathological changes characteristic of the disease and those that predict risk for clinical expression of disease.[17,36] This paradigm reflects current hypotheses of "cognitive reserve," the seemingly protective effect of increased formal education in delaying the onset of AD symptoms, irrespective of neuropathological changes consistent with the diagnosis of AD. [37,38] Although previously thought to reflect a bias in neuropsychological screening tests,[39] prospective cohort studies confirm that lower educational attainment is associated with a higher risk of developing AD.[40–42]

Furthermore, subjects with more years of formal education may decline more rapidly following diagnosis of probable AD.[43] These observations, coupled with discrepancies in AD neuropathological burden and clinical signs and symptoms in highly educated subjects, have been deemed supportive of the "cognitive reserve" hypothesis. Such reserve is conceptualized as the ability to engage in alternative cognitive strategies and enlist parallel brain networks to compensate for deficits resulting from AD pathology.[44] However, the precision of the model remains somewhat controversial as it is possible that years of formal education is merely a surrogate for intelligence or IQ, which is known to have a genetic component and be predictive for late-life cognitive performance,[45] or rather, simply to reflect socioeconomic variables.

Recently, less-contentious environmental risk modifiers encountered in midlife have been considered in large cohorts, suggesting that regional variability in diet and exercise may influence the risk of the development of AD. While there has been the suggestion that high intake of vitamins C, E, B_6, B_{12} and folate may lead to a lower risk of developing AD, these results have been inconsistent.[46] Modest to moderate intake of alcohol has been suggested to lower the risk of AD,[47–48] while moderate intake of saturated fats may increase the risk for developing AD.[50–52] Likewise, a diet high in unsaturated fat, fish, vegetables, fruits, legumes and cereals, the so-called "Mediterranean diet," has been associated with a reduction in AD risk.[52] Physical exercise in midlife has also been associated with a reduced risk for the development of AD, independent of other risk factors.[53,54] Theoretically, "cognitive exercise" could also reduce the risk for developing AD;[55,56] however, this construct has been difficult to dissociate from education, IQ and other environmental confounds.[57]

Genetic factors

Family history is the second greatest risk factor for the development of AD.[58] Twin studies confirm the role of genetics in the development of the disease, [59] although the identified Mendelian genetic mutations account for only a small fraction of AD cases, approximately 5%, with most of these demonstrating autosomal dominant transmission and disease onset prior to age 65. Three genes with over 160 different mutations have been identified and share a common biochemical pathway that leads to abnormal production of β-amyloid, a protein to be discussed further in descriptions of the pathophysiology of AD (Table 5.1). The currently identified AD genes include those for amyloid precursor protein (APP) on chromosome 21, [60] presenilin 1 (*PSEN1*) on chromosome 14,[61] and presenilin 2 (*PSEN2*) on chromosome 1.[62] The most common mutation is *PSEN1*, observed in more than 10% of cases referred for genetic testing [63] and accounting for the majority of AD cases with onset prior to age 50.[58]

Down syndrome (trisomy 21) also leads to the development of neuropathological changes consistent with the diagnosis of AD, with such changes demonstrable by the age of 40 in nearly all patients.[64] Although not all those with Down syndrome become demented, the prevalence of dementia in Down syndrome has been estimated to reach 50% by the sixth decade of life.[65] Furthermore, there is an increased risk for development of AD in mothers of those with Down syndrome if the mother gave birth before age 35.[66]

Another genetic factor that has been strongly associated with both familial and sporadic AD is found on chromosome 19, the allelic variant ε4 of the gene for apolipoprotein E (APOE 4).[67,68] The exact mechanism by which its protein product, ApoE,

Table 5.1. Alzheimer's disease: identified genetic loci

Chromosome	Gene coding for:	% of those with AD
21	APP	<1
14	PS1	1–5
1	PS2	<1
19	APOE	50
11	SORL1	?

Notes:
AD, Alzheimer's disease; APP, amyloid precursor protein;
PS1, presenilin 1; *PS2*, presenilin 2; APOE, apolipoprotein E;
SORL1, neuronal sortilin-related receptor.

involved with cholesterol transport, promotes disease at the molecular level has remained elusive. However, the proportion of AD estimated to be related to the ε4 allele is nearly 20%, rendering it the most important currently identified genetic contributor to the development of AD. A single ε4 allele increases the risk of disease two- to three-fold, while a homozygous presentation (ε4/ε4) increases the risk by a factor of five to fifteen.[69,70] It appears that the ε4 allele modifies the age of illness onset [71] by approximately 10 years per copy.[67]

Using converging evidence from inherited forms of AD and neuropathological studies, investigators have recently described a compelling genetic association between AD and variation in the neuronal sortilin-related receptor (SORL1) in families with late-onset AD. Unlike the ε4 allele of *APOE*, there is no single *SORL1* haplotype implicated in the development of AD, but the gene, found on chromosome 11, was associated with disease development in several unique datasets. This receptor is known to be involved in the processing of APP and also functions as a lipoprotein receptor, although the exact mechanism of its contribution to the development of AD remains to be more clearly defined.[72–74]

Pathology

Microscopically, brains of patients with AD demonstrate neuronal loss and shrinkage of large cortical neurons. Synaptic loss is considered by many investigators to be the critical pathological change, owing to its high correlation with dementia severity as assessed by clinical measures.[75] Such cell loss is reflected in the generalized cortical atrophy observed in gross tissue specimens. Sulcal widening and corresponding gyral atrophy secondary to thinning of the cortical ribbon, with compensatory ventricular dilatation, is observed throughout the brain in late stages of the disease. Typically, there is relative sparing of the occipital pole and a more obvious dilatation of the temporal horn of the lateral ventricle owing to preferential hippocampal and amygdalar atrophy.[75]

Histological hallmarks beyond cell loss include those initially described by Alzheimer as miliary bodies and dense tangles of fibrils,[76] now commonly referred to as senile or neuritic plaques and NFT, respectively. Other microscopic pathology includes granulovacuolar degeneration and amyloid angiopathy. The relationship of these histological changes to the pathogenesis of AD is under active study.

Neuritic plaques are extracellular structures composed of an amyloid core surrounded by swollen neuritic processes which stain strongly with silver. These plaques contain β-amyloid protein, a peptide of 40–42 amino acid residues that is derived from the proteolytic cleavage of the large transmembrane APP. Initially, β-amyloid was thought to be an abnormal protein; however, subsequent evidence suggests that it is produced during normal cell metabolism [77] via the action of two proteases, designated β-secretase and γ-secretase.

While neuritic plaque burden was previously thought to correlate with disease severity,[78] pathological changes are now hypothesized by some investigators to be referable to an imbalance in production and clearance of β-amyloid, particularly the more toxic oligomers of Aβ42.[79] Increased production of toxic β-amyloid isoforms is implicated in familial disease with decreased clearance implicated in sporadic AD.[80] Beta-amyloid 42 contributes to the misfolding of other β-amyloid isoforms, with soluble β-amyloid presumed to undergo a conformational change. This conformational change leads to aggregation as both insoluble fibrils in plaques, which presumably initiate an inflammatory cascade and lead to neuronal death, and soluble oligomers, which have more recently been implicated in AD symptomatology.[81]

Neurofibrillary tangles are intraneuronal cytoplasmic inclusions composed predominantly of hyperphosphorylated tau, a normal axonal protein associated with microtubule binding.[82] Ubiquitin and neurofilament protein make less-prominent contributions to tangle formation. Like neuritic plaques, NFTs also represent an abnormal process of aggregation. Selective regional vulnerability to this pathological change is evidenced early in the disease by a predictable distribution of NFTs beginning transentorhinally, with subsequent spread to the hippocampus, amygdalae, and neocortex.[83] The evolution of NFT pathology appears to be independent of plaque formation; yet, the exact relationship of both to disease onset and progression remains to be further elucidated. [84] Unlike amyloid plaque burden, NFT formation appears to correlate well with specific deficits such as memory loss.[85]

Granuovacuolar degeneration has the appearance of a small, intraneuronal, cytoplasmic vacuole containing a single argyrophilic granule and represents an additional pathological hallmark of AD. Neuropil threads and amyloid angiopathy may also be observed. Amyloid angiopathy is characterized by amyloid deposition in small and medium-sized leptomeningeal and cortical arteries, leading to a predisposition for hemorrhage.[86]

In addition to these cellular changes, the most notable neurochemical alteration associated with AD is depletion of cortical acetylcholine in association with cell loss in the nucleus basalis of Meynert, the basal forebrain structure responsible for the majority of cortical cholinergic projections.[87] Further neurochemical deficiencies in AD brains have been described for dopamine, norepinephrine and serotonin.[88–90]

Neuropathological diagnosis

Prompted by the recognition that non-demented older adults may have neuropathological changes associated with AD,[91] guidelines for the neuropathological diagnosis of AD have evolved in recent years. The Khachaturian criteria were proposed in 1985 as a means to provide uniform guidelines for the diagnosis of AD; these criteria are the most sensitive and least stringent, requiring minimal plaque densities, which are age adjusted but not region specific.[92] The Consortium to Establish a Registry for Alzheimer's Disease (CERAD) was subsequently established, proposing criteria for *definite*, *probable* or *possible* AD based on clinical information, age groupings and the quantification of neuritic plaques in specified cortical regions.[93]

In parallel, Braak and Braak [94] provided compelling evidence that quantification of NFTs in transentorhinal cortex, limbic regions and isocortex may also be relevant to the neuropathological staging and diagnosis of AD.[94] Most recently, the National Institute on Aging (NIA)-Reagan criteria were formulated to account for both CERAD neuritic plaque scores and quantification of NFT pathology by region. *Probable AD*, according to NIA-Reagan neuropathological criteria, requires NFTs in the neocortex and frequent neuritic plaques. Likewise, a diagnosis of *possible AD* requires moderate neuritic plaques and hippocampal NFTs.[95]

Depending on the neuropathological criteria used for diagnosis, elderly subjects without symptoms of dementia may actually possess levels of pathological change that would be sufficient to diagnose AD.[91] While such findings are consistent with the observation that age is the primary risk factor for AD, they also reflect the need for improving sensitivity and specificity of clinical criteria for AD diagnosis as a complement to the expanding biochemical and neuropathological knowledge of the disease.

Clinical diagnosis

Alzheimer's disease is a slowly progressive disorder with a broad spectrum of symptoms, reflecting the wide array of cortical regions that may be impacted by the disease. Insidious in onset, the most common presenting complaint is episodic memory impairment, often involving names of persons or objects. Patients frequently describe a relative inability to recollect recent as compared with remote events.[1] These complaints reflect involvement of the neuroanatomically vulnerable basal forebrain and medial temporal structures. Additional clinical features likewise reflect the characteristic spread of pathology to involve the posterior cingulate gyrus and the temporal and parietal cortices.

In the language domain, reduced spontaneous verbal output often accompanies early memory symptoms, but many patients develop increasing anomia and non-fluency, with prominent word-finding problems, hesitancy and occasional paraphasic errors. Grammar and syntax may also become progressively less complex. Many patients have a period when comprehension is impaired but repetition is normal, so-called transcortical sensory aphasia; this, in turn, progresses to Wernicke's aphasia with poor comprehension and repetition. Patients with asymmetric involvement of the left posterior temporal and parietal regions can show word-finding difficulty, problems with repetition and anomia – a constellation of symptoms consistent with logopenic aphasia.[96] In severe AD, patients may eventually develop global aphasia or mutism. The speech and language disturbances seen with AD strongly correlate with the severity of left posterior parietal and temporal lobe disease.

Visuospatial deficits often manifest, with patients becoming lost or disoriented while navigating. Misplacement of personal objects may also reveal a visual memory deficit. Inability to navigate correlates strongly with the severity of right posterior hippocampal and parietal dysfunction. Owing to the involvement of the temporal and parietal lobes as the disease advances, the ventral "what" and dorsal "where" visual pathways may both be rendered deficient by AD, although the occipitotemporal "what" network appears to be more often affected.[97] Other cognitive symptoms such as executive dysfunction (difficulty planning, sequencing or abstracting), agnosia (difficulty recognizing objects) and apraxia (an inability to perform a learned motor act) occur with variable frequency in patients with AD, most often in the moderate to late stages of the illness.

Table 5.2. Alzheimer's disease: diagnostic criteria

NINCDS-ARDA (110)	DSM-IV (109)
Probable AD • Dementia established by clinical examination • Dementia confirmed with cognitive testing • Deficits in two or more domains of cognition • Progressive decline in memory and other cognitive functions • Preserved consciousness • Onset between ages 40 and 90 years • Absence of systemic or other brain disease that accounts for symptoms *Possible AD* • Atypical onset, presentation or clinical course of dementia • Another illness capable of producing dementia is present but is not considered to be the primary cause *Definite AD* • Tissue diagnosis by autopsy or biopsy • Clinical criteria for probable AD	Insidious onset with progressive decline of cognitive function resulting in impairment of social or occupational functioning from a previously higher level Impairment in recent memory Disturbance in at least one of the following cognitive domains: • aphasia • apraxia • agnosia Executive functioning (planning, organizing, sequencing, abstracting) Cognitive deficits are NOT due to other neurologic, psychiatric, toxic, metabolic, or systemic diseases Cognitive deficits do not occur solely in the setting of delirium

Notes:
AD, Alzheimer's desease; NINCDS-ARDA, National Institute of Neurological and Communicative Disorders and Stroke–Alzheimer's Disease and Related Disorders Association; DSM-IV, *Diagnostic and Statistical Manual of Mental Disorders,* 4th edn, text revision; reprinted with permission from the American Psychiatric Association (copyright 2000).

Equally important, behavioral symptoms are common in AD and change as the disease progresses. [98,99] Neuropsychiatric symptoms are reported in up to 80% of patients with AD.[100] Depression, apathy and agitation are most commonly noted by caregivers as behavioral manifestations.[101–103] Anxiety and delusions, often paranoid, also become more common as the illness progresses.[99]

Focal variants of AD are well described in the literature and present with an alteration in the typical constellation and chronology of symptoms, presumably reflecting the region of the brain most affected with disease burden. Some of these syndromes include posterior cortical atrophy, corticobasal syndrome, primary progressive aphasia, progressive apraxia and frontal variant AD.[104–108] Detailed discussion of these clinical syndromes is addressed elsewhere in this volume.

Criteria that are commonly used for the diagnosis of AD may be found in the *Diagnostic and Statistical Manual of Mental Disorders,* 4th edition (DSM-IV). [109] Dementia of the Alzheimer's type, according to this standard, is a gradual and progressive decline in cognitive function with impairments in recent memory and one other cognitive domain, not caused by other identified medical or psychiatric illness, and resultant in a functional impairment socially or occupationally. Other specified cognitive domains are detailed in Table 5.2.

Also widely used, the National Institute of Neurological and Communicative Disorders and Stroke and the Alzheimer's Disease and Related Disorders Association Joint Task Force (NINCDS-ARDA) issued criteria for the classification of AD as *possible, probable* or *definite.*[110] NINCDS-ARDA *definite AD* requires neuropathological confirmation at autopsy or brain biopsy such that DSM-IV-diagnosed AD most closely resembles NINCDS-ARDA *probable AD.* By the NINCDS-ARDA diagnostic standard, *probable AD* is dementia with cognitive deficits in at least two cognitive domains including progressive memory loss, with onset between 40 and 90 years of age in the absence of another plausible medical cause. If a potentially contributing medical condition coexists or if the clinical syndrome demonstrates focal features, then a diagnosis of *possible AD* may be appropriate.

History and neurological examination

Obtaining a detailed history from the patient and a close informant are of primary importance in diagnosing AD. The most common first symptom is memory loss, and this often distinguishes AD from other neurodegenerative conditions.[111] Nearly one-half of those with AD have other symptoms, including executive loss, acalculia or alexia, visuospatial disturbance or depression. Past medical history and medication use influence the expression of symptoms and may modify risk, and a positive family history is common, even in those without an identified genetic cause. Social history may reveal AD risk modifiers of ethnicity, education and socioeconomic environment, as well as alcohol and tobacco use or abuse.

The general neurological examination is typically unremarkable in mild to moderate AD. Focal abnormalities may suggest an alternative cause for memory impairment. Later in the illness, patients may develop pyramidal signs with hyper-reflexia or extrapyramidal parkinsonism, although these findings may be referable to concomitant vascular or Lewy body pathology. [112] Myoclonus is also observed in up to 50% of those with AD as the illness progresses, although it is more often reported in early-onset and familial cases and is often seen later in the illness.[113] Dysphagia is an important late symptom of the disease and likely a contributing factor to the observation that the majority of AD deaths result from bronchopneumonia.[114]

Bedside mental status testing is crucial for determining domains of cognitive deficit. Standardized screening tests such as the Folstein Mini-Mental Status Examination (MMSE) [115] or the Kokmen Short Test of Mental Status [116] assess, at minimum, orientation, attention, learning, memory, language and constructional praxis. A poor performance compared with normative data on one of these screening instruments (factoring in age, education, ethnicity and language [117]) may prompt a more detailed cognitive assessment. Additional neuropsychological testing may be better structured to reveal a pattern of deficits consistent with AD and to quantify the severity of the illness more accurately.

Neuropsychological testing

Based on the characteristic clinical history and neuroanatomic locations selectively vulnerable to AD pathologic changes, it is not surprising that neuropsychological tests of delayed verbal memory successfully differentiate AD from other neurodegenerative conditions, including frontotemporal, vascular and Lewy body dementias.[118,119] Tests of naming and verbal fluency also demonstrate discriminative capacity when the clinical syndrome reflects overlapping diagnostic considerations.[118,120,121] However, the regional variability in neuropsychological testing protocols and in the relative influence of various portions of the dementia evaluation on determining the clinical diagnosis have been recognized as a limiting factor in more effectively characterizing and treating AD.

To this end, CERAD developed and administered a standard battery of neuropsychological tests to 350 AD patients and 275 controls in order to demonstrate reliability in diagnosis.[122] The neuropsychological tests included a 6-item Short Blessed Test,[123] MMSE,[115] animal category fluency, modified Boston Naming Test,[124] Word List Memory (learning), Word List Recall, Word List Recognition and Constructional Praxis. Additional information is obtained through informant measures, the Blessed Dementia Scale (BDS) [78] and the Clinical Dementia Rating (CDR),[125] both of which assess functional impairment. Such standardization has been recognized as advantageous to the advancement of neuroscience and patient care and has prompted further iterations of standardized assessment in the form of the NIA Minimum Data Set and, more recently, the United States Alzheimer Disease Centers Uniform Data Set (UDS).[126]

The UDS not only expands the neuropsychological test battery used to characterize the cognitive deficits to include digit spans,[127] trailmaking [128] and a digit-symbol task [129] but also broadens the functional and behavioral assessment with the inclusion of the Neuropsychiatric Inventory-Questionnaire,[130] Functional Assessment Questionnaire [131] and the Geriatric Depression Scale.[132] Validation of this specific battery awaits further study, but the combination of functional scales and standardized assessment of multiple cognitive domains is certain to contribute to diagnostic accuracy, and longitudinal evaluation with such tools will better delineate the trajectory of decline in AD.

Laboratory evaluation

In 2001, the American Academy of Neurology (AAN) Practice Parameter for the diagnosis of dementia updated guidelines regarding the usefulness of laboratory testing in the initial clinical assessment of dementia using an evidence-based approach.[133] This review concluded with recommendations to screen for depression, hypothyroidism, electrolyte imbalance and vitamin B_{12} deficiency as potentially treatable causes of cognitive impairment. Notably, syphilis screening was recommended only in the context of a clinical suspicion of neurosyphilis. Depending on the clinical scenario, several other laboratory tests were recommended in the initial version of the guidelines, including those meant to assess for metabolic derangement, such as complete blood count, serum electrolytes, fasting blood glucose, blood urea nitrogen/creatinine and liver function tests. In more highly select patients, an erythrocyte sedimentation rate, testing for the human immunodeficiency virus, toxicology screen, urine heavy metals testing, chest radiograph, serum homocysteine or serum folate levels may be indicated.[134]

Electroencephalography (EEG) is not recommended for routine use in the diagnosis of dementia, and is often normal in AD. If the study is abnormal, it may reveal non-specific generalized slowing. However, EEG may be useful in distinguishing dementia from delirium and for diagnosing seizures, which accompany AD pathology in up to 17% of patients [135] and may be present at the time of diagnosis in up to 6%.[136]

Cerebrospinal fluid (CSF) studies were also not recommended by the AAN for routine use in the diagnostic evaluation of patients with suspected AD. However, in certain scenarios, CSF studies may help to differentiate AD from inflammatory, infectious or neoplastic causes of cognitive dysfunction. With respect to AD specifically, at the time of the 2001 structured review of the literature, there was considerable evidence to support a CSF profile associated with AD.[133] Reduction in the CSF $A_{\beta-42}$ and elevation in the CSF tau protein combined yielded a reported sensitivity and specificity of approximately 80–90% in comparing AD patients and controls,[137,138] although there is some overlap with other syndromes.[139,140] This diagnostic overlap may be limited with the use of assays for both total tau (T-tau) and phosphorylated tau (P-tau), with high levels of P-tau increasing specificity for AD.[141] There remains continued uncertainty as to how CSF biomarkers may prospectively contribute to AD diagnostic strategies beyond the standard clinical assessment.[133] However, CSF studies continue to be investigated as a potential surrogate marker of disease, with a recent investigation revealing that CSF biomarkers may accurately predict incipient AD in patients with mild cognitive impairment (MCI).[142] An additional predictive utility of CSF biomarkers has been suggested by another recent investigation, which reported that CSF $A_{\beta42}$ deficits correlated with earlier death, while increased CSF tau levels may correlate with dementia severity.[143]

Neuroimaging

Structural neuroimaging with magnetic resonance imaging (MRI) or non-contrast computed tomography (CT) allows the clinician to assess for structural pathology that may present with cognitive decline, including neoplasms, cerebrovascular lesions and hydrocephalus, while confirming the typical changes associated with AD. The use of neuroimaging as part of an initial evaluation for possible dementia is currently recommended by the AAN.[133] In AD, MRI and CT most often demonstrate non-specific, generalized atrophy, which is more pronounced in the medial temporal structures.[144] As expected based on the known distribution of neuropathological change in AD,[94] the hippocampus [145,146] and entorhinal cortex [147] are subject to relatively greater atrophy when studied with volumetric measures; unfortunately, this pattern is sensitive but not specific for AD,[148] demonstrating considerable overlap with other dementia subtypes and normal aging. Medial temporal volumetric imaging studies are not routinely recommended in the clinical setting,[133] in part owing to the known hippocampal volume loss associated with aging; [149] however, there is increasing evidence that volumetric imaging may be useful in predicting incipient AD in patients with MCI.[150,151]

Functional imaging with single-photon emission tomography (SPECT) and [^{18}F]-fluorodeoxyglucose positron emission tomography (FDG-PET) have been considered extensively as methods to differentiate AD from other dementias, and also as a tool to predict the evolution of MCI to AD. The use of SPECT had a lower sensitivity than clinical criteria for AD diagnosis in a prospective study, and variable sensitivities and specificities when used to differentiate dementia subtypes;[152–154] it is not recommended for use in routine clinical practice.[133]

However, FDG-PET has demonstrated greater promise in recent years, differentiating AD from normal aging,[155] differentiating AD from other dementias [156] and predicting AD pathology in MCI,[157] using an identifiable pattern of deficient regional glucose metabolism in the posterior temporoparietal regions, precuneus and posterior cingulate cortex (Fig. 5.1). Although FDG-PET functional imaging is not currently recommended by any consensus guidelines for diagnosing AD,[84,133] the US Center for Medicare and Medicaid recently approved payment for this imaging modality for use in differentiating frontotemporal dementia from AD,[111] which will potentially increase the clinical correlational data available beyond that obtained in the research environment. Similar patterns of hypometabolism are seen in the same regions with functional MRI.

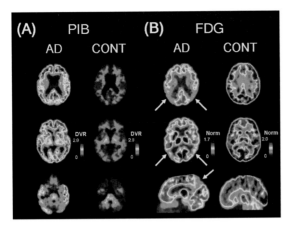

Fig. 5.1. Protein and functional imaging in Alzheimer's disease. (A) Pittsburgh compound B (PIB) binds to brain amyloid in a patient clinically diagnosed with Alzheimer's disease (AD) compared with a control subject (CONT). (B) Fluorodeoxyglucose positron emission tomography (FDG) demonstrates markedly reduced glucose metabolism in the region of the posterior cingulate gyrus and bilateral parietal lobes in a patient clinically diagnosed with AD compared with a control subject on selected axial and sagittal cuts. (Images courtesy of Dr. Gil Rabinovici.)

Assessment of fibrillar amyloid deposition, a neuropathological signature of AD, may now be obtained in vivo using experimental PET radiotracer ligands, including a thioflavin analogue Pittsburgh compound B (PIB; Fig. 5.1),[158] fluoro-dicyano-dimethylamino-naphthalenyl-propene (FDDNP) [159] and N-methylamino-hydroxystilbene (SB-13).[160] Potential clinical applications of these techniques await further characterization of longitudinal trends in ligand-related imaging patterns,[161] as well as further description of the imaging patterns obtained in normal aging and other dementia subtypes.[162] Likewise, a better understanding of the precise role of amyloid in the pathogenesis of AD will presumably make such imaging strategies more useful in the design of therapeutic interventions.[163]

Treatment

Symptomatic treatment

Based on the known neurochemical derangements in AD, two classes of medication have been approved for treatment of cognitive symptoms: cholinesterase inhibitors, including donepezil, galantamine, and rivastigmine, and an N-methyl-D-aspartate (NMDA) receptor antagonist, memantine (Table 5.3). Cholinesterase inhibition is predicted to enhance cholinergic transmission which is recognized as deficient because

of basal forebrain AD pathology. These agents have demonstrated modest effects on cognition, activities of daily living and global function versus placebo in a large number of randomized, double-blind trials,[164] with efficacy demonstrated for up to 2 to 5 years.[165,166] Rivastigmine differs from the other cholinesterase inhibitors in its inhibition of butyl-cholinesterase and its non-hepatic metabolism.[167] Galantamine also modulates presynaptic nicotinic receptors.[168] The clinical significance of these and other pharmacodynamic differences is unknown, as there is no evidence suggesting that the agents differ in efficacy.[164] Medication side-effects are generally mild and may be limited with a gradual titration to the recommended dosage. Commonly reported complaints include gastrointestinal symptoms, which are limited if medication is taken with food, and insomnia or vivid dreams, which is avoided with a morning dosing schedule. Other less common side-effects include leg cramps and symptomatic bradycardia. The latter may prompt a baseline electrocardiogram before initiation of cholinesterase inhibition in a patient with cardiovascular risk factors. The US Food and Drug Administration (FDA) has approved all cholinesterase inhibitors for the treatment of mild to moderate AD, with an indication for severe AD recently granted to donepezil. These medications are recommended as standard therapy for AD by the AAN.[169] Internationally, there may be less enthusiasm for continuing therapy without demonstrable benefit.[170]

Memantine is a non-competitive NMDA-receptor antagonist thought to protect neurons from excitotoxicity associated with glutamatergic activity. Its precise mechanism of action in AD is not clearly defined; however, the glutamate transporter is known to be downregulated in AD, leading to changes in β-amyloid and tau burden.[171–173] Clinical trials of memantine in AD suggest improvement in cognition, behavior and activities of daily living in moderate to severe disease.[174] Furthermore, added benefit was observed when used in combination with cholinesterase inhibition.[175] The medication is well tolerated with a side-effect profile similar to placebo in randomized studies and is currently approved by the FDA for use in moderate to severe AD.

The treatment of commonly encountered behavioral signs and symptoms is paramount in AD. Strategies to adequately manage depression, anxiety, sleep disturbances and psychosis continue to evolve, but these symptoms remain a considerable challenge for caregivers, in the home and in the medical community.

Table 5.3. Alzheimer's disease: clinical pharmacology of selected agents

	Donepezil	Galantamine	Rivastigmine	Memantine
Mechanism of action	Cholinesterase inhibitor	Cholinesterase inhibitor	Cholinesterase inhibitor	NMDA-receptor antagonist
Dose (initial/maximal)	5 mg daily/10 mg daily	4 mg twice daily/12 mg twice daily	1.5 mg twice daily/6 mg twice daily	5 mg daily/10 mg twice daily
Absorption affected by food	No	Yes	Yes	No
Hours to maximum serum concentration	3–5	0.5–1	0.5–2	3–7
Serum half-life (h)	70–80	5–7	2–8	60–80

Depression is common in AD, and several placebo-controlled treatment trials have demonstrated mixed results with both selective serotonin-reuptake inhibitors (SSRIs) and tricyclic antidepressants.[176,177] Owing to the anticholinergic side-effect profile of the tricyclic antidepressants, SSRIs (with combination noradrenergic-reuptake inhibitor activity) are chosen by most clinicians. In patients with AD, anxiety often manifests as a fear of being left unattended, a symptom that may also respond to SSRIs, although evidence is anecdotal.[178] Alternative anxiolytics such as benzodiazepines are less-attractive candidates for long-term management because of their cognitive side-effects. Sleep disturbance may also respond to antidepressant medications such as mirtazapine.[100]

Psychotic symptoms associated with AD include hallucinations, delusions and agitation/aggression. It is important to rule out delirium as a result of a common medical illness, such as a urinary tract infection, as a mimicker of dementia-related psychosis. If pharmacotherapy is needed to treat psychotic symptoms, then most clinicians prefer newer generation antipsychotic medications,[179] although this practice is not approved by the FDA. A recent double-blind, placebo-controlled trial observed only a small difference in perceived change in patients with AD-related psychosis treated with second-generation antipsychotic medications, such as olanzepine, quetiapine and risperidone, when compared with placebo.[180] This coupled with a recent black box warning label requirement from the FDA, suggesting increased mortality associated with these medications,[111] led investigators to conclude that, "Adverse effects offset advantages in the efficacy of atypical antipsychotic drugs for treatment of psychosis, aggression, or agitation in patients with Alzheimer's disease." [180] Unfortunately, clinicians have limited options in treating psychotic symptoms, as more traditional antipsychotic medications, such as haloperidol, are known to produce or exacerbate parkinsonism and may be more likely than newer antipsychotic drugs to increase mortality.[181] Notably, neuropsychiatric symptoms may respond to initiation of cholinesterase inhibition, memantine or a combination of these approved AD medications.[182]

Following a diagnosis of AD, interventions that are non-pharmacological will likely be required, emphasizing patient and caregiver safety. One issue that may dramatically change the lifestyle of a patient with AD is restriction or revocation of driving privileges. Current physician reporting standards vary by US state and country, and assorted medical governing bodies have determined different standards, as well. For example, the AAN recommends that patients with a functional measure signifying mild dementia with memory predominance be advised to discontinue driving,[183] while the American Medical Association bases its recommendations on performance on two office-based cognitive tasks.[184] While the up to eight-fold increase in collisions involving patients with AD who continue to operate a motor vehicle [185] must be addressed as a public health concern, current predictors of driver fitness may be inadequate and warrant further study.[186,187]

Investigational treatments

Currently available interventions improve symptoms associated with AD, but strategies to halt disease progression or prevent disease development are the major candidates for affecting change on the natural history and epidemiology of AD, as a uniformly fatal illness with an increasing prevalence worldwide. Several investigational treatments and preventive strategies are currently in clinical trials or development:

- secretase modulation
- amyloid anti-aggregation
- kinase modulation

- neurotransmitter modulation
- heavy metal modulation
- β-amyloid immunotherapy
- lipid metabolism modulation
- anti-oxidative measures
- hormone modulation
- increased β-amyloid elimination.

Therapeutic targets for disease modification include both β-amyloid and tau.

Several approaches to modify the pathogenicity of β-amyloid have been undertaken, from reducing production to reducing aggregation to increasing clearance. Sequential cleavage of APP by β- and γ-secretase generate β-amyloid, rendering secretase modulators prime targets for drug development, with γ-secretase inhibitors in both phase II (efficacy) and phase III (clinical) trials.[188] Beta-, secretase inhibitors have reduced β-amyloid concentrations in AD transgenic mice.[189] Also in a transgenic mouse model of AD, an α-secretase enhancer, which shifts APP processing toward a non-amyloid generating pathway, has demonstrated efficacy in reducing brain β-amyloid.[190]

Active immunization with a vaccine of pre-aggregated Aβ-42, hypothesized to induce an efflux of β-amyloid from the brain by activity of antibodies in the periphery or the activation of microglial clearance of plaques by antibody activity in the central nervous system, [191,192] was halted in a phase II trial as a result of the development of presumably T-cell-mediated encephalitis.[193] However, passive immunization, currently in phase II trials, remains as a potential therapy for reducing amyloid burden, while a modified active immunization is also being investigated.[188] Several small molecules that interfere with β-amyloid aggregation via different mechanisms are also being studied, including a glycosaminoglycan mimetic [194] and a metal chelator.[195]

Tau pathology represents another target for drug design, with molecules interfering with tau phosphorylation under preclinical investigation [84]; however, redundancy in tau kinases may render a single molecule clinically ineffective. Lithium, a known inhibitor of tau phosphorylation,[196] is currently in clinical trials for the treatment of AD.

Other therapeutic interventions currently under investigation are largely based on observational data, which are often difficult to reproduce with prospective study. Anti-inflammatory agents have been recognized to reduce risk of AD in epidemiological studies,[197,198] yet, both steroids and non-steroidal anti-inflammatory drugs (NSAIDs) have demonstrated no effect on cognitive outcomes in AD clinical trials so far.[199] One NSAID currently in clinical trials, flurbiprofen, has demonstrated selective lowering of Aβ42 as a potential mechanism of action.[200] Estrogen replacement therapy in postmenopausal women was also associated with reduced risk for AD in epidemiological studies,[201] although clinical trials have not supported the use of estrogen for AD risk reduction.[202]

Antioxidants, including vitamins E and C, may reduce the risk of AD according to large observational studies,[203] although treatment trials with vitamin E have yielded mixed results,[194,204] and recent evidence that high-dose vitamin E may increase cardiac risks [205] has tempered enthusiasm for supplementation above 400 IU daily. Alternatively, lipid-lowering agents are presently in large clinical trials after retrospective case–control data suggested that statins may modify risk for disease development.[206]

Novel naturopathic intervention strategies such as ginkgo biloba and huperzine A may show marginal benefit in the treatment of AD [100] and warrant further investigation. Such interventions may demonstrate activity against AD pathology via multiple mechanisms. For example, curcumin (curry spice) is currently in clinical trials [84] and reportedly acts as an anti-inflammatory, anti-oxidant, and anti-amyloid aggregant.[207]

Future directions

Over 100 years after Alzheimer's initial clinicopathological presentation, much has been learned about the neurodegenerative disorder which bears his name, with more than 50 000 articles on the topic currently accessible through public electronic medical reference. However, there are many exciting scientific discoveries on the horizon. New microarray technologies offer the opportunity to better understand the complicated genetic susceptibilities and cellular pathways that may lead to the development of AD.[208] Concomitantly, proteome-based studies of CSF [209] and serum [210] promise new biomarkers for AD that will potentially serve as surrogate markers for diagnosis or disease progression and drive therapeutic intervention studies forward. Furthermore, a cooperative neuroimaging study seeks to identify imaging and associated biomarkers through a longitudinal, multicenter, prospective study of normal aging, MCI and AD.[211]

Of equal importance is a pressing need for accurate clinical characterization of AD in its early stages in an effort to initiate interventions strategically. Likewise, diagnosis and treatment of patients already demonstrating signs and symptoms of AD demand improvement. In primary care settings, less than 50% of patients with dementia are diagnosed,[212] with a consequential lack of screening for potentially treatable conditions.[213] Equally surprising, only half of patients diagnosed with AD are treated with currently available therapies.[100] With promising new treatments already in clinical trials, it is necessary to advocate for accurate and early diagnosis or referral. To maintain quality of life for those already diagnosed with AD, appropriate symptom management with approved medications and perhaps less-conventional interventions such as music therapy [214] and exercise [215] should also be emphasized. While many challenges remain in AD scientific discovery and patient management, recent advances and continued collaborative efforts are encouraging for a successful preventative strategy to be developed in the near future.

References

1. Morris J. Clinical presentation and course of Alzheimer disease. In Terry R, Katzman R, Bick K, Sisodia S (eds.) *Alzheimer Disease*. Philadelphia, PA: Lippincott Williams & Wilkins; 1999:11–24.

2. Moller HJ, Graeber MB. The case described by Alois Alzheimer in 1911. Historical and conceptual perspectives based on the clinical record and neurohistological sections. *Eur Arch Psychiatry Clin Neurosci* 1998;**248**(3):111–22.

3. Ernst RL, Hay JW. Economic research on Alzheimer disease: a review of the literature. *Alzheimer Dis Assoc Disord* 1997;**11**(Suppl 6):135–45.

4. Ferri CP, Prince M, Brayne C *et al.* Global prevalence of dementia: a Delphi consensus study. *Lancet* 2005;**366**(9503):2112–17.

5. Mayeux R. Epidemiology of neurodegeneration. *Annu Rev Neurosci* 2003;**26**:81–104.

6. Brookmeyer R, Gray S, Kawas C. Projections of Alzheimer's disease in the United States and the public health impact of delaying disease onset. *Am J Public Health* 1998;**88**(9):1337–42.

7. Kukull WA, Ganguli M. Epidemiology of dementia: concepts and overview. *Neurol Clin* 2000;**18**(4):923–50.

8. Bachman DL, Wolf PA, Linn R *et al.* Prevalence of dementia and probable senile dementia of the Alzheimer type in the Framingham Study. *Neurology* 1992;**42**(1):115–19.

9. Kokmen E, Beard CM, Offord KP, Kurland LT. Prevalence of medically diagnosed dementia in a defined United States population: Rochester, Minnesota, January 1, 1975. *Neurology* 1989;**39**(6):773–6.

10. Miech RA, Breitner JC, Zandi PP *et al.* Incidence of AD may decline in the early 90s for men, later for women: the Cache County study. *Neurology* 2002; **58**(2):209–18.

11. Ruitenberg A, Ott A, van Swieten JC, Hofman A, Breteler MM. Incidence of dementia: does gender make a difference? *Neurobiol Aging* 2001;**22**(4): 575–80.

12. Tang MX, Cross P, Andrews H *et al.* Incidence of AD in African-Americans, Caribbean Hispanics, and Caucasians in northern Manhattan. *Neurology* 2001; **56**(1):49–56.

13. Perkins P, Annegers JF, Doody RS *et al.* Incidence and prevalence of dementia in a multiethnic cohort of municipal retirees. *Neurology* 1997;**49**(1):44–50.

14. Wolfson C, Wolfson DB, Asgharian M *et al.* A reevaluation of the duration of survival after the onset of dementia. *N Engl J Med* 2001;**344**(15):1111–16.

15. Helmer C, Joly P, Letenneur L, Commenges D, Dartigues JF. Mortality with dementia: results from a French prospective community-based cohort. *Am J Epidemiol* 2001;**154**(7):642–8.

16. Waring SC, Doody RS, Pavlik VN, Massman PJ, Chan W. Survival among patients with dementia from a large multi-ethnic population. *Alzheimer Dis Assoc Disord* 2005;**19**(4):178–83.

17. Borenstein AR, Copenhaver CI, Mortimer JA. Early-life risk factors for Alzheimer disease. *Alzheimer Dis Assoc Disord* 2006;**20**(1):63–72.

18. Mayeux R, Ottman R, Maestre G *et al.* Synergistic effects of traumatic head injury and apolipoprotein-epsilon 4 in patients with Alzheimer's disease. *Neurology* 1995;**45**(Pt 1):555–7.

19. Jordan BD, Relkin NR, Ravdin LD *et al.* Apolipoprotein E epsilon4 associated with chronic traumatic brain injury in boxing. *JAMA* 1997;**278**(2):136–40.

20. Plassman BL, Havlik RJ, Steffens DC *et al.* Documented head injury in early adulthood and risk of Alzheimer's disease and other dementias. *Neurology* 2000;**55**(8): 1158–66.

21. Guo Z, Cupples LA, Kurz A *et al.* Head injury and the risk of AD in the MIRAGE study. *Neurology* 2000; **54**(6):1316–23.

22. Luchsinger JA, Tang MX, Shea S, Mayeux R. Hyperinsulinemia and risk of Alzheimer disease. *Neurology* 2004;**63**(7):1187–92.

23. Craft S. Insulin resistance syndrome and Alzheimer disease: pathophysiologic mechanisms and therapeutic implications. *Alzheimer Dis Assoc Disord* 2006;**20**(4): 298–301.

24. Decarli C. Vascular factors in dementia: an overview. *J Neurol Sci* 2004;**226**(1–2):19–23.

25. Breteler MM. Vascular risk factors for Alzheimer's disease: an epidemiologic perspective. *Neurobiol Aging* 2000;**21**(2):153–60.

26. Kivipelto M, Helkala EL, Hanninen T *et al.* Midlife vascular risk factors and late-life mild cognitive impairment: a population-based study. *Neurology* 2001;**56**(12):1683–9.

27. Petrovitch H, White LR, Izmirilian G *et al.* Midlife blood pressure and neuritic plaques, neurofibrillary tangles, and brain weight at death: the HAAS. Honolulu-Asia Aging Study. *Neurobiol Aging* 2000;**21**(1):57–62.

28. Wolf H, Julin P, Gertz HJ, Winblad B, Wahlund LO. Intracranial volume in mild cognitive impairment, Alzheimer's disease and vascular dementia: evidence for brain reserve? *Int J Geriatr Psychiatry* 2004;**19**(10):995–1007.

29. Beeri MS, Davidson M, Silverman JM *et al.* Relationship between body height and dementia. *Am J Geriatr Psychiatry* 2005;**13**(2):116–23.

30. Abbott RD, White LR, Ross GW *et al.* Height as a marker of childhood development and late-life cognitive function: the Honolulu-Asia Aging Study. *Pediatrics* 1998;**102**(Pt 1):602–9.

31. Wilson RS, Scherr PA, Bienias JL *et al.* Socioeconomic characteristics of the community in childhood and cognition in old age. *Exp Aging Res* 2005;**31**(4):393–407.

32. Hall KS, Gao S, Unverzagt FW, Hendrie HC. Low education and childhood rural residence: risk for Alzheimer's disease in African Americans. *Neurology* 2000;**54**(1):95–9.

33. Moceri VM, Kukull WA, Emanuel I, van Belle G, Larson EB. Early-life risk factors and the development of Alzheimer's disease. *Neurology* 2000;**54**(2):415–20.

34. Wilson RS, Scherr PA, Hoganson G *et al.* Early life socioeconomic status and late life risk of Alzheimer's disease. *Neuroepidemiology* 2005;**25**(1):8–14.

35. Kaplan GA, Turrell G, Lynch JW *et al.* Childhood socioeconomic position and cognitive function in adulthood. *Int J Epidemiol* 2001;**30**(2):256–63.

36. Mortimer JA. Brain reserve and the clinical expression of Alzheimer's disease. *Geriatrics* 1997;**52**(Suppl 2):S50–3.

37. Qiu C, Backman L, Winblad B, Aguero-Torres H, Fratiglioni L. The influence of education on clinically diagnosed dementia incidence and mortality data from the Kungsholmen Project. *Arch Neurol* 2001;**58**(12):2034–9.

38. Roe C, Xiong C, Miller J, Morris J. Education and Alzheimer disease without dementia: support for the cognitive reserve hypothesis. *Neurology* 2007;**68**(3):223–8.

39. Kittner SJ, White LR, Farmer ME *et al.* Methodological issues in screening for dementia: the problem of education adjustment. *J Chronic Dis* 1986;**39**(3):163–70.

40. Zhang MY, Katzman R, Salmon D *et al.* The prevalence of dementia and Alzheimer's disease in Shanghai, China: impact of age, gender, and education. *Ann Neurol* 1990;**27**(4):428–37.

41. Stern Y, Gurland B, Tatemichi TK *et al.* Influence of education and occupation on the incidence of Alzheimer's disease. *JAMA* 1994;**271**(13):1004–10.

42. Karp A, Kareholt I, Qiu C *et al.* Relation of education and occupation-based socioeconomic status to incident Alzheimer's disease. *Am J Epidemiol* 2004;**159**(2):175–83.

43. Stern Y, Albert S, Tang MX, Tsai WY. Rate of memory decline in AD is related to education and occupation: cognitive reserve? *Neurology* 1999;**53**(9):1942–7.

44. Stern Y, Habeck C, Moeller J *et al.* Brain networks associated with cognitive reserve in healthy young and old adults. *Cereb Cortex* 2005;**15**(4):394–402.

45. Plassman BL, Welsh KA, Helms M *et al.* Intelligence and education as predictors of cognitive state in late life: a 50-year follow-up. *Neurology* 1995;**45**(8):1446–50.

46. Luchsinger JA, Mayeux R. Dietary factors and Alzheimer's disease. *Lancet Neurol* 2004;**3**(10):579–87.

47. Deng J, Zhou DH, Li J *et al.* A 2-year follow-up study of alcohol consumption and risk of dementia. *Clin Neurol Neurosurg* 2006;**108**(4):378–83.

48. Ruitenberg A, van Swieten JC, Witteman JC *et al.* Alcohol consumption and risk of dementia: the Rotterdam Study. *Lancet* 2002;**359**(9303):281–6.

49. Mukamal KJ, Kuller LH, Fitzpatrick AL *et al.* Prospective study of alcohol consumption and risk of dementia in older adults. *JAMA* 2003;**289**(11):1405–13.

50. Laitinen MH, Ngandu T, Rovio S *et al.* Fat intake at midlife and risk of dementia and Alzheimer's disease: a population-based study. *Dement Geriatr Cogn Disord* 2006;**22**(1):99–107.

51. Morris MC, Evans DA, Bienias JL *et al.* Dietary fats and the risk of incident Alzheimer disease. *Arch Neurol* 2003;**60**(2):194–200.

52. Morris MC, Evans DA, Bienias JL *et al.* Consumption of fish and n-3 fatty acids and risk of incident Alzheimer disease. *Arch Neurol* 2003;**60**(7):940–6.

53. Rovio S, Kareholt I, Helkala EL *et al.* Leisure-time physical activity at midlife and the risk of dementia and Alzheimer's disease. *Lancet Neurol* 2005;**4**(11):705–11.

54. Larson EB, Wang L, Bowen JD *et al.* Exercise is associated with reduced risk for incident dementia

67

among persons 65 years of age and older. *Ann Intern Med* 2006;**144**(2):73–81.

55. Fratiglioni L, Paillard-Borg S, Winblad B. An active and socially integrated lifestyle in late life might protect against dementia. *Lancet Neurol* 2004; **3**(6):343–53.

56. Wilson RS, Bennett DA, Bienias JL *et al.* Cognitive activity and incident AD in a population-based sample of older persons. *Neurology* 2002;**59**(12):1910–14.

57. Gatz M. Educating the brain to avoid dementia: can mental exercise prevent Alzheimer disease? *PLoS Med* 2005;**2**(1):e7.

58. Bertram L, Tanzi RE. The genetic epidemiology of neurodegenerative disease. *J Clin Invest* 2005; **115**(6): 1449–57.

59. Gatz M, Reynolds CA, Fratiglioni L *et al.* Role of genes and environments for explaining Alzheimer disease. *Arch Gen Psychiatry* 2006;**63**(2):168–74.

60. Goate A, Chartier-Harlin MC, Mullan M *et al.* Segregation of a missense mutation in the amyloid precursor protein gene with familial Alzheimer's disease. *Nature* 1991;**349**(6311):704–6.

61. Sherrington R, Rogaev EI, Liang Y *et al.* Cloning of a gene bearing missense mutations in early-onset familial Alzheimer's disease. *Nature* 1995;**375** (6534):754–60.

62. Levy-Lahad E, Wasco W, Poorkaj P *et al.* Candidate gene for the chromosome 1 familial Alzheimer's disease locus. *Science* 1995;**269**(5226):973–7.

63. Rogaeva EA, Fafel KC, Song YQ *et al.* Screening for PS1 mutations in a referral-based series of AD cases: 21 novel mutations. *Neurology* 2001;**57**(4):621–5.

64. Wisniewski K, Wisniewski H, Wen G. Occurrence of neuropathological changes and dementia of Alzheimer's disease in Down's syndrome. *Ann Neurol* 1985;**17**:278–82.

65. Evenhuis HM. The natural history of dementia in Down's syndrome. *Arch Neurol* 1990;**47**(3):263–7.

66. Schupf N, Kapell D, Nightingale B *et al.* Specificity of the fivefold increase in AD in mothers of adults with Down syndrome. *Neurology* 2001;**57**(6):979–84.

67. Corder EH, Saunders AM, Strittmatter WJ *et al.* Gene dose of apolipoprotein E type 4 allele and the risk of Alzheimer's disease in late onset families. *Science* 1993;**261**(5123):921–3.

68. Poirier J, Davignon J, Bouthillier D *et al.* Apolipoprotein E polymorphism and Alzheimer's disease. *Lancet* 1993; **342**(8873):697–9.

69. Slooter AJ, Cruts M, Kalmijn S *et al.* Risk estimates of dementia by apolipoprotein E genotypes from a population-based incidence study: the Rotterdam Study. *Arch Neurol* 1998;**55**(7):964–8.

70. Farrer LA, Cupples LA, Haines JL *et al.* Effects of age, sex, and ethnicity on the association between apolipoprotein E genotype and Alzheimer disease. A meta-analysis. APOE and Alzheimer Disease Meta Analysis Consortium. *JAMA* 1997;**278**(16): 1349–56.

71. Meyer MR, Tschanz JT, Norton MC *et al.* APOE genotype predicts when – not whether – one is predisposed to develop Alzheimer disease. *Nat Genet* 1998;**19**(4):321–2.

72. Rogaeva E, Meng Y, Lee JH *et al.* The neuronal sortilin-related receptor SORL1 is genetically associated with Alzheimer disease. *Nat Genet* 2007;**39**(2):168–77.

73. Scherzer CR, Offe K, Gearing M *et al.* Loss of apolipoprotein E receptor LR11 in Alzheimer disease. *Arch Neurol* 2004;**61**(8):1200–5.

74. Dodson SE, Gearing M, Lippa CF *et al.* LR11/SorLA expression is reduced in sporadic Alzheimer disease but not in familial Alzheimer disease. *J Neuropathol Exp Neurol* 2006;**65**(9):866–72.

75. Corey-Bloom J. Alzheimer's Disease. In Miller A (ed.) *Continuum: Dementia.* Philadelphia, PA: Lippincott, Williams & Wilkins; 2004:29–57.

76. Graeber MB, Mehraein P. Reanalysis of the first case of Alzheimer's disease. *Eur Arch Psychiatry Clin Neurosci* 1999;**249** (Suppl 3):10–13.

77. Haass C, Schlossmacher MG, Hung AY *et al.* Amyloid beta-peptide is produced by cultured cells during normal metabolism. *Nature* 1992;**359**(6393):322–5.

78. Blessed G, Tomlinson B, Roth M. The association between quantitative measures of dementia and of senile change in the cerebral grey matter of elderly subjects. *Br J Psychiatry* 1968;**114**:797–811.

79. Bayer TA, Wirths O, Majtenyi K *et al.* Key factors in Alzheimer's disease: beta-amyloid precursor protein processing, metabolism and intraneuronal transport. *Brain Pathol* 2001;**11**(1):1–11.

80. Hardy J, Selkoe DJ. The amyloid hypothesis of Alzheimer's disease: progress and problems on the road to therapeutics. *Science* 2002;**297**(5580):353–6.

81. Walsh DM, Selkoe DJ. Deciphering the molecular basis of memory failure in Alzheimer's disease. *Neuron* 2004;**44**(1):181–93.

82. Iqbal K, Alonso Adel C, Chen S *et al.* Tau pathology in Alzheimer disease and other tauopathies. *Biochim Biophys Acta* 2005;**1739**(2–3):198–210.

83. Braak E, Griffing K, Arai K *et al.* Neuropathology of Alzheimer's disease: what is new since A. Alzheimer. *Eur Arch Psychiatry Clin Neurosci* 1999;**249**(Suppl 3): 14–22.

84. Blennow K, de Leon MJ, Zetterberg H. Alzheimer's disease. *Lancet* 2006;**368**(9533):387–403.

85. Hyman BT, van Hoesen GW, Damasio AR, Barnes CL. Alzheimer's disease: cell-specific pathology isolates the hippocampal formation. *Science* 1984;**225**(4667): 1168–70.

86. Fuller G, Goodman J. Neurodegenerative disorders. *Practical Review of Neuropathology*. Philadelphia, PA: Lippincott, Williams & Wilkins; 2001:257–264.

87. Mesulam M, Shaw P, Mash D, Weintraub S. Cholinergic nucleus basalis tauopathy emerges early in the aging-MCI-AD continuum. *Ann Neurol* 2004; **55**(6):815–28.

88. Storga D, Vrecko K, Birkmayer JG, Reibnegger G. Monoaminergic neurotransmitters, their precursors and metabolites in brains of Alzheimer patients. *Neurosci Lett* 1996;**203**(1):29–32.

89. Reinikainen KJ, Paljarvi L, Huuskonen M *et al.* A post-mortem study of noradrenergic, serotonergic and GABAergic neurons in Alzheimer's disease. *J Neurol Sci* 1988;**84**(1):101–16.

90. Reinikainen KJ, Soininen H, Riekkinen PJ. Neurotransmitter changes in Alzheimer's disease: implications to diagnostics and therapy. *J Neurosci Res* 1990;**27**(4):576–86.

91. Keller JN. Age-related neuropathology, cognitive decline, and Alzheimer's disease. *Ageing Res Rev* 2006; **5**(1):1–13.

92. Khachaturian ZS. Diagnosis of Alzheimer's disease. *Arch Neurol* 1985;**42**(11):1097–105.

93. Mirra SS, Heyman A, McKeel D *et al.* The Consortium to Establish a Registry for Alzheimer's Disease (CERAD). Part II. Standardization of the neuropathologic assessment of Alzheimer's disease. *Neurology* 1991; **41**(4):479–86.

94. Braak H, Braak E. Neuropathological staging of Alzheimer-related changes. *Acta Neuropathol (Berl)* 1991;**82**(4):239–59.

95. The National Institute on Aging, and Reagan Institute Working Group on Diagnostic Criteria for the Neuropathological Assessment of Alzheimer's Disease. Consensus recommendations for the postmortem diagnosis of Alzheimer's disease. *Neurobiol Aging* 1997;**18**(4 Suppl):S1–2.

96. Gorno-Tempini ML, Dronkers NF, Rankin KP *et al.* Cognition and anatomy in three variants of primary progressive aphasia. *Ann Neurol* 2004; **55**(3):335–46.

97. McMonagle P, Deering F, Berliner Y, Kertesz A. The cognitive profile of posterior cortical atrophy. *Neurology* 2006;**66**(3):331–8.

98. Lyketsos CG, Lopez O, Jones B *et al.* Prevalence of neuropsychiatric symptoms in dementia and mild cognitive impairment: results from the cardiovascular health study. *JAMA* 2002;**288**(12):1475–83.

99. Tatsch MF, Bottino CM, Azevedo D *et al.* Neuropsychiatric symptoms in Alzheimer disease and cognitively impaired, nondemented elderly from a community-based sample in Brazil: prevalence and relationship with dementia severity. *Am J Geriatr Psychiatry* 2006;**14**(5):438–45.

100. Cummings JL. Alzheimer's disease. *N Engl J Med* 2004;**351**(1):56–67.

101. Ortiz F, Fitten LJ, Cummings JL, Hwang S, Fonseca M. Neuropsychiatric and behavioral symptoms in a community sample of Hispanics with Alzheimer's disease. *Am J Alzheimers Dis Other Demen* 2006; **21**(4):263–73.

102. Chow TW, Liu CK, Fuh JL *et al.* Neuropsychiatric symptoms of Alzheimer's disease differ in Chinese and American patients. *Int J Geriatr Psychiatry* 2002; **17**(1):22–8.

103. Cummings JL, Mega M, Gray K *et al.* The Neuropsychiatric Inventory: comprehensive assessment of psychopathology in dementia. *Neurology* 1994;**44**(12):2308–14.

104. Tang-Wai DF, Graff-Radford NR, Boeve BF *et al.* Clinical, genetic, and neuropathologic characteristics of posterior cortical atrophy. *Neurology* 2004; **63**(7):1168–74.

105. Boeve BF, Maraganore DM, Parisi JE *et al.* Pathologic heterogeneity in clinically diagnosed corticobasal degeneration. *Neurology* 1999;**53**(4):795–800.

106. Caselli RJ, Stelmach GE, Caviness JN *et al.* A kinematic study of progressive apraxia with and without dementia. *Mov Disord* 1999;**14**(2):276–87.

107. Johnson JK, Head E, Kim R, Starr A, Cotman CW. Clinical and pathological evidence for a frontal variant of Alzheimer disease. *Arch Neurol* 1999;**56**(10):1233–9.

108. Kramer JH, Miller BL. Alzheimer's disease and its focal variants. *Semin Neurol* 2000;**20**(4):447–54.

109. American Psychiatric Association. *Diagnostic and Statistical Manual of Mental Disorders, 4th edn.* Washington, DC: American Psychiatric Press; 1994.

110. McKhann G, Drachman D, Folstein M *et al.* Clinical diagnosis of Alzheimer's disease: report of the NINCDS–ADRDA Work Group under the auspices of Department of Health and Human Services Task Force on Alzheimer's Disease. *Neurology* 1984; **34**(7):939–44.

111. Caselli RJ, Beach TG, Yaari R, Reiman EM. Alzheimer's disease a century later. *J Clin Psychiatry* 2006;**67**(11):1784–800.

112. Barker WW, Luis CA, Kashuba A *et al.* Relative frequencies of Alzheimer disease, Lewy body, vascular and frontotemporal dementia, and hippocampal sclerosis in the State of Florida Brain Bank. *Alzheimer Dis Assoc Disord* 2002;**16**(4):203–12.

113. Caviness JN. Myoclonus and neurodegenerative disease: what's in a name? *Parkinsonism Relat Disord* 2003;**9**(4):185–92.

114. Attems J, Konig C, Huber M, Lintner F, Jellinger KA. Cause of death in demented and non-demented elderly inpatients; an autopsy study of 308 cases. *J Alzheimer's Dis* 2005;**8**(1):57–62.

115. Folstein MF, Folstein SE, McHugh PR. "Mini-mental state." A practical method for grading the cognitive state of patients for the clinician. *J Psychiatr Res* 1975;**12**(3):189–98.

116. Kokmen E, Smith GE, Petersen RC, Tangalos E, Ivnik RC. The short test of mental status. Correlations with standardized psychometric testing. *Arch Neurol* 1991;**48**(7):725–8.

117. Mungas D, Marshall SC, Weldon M, Haan M, Reed BR. Age and education correction of Mini-Mental State Examination for English and Spanish-speaking elderly. *Neurology* 1996;**46**(3):700–6.

118. Braaten AJ, Parsons TD, McCue R, Sellers A, Burns WJ. Neurocognitive differential diagnosis of dementing diseases: Alzheimer's dementia, vascular dementia, frontotemporal dementia, and major depressive disorder. *Int J Neurosci* 2006;**116**(11):1271–93.

119. Crowell TA, Luis CA, Cox DE, Mullan M. Neuropsychological comparison of Alzheimer's disease and dementia with Lewy bodies. *Dement Geriatr Cogn Disord* 2007;**23**(2):120–5.

120. Diehl J, Monsch AU, Aebi C et al. Frontotemporal dementia, semantic dementia, and Alzheimer's disease: the contribution of standard neuropsychological tests to differential diagnosis. *J Geriatr Psychiatry Neurol* 2005;**18**(1):39–44.

121. Rascovsky K, Salmon DP, Hansen LA, Thal LJ, Galasko D. Disparate letter and semantic category fluency deficits in autopsy-confirmed frontotemporal dementia and Alzheimer's disease. *Neuropsychology* 2007;**21**(1):20–30.

122. Morris JC, Heyman A, Mohs RC et al. The Consortium to Establish a Registry for Alzheimer's Disease (CERAD). Part I. Clinical and neuropsychological assessment of Alzheimer's disease. *Neurology* 1989;**39**(9):1159–65.

123. Katzman R, Brown T, Fuld P et al. Validation of a short Orientation–Memory–Concentration Test of cognitive impairment. *Am J Psychiatry* 1983;**140**(6):734–9.

124. Kaplan E, Goodglass H, Weintraub S. *The Boston Naming Test*. Boston, MA: Veterans Administration Medical Center; 1978.

125. Berg L. Clinical Dementia Rating (CDR). *Psychopharmacol Bull* 1988;**24**(4):637–9.

126. Morris JC, Weintraub S, Chui HC et al. The Uniform Data Set (UDS): clinical and cognitive variables and descriptive data from Alzheimer Disease Centers. *Alzheimer Dis Assoc Disord* 2006;**20**(4):210–16.

127. Wechsler D, Stone C. *Manual: Wechsler Memory Scale.* New York: Psychological Corporation; 1973.

128. Armitage S. An analysis of certain psychological tests used in evaluation of brain injury. *Psych Mono* 1946;**60**:1–48.

129. Wechsler D. *Manual: Wechsler Adult Intelligence Scale.* New York: Psychological Corporation; 1955.

130. Kaufer DI, Cummings JL, Ketchel P et al. Validation of the NPI-Q, a brief clinical form of the Neuropsychiatric Inventory. *J Neuropsychiatry Clin Neurosci* 2000;**12**(2):233–9.

131. Pfeffer RI, Kurosaki TT, Harrah CH, Jr., Chance JM, Filos S. Measurement of functional activities in older adults in the community. *J Gerontol* 1982;**37**(3):323–9.

132. Sheikh J, Yesavage J. Geriatric Depression Scale (GDS): recent evidence and development of a shorter version. In Brink T (ed.) *Clinical Gerontology: A Guide to Assessment and Intervention.* New York: Haworth Press; 1986:165–173.

133. Knopman DS, DeKosky ST, Cummings JL et al. Practice parameter: diagnosis of dementia (an evidence-based review). Report of the Quality Standards Subcommittee of the American Academy of Neurology. *Neurology* 2001;**56**(9):1143–53.

134. American Academy of Neurology. Report of the Quality Standards Subcommittee of the American Academy of Neurology. Practice parameter for diagnosis and evaluation of dementia. [Summary statement.] *Neurology* 1994;**44**(11):2203–6.

135. Mendez MF, Catanzaro P, Doss RC et al. Seizures in Alzheimer's disease: clinicopathologic study. *J Geriatr Psychiatry Neurol* 1994;**7**(4):230–3.

136. Lozsadi DA, Larner AJ. Prevalence and causes of seizures at the time of diagnosis of probable Alzheimer's disease. *Dement Geriatr Cogn Disord* 2006;**22**(2):121–4.

137. Hulstaert F, Blennow K, Ivanoiu A et al. Improved discrimination of AD patients using beta-amyloid (1–42) and tau levels in CSF. *Neurology* 1999;**52**(8):1555–62.

138. Shoji M, Matsubara E, Kanai M et al. Combination assay of CSF tau, A beta 1–40 and A beta 1–42(43) as a biochemical marker of Alzheimer's disease. *J Neurol Sci* 1998;**158**(2):134–40.

139. Gomez-Tortosa E, Gonzalo I, Fanjul S et al. Cerebrospinal fluid markers in dementia with Lewy bodies compared with Alzheimer disease. *Arch Neurol* 2003;**60**(9):1218–22.

140. Sunderland T, Linker G, Mirza N et al. Decreased beta-amyloid 1–42 and increased tau levels in cerebrospinal fluid of patients with Alzheimer disease. *JAMA* 2003;**289**(16):2094–103.

141. Hampel H, Buerger K, Zinkowski R *et al.* Measurement of phosphorylated tau epitopes in the differential diagnosis of Alzheimer disease: a comparative cerebrospinal fluid study. *Arch Gen Psychiatry* 2004;**61**(1):95–102.

142. Hansson O, Zetterberg H, Buchhave P *et al.* Association between CSF biomarkers and incipient Alzheimer's disease in patients with mild cognitive impairment: a follow-up study. *Lancet Neurol* 2006;**5**(3):228–34.

143. Wallin AK, Blennow K, Andreasen N, Minthon L. CSF biomarkers for Alzheimer's disease: levels of beta-amyloid, tau, phosphorylated tau relate to clinical symptoms and survival. *Dement Geriatr Cogn Disord* 2006;**21**(3):131–8.

144. Zakzanis KK, Graham SJ, Campbell Z. A meta-analysis of structural and functional brain imaging in dementia of the Alzheimer's type: a neuroimaging profile. *Neuropsychol Rev* 2003;**13**(1):1–18.

145. Yavuz BB, Ariogul S, Cankurtaran M *et al.* Hippocampal atrophy correlates with the severity of cognitive decline. *Int Psychogeriatr* 2006;**19**:767–77.

146. Laakso MP, Partanen K, Riekkinen P *et al.* Hippocampal volumes in Alzheimer's disease, Parkinson's disease with and without dementia, and in vascular dementia: an MRI study. *Neurology* 1996;**46**(3):678–81.

147. Frisoni GB, Laakso MP, Beltramello A *et al.* Hippocampal and entorhinal cortex atrophy in frontotemporal dementia and Alzheimer's disease. *Neurology* 1999;**52**(1):91–100.

148. Nagy Z, Hindley NJ, Braak H *et al.* Relationship between clinical and radiological diagnostic criteria for Alzheimer's disease and the extent of neuropathology as reflected by "stages": a prospective study. *Dement Geriatr Cogn Disord* 1999;**10**(2):109–14.

149. van de Pol LA, Hensel A, Barkhof F *et al.* Hippocampal atrophy in Alzheimer disease: age matters. *Neurology* 2006;**66**(2):236–8.

150. Jack CR, Jr., Petersen RC, Xu YC *et al.* Prediction of AD with MRI-based hippocampal volume in mild cognitive impairment. *Neurology* 1999;**52**(7):1397–403.

151. deToledo-Morrell L, Stoub TR, Bulgakova M *et al.* MRI-derived entorhinal volume is a good predictor of conversion from MCI to AD. *Neurobiol Aging* 2004;**25**(9):1197–203.

152. Mattman A, Feldman H, Forster B *et al.* Regional HmPAO SPECT and CT measurements in the diagnosis of Alzheimer's disease. *Can J Neurol Sci* 1997;**24**(1):22–8.

153. Van Gool WA, Walstra GJ, Teunisse S *et al.* Diagnosing Alzheimer's disease in elderly, mildly demented patients: the impact of routine single photon emission computed tomography. *J Neurol* 1995;**242**(6):401–5.

154. Bonte FJ, Weiner MF, Bigio EH, White CL, III. Brain blood flow in the dementias: SPECT with histopathologic correlation in 54 patients. *Radiology* 1997;**202**(3):793–7.

155. Herholz K, Salmon E, Perani D *et al.* Discrimination between Alzheimer dementia and controls by automated analysis of multicenter FDG PET. *Neuroimage* 2002;**17**(1):302–16.

156. Hoffman JM, Welsh-Bohmer KA, Hanson M *et al.* FDG PET imaging in patients with pathologically verified dementia. *J Nucl Med* 2000;**41**(11):1920–8.

157. Chetelat G, Desgranges B, de la Sayette V *et al.* Mild cognitive impairment: can FDG-PET predict who is to rapidly convert to Alzheimer's disease? *Neurology* 2003;**60**(8):1374–7.

158. Klunk WE, Engler H, Nordberg A *et al.* Imaging brain amyloid in Alzheimer's disease with Pittsburgh Compound-B. *Ann Neurol* 2004;**55**(3):306–19.

159. Shoghi-Jadid K, Small GW, Agdeppa ED *et al.* Localization of neurofibrillary tangles and beta-amyloid plaques in the brains of living patients with Alzheimer disease. *Am J Geriatr Psychiatry* 2002;**10**(1):24–35.

160. Kung MP, Hou C, Zhuang ZP, Skovronsky D, Kung HF. Binding of two potential imaging agents targeting amyloid plaques in postmortem brain tissues of patients with Alzheimer's disease. *Brain Res* 2004;**1025**(1–2):98–105.

161. Engler H, Forsberg A, Almkvist O *et al.* Two-year follow-up of amyloid deposition in patients with Alzheimer's disease. *Brain* 2006;**129**(Pt 11):2856–66.

162. Small GW, Kepe V, Barrio JR. Seeing is believing: neuroimaging adds to our understanding of cerebral pathology. *Curr Opin Psychiatry* 2006;**19**(6):564–9.

163. Lockhart A. Imaging Alzheimer's disease pathology: one target, many ligands. *Drug Discov Today* 2006;**11**(23–24):1093–9.

164. Birks J. Cholinesterase inhibitors for Alzheimer's disease. *Cochrane Database Syst Rev* 2006;**1**:CD005593.

165. Bullock R, Touchon J, Bergman H *et al.* Rivastigmine and donepezil treatment in moderate to moderately-severe Alzheimer's disease over a 2-year period. *Curr Med Res Opin* 2005;**21**(8):1317–27.

166. Bullock R, Dengiz A. Cognitive performance in patients with Alzheimer's disease receiving cholinesterase inhibitors for up to 5 years. *Int J Clin Pract* 2005;**59**(7):817–22.

167. Rosler M, Anand R, Cicin-Sain A *et al.* Efficacy and safety of rivastigmine in patients with Alzheimer's disease: international randomised controlled trial. *BMJ* 1999;**318**(7184):633–8.

71

168. Raskind MA, Peskind ER, Wessel T, Yuan W. Galantamine in AD: a 6-month randomized, placebo-controlled trial with a 6-month extension. The Galantamine USA-1 Study Group. *Neurology* 2000; **54**(12):2261–8.

169. Doody RS, Stevens JC, Beck C *et al.* Practice parameter: management of dementia (an evidence-based review). Report of the Quality Standards Subcommittee of the American Academy of Neurology. *Neurology* 2001;**56**(9):1154–66.

170. Kmietowicz Z. NICE proposes to withdraw Alzheimer's drugs from NHS. *BMJ* 2005;**330** (7490):495.

171. Harkany T, Abraham I, Timmerman W *et al.* Beta-amyloid neurotoxicity is mediated by a glutamate-triggered excitotoxic cascade in rat nucleus basalis. *Eur J Neurosci* 2000;**12**(8):2735–45.

172. Topper R, Gehrmann J, Banati R *et al.* Rapid appearance of beta-amyloid precursor protein immunoreactivity in glial cells following excitotoxic brain injury. *Acta Neuropathol (Berl)* 1995;**89**(1):23–8.

173. Couratier P, Lesort M, Sindou P *et al.* Modifications of neuronal phosphorylated tau immunoreactivity induced by NMDA toxicity. *Mol Chem Neuropathol* 1996;**27**(3):259–73.

174. Wilcock GK. Memantine for the treatment of dementia. *Lancet Neurol* 2003;**2**(8):503–5.

175. Tariot PN, Farlow MR, Grossberg GT *et al.* Memantine treatment in patients with moderate to severe Alzheimer disease already receiving donepezil: a randomized controlled trial. *JAMA* 2004;**291**(3): 317–24.

176. Lyketsos CG, Sheppard JM, Steele CD *et al.* Randomized, placebo-controlled, double-blind clinical trial of sertraline in the treatment of depression complicating Alzheimer's disease: initial results from the Depression in Alzheimer's Disease Study. *Am J Psychiatry* 2000;**157**(10):1686–9.

177. Taragano FE, Lyketsos CG, Mangone CA, Allegri RF, Comesana-Diaz E. A double-blind, randomized, fixed-dose trial of fluoxetine vs. amitriptyline in the treatment of major depression complicating Alzheimer's disease. *Psychosomatics* 1997;**38**(3):246–52.

178. Alexopoulos GS, Jeste DV, Chung H *et al.* The expert consensus guideline series. Treatment of dementia and its behavioral disturbances. Introduction: methods, commentary, and summary. *Postgrad Med* 2005; (Spec No):6–22.

179. Sink KM, Holden KF, Yaffe K. Pharmacological treatment of neuropsychiatric symptoms of dementia: a review of the evidence. *JAMA* 2005;**293**(5):596–608.

180. Schneider LS, Tariot PN, Dagerman KS *et al.* Effectiveness of atypical antipsychotic drugs in patients with Alzheimer's disease. *N Engl J Med* 2006;**355** (15):1525–38.

181. Wang PS, Schneeweiss S, Avorn J *et al.* Risk of death in elderly users of conventional vs. atypical antipsychotic medications. *N Engl J Med* 2005; **353**(22):2335–41.

182. Beier MT. Treatment strategies for the behavioral symptoms of Alzheimer's disease: focus on early pharmacologic intervention. *Pharmacotherapy* 2007; **27**(3):399–411.

183. Dubinsky RM, Stein AC, Lyons K. Practice parameter: risk of driving and Alzheimer's disease (an evidence-based review): report of the quality standards subcommittee of the American Academy of Neurology. *Neurology* 2000;**54**(12):2205–11.

184. Wang C, Kosinski C, Schwartzberg J. *Physician's Guide to Assessing and Counseling Older Drivers.* Washington, DC: National Highway Traffic Safety Administration; 2003.

185. Friedland RP, Koss E, Kumar A *et al.* Motor vehicle crashes in dementia of the Alzheimer type. *Ann Neurol* 1988;**24**(6):782–6.

186. Carr DB, Duchek J, Morris JC. Characteristics of motor vehicle crashes of drivers with dementia of the Alzheimer type. *J Am Geriatr Soc* 2000;**48**(1):18–22.

187. Molnar FJ, Patel A, Marshall SC, Man-Son-Hing M, Wilson KG. Clinical utility of office-based cognitive predictors of fitness to drive in persons with dementia: a systematic review. *J Am Geriatr Soc* 2006;**54** (12):1809–24.

188. Roberson ED, Mucke L. 100 years and counting: prospects for defeating Alzheimer's disease. *Science* 2006;**314**(5800):781–4.

189. Chang WP, Koelsch G, Wong S *et al.* In vivo inhibition of Abeta production by memapsin 2 (beta-secretase) inhibitors. *J Neurochem* 2004;**89**(6):1409–16.

190. Etcheberrigaray R, Tan M, Dewachter I *et al.* Therapeutic effects of PKC activators in Alzheimer's disease transgenic mice. *Proc Natl Acad Sci USA* 2004;**101**(30):11141–6.

191. Schenk D, Hagen M, Seubert P. Current progress in beta-amyloid immunotherapy. *Curr Opin Immunol* 2004;**16**(5):599–606.

192. Weiner HL, Frenkel D. Immunology and immunotherapy of Alzheimer's disease. *Nat Rev Immunol* 2006;**6**(5):404–16.

193. Orgogozo JM, Gilman S, Dartigues JF *et al.* Subacute meningoencephalitis in a subset of patients with AD after Abeta42 immunization. *Neurology* 2003; **61**(1):46–54.

194. Geerts H. NC-531 (Neurochem). *Curr Opin Investig Drugs* 2004;**5**(1):95–100.

195. Crouch PJ, Barnham KJ, Bush AI, White AR. Therapeutic treatments for Alzheimer's disease based on metal bioavailability. *Drug News Perspect* 2006;**19** (8):469–74.

196. Engel T, Goni-Oliver P, Lucas JJ, Avila J, Hernandez F. Chronic lithium administration to FTDP-17 tau and GSK-3beta overexpressing mice prevents tau hyperphosphorylation and neurofibrillary tangle formation, but pre-formed neurofibrillary tangles do not revert. *J Neurochem* 2006;**99**(6):1445–55.

197. Delanty N, Vaughan C. Risk of Alzheimer's disease and duration of NSAID use. *Neurology* 1998;**51**(2):652.

198. Szekely CA, Thorne JE, Zandi PP *et al.* Nonsteroidal anti-inflammatory drugs for the prevention of Alzheimer's disease: a systematic review. *Neuroepidemiology* 2004;**23**(4):159–69.

199. Aisen PS. The potential of anti-inflammatory drugs for the treatment of Alzheimer's disease. *Lancet Neurol* 2002;**1**(5):279–84.

200. Eriksen JL, Sagi SA, Smith TE *et al.* NSAIDs and enantiomers of flurbiprofen target gamma-secretase and lower Abeta 42 in vivo. *J Clin Invest* 2003;**112**(3):440–9.

201. Tang MX, Jacobs D, Stern Y *et al.* Effect of oestrogen during menopause on risk and age at onset of Alzheimer's disease. *Lancet* 1996;**348**(9025):429–32.

202. Henderson VW, Paganini-Hill A, Miller BL *et al.* Estrogen for Alzheimer's disease in women: randomized, double-blind, placebo-controlled trial. *Neurology* 2000;**54**(2):295–301.

203. Engelhart MJ, Geerlings MI, Ruitenberg A *et al.* Dietary intake of antioxidants and risk of Alzheimer disease. *JAMA* 2002;**287**(24):3223–9.

204. Sano M, Ernesto C, Thomas RG *et al.* A controlled trial of selegiline, alpha-tocopherol, or both as treatment for Alzheimer's disease. The Alzheimer's Disease Cooperative Study. *N Engl J Med* 1997;**336**(17):1216–22.

205. Lonn E, Bosch J, Yusuf S *et al.* Effects of long-term vitamin E supplementation on cardiovascular events and cancer: a randomized controlled trial. *JAMA* 2005;**293**(11):1338–47.

206. Jick H, Zornberg GL, Jick SS, Seshadri S, Drachman DA. Statins and the risk of dementia. *Lancet* 2000;**356**(9242):1627–31.

207. Yang F, Lim GP, Begum AN *et al.* Curcumin inhibits formation of amyloid beta oligomers and fibrils, binds plaques, and reduces amyloid in vivo. *J Biol Chem* 2005;**280**(7):5892–901.

208. Reddy PH, McWeeney S. Mapping cellular transcriptosomes in autopsied Alzheimer's disease subjects and relevant animal models. *Neurobiol Aging* 2006;**27**(8):1060–77.

209. Davidsson P, Sjogren M. Proteome studies of CSF in AD patients. *Mech Ageing Dev* 2006;**127**(2):133–7.

210. Hye A, Lynham S, Thambisetty M *et al.* Proteome-based plasma biomarkers for Alzheimer's disease. *Brain* 2006;**129**(Pt 11):3042–50.

211. Mueller SG, Weiner MW, Thal LJ *et al.* The Alzheimer's disease neuroimaging initiative. *Neuroimaging Clin N Am* 2005;**15**(4):869–77, xi–xii.

212. Lopponen M, Raiha I, Isoaho R, Vahlberg T, Kivela SL. Diagnosing cognitive impairment and dementia in primary health care: a more active approach is needed. *Age Ageing* 2003;**32**(6):606–12.

213. Callahan CM, Hendrie HC, Tierney WM. Documentation and evaluation of cognitive impairment in elderly primary care patients. *Ann Intern Med* 1995;**122**(6):422–9.

214. Svansdottir HB, Snaedal J. Music therapy in moderate and severe dementia of Alzheimer's type: a case-control study. *Int Psychogeriatr* 2006;**18**(4):613–21.

215. Rolland Y, Pillard F, Klapouszczak A *et al.* Exercise program for nursing home residents with Alzheimer's disease: a 1-year randomized, controlled trial. *J Am Geriatr Soc* 2007;**55**(2):158–65.

Chapter 6

Mental status examination

Casey E. Krueger and Joel H. Kramer

Introduction

One of the challenges facing behaviorally oriented neurologists is that many patients' symptoms fall beyond the scope of a physical neurological evaluation. Frequently, patients with neurodegenerative disease, particularly in the early stages, present with intact cranial nerves, reflexes, eye movements, and sensory-motor function. Accordingly, clinicians need tools to formally assess the cognitive, psychiatric and behavioral abnormalities that define many dementing disorders. The mental status examination is the part of the neurological examination that assesses current mental capacity through evaluation of appearance, mood, perceptions (e.g. delusions, hallucinations) and all aspects of cognition (e.g. attention, orientation, memory).

According to Frey (2002), a comprehensive mental status examination evaluates 10 areas of functioning: (1) overall appearance, (2) movement and behavior (gait, coordination, eye contact and facial expressions), (3) mood (underlying emotional tone of person's answers), (4) affect (outwardly observable emotional reactions), (5) speech (volume, rate, tone, appropriateness and clarity), (6) thought content (hallucinations, delusions, obsessions, dissociative symptoms and thoughts of suicide), (7) thought process (repeated words or phrases, thought blocking, illogical connections), (8) cognition, (9) judgement (what to do about a common sense problem) and (10) insight (ability to recognize a problem and understand its nature and severity). This chapter will describe some widely used approaches for assessing mental status, with a particular emphasis on the cognitive changes typically seen in neurodegenerative disease.

Several standardized mental status examinations exist that enable quantification of cognitive impairment, typically yielding a single composite score that reflects disease severity. Some examples include the

Mini-Mental State Examination (MMSE; Folstein et al., 1975), Modified Mini-Mental State Examination (Teng and Chui, 1987), Short Portable Mental Status Questionnaire (Pfeiffer, 1975), Cognitive Abilities Screening Test (Teng et al., 1994), Cognistat (or Neurobehavioral Cognitive Status Examination; Kiernan et al., 1987), 7 Minute Screen (Solomon et al., 1998), and Geriatric Mental State Schedule (Copeland et al., 1976). Perhaps the most widely used measure in behavioral neurology and dementia is the MMSE. Typically taking about 10 minutes, the MMSE evaluates orientation to time and place, registration, attention, working memory, recall, language and visuoconstruction. This 30-point scale was originally designed to facilitate differential diagnosis of hospitalized psychiatric patients, but it is now routinely used to assess cognitive abilities in a broad range of diagnoses. Folstein et al. (1975) reported high test–retest reliability in the original standardization sample of 22 non-demented psychiatric inpatients over a 24-hour period, whether the examiner was the same both times ($r = 0.89$) or different ($r = 0.83$). Test–retest reliability over a 4 week period was nearly perfect for 23 patients with dementia ($r = 0.99$). Studies have demonstrated considerable incremental validity of the MMSE in comparison with routine clinical evaluation (Mitrushina and Satz, 1991). Additionally, significant correlations have been found with many neuropsychological measures, suggesting high convergent validity (Mitrushina and Satz, 1991).

Crum et al. (1993) examined the distribution of MMSE scores in 18 056 adult participants. They found that cognitive performance as measured by the MMSE scores varied by both age and education level. There was an inverse relationship between age and MMSE scores and a positive relationship between years of education and MMSE scores. For example, the median MMSE score of those aged 18 to 24 was 29, while the median score for individuals 80 years old and above was 25. Furthermore, the median MMSE score for participants with at least 9 years of formal education was 29, while the median score for those with 0–4 years of education was 22. These data highlight the need to consider age and education when interpreting MMSE scores.

The strength of tests like the MMSE is that they provide composite scores that can be used as markers of disease severity over time. The MMSE performance of healthy older adults is reasonably stable over time, while MMSE scores of patients with Alzheimer's disease (AD) decreases over time at an average rate of around 3 points per year (Wilson *et al.*, 2000). In addition, patterns of performance on individual items on the MMSE may help to distinguish patients with different dementia etiologies (Brandt *et al.*, 1988; Lezak *et al.*, 2004). For example, Ala *et al.* (2001) found that patients with dementia with Lewy bodies (DLB) performed worse than patients with AD on attention and construction items, whereas patients with AD performed worse on the MMSE memory items. Patients with AD tend to perform poorly on temporal orientation items and delayed recall (Jefferson *et al.*, 2002).

However, tests like the MMSE are not particularly sensitive indicators of early disease manifestations (Mungas *et al.*, 2003). Also, it is important to remember that the MMSE was designed primarily for quantifying dementia severity and not for differential diagnosis. Therefore, in some instances, the behavioral neurologist will need to assess skills such as episodic memory, working memory, executive functions, language and visuospatial abilities in greater detail. This chapter will elaborate upon the mental status examination of each of these domains. Then, it will provide typical neuropsychological profiles of various dementia types (AD, frontotemporal dementia [FTD], semantic dementia [SD], DLB and progressive supranuclear palsy [PSP]) in order to aid in differential diagnosis.

Cognitive mental status examination
Memory
Most patients with dementia show memory problems early in the course of their disease (Strub and Black, 2000). Memory is a general term for a mental process that allows the individual to store information for later recall (Squire and Butters, 1984). Importantly, memory is not a unitary construct, but rather an alliance of inter-related subsystems (Baddeley, 1995). Episodic memory refers to the system involved in remembering particular experiences or episodes, such as what you had for breakfast or where you went on vacation last summer. These memories are context dependent and are associated with a particular time,

place and feelings. Episodic memory depends on a neural network that includes the temporal lobes, hippocampus and frontal lobes (Baddeley, 1995). The hippocampus is a structure within the temporal lobes that is crucial for consolidating information into long-term storage. Focal hippocampal injury produces impaired new learning in the context of intact immediate and remote memory (Squire and Butters, 1984)

When assessing episodic memory in the clinic, examiners should use enough information to exceed immediate memory span, and to consider separately initial learning versus retention, and recall versus recognition. Cullum *et al.* (1993) examined the utility of using three-word recall tasks (such as the task in the MMSE) for assessing recall performance. They found substantial variability within their subjects, and a significant proportion of normal subjects recalled zero or one word. They noted that caution must be used when interpreting simple recall performance as an index of memory. Supraspan list-learning tasks with delayed recall and recognition conditions (e.g. California Verbal Learning Test-II [CVLT-II; Delis *et al.*, 2000] and Rey Auditory Verbal Learning Test [Rey, 1941; Lezak *et al.*, 2004] are better suited for bedside evaluation of memory.

Different neurodegenerative conditions can affect memory functioning in different ways. Patients with fronto-subcortical atrophy have problems with encoding and initial learning, but relatively intact retention. In addition, recognition memory is often within normal limits (Albert *et al.*, 1974; Massman *et al.*, 1990). In contrast, patients with AD may show normal immediate recall but have difficulty retaining information over delays as brief as a few minutes and tend to have poor recognition.

Kramer *et al.* (2004) demonstrated the importance of examining delayed episodic memory and not just immediate memory when conducting a dementia evaluation. They found that delayed recall was best predicted by hippocampal volume, even after controlling for levels of initial acquisition. These results suggest that impaired delayed recall may be used as an indictor of hippocampal dysfunction, while difficulty with immediate recall may reflect problems in other brain regions involved in attention and organization.

Executive functions
Executive functioning has been called the most subtle and central realm of human activity (Barkley, 2000). It is particularly important to assess because it is affected in most types of dementia. Executive function

75

is the process of bringing together and coordinating information for a purpose, such as decision making, and it includes skills such as mental flexibility and response inhibition. Lesion studies and structural and functional neuroimaging studies have implicated the prefrontal cortex as critical for performing executive function tasks (Anderson *et al.*, 1995; Baker *et al.*, 1996; Walker *et al.*, 1998; McMillan *et al.*, 2004). However, poor performance on executive function tasks should not always be construed as evidence for frontal pathology because many such tasks are cognitively complex, and other brain regions, including subcortical structures, play an important role in task completion (Tekin and Cummings, 2002; Kramer and Quitania, 2007).

Several clinical tasks have been developed to assess different aspects of executive function, including novel verbal and non-verbal problem-solving tasks, maze tracing, tower tests, card or object sorting, and set-shifting. Common areas assessed under the rubric of executive function include working memory, mental flexibility, inhibition, fluency and abstract reasoning.

Working memory

Working memory is a functional system that works to register, recall and mentally manipulate information within short-term memory (Baddeley, 1995); it is a common substrate to patients' difficulty with multi-tasking. Digit span tests are widely used, with the forward digit span component used to assess immediate auditory memory, and the backward span component evaluating working memory (i.e. the capacity to juggle information mentally). Research has shown that, on average, people can keep 7 ± 2 items in their short-term memory (which is why the US Federal Government made phone numbers seven digits long). Working memory is also assessed on the MMSE when the patient carries out serial 7's or spells "WORLD" backward. Other bedside techniques include reciting the months of the year in reverse order.

Mental flexibility

The Trail Making Test (Reitan and Wolfson, 1985) is a widely administered test of attention and cognitive flexibility. In Part A of the Trails, patients connect a series of numbered circles distributed arbitrarily on a page. In Part B, the subject is asked to alternate serially between connecting numbers and letters. The scores are the time taken to complete each part. This test is particularly sensitive to the progressive cognitive decline in dementia (Greenlief *et al.*, 1985).

Elderly persons who perform poorly on Part B are likely to have problems with complex activities of daily living (Bell-McGinty *et al.*, 2002).

Inhibition

Response inhibition requires the patient to suppress an overlearned response or a salient environmental stimulus. Stroop interference tests are widely used to assess inhibition. In this paradigm, patients are shown a series of color names printed in different color ink (e.g. the word "RED" printed in blue ink). The patient has to inhibit the overlearned tendency to read the words and instead name the color of the ink in which the words are printed. Other tasks, such as opposite responding, require the patient to inhibit their response to a salient stimulus while providing a competing response. For example, the evaluator tells the patient, "When I tap once, you tap twice, but when I tap twice, you tap once." Similarly, the evaluator may ask the patient to point to his/her chin while the evaluator points to his/her nose.

Fluency

Fluency is another aspect of executive function because it requires organized search and retrieval strategies. Fluency can be assessed by having the patient generate words beginning with specified letters or belonging to semantic categories. Relative difficulty with semantic categories often suggests AD or SD, whereas relative difficulty with letter prompts (phonemic cueing) suggests frontal and/or subcortical deficits (Rascovsky *et al.*, 2007). The Controlled Oral Word Association (Benton and Hamsher, 1989) consists of three word-naming trials using the letters F-A-S. Semantic fluency is often evaluated using the category of animals (Troyer, 2000). Non-verbal fluency tasks (e.g. Design Fluency [Delis *et al.*, 2001], Ruff Figural Fluency Test [Ruff *et al.*, 1987]) typically present patients with boxes containing dots and asks them to generate as many novel designs as possible.

Abstract reasoning

Abstract reasoning can be evaluated by asking patients to describe conceptual similarities or differences between word pairs (e.g. "dog–lion"), give opposites (e.g. "healthy–sick"), find analogies (e.g. "table is to leg as bicycle is to?") (Lezak *et al.*, 2004) or interpret proverbs (e.g. "An old ox plows a straight row").

Language

Several aspects of language should be screened during mental status testing, including articulatory agility, repetition of high- and low-frequency word combinations (e.g. "No ifs, ands or buts", "Methodist Episcopal"), comprehension of single words (give the subject simple commands, such as "Show me your chin," or have the patient say the word that a picture is illustrating), comprehension of complex syntax (e.g. "Put your left hand on your right ear"), reading of regular and irregular words, and naming (point to objects in the room; name colors, letters, numbers and actions [Strub and Black, 2000]; the Boston Naming Test [Kaplan et al., 1983]). Examiners should also pay close attention to several features of the patient's spontaneous and conversational speech, including intonation, prosody, typical phrase length, the presence of grammatical terms, the presence and type of paraphasia, word-finding ability and how well the patient seems to understand what is being said. Reading and writing should also be assessed.

Strub and Black (2000) have explained some typical terminology used to describe language impairments. *Agraphia* is an acquired disturbance in writing. *Alexia* is the term used to describe a loss of reading ability in a previously literate person. *Aphasia* is a true language disturbance in which the patient demonstrates an impaired production and/or comprehension of spoken language. *Dysprosody* is an interruption of speech melody, inflection and rhythm.

Visuospatial abilities

Constructional tasks are extremely useful in detecting organic brain disease and should be included in every mental status examination (Strub and Black, 2000). Constructional abilities require complex non-verbal cognitive functions and involve the integration of occipital, parietal and frontal lobe functions. Nevertheless, the parietal lobes are the principal cortical areas involved in visual-motor integration (Strub and Black, 2000). Design copying (e.g. interlocking pentagons or hexagons, cube, clock, Rey–Osterrieth Complex Figure) is commonly used to examine visuoconstructional abilities at the bedside. Noticing how the patient approaches his/her copy can be an extremely useful part of the evaluation. For example, working from right to left, omitting parts of the left side, missing the overall configuration and directional confusion all raise the possibility of right-hemisphere injury, regardless of how good the final copy is. Basic perceptual skills should also be assessed in patients who fail constructional tasks. Widely used bedside measures include line bisection tasks, matching faces

or designs, or even having patients describe complex pictures (assuming intact language).

Psychiatric symptoms

Personality or emotional changes are often present in patients with dementia. These changes may be a direct product of the illness itself or the patient's reaction to their experiences of loss, frustration and changes in lifestyle. It is important to distinguish personality changes that are a result of the disease from comorbid psychiatric symptoms. Common personality changes and behavioral problems include irritability, low frustration tolerance, apathy, disinhibition, emotional dulling and hoarding. Depression is likely the most common comorbid psychiatric symptom that follows a diagnosis of dementia, with pervasive anxiety following closely (Lezak et al., 2004). It is important to assess for psychiatric disorders, such as depression, bipolar disorder, generalized anxiety disorder, anxiety disorder caused by a general medical condition, somatization disorder, conversion disorder and obsessive–compulsive disorder. Therefore, it is important to ask about domains related to a patient's emotional status, including mood, appetite, sleep, pleasurable activities they partake in, anxiety, energy level and obsessions. The Geriatric Depression Scale (Yesavage et al., 1983) is useful in assessing for depression in elderly patients, and the Neuropsychiatric Inventory (Cummings et al., 1994) allows informants to rate the patient's behaviors and psychiatric symptoms.

Functional status

A diagnosis of dementia requires impairment both in cognition and in everyday functioning. Functional status refers to the capacity to carry out instrumental activities of daily living, such as food preparation, medication management, driving, housekeeping, financial management and shopping (Jefferson et al., 2006). It can be informally assessed by asking the patient if they are having difficulty carrying out these daily activities. Functional abilities can also be assessed by having caregivers complete questionnaires, such as the Functional Activities Questionnaire (Pfeffer et al., 1982) and the Clinical Dementia Rating Scale (Hughes et al., 1982). Evaluating functional status is crucial in the diagnosis of dementia, and also in determining the practical effects of dementia on patients and their families (Cahn-Weiner et al., 2003).

Components of the mental status examination that bear the strongest relationship to functional abilities are memory and executive functioning (Sunderland *et al.*, 1986; Wilson *et al.*, 1989; Wilson, 1991; Cahn-Weiner *et al.*, 2000, 2002, 2003; Boyle *et al.*, 2003). Executive dysfunction often results in impairments in planning, organization and insight, all of which are likely to affect the ability to care for one's self (Cahn-Weiner *et al.*, 2000). Jefferson and colleagues (2006) determined that out of the elements of executive functioning (e.g. working memory, generation, inhibition, planning and sequencing), inhibition was most strongly related to impairments in instrumental activities of daily living in patients at risk for future cognitive and functional decline. In addition to executive dysfunction, apathy (a frontally mediated behavior) was also found to be associated with impairment in instrumental activities of daily living (Boyle *et al.*, 2003). Sunderland and colleagues (1986) demonstrated that a story-recall test reported everyday memory problems. Wilson and colleagues (1989) found that the Rivermead Behavioural Memory Test (RBMT; Wilson *et al.*, 1985) was sensitive and correlated highly with lapses in everyday memory. A follow-up study by Wilson (1991) determined that the RBMT predicted whether or not a patient would be capable of living independently.

Suggested mental status examination

An example of a comprehensive bedside mental status examination includes the following: MMSE, a supra-span memory test with delayed recall and recognition (e.g. CVLT-II short form), design copy and recall, high- and low-frequency object naming (e.g. jacket, lapel, sleeve and cuff; shoe, sole, heel and tongue), naming to descriptions (e.g. "What is the name of a small lizard noted for its ability to change color"), comprehension of single words and syntax (e.g. "A lion and tiger were fighting. If the lion was killed by the tiger, which animal is dead?"), forward and backward digit span, verbal fluency (words beginning with the letter D, animals), opposite responding, similarities and proverbs, and the Geriatric Depression Scale. It is recommended that clinicians develop items they use in a standardized way. Clinicians interested in specific standardized instruments should refer to Strub and Black (2000) and Lezak *et al.* (2004).

Differential diagnosis

Typical cognitive changes associated with several neurodegenerative diseases are characterized below. Although not all patients with these dementias exhibit prototypical patterns of impairment, comprehensive mental status testing can often help with differential diagnosis.

Alzheimer's disease

Alzheimer's disease is the single most common cause of dementia, accounting for at least 65% of cases (Berg *et al.*, 1994). Strub and Black (2000) described the early features of AD as apathy, vague subjective complaints, decreased verbal fluency, memory difficulties, constructional impairments, dyscalculia and problems with abstract reasoning. Social skills tend to be relatively well preserved. The most frequent first symptom in AD is memory difficulties, but changes in naming, visuospatial abilities and executive functions are also commonly reported (Fig. 6.1). Numerous studies have found that patients with AD have greater memory impairments than other diagnostic cohorts (Perry and Hodges, 2000; Ala *et al.*, 2002; Kramer *et al.*, 2003; Diehl *et al.*, 2005).

Although diffuse cognitive changes are typical, particularly in the middle and later stages, AD is associated with two particularly distinct findings on mental status testing: rapid forgetting on tasks of episodic memory and decreased category fluency compared with lexical fluency.

Rapid forgetting reflects impairment in consolidating new information into long-term memory. Thus, even though patients with AD can demonstrate relatively intact immediate recall, much of the information is lost after delays as brief as a few minutes (Kramer *et al.*, 2004; Wicklund *et al.*, 2006). Figure 6.2, for example, displays the verbal learning data from well-matched samples of 92 AD subjects (mean age,

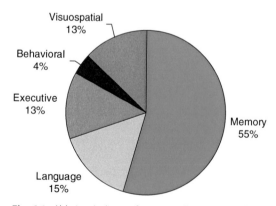

Fig. 6.1. Alzheimer's disease: frequency of symptoms as first symptom. (With Permission from Johnson UCSF Memory and Aging Center.)

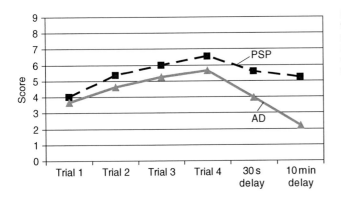

Fig. 6.2. Free recall in Alzheimer's disease (AD) compared with progressive supranuclear palsy (PSP). This graph shows the poorer performance on the Californian Verbal Learning Test in patients with AD compared with patients with PSP. A prominent feature of AD is the rapid rate of forgetting.

68.4 years; MMSE score, 26.3) and 35 PSP subjects (mean age, 67.4 years; MMSE score, 26.8). Subjects were given a nine-word list over four learning trials; free recall was elicited after 30 second and 10 minute delays. As can be seen, both groups showed increased recall over the four learning trials. After delays, however, recall levels in the AD subjects dropped off rapidly, whereas PSP subjects tended to recall the words they had initially learned.

Decreased category fluency in the context of preserved letter fluency is another prominant feature of AD on mental status testing. Rascovsky and colleages (2007) compared verbal fluency results from 32 patients whose AD was confirmed at autopsy with those of 16 patients with autopsy-confirmed FTD. They found that those with AD were more impaired on semantic fluency than letter fluency, while those with FTD displayed the reverse pattern of impairment. Results suggest that the disparity between letter and semantic category fluency is effective in differentiating AD from FTD. Semantic category fluency deficits in AD may reflect the gradual progression of AD pathology in the temporal association areas that underlie semantic memory (Terry and Katzman, 1983; Rascovsky et al., 2007).

Frontotemporal lobar degeneration

Frontotemporal lobar degeneration (FTLD) is a heterogeneous group of disorders that display involvement of frontal and anterior temporal structures. Neary et al. (1999) recognized three distinct subtypes of FTLD; FTD, SD and progressive non-fluent aphasia (PNFA). Each subtype is associated with distinct changes on mental status testing (Libon et al., 2007).

Frontotemporal dementia is characterized by a decline in personal and social conduct. Patients are often described as lacking empathy, being rude and inappropriate. First symptoms also include lack of insight, hyperorality, apathy, irritability and disinhibition. Patients with FTD also show stimulus-boundedness and environmental dependency. Questionnaires for caregivers, such as the Neuropsychiatric Inventory and Functional Activities Questionnaire, are helpful in noting the behavioral and functional changes in patients with FTD.

Executive functioning impairments may distinguish FTD from other neurodegenerative disorders. Patients with FTD performed worse on backward digit span than patients with AD or SD (Kramer et al., 2003), and worse on letter fluency than patients with AD (Mathuranath et al., 2000; Rascovsky et al., 2007). In addition, patients with FTD are more prone to making repetition errors and deviating from standard test instructions (e.g. on Stroop interference tasks, they read the words instead of naming the ink colors (Kramer et al., 2003; Thompson et al., 2005). In contrast, those with FTD generally perform relatively better on tests of spatial ability, episodic memory and semantic tasks (Hodges et al., 1999; Perry and Hodges, 2000).

Semantic dementia

Semantic dementia is known as the temporal variant of FTLD (Hodges et al., 1999; Johnson et al., 2005b) because atrophy is most severe in the anterior temporal cortex, particularly in the left hemisphere (Rosen et al., 2002; Diehl-Schmid et al., 2006). Semantic dementia is predominantly characterized by a progressive semantic impairment that affects the meaning of words. Verbal output is fluent, effortless and grammatically correct, but because of severe word-finding difficulties may have an empty quality. On formal mental status testing, patients with SD demonstrate severe naming deficits and loss of word knowledge,

79

but visual memory and visuocontructional abilities are typically intact (Hodges and Miller, 2001) and activities of daily living are often maintained. Reflecting their underlying semantic deficit, category fluency is particularly impaired. Mental status testing will also reveal deficits in picture naming, with semantic errors being particularly noteworthy (e.g. "dog" for a picture of a hippopotamus). These patients also have agnosia for faces and objects but preserved ability to repeat single words and read orthographically regular (but not irregular) words.

Over time, patients with SD may exhibit behavioral manifestations similar to patients with FTD. They may demonstrate narrowed preoccupations, financial parsimony and loss of sympathy or empathy. Behavioral and social changes often suggest significant right temporal involvement (Miller *et al.* 2001).

Dementia with Lewy bodies

Dementia with Lewy bodies is believed to be the second most common form of dementia in old age (McKeith *et al.*, 1996). Hallmarks of DLB include recurrent visual hallucinations, fluctuations in attention and alertness, parkinsonian features and visuospatial impairments.

Ferman and colleagues (2004) found that four symptoms differentiated DLB from AD. These symptoms include daytime drowsiness and lethargy all the time or several times per day, daytime sleep greater than 2 hours before 7 p.m., staring into space for a long period, and episodes of disorganized or illogical speech. Perseverative behaviors are also common. Bradshaw *et al.* (2004) noted that qualitative descriptions from caregivers of patients with DLB differ from those of caregivers of patients with AD. Caregivers in DLB describe an interruption in flow of awareness or attention, which is associated with transient episodes of confusion. For example, a caregiver described a patient with DLB as, "One day telling me she's been to NY, next day she is lucid," and "Some days she thinks there are extra people for dinner." These episodes are followed by a return to near normal level of functioning. Caregivers of those with AD describe repetitiveness in conversation and forgetfulness in relation to a recent task. Examples include the patient forgetting what he/she was going to do and then starting something else. Fluctuations are described more as good days and bad days rather than spontaneous short-lived alterations in awareness.

A study by Ala and colleagues (2002) examined whether the MMSE could be used to differentiate DLB from AD. Consistent with previous literature, patients with DLB had relatively greater impairment of attention and construction while those with AD had relatively greater impairment of memory. Johnson *et al.* (2005a) also found that patients with DLB performed worse than patients with AD on visuospatial tasks, while patients with AD performed worse than patients with DLB on verbal memory. They noted that the rate of cognitive decline was equivalent in both groups. Similarly, Mori and colleagues (2000) found that patients with DLB performed worse on visuospatial tasks than those with AD. They believed that malfunctioning visual perception may result in the development of the visual hallucinations and delusional misidentifications that are common in patients with DLB. Neuropsychological features are similar to AD, but patients with DLB frequently display relatively greater deficits in attention, executive functions, visuospatial and constructional capacities, psychomotor speed and verbal fluency (Fields, 1998; Kraybill *et al.*, 2005). These results indicate that neuropsychological variables can be used to support other clinical findings in the diagnostic process.

Progressive supranuclear palsy

Progressive supranuclear palsy is generally classified as a movement disorder characterized by extrapyramidal symptoms, axial rigidity, falls and the appearance of supranuclear gaze palsy. Cognitive impairments are also evident on mental status testing, however, and have a predominately frontal executive pattern. Patients with PSP display impairments in tasks of executive function, including abstract thought, speed of information processing, planning, set-shifting and response initiation (Millar *et al.*, 2006). Bak and colleagues (2005) found that PSP was characterized by a disproportionate impairment in verbal fluency, particularly letter fluency. The memory pattern of PSP is also distinct from AD (Fig. 6.2). Although initial acquisition of information may be slow, retention over time is good and patients with PSP often exhibit significant improvements when their memory is tested using recognition relative to free recall.

Mental status testing also typically reveals behavioral features. Patients with PSP utilize imitation behavior and demonstrate frontal release signs. Apathy is typical, and disinhibition is sometimes reported. Millar *et al.* (2006) found that patients with PSP demonstrated changes in apathy, social withdrawal and independence, but they displayed little change in belligerence, social irresponsibility, unco-operativeness, obstreperousness, anxiety and depression. Behavioral features are distinguishable from conditions such as AD by the presence of bradyphrenia, gait and balance disturbance, movement disorder, dysarthria and apathy (Fields, 1998).

Summary

Performing a systematic and complete mental status examination is crucial when working with patients with dementia and should include level of consciousness, physical appearance and emotional status, attention, expressive and receptive language, memory, constructional ability, executive functioning and abstract reasoning (Strub and Black, 2000). A systematic mental status examination can help to differentiate between patients with neurodegenerative diseases and changes of normal aging and help to ascertain dementia severity. Importantly, noting the patterns of performance on mental status testing can be a helpful part of the process of differentiating between the different neurodegenerative disorders.

References

Ala, T. A., Hughes, L. F., Kyrouac, G. A., Ghobrial, M. W., and Elble, R. J. (2001). Pentagon copying is more impaired in dementia with Lewy bodies than in Alzheimer's disease. *Journal of Neurology, Neurosurgery, and Psychiatry*, **72**, 129–130.

Ala, T. A., Hughes, L. F., Kyrouac, G. A., Ghobrial, M. W., and Elble, R. J. (2002). The mini-mental state exam may help in the differentiation of dementia with Lewy bodies and Alzheimer's disease. *International Journal of Geriatric Psychiatry*, **17**, 503–509.

Albers, D. S., Augood, S. J., Park, L. C. H. et al. (2000). Frontal lobe dysfunction in progressive supranuclear palsy. *Journal of Neurochemistry*, **74**, 878–881.

Albert, M. L., Feldman, R. G., and Willis, A. L. (1974). The "subcortical dementia" of progressive supranuclear palsy. *Journal of Neurology, Neurosugery, and Psychiatry*, **37**, 121–130.

Anderson, C. V., Bigler, E. D. and Blatter, D. D. (1995). Frontal lobe lesions, diffuse damage, and neuropsychological functioning in traumatic brain-injured patients. *Journal of Clinical and Experimental Neuropsychology*, **17**, 900–908.

Baddeley, A. D. (1995). The psychology of memory. In A. D. Baddeley, B. A. Wilson and F. N. Watts (eds.), *Handbook of Memory Disorder*. Cambridge, UK: John Wiley, pp. 3–25.

Bak, T. H., Crawford, L. M., Hearn, V. C., Mathuranath, P. S., and Hodges, J. R. (2005). Subcortical dementia revisited: similarities and differences in cognitive function between progressive supranuclear palsy (PSP), corticobasal degeneration (CBD) and multiple system atrophy (MSA). *Neurocase*, **11**, 268–273.

Baker, S., Roger, R., Owen, A. et al. (1996). Neural systems engaged by planning: a PET study of the Tower of London Task. *Neuropsychologia*, **34**, 515–526.

Barkley, R. A. (2000). Genetics of childhood disorders. *Journal of the American Academy of Child Adolescent Psychiatry*, **39**, 1064–1070.

Bell-McGinty, S., Podell, K., Franzen M. et al. (2002). Standard measures of executive function in predicting instrumental activities of daily living in older adults. *International Journal of Geriatric Psychiatry*, **17**, 828–834.

Benton, A. L. and de Hamsher, K. S. (1989). *Multilingual Aphasia Examination*. Iowa City, IA: AJA Associates.

Benton, A. L., Hannay, H. J., and Varney, N. R. (1975). Visual perception of line direction in patients with unilateral brain disease. *Neurology*, **25**, 907–910. [Reprinted in L. Costa and O. Spreen (eds.) (1985). *Studies in Neuropsychology. Selected Papers of Arthur Benton*. New York: Oxford University Press.]

Berg, R. A., Franzen, M., and Wedding, D. (1994). *Screening for Brain Impairment: A Manual for Mental Health Practice*, 2nd edn. New York: Springer.

Boyle, P. A., Malloy, P. F., Salloway, S. et al. (2003). Executive dysfunction and apathy predict functional impairment in Alzheimer's disease. *American Journal of Geriatric Psychiatry*, **11**, 214–221.

Bradshaw, J., Saling, M., Hopwood, M., Anderson, V., and Brodtmann, A. (2004). Fluctuating cognition in dementia with Lewy bodies and Alzheimer's disease is qualitatively distinct. *Journal of Neurology, Neurosurgery, and Psychiatry*, **75**, 382–387.

Brandt, J., Folstein, S. E., and Folstein, M. F. (1988). Differential cognitive impairments in Alzheimer's disease and Huntington's disease. *Annals of Neurology*, **23**, 555–561.

Cahn-Weiner, D. A., Malloy, P. F., Boyle, P. A., Marran, M., and Salloway, S. (2000). Prediction of functional status from neuropsychological tests in community-dwelling elderly individuals. *Clinical Neuropsychology*, **14**, 187–195.

Cahn-Weiner, D. A., Boyle, P. A., and Malloy, P. F. (2002). Tests of executive function predict instrumental activities of daily living in community-dwelling older individuals. *Applications of Neuropsychology*, **9**, 187–191.

Cahn-Weiner, D. A., Ready, R. E., and Malloy, P. F. (2003). Neuropsychological predictors of everyday memory and everyday functioning in patients with mild Alzheimer's disease. *Journal of Geriatric Psychiatry and Neurology*, **16**, 84–89.

Copeland, J. R., Kelleher, M. J., Kellett, J. M. et al. (1976). A semi-structured clinical interview for the assessment of diagnosis and mental state in the elderly: the Geriatric Mental State Schedule. I. Development and reliability. *Psychological Medicine*, **6**, 439–449.

Crum, R. M., Anthony, J. C., Bassett, S. S., and Folstein, M. F. (1993). Population-based norms for the Mini-Mental State Examination by age and educational level. *Journal of the American Medical Association*, **269**, 2386–2391.

Cullum, C. M., Thompson, L. L., and Smernoff, E. N. (1993). Three-word recall as a measure of memory. *Journal of Clinical and Experimental Neuropsychology*, **15**, 321–329.

Cummings, J. L., Mega, M., Gray, K. *et al.* (1994). The Neuropsychiatric Inventory: comprehensive assessment of psychopathology in dementia. *Neurology*, **44**, 2308–2314.

Delis, D. C., Kramer, J. H., Kaplan, E., and Ober, B. A. (2000). *California Verbal Learning Test-Second Edition (CVLT-II)*. San Antonio, TX: Psychological Corporation.

Delis, D., Kaplan, E., and Kramer, J. (2001). *Delis–Kaplan Executive Function Scale*. San Antonio, TX: Psychological Corporation.

Diehl, J., Monsch, A. U., Aebi, C. *et al.* (2005). Frontotemporal dementia, semantic dementia, and Alzheimer's disease: the contribution of standard neuropsychological tests to differentiate diagnosis. *Journal of Geriatric Psychiatry and Neurology*, **18**, 39–44.

Diehl-Schmid, J., Grimmer, T., Drzezga, A. *et al.* (2006). Longitudinal changes of cerebral glucose metabolism in semantic dementia. *Dementia and Geriatric Cognitive Disorders*, **22**, 346–351.

Eslinger, P. J. and Benton, A. L. (1983). Visuoperceptual performances in aging and dementia: clinical and theoretical implications. *Journal of Clinical Neuropsychology*, **5**, 213–220.

Farias, S. T., Harrell, E., Neumann, C., and Houtz, A. (2003). The relationship between neuropsychological performance and daily functioning in individuals with Alzheimer's disease: ecological validity of neuropsychological tests. *Archives of Clinical Neuropsychology*, **18**, 655–672.

Ferman, T. J., Smith, G. E., Boeve, B. F. *et al.* (2004). DLB fluctuations: specific features that reliably differentiate DLB from AD and normal aging. *Neurology*, **62**, 181–187.

Fields, R. (1998). The dementias. In P. J. Snyder and P. D. Nussbaum (eds.), *Clinical Neuropsychology*. Washington, DC: American Psychological Association, pp. 211–242.

Folstein, M. Folstein, S., and McHugh, P. (1975). Mini-mental state: a practical method for grading the cognitive state of patients for the clinician. *Journal of Psychiatric Research*, **12**, 189–198.

Frey, R. J. (2002). Mental status examination. In D. Olendorf, C. Jervan, and K. Boyden (eds.), *The Gale Encyclopedia of Medicine*. New York: Thomson Gale.

Greenlief, C. L., Margolis, R. B., and Erker, G. J. (1985). Application of the Trail Making Test in differentiating neuropsychological impairment of elderly persons. *Perceptual and Motor Skills*, **61**, 1283–1289.

Hodges, J. and Miller, B. (2001). The neuropsychology of frontal variant frontotemporal dementia and semantic dementia. Introduction to the special topic papers: part II. *Neurocase*, **7**, 113–121.

Hodges J., Patterson, K., Ward, R. *et al.* (1999). The differentiation of semantic dementia and frontal lobe dementia (temporal and frontal variance of frontotemporal dementia) from early Alzheimer's disease: a comparative neuropsychological study. *Neuropsychology*, **13**, 31–40.

Hughes, C. P., Berg, L., Danziger, W. L., Coben, L. A., and Martin, R. L. (1982). A new clinical scale for the staging of dementia. *British Journal of Psychiatry*, **140**, 566–572.

Jefferson, A. L., Cosentino, S. A., Ball, S. K. *et al.* (2002). Errors produced on the mini-mental state examination and neuropsychological test performance in Alzheimer's disease, ischemic vascular dementia, and Parkinson's disease. *Journal of Neuropsychiatry and Clinical Neuroscience*, **14**, 311–320.

Jefferson, A. L., Paul, R. H., Ozonoff, A. and Cohen, R. A. (2006). Evaluating elements of executive functioning as predictors of instrumental activities of daily living (IADLs). *Archives of Clinical Neuropsychology*, **21**, 311–320.

Johnson, D. K., Morris, J. C., and Galvin, J. E. (2005a). Verbal and visuospatial deficits in dementia with Lewy bodies. *Neurology*, **65**, 1232–1238.

Johnson, J. K., Diehl, J. M., Neuhaus, J. *et al.* (2005b). Frontotemporal lobar degeneration demographic characteristics of 353 patients. *Archives of Neurology*, **62**, 925–930.

Kaplan, E. F., Goodglass, H., and Weintraub, S. (1983). *The Boston Naming Test, 2nd edn*. Philadelphia, PA: Lea and Febiger.

Kiernan, R. J., Mueller, J., Langston, J. W., and van Dyke, C. (1987). The Neurobehavioral Cognitive Status Examination: a brief but quantitative approach to cognitive assessment. *Annuls of International Medicine*, **107**, 481–485.

Kramer, J. H. and Quitania, L. (2007). Bedside frontal lobe testing. In B. L. Miller and J. L. Cummings (eds.), *The Human Frontal Lobes: Functions and Disorders, 2nd edn*. New York: The Guilford Press, pp. 279–291.

Kramer, J. H., Jurik, J., Sha, S. J. *et al.* (2003). Distinctive neuropsychological patterns in frontotemporal dementia, semantic dementia, and alzheimer disease. *Cognitive and Behavioral Neurology*, **16**, 211–218.

Kramer, J. H., Schuff, N., Reed, B. R. *et al.* (2004). Hippocampal volume and retention in Alzheimer's disease. *Journal of the International Neuropsychological Society*, **10**, 639–643.

Kraybill, M. L., Larson, E. B., Tsuang, D. W. *et al.* (2005). Cognitive differences in dementia patients with autopsy-verified AD, Lewy body pathology, or both. *Neurology*, **64**, 2069–2073.

Lezak, M., Howieson, D., and Loring, D. (2004). *Neuropsychological Assessment*, 4th edn. New York: Oxford University Press.

Libon, D. J., Xie, S. X., Moore, P. *et al.* (2007). Patterns of neuropsychological impairment in frontotemporal dementia. *Neurology*, **68**, 369–375.

Luis, C. A., Mittenberg, W., Gass, C. S., and Durara, R. (1999). Diffuse Lewy body disease: clinical, pathological, and neuropsychological review. *Neuropsychology Review*, **9**, 137–150.

Massman, P. J., Delis, D. C., Butters, N., Levin, B. E., and Salmon, D. P. (1990). Are all subcortical dementias alike? Verbal learning and memory in Parkinson's and Huntington's disease patients. *Journal of Clinical and Experimental Neuropsychology*, **12**, 729–744.

Mathuranath, P. S., Neston, P. J., Berrios, G. E., Rakowicz, W., and Hodges, J. R. (2000). A brief cognitive test battery to differentiate Alzheimer's disease and frontotemporal dementia. *American Academy of Neurology*, **55**, 1613–1620.

McKeith, I. G., Galasko, D., Kosaka, K. *et al.* (1996). Consensus guidelines for the clinical and pathologic diagnosis of dementia with Lewy bodies (DLB): report of the Consortium of DLB International Workshop. *Neurology*, **47**, 1113–1124.

McKeith, I. G., Dickson, D. W., Lowe, J. *et al.* (2005). Diagnosis and management of dementia with Lewy bodies: third report of the DLB Consortium. *Neurology*, **65**, 1863–1872.

McMillan, C., Gee, J., Moore, P. *et al.* (2004). Confrontation naming and morphometric analyses of structural MRI in frontotemporal dementia. *Dementia and Geriatric Cognitive Disorders*, **17**, 320–323.

Millar, D., Griffiths, P., Zermansky, A. J., and Burn, D. J. (2006). Characterizing behavioral and cognitive dysexecutive changes in progressive supranuclear palsy. *Movement Disorders*, **21**, 199–207.

Miller, B. L., Seeley, W. W., Mychack, P. *et al.* (2001). Neuroanatomy of the self: evidence from patients with frontotemporal dementia. *Neurology*, **57**, 817–821.

Mitrushina, M. and Satz, P. (1991). Reliability and validity of the Mini-Mental State Exam in neurologically intact elderly. *Journal of Clinical Psychology*, **47**, 537–543.

Mori, E., Shimomura, T., Fujimori, M. *et al.* (2000). Visuoperceptual impairment in dementia with Lewy bodies. *Archives of Neurology*, **57**, 489–493.

Mungas, D., Reed, B. R., and Kramer J. H. (2003). Psychometrically matched measures of global cognition,

memory and executive function for assessment of cognitive decline in older persons. *Neuropsychology*, **17**, 380–392.

Neary D., Snowden, J. S., Gustafson, L. *et al.* (1999). Frontotemporal lobar degeneration: a consensus on clinical diagnostic criteria. *Neurology*, **51**, 1546–1554,

Osterrieth, P. A. (1944). Le test de copie d'une figure complexe. *Archives de Psychologie*, 30, 206–356 [Trans. J. Corwin and F. W. Bylsma (1993) *The Clinical Neuropsychologist*, 7, 9–15].

Perry, R. and Hodges, J. (2000). Differentiating frontal and temporal variant frontotemporal dementia from Alzheimer's disease. *Neurology*, **54**, 2277–2284.

Pfeffer, R. I., Kurosaki, T. T., Harrah, C. H. Jr., Chance, J. M., and Filos, S. (1982). Measurement of functional activities in older adults in the community. *Journal of Gerontology*, 37, 323–329.

Pfeiffer, E. (1975). A short portable mental status questionnaire for the assessment of organic brain deficit in elderly patients. *Journal of the American Geriatric Society*, **23**, 433–441.

Rascovsky, K., Salmon, D. P., Hansen, L. A., Thal, L. J., and Galasko, D. (2007). Disparate letter and semantic category fluency deficits in autopsy-confirmed frontotemporal dementia and Alzheimer's disease. *Neuropsychology*, **21**, 20–30.

Reitan, R. M., and Wolfson, D. (1985). *The Halstead–Reitan Neuropsychological Test Battery*. Tucson, AZ: Neuropsychological Press.

Rey, A. (1941). L'examen psychologique dans les cas d' encephalopathie traumatique. *Archives de Psychologie*, **28**, 21.

Rosen, H. J., Gorno-Tempini, M. L., Goldman, W. P. *et al.* (2002). Patterns of brain atrophy in frontotemporal dementia and semantic dementia. *Neurology*, **22**, 198–208.

Ruff, R. M., Light, R. H., and Evans, R. W. (1987). The Ruff Figural Fluency Test: a normative study with adults. *Developmental Neuropsychology*, **3**, 37–52.

Solomon, P. R., Hirschoff, A., Kelly, B. *et al.* (1998). A 7 minute neurocognitive screening battery highly sensitive to Alzheimer's disease. *Archives of Neurology*, **55**, 349–355.

Squire, L. R. and Butters, N. (eds.) (1984). *Neuropsychology of Memory*. New York: The Guilford Press.

Stroop, J. R. (1935). Studies of interference in serial verbal reactions. *Journal of Experimental Psychology*, **18**, 643–662.

Strub, R. L. and Black, F. W. (2000). *The Mental Status Examination in Neurology*, 4th edn. Philadelphia, PA: F. A. Davis.

Sunderland, A., Watts, K., Baddeley, A. D., and Harris, J. E. (1986). Subjective memory assessment and test performance in elderly adults. *Journal of Gerontology*, **41**, 376–384.

Tekin, S., and Cummings., J. L. (2002). Frontal–subcortical neuronal circuits and clinical neuropsychiatry: an update. *Journal of Psychosomatic Research*, **53**, 647–654.

Teng, E. L. and Chiu, H. C. (1987). The modified mini-mental state (3MS) examination. *Journal of Clinical Psychiatry*, **48**, 314–318.

Teng, E. L., Hasegawa, K., Homma, A. *et al.* (1994). The Cognitive Abilities Screening Instrument (CASI): a practical test for cross-cultural epidemiological studies of dementia. *International Psychogeriatrics*, **6**, 45–58.

Terry, R. D., and Katzman R. (1983). Senile dementia of the Alzheimer type. *Annals of Neurology*, **14**, 497–506.

Thompson, J. C., Stopford, C. L., Snowden, J. S., and Neary, D. (2005). Qualitative neuropsychological performance characteristics in frontotemporal dementia and Alzheimer's disease. *Journal of Neurology, Neurosurgery and Psychiatry*, **76**, 920–927.

Troyer, A. K. (2000). Normative data for clustering and switching on verbal fluency tasks. *Journal of Clinical and Experimental Neuropsychology*, **22**, 29–39.

Walker, R., Husain, M., Hodgson, T. L., Harrison, J., Kennard, C. (1998). Saccadic eye movement and working memory deficits following damage to human prefrontal cortex. *Neuropsychologia*, **36**, 1141–1159.

Walker, Z., Allen, R. L., Shergill, S., and Katona, C. L. E. (1997). Neuropsychological performance in Lewy body dementia and Alzheimer's disease. *British Journal of Psychiatry*, **170**, 156–158.

Warrington, E. K. and James, M. (1991). *Visual Object and Space Perception Battery*. Bury St. Edmunds, UK: Thames Valley Test.

Wechsler, D. (1997). *Wechsler Adult Intelligence Scale, 3rd edn, (WAIS-III) Administration and Scoring Manual*. San Antonio, TX: The Psychological Corporation.

Wicklund, A. H., Johnson, H., Rademaker A., Weitner, B. B., and Weintraub, S. (2006). Word list versus story memory in Alzheimer disease and frontotemporal dementia. *Alzheimer Disease and Associated Disorders*, **20**, 86–92.

Wilson, B. A. (1991). Long-term prognosis of patients with severe memory disorder. *Neuropsychological Rehabilitation*, **1**, 117–134.

Wilson, B. A., Cockburn, J., and Baddeley, A. (1985). *The Rivermead Behavioural Memory Test*. Bury St. Edmunds, UK: Thames Valley Test.

Wilson, B. A., Cockburn, J., Baddeley, A. D., and Hiorns, R. (1989). The development and validation of a test battery for detecting and monitoring everyday memory problems. *Journal of Clinical and Experimental Neuropsychology*, **11**, 855–870.

Wilson, R. S., Gilley, D. W., Bennett, D. A., Beckett, L. A., and Evans, D. A. (2000). Person-specific paths of cognitive decline in Alzheimer's disease and their relation to age. *Psychology and Aging*, **15**, 18–28.

Yesavage, J. A., Brink, T. L., Rose, T. L. *et al.* (1983). Development and validation of a geriatric depression screening scale: a preliminary report. *Journal of Psychiatric Research*, **17**, 37–49.

Chapter 7

Neuropsychiatric features of dementia

Edmond Teng, Gad A. Marshall and Jeffrey L. Cummings

Introduction

Neuropsychiatric symptoms are a common problem in dementia. Epidemiological studies indicate that approximately 60% of demented subjects in the community exhibit some degree of psychopathology.[1] Among specific populations of subjects diagnosed with frontotemporal dementia (FTD) or advanced Alzheimer's disease (AD), the prevalence of behavioral pathology increases to 95%.[2,3] The most frequently reported behavioral symptoms include apathy, agitation and depression.[1]

The significant contributions of neuropsychiatric symptoms to the more common dementia syndromes are reflected by their prominent role in the diagnosis of these conditions. Behavioral symptoms are primary components of the diagnostic criteria for FTD[4] and dementia with Lewy bodies (DLB)[5] and are among the secondary supportive factors in the diagnostic criteria for AD[6] and vascular dementia (VaD).[7] Disturbances in behavior have also been reported in mild cognitive impairment (MCI),[8] Parkinson's disease with dementia (PDD),[9] progressive supranuclear palsy (PSP)[10] and corticobasal degeneration (CBD).[11]

While the severity of a dementing illness is often determined using cognitive criteria, behavioral disturbances are responsible for a substantial proportion of the morbidity caused by different dementia syndromes. Caregivers for patients with dementia find behavioral abnormalities significantly more troubling than cognitive deficits.[12] The presence of neuropsychiatric symptoms correlates with increased rates of institutionalization,[13] cost of care[14] and caregiver stress and burden.[15,16]

The behavioral disruptions seen in dementia are not simply an inevitable consequence of worsening cognitive impairment. Although neuropsychiatric symptoms are often seen with greater frequency and severity in the later stages of dementing illnesses,[2] the clinical course of different behavioral symptoms is often heterogeneous and does not correlate closely with the severity of cognitive or functional impairment.[17,18] Longitudinal studies suggest that while cognitive and functional declines in dementia are gradually but inexorably progressive, individual behavioral symptoms may wax and wane, with a high rate of recurrence after onset.[17,19] Neuropathological and functional neuroimaging studies demonstrate that behavioral abnormalities correlate with degenerative changes and dysfunction in specific brain regions.[20,21] Taken together, these findings indicate that neuropsychiatric disturbances in dementia are independent from concurrently worsening cognitive deficits and represent separate manifestations of the underlying disease processes.

Assessment

While clinical assessments of the wide range of neuropsychiatric symptoms seen in dementia incorporate the patient's subjective impressions and the physician's behavioral observations, many of the more reliable standardized instruments for measuring psychopathology rely primarily upon caregiver interviews. Most of these rating tools have been specifically developed for use with dementia patients, but a few, such as the Hamilton Depression Rating Scale,[22] were originally devised for use with other psychiatric populations. A number of the most frequently used scales are listed in Table 7.1. Behavioral rating scales typically fall into two different categories. Some focus on evaluating specific categories of abnormal behaviors with precise detail, such as the Cohen–Mansfield Agitation Inventory,[23] the Cornell Scale for Depression in Dementia[24] and the Apathy Inventory.[25] Other commonly used instruments, including the Behavioral Pathology in Alzheimer's Disease Rating Scale (BEHAVE-AD),[26] the Neuropsychiatric Inventory (NPI)[27,28] and the Behavioral Rating Scale for Dementia (BRSD),[29] are

The Behavioral Neurology of Dementia, eds. Bruce L. Miller and Bradley F. Boeve. Published by Cambridge University Press.
© Cambridge University Press 2009.

Table 7.1. Rating scales used for the evaluation of neuropsychiatric symptoms in dementia

Behavior	Rating scale
Specific behaviors	Agitated Behavior Inventory for Dementia
	Agitation–Calmness Evaluation Scale
	Apathy Inventory
	Apathy Scale
	Bech–Rafaelsen Mania Scale
	Cohen–Mansfield Agitation Inventory
	Cornell Scale for Depression in Dementia
	Dementia Psychosis Scale
	Disinhibition Scale
	Frontal Behavior Inventory
	Frontal Systems Behavior Scale
	Geriatric Depression Scale
	Hamilton Rating Scale for Depression
	Hamilton Rating Scale for Anxiety
	Irritability Scale
	Middelheim Frontality Scale
	Overt Aggression Scale
	Social Dysfunction and Aggression Scale
Multiple behaviors	Alzheimer's Disease Assessment Scale: Noncognitive Subscale
	Behavior Observation Scale for Intramural Psychogeriatric Patients
	Behavior and Emotional Activities Manifested in Dementia
	Behavioral Pathology in Alzheimer's Disease Rating Scale
	Behavioral Rating Scale for Dementia
	Behavioral Symptoms Scale for Dementia
	Brief Psychiatric Rating Scale
	Columbia University Scale for Psychopathology in Alzheimer's Disease
	Comprehensive Psychopathological Rating Scale
	Dementia Behavior Disturbance Scale
	Manchester and Oxford Universities Scale for Psychopathological Assessment of Dementia
	Neurobehavioral Rating Scale
	Neuropsychiatric Inventory
	Positive and Negative Syndrome Scale
	Present Behavior Examination
	Revised Memory and Behavior Problem Checklist
	Troublesome Behavior Scale

designed to capture a broad cross-section of different varieties of behavioral disturbances.

The BEHAVE-AD examines 25 symptoms arranged in seven clusters: paranoid and delusional ideation, hallucinations, aggressiveness, activity disturbances, diurnal rhythm disturbances, affective disturbances, and anxiety and phobias.[26] The NPI evaluates 12 categories of psychopathology: delusions, hallucinations, agitation/aggression, depression/dysphoria, anxiety, elation/euphoria, apathy/indifference, disinhibition, irritability, aberrant motor behavior, nighttime behaviors, and appetite/eating behaviors.[28] The BRSD assesses 46 behaviors grouped into six subscales: depressive symptoms, inertia, vegetative symptoms, irritability and aggression, behavioral dysregulation, and psychotic symptoms.[29] The BEHAVE-AD and NPI have been particularly useful for monitoring the longitudinal course of behavioral symptoms and their response to various treatments.

Behavioral syndromes

Individual patients often exhibit multiple behavioral disturbances simultaneously. A number of studies have employed factor analysis to identify abnormal behaviors that group together into specific symptom clusters. Five distinct behavioral syndromes emerge from a survey of this literature: aggression, depression, apathy, motor hyperactivity and psychosis.[30] This section will describe the individual symptoms that make up these syndromes as well as other commonly reported behavioral symptoms that do not fit neatly into this classification scheme. It will also review the functional imaging and neuropathological evidence for the localization of the underlying neurological substrates for these behaviors.

Aggression

This syndrome encompasses physically and verbally aggressive behaviors, irritability and disinhibition. Physically aggressive behavior includes such actions as hitting, biting, spitting and throwing of objects, while verbally aggressive behavior involves cursing or other forms of verbal abuse.[23] Increased irritability typically manifests with frequent arguments, pouting, sulking and angry loud outbursts.[31] Disinhibited behavior is most commonly seen in FTD, with reported prevalences as high as 75%,[3,32] but it can also be seen in over 50% of patients with PSP.[33] Disinhibition frequently impacts social behavior, resulting in excessive friendliness, inappropriate comments and violation of interpersonal norms.[28] Sexual behaviors can also be exaggerated by disinhibition, giving rise to compulsive masturbation, self-exposure of genitalia or inappropriate sexual advances and touching. These behavioral disturbances may be extremely disturbing for caregivers and family members and can result in legal consequences for the patient.[34,35] The frequency and severity of aggressive behavior among demented patients are strongly correlated with overall levels of caregiver burden and stress.[16,36]

Single-photon emisson computed tomography (SPECT) and positron emission tomography (PET) studies have revealed relative hypoperfusion and hypometabolism in the frontal and temporal lobes among demented subjects who exhibit symptoms of aggression or disinhibition.[37–40] Neuropathological data corroborate some of these findings. Autopsy studies of patients with AD who had been aggressive have found increased neurofibrillary tangle deposition in the orbitofrontal and anterior cingulate cortices.[21]

Depression

Depressive symptoms are highly prevalent in dementia, particularly in CBD, where over 70% of patients exhibit some degree of dysphoria.[11] The depressive symptomatology experienced by demented subjects is similar to that seen in depressed elderly control subjects and is significantly different from that reported by younger depressed subjects.[41] Anhedonia, difficulty initiating and sustaining activities and decreased confidence and self-esteem are more common among patients with dementia, while sadness, feelings of guilt and suicidality are less prominent.[42] Overall, depression in elderly and demented populations is more transient and less intense than that seen in younger populations.[43] These differences have spurred the development of formal diagnostic criteria that are specific for depression in AD. The primary differences between these criteria and the conventional criteria for major depression are the fewer total symptoms required and the inclusion of depressive symptoms that are more prevalent in dementia, such as irritability, withdrawal, social isolation and decreased pleasure with social contact.[44]

Among demented subjects, the presence of depression correlates strongly with the presence of anxiety.[16,45] The most common manifestations are excessive worrying, apprehension and fearfulness, particularly the fear of being left alone.[45,46] While depression and anxiety both engender moderate levels of caregiver distress in AD,[47] depressive symptoms

are far more distressing for caregivers of patients with FTD.[16]

The specific functional localization of depression in dementia remains uncertain. One PET study in patients with AD has identified relative hypometabolism in the frontal and anterior cingulate cortices, a finding that is consistent with other reports of cerebral metabolic dysfunction in primary and secondary depressive syndromes.[20] However, SPECT studies in AD and PET studies in FTD have implicated other regions, including parietal and right temporal regions.[37,40] Autopsy studies have not revealed any correlations between cortical neuropathology and depressive symptomatology. Instead, the primary degenerative changes associated with depression in dementia are found among the aminergic neurons of the substantia nigra and the dorsal raphe nucleus. The cholinergic neurons in the nucleus basalis of Meynert are relatively spared. These findings are reinforced by neurochemical evidence of decreased norepinephrine and serotonin levels and relatively preserved choline acetyltransferase levels in the cortical and subcortical regions of depressed dementia patients.[48] These results suggest that the degenerative changes seen in the brainstem are likely to modulate the metabolic abnormalities seen in the cortical regions. The divergent conclusions generated by different SPECT and PET studies may reflect differences between the assessment tools used to quantify the frequency and severity of depressive symptoms and the transitory nature of depression in dementia.

Apathy

Apathy has been identified as the most common behavioral disturbance across multiple dementia syndromes. Over 25% of all demented subjects in a community-based epidemiological study[1] and over 70% of subjects with AD,[2] FTD,[3] DLB[32] or PSP[10] recruited from subspecialty clinics exhibited symptoms of apathy. Although the neurovegetative features of apathetic and depressive syndromes appear to overlap, apathy in dementia has been shown to be a separate behavioral entity.[49] Symptoms that are particularly useful for distinguishing between apathy and depression include decreased emotional responsiveness, increased indifference and the lack of social engagement.[50]

Converging data from the examination of the neuroanatomical correlates of apathy in dementia further reinforce the concept that apathy represents a discrete behavioral syndrome. Several investigators using SPECT and PET techniques have reported that increasing levels of apathy in AD and FTD correlate with hypoperfusion and hypometabolism in the anterior cingulate and frontal cortices.[39,51-53] Further subdivision of apathy in AD into discrete types of apathetic behavior has yielded additional insights into the localization of these symptoms. Emotional blunting corresponds with left superior frontal hypoperfusion; lack of interest correlates with bilateral middle frontal gyrus hypoperfusion; and lack of initiative correlates with right anterior cingulate hypoperfusion.[54] These findings are also supported by neuropathological investigations of apathy in AD, which show significant correlations between neurofibrillary tangle density in the anterior cingulate cortex and increased frequency and severity of apathetic symptoms.[55]

Motor hyperactivity

A wide variety of aberrant motor behaviors can be seen with progressive dementia. Non-aggressive agitated behaviors such as inappropriate dressing and disrobing and constant requests for attention are a frequent cause of frustration among caregivers.[23] Wandering and other forms of motor restlessness may also become increasingly problematic as dementia severity increases; these appear to correlate with diminishing visuospatial abilities. Excessive pacing, nocturnal ambulation, attempts to leave the house or nursing home, walking with an inappropriate purpose or frequency and walking off during meals are examples of such activities.[56] An assortment of stereotyped behaviors may also be observed, particularly in patients with FTD, which can involve the repeated use of identical phrases, obsessive hoarding and collecting or a strict adherence to customary routines.[57]

Our understanding of the neurological substrates of motor hyperactivity in dementia remains underdeveloped. A single SPECT study of wandering behavior in AD produced the counterintuitive finding of left parietotemporal hypoperfusion.[58] Increases in aberrant motor activity correlate with higher neurofibrillary tangle counts in the left orbitofrontal cortex, which may reflect a component of disinhibition driving such behaviors.[21] Additional research will be required to unravel the clinicopathological correlates for this constellation of neuropsychiatric symptoms.

Psychosis

Hallucinations and delusions are most common in DLB, with each of these disturbances occurring in over 50% of patients. However, these disturbances are also present in AD and other dementias.[59] Psychotic symptoms, particularly delusions, contribute disproportionately to the overall morbidity of a dementing illness and increase the likelihood of institutionalization.[13] Delusional thinking is often non-bizarre in content and consists primarily of misidentifications and paranoid ideation. Frequently reported misidentifications include the belief that images seen on the television are occurring in the patient's home (picture sign), that imposters have replaced the patient's family and friends (Capgras syndrome) and that the patient's house is not their home. Paranoid delusions can involve the belief that the patient's spouse is having an affair (infidelity), that someone is stealing the patient's things (theft) or that a stranger is living in the patient's house (phantom boarder syndrome). Hallucinations are most often visual or auditory in nature; olfactory and tactile phenomena are distinctly less common.[59] Visual hallucinations are typically complex, well formed and in color; they can depict familiar or anonymous people, animals or parts of the body.[60,61] Auditory hallucinations commonly consist of hearing the voices of persons who are either deceased or not in the room.[60]

Functional imaging of psychotic behavior in demented subjects has implicated a wide swath of potentially dysfunctional areas in the frontal, cingulate and parietal regions of the brain.[37,62] Specific studies of visual hallucinations in AD and DLB using SPECT techniques have revealed more focal regions of hypoperfusion in the posterior portions of the brain, including the occipital, parietal and posterior cingulate cortices.[63-65] Likewise, while SPECT studies that combined different types of delusion found broader abnormalities in the frontal and temporal lobes,[63,66] investigations with SPECT and PET limited to specific categories of delusional thinking have yielded more circumscribed areas of hypoperfusion and hypometabolism, concentrated primarily in the frontal lobes.[67,68] These findings suggest that individual psychotic phenomena result from discrete patterns of cortical dysfunction. Neuropathological and neurochemical analyses of psychotic psychopathology in AD and DLB have also reported abnormalities in the frontal and medial temporal lobes that, in some cases, can distinguish between different types of delusion and hallucination.[69-72]

Other symptoms

A number of the neuropsychiatric symptoms seen in demented patients do not fit neatly into this classification scheme. These include euphoria, appetitive disturbances and sleep abnormalities.

Symptoms of abnormally elevated mood are relatively rare in most dementia syndromes. Common manifestations include inappropriate happiness, humor and laughter. Clinically significant mania is only slightly more prevalent in the overall demented population than the general elderly population.[73,74] Euphoria and mania/hypomania are seen most often in patients with FTD[32] as up to 40% of subjects exhibit such behaviors.[3] Studies in the FTD population using SPECT have demonstrated that hypomanic behavior correlates with bilateral temporal lobe hypoperfusion,[53] whereas case reports of secondary mania in neurological disorders have implicated frontal lobe pathology.[75]

A variety of disturbances in appetite and eating behaviors frequently emerges with dementia progression, particularly in AD and FTD. Early in the course of AD, a small proportion of patients may experience significant weight gain as a result of hyperorality, insatiable cravings for sweets and gorging behavior. Later in the disease, most patients experience weight loss, which is most often multifactorial in etiology. Depressive symptoms can lead to decreased nutritional intake and anorexia, while increased motor activity and restlessness can generate increased caloric requirements.[76] Among those with FTD, the most common appetitive disorders include gluttony and indiscriminate eating. Patients with semantic dementia (SD) become significantly more selective in the foods that they are willing to consume.[77] In end-stage dementia, patients may develop visual agnosias, which can interfere with their ability to identify food items, or motor apraxias, which can interfere with the functional skills required for self-feeding or the coordination necessary to synchronize chewing and swallowing. These patients may require the placement of a gastric tube to achieve adequate nutritional support.[76]

Sleep disturbances are a common and difficult problem in dementia, and these can be a major factor leading to increased caregiver distress and rates of institutionalization.[78] Sleep/wake rhythms are frequently disrupted among demented subjects, resulting in frequent daytime napping, prolonged night-time wakefulness and multiple nocturnal awakenings.[79] Rapid eye movement (REM) sleep-behavior disorder is reported in over 50% of all patients with DLB or PDD but is rarely seen in other dementing conditions. It is characterized by the expression of bodily movements associated with dream re-enactment and is linked to the loss of the normal skeletal muscle atonia that is usually present during REM sleep. Neuropathological studies have found that the symptoms of REM sleep-behavior disorder correlate with the presence of Lewy bodies and degeneration of brainstem nuclei.[80]

Neuropsychiatric profiles of specific dementia syndromes

There is significant overlap in the manifestation of individual neuropsychiatric symptoms among the different dementia syndromes. However, the overall patterns of behavioral disturbances for each dementing disorder can be quite distinctive. The different behavioral patterns seen with different dementia etiologies reflect the different patterns of regional degeneration and cerebral dysfunction across diseases. This section reviews the most prominent psychopathological features of each of the common degenerative and vascular dementia syndromes.

Alzheimer's disease

Neuropsychiatric symptoms have been most intensively studied in patients with AD. The most common symptoms in this population include apathy, aggression and anxiety.[2] The prevalence of these symptoms varies according to the specific population studied. Community-based epidemiological studies report lower levels of psychopathology, while convenience samples based in memory disorder clinics exhibit a higher prevalence of behavioral symptomatology.[1,2] Cross-sectional studies suggest that the qualitative and quantitative characteristics of neuropsychiatric disturbances evolve over the course of the disease (Fig. 7.1). In mild AD and putative preclinical AD conditions such as MCI, apathy, depression, irritability and anxiety are typically the most prominent symptoms, but fewer behavioral abnormalities are reported overall.[2,8] Among patients with moderate to severe AD, virtually all subjects exhibit some behavioral abnormalities, and symptoms such as agitation, anxiety and motor hyperactivity become increasingly prominent.[2] While the overall frequency of symptoms is greatest in patients with severe AD,[2] it appears to decrease among patients with end-stage AD, perhaps because their increasing functional impairments limit their ability to exhibit behavioral pathology.[81]

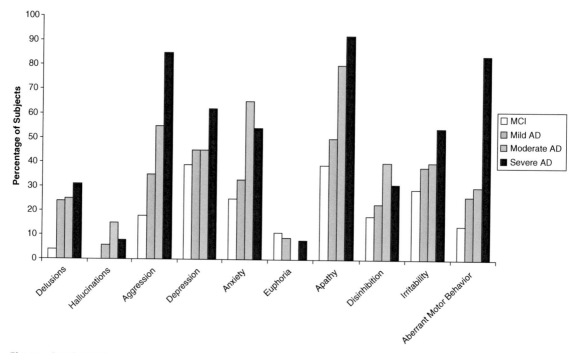

Fig. 7.1. Prevalence of neuropsychiatric symptoms in subjects with mild cognitive impairment (MCI) and subjects with mild, moderate, or severe Alzheimer's disease (AD). (Data derived from Mega *et al.* [1996][2] and Hwang *et al.* [2004].[8])

These cross-sectional studies suggest that the frequency and severity of behavioral symptoms progressively increase as cognitive function declines in AD. However, longitudinal assessments indicate that the evolution of neuropsychiatric symptoms is much more variable than the decline seen in cognitive and functional domains.[18] Behavioral abnormalities fluctuate over time in both frequency and severity, and individual symptoms often demonstrate an episodic course rather than a progressive deterioration.[17] Once a specific symptom emerges, it is likely to be recurrent rather than continuously present.[19]

Vascular dementia

The neuropsychological deficits produced by VaD can be quite variable, depending upon the specific brain regions that are affected by cerebrovascular disease. The neuropsychiatric symptoms seen in VaD are similarly diverse. Across studies, depression, apathy and irritability are among the most consistently problematic behavioral abnormalities.[82–84] Quantitative comparisons of overall psychopathology between VaD and AD have produced conflicting results, with some studies suggesting that behavioral disturbances are more problematic in VaD,[82] and

others reporting a similar frequency and severity of symptoms in VaD and AD.[83,84] Likewise, although some investigators have found that depression, apathy and anxiety are more common in VaD and delusions are more prevalent in AD,[1,83,85] others have not found significant differences in the frequencies of individual behaviors.[84,86]

The specific profile of neuropsychiatric deficits for a given patient may depend on the underlying pattern of cerebrovascular disease present in the brain. Imaging studies in non-demented elderly populations have demonstrated a greater prevalence of deep white matter microvascular ischemic changes in the frontal lobes of depressed subjects relative to non-depressed controls.[87] However, a recent analysis of behavioral symptoms in demented subjects with cortical versus subcortical loci of ischemic changes did not reveal distinctive patterns of psychopathology between these two groups (Fig. 7.2). Although subjects with cortical VaD exhibited more frequent and severe behavioral abnormalities, these differences appeared to be related to their more profound cognitive impairments.[84] More precise characterization of the association between the localization of ischemic disease and specific behavioral syndromes may be needed to develop

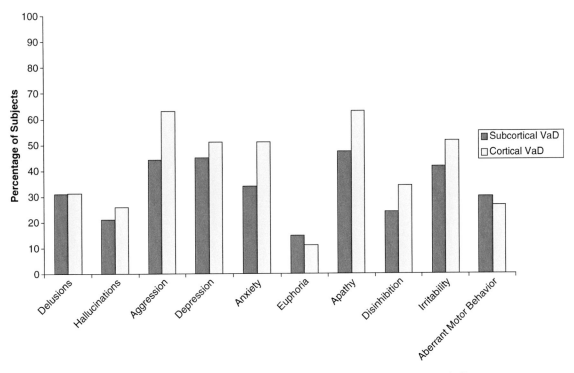

Fig. 7.2. Prevalence of neuropsychiatric symptoms in subjects with subcortical or cortical vascular dementia (VaD). (Data derived from Fuh *et al.* [2005].[84])

a better understanding of the variability of neuropsychiatric symptoms in VaD.

Frontotemporal lobar degeneration

Frontotemporal lobar degeneration (FTLD) encompasses a spectrum of cognitive and behavioral disorders that result from selective deterioration in regions of the frontal and temporal lobes. Three discrete clinical syndromes have been described: FTD, which is associated with predominantly frontal lobe degeneration; SD, which is correlated with predominantly anterior temporal lobe degeneration; and progressive non-fluent aphasia (PNFA), which is more specifically related to left posterior frontal lobe degeneration.[77,88]

Personality, emotional and behavioral changes are among the core diagnostic criteria for FTD.[4] Apathy, motor hyperactivity, disinhibition and hyperphagia are consistently among the most commonly reported behavioral disturbances in FTD.[3,16,77] Other distinctive behavioral features of FTD include diminished ability to demonstrate basic emotions, loss of insight and social awareness, complex ritualized activity and overtly sociopathic behavior.[35,57,77] Comparisons of the neuropsychiatric features of FTD and AD indicate

that significantly more behavioral pathology is seen in FTD.[89] Symptoms such as disinhibition, apathy, euphoria and aberrant motor activity are seen more commonly in FTD, while depression and delusions are more characteristic of AD.[3,32,89,90]

The cognitive dimensions of SD that distinguish it from the other syndromes of frontotemporal lobar degeneration include progressive fluent aphasia and associative visual agnosia. Clinically, the cognitive features of SD are more prominent than the behavioral symptoms. However, the overall frequency and severity of neuropsychiatric features are relatively similar between SD and FTD.[3,90] When specific categories of behavioral disturbances are compared (Fig. 7.3), patients with SD are more likely to be depressed, while patients with FTD are more likely to be apathetic.[3] Other investigators, using different methodologies, have found other differences between SD and FTD that are not reflected in Fig. 7.3. These include increased levels of mental rigidity and repetitive/compulsive behaviors in SD, and higher frequencies of disinhibition and gluttony in FTD.[77,90]

Patients with PNFA present with an expressive language deficit but initially have otherwise preserved

91

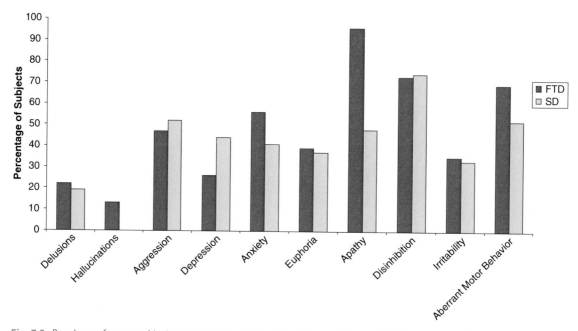

Fig. 7.3. Prevalence of neuropsychiatric symptoms in subjects with frontotemporal dementia (FTD) or semantic dementia (SD). (Data derived from Liu *et al.* [2004].[3])

cognitive and social functioning. The neuropsychiatric features of PNFA have been less well characterized than the other disorders of FTLD. At disease onset, subjects with PNFA display significantly fewer behavioral symptoms than subjects with FTD. However, longitudinal follow-up of these subjects indicates that, over a span of 3 years, there are significant increases in apathy, disinhibition, restlessness and aggression in the PNFA group. As FTD and PNFA progress in severity, their cognitive and behavioral profiles become increasingly similar.[91]

Dementia with Lewy bodies and Parkinson's disease with dementia

Both DLB and PDD are characterized by dementia, parkinsonism and the presence of cortical and brain-stem Lewy bodies, which represent pathologic accumulations of α-synuclein protein. These two nosological entities differ in their initial presentation: cognitive symptoms appear prior to or concurrent with parkinsonian symptoms in DLB, while Parkinson's disease is well established prior to the onset of dementia in PDD.[5] However, clinical and neuropathological findings in DLB and PDD show significant convergence with disease progression, raising the possibility that they are different manifestations of a common neurodegenerative process.[92]

Particularly distinctive features of DLB include the presence of fluctuating levels of alertness, frequent visual hallucinations, marked sensitivity to neuroleptic medications and REM sleep-behavior disorder.[5] Other significant neuropsychiatric symptoms that are often identified among those with DLB include delusions, auditory hallucinations, apathy and aberrant motor behavior.[32,59] The overall prevalence of behavioral abnormalities is higher among patients with DLB than among patients with AD.[32] Psychotic features most consistently differentiate the behavioral syndromes seen in DLB and AD. In particular, delusions of misidentification and hallucinations in both visual and auditory modalities are significantly more common in DLB than AD.[32,59]

Patients with PDD initially present with extrapyramidal motor symptoms typical of idiopathic Parkinson's disease but subsequently develop a subcortical dementia syndrome. The neuropsychiatric features of PDD resemble those of DLB in that hallucinations, depression and anxiety are among the most frequently reported behavioral abnormalities.[9] Psychosis is significantly more common in PDD than Parkinson's disease without dementia.[92] As the severity of PDD progresses, subjects experience more delusions but become less apathetic. Quantitative assessments have suggested that similar overall levels of psychopathology

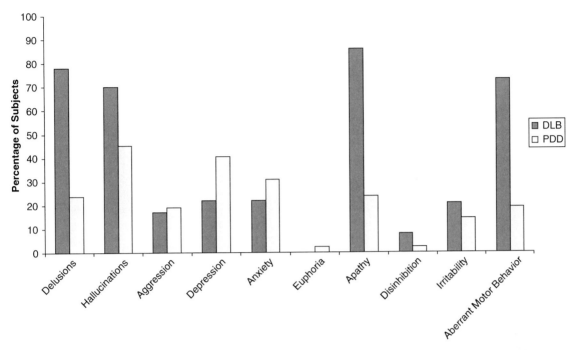

Fig. 7.4. Prevalence of neuropsychiatric symptoms in subjects with dementia with Lewy bodies (DLB) or Parkinson's disease with dementia (PDD). (Data derived from Hirono *et al.* [1999][32] and Aarsland *et al.* [2001].[9])

are found in PDD and AD. Hallucinations are more likely to be reported in PDD, while apathy, agitation, disinhibition and irritability are more likely to be reported in AD.[9]

Comparisons of behavioral pathology between DLB and PDD (Fig. 7.4) reveal that the prevalence of hallucinations and delusions is significantly greater in DLB than PDD. However, the qualitative features of the psychotic symptoms are similar across the two groups.[92] Other behavioral abnormalities that are seen more commonly in DLB than PDD include apathy and aberrant motor behavior.[32,92] Depressive symptoms occur with equal frequency in both DLB and PDD but are particularly common among subjects experiencing hallucinations.[92]

Progressive supranuclear palsy and corticobasal degeneration

Both PSP and CBD are degenerative dementing conditions that present with prominent extrapyramidal symptoms. Typical motor manifestations of PSP include symmetrical axial rigidity, supranuclear gaze palsy and early falls. However, CBD can be distinguished from PSP by its asymmetric rigidity and

dystonia, and the presence of cortical symptoms such as apraxia, alien limb phenomena or myoclonus. Although PSP and CBD are both tauopathies, they produce different patterns of abnormal tau deposition. Subcortical globose neurofibrillary tangles and tufted astrocytes are characteristic of PSP, while cortical ballooned neurons, astrocytic plaques and coiled bodies are characteristic of CBD. Magnetic resonance imaging studies reveal widespread midbrain and pontine atrophy in PSP, and asymmetric atrophy of the basal ganglia and frontoparietal cortex in CBD.[93] Despite these clinical and pathological distinctions, patients with either disorder often exhibit similar subcortical dementia syndromes, with deficits in frontal and executive functioning.

The most prominent behavioral abnormalities in subjects with PSP are apathy and disinhibition. Psychotic symptoms are exceedingly rare, particularly relative to other parkinsonian dementia syndromes such as DLB and PDD.[33] While similar overall levels of psychopathology have been found in PSP and AD, patients with PSP have a significantly higher prevalence of apathy, while patients with AD are more likely to exhibit delusions, agitation, anxiety and irritability.[10]

93

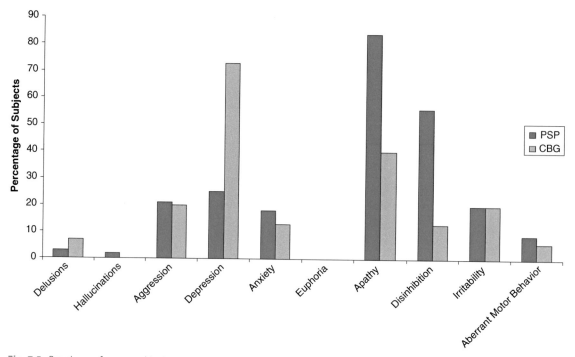

Fig. 7.5. Prevalence of neuropsychiatric symptoms in patients with progressive supranuclear palsy (PSP) or corticobasal degeneration (CBG). (Data derived from Aarsland *et al.* [2001][33] and Litvan *et al.* [1998].[11])

Corticobasal degeneration is characterized by a high frequency of depressive symptomatology. Other categories of behavioral disruptions often reported by caregivers include apathy, irritability and agitation.[11] The frequency and severity of behavioral symptoms in CBD is similar to that seen in mild AD. However, in CBD, much like in PSP, the frequencies of anxiety, agitation and delusions are lower than those reported for AD.[2,11] While the neuropsychological profiles of CBD and PSP may be similar, the neuropsychiatric profiles are distinct (Fig. 7.5). Patients with CBD are much more likely to be depressed compared with patients with PSP, who are often significantly more apathetic or disinhibited.[11,33]

Treatment

Mild to moderate reductions in the neuropsychiatric symptoms associated with dementia have been achieved with both pharmacological and non-pharmacological treatments. Given the wide spectrum of behavioral disturbances seen in demented subjects, it is perhaps not surprising that different classes of abnormal behavior are likely to respond to different treatment modalities. Successful management strategies often must be individualized for each patient and may require a combination of pharmacological and non-pharmacological approaches.[94,95]

Non-pharmacological therapies should be instituted either prior to or in conjunction with pharmacological therapies. These strategies often seek to ameliorate the psychosocial and environmental factors that contribute to the frequency or severity of neuropsychiatric symptomatology. A broad range of different approaches has been investigated, including sensory enhancement and relaxation techniques such as massage, music or white noise; increased social contact, including one-to-one interactions and simulated family videos; behavior therapy, which encompasses differential reinforcement and stimulus control techniques; caregiver education; structured activities such as formal recreation and physical exercise routines; environmental enhancement, with decreased stimulation levels and more familiar surroundings; and specific medical and nursing interventions involving light therapy, minimization of restraints or optimized pain management. Although most studies report some improvement in behavioral symptoms, many are neither rigorously blinded nor well controlled. Direct comparisons of different protocols often favor those that emphasize increased social interaction.[96]

Several classes of medication have been shown to be effective in reducing abnormal behaviors in dementia, including cholinesterase inhibitors, antidepressants and antipsychotics. The selection of the appropriate pharmacological treatment should be tailored to the specific symptoms that are the most problematic. Since elderly patients are often taking multiple drugs and can be very sensitive to medication effects, new agents often need to be started at low doses and escalated slowly.

Cholinesterase inhibitors, such as donepezil, rivastigmine and galantamine, are appealing treatments as they are effective for delaying cognitive and functional decline as well as for reducing psychopathology. The use of cholinesterase inhibitors has consistently been shown to produce modest reductions in the overall frequency and severity of neuropsychiatric symptoms in AD, VaD, DLB and PDD.[97,98] The most robust improvements have been seen with apathy and hallucinations.[99] Memantine, a non-competitive N-methyl-D-aspartate (NMDA) receptor antagonist approved for the treatment of cognitive and functional deterioration in moderate-to-severe AD, may also further delay the progression of behavioral disturbances when used alone or in conjunction with donepezil.[100]

When studied in AD populations, serotonin selective-reuptake inhibitors (SSRIs) such as citalopram and sertraline are effective primarily for depressive symptoms.[98] Tricyclic antidepressants, including imipramine and amitryptiline, demonstrate similar efficacy for treating depression in patients with AD, but their less favorable side-effect profiles, especially their anticholinergic effects, may preclude their use as first-line agents.[101,102] When used in FTD, SSRIs and other antidepressants such as trazodone and selegiline may provide more substantial benefits across a wider array of behavioral disturbances. However, the interpretation of these more preliminary studies is limited by their small size and predominantly open-label designs.[103] Mood-stabilizing agents such as carbamazepine and valproate may be helpful for the control of agitation, but their utility is complicated by multiple drug–drug interactions and a relatively high incidence of adverse events.[98]

Antipsychotic agents have frequently been used to treat behavioral disturbances in dementia. Typical antipsychotic drugs, particularly haloperidol, demonstrate specific efficacy for the treatment of aggression. Atypical antipsychotic drugs, such as olanzapine, quietiapine and risperidone, have been shown to decrease the frequency and severity of a wider spectrum of symptoms, including agitation, aggression, hallucinations and delusions.[98] Despite the wide range of efficacy that has been demonstrated with this group of medications, there are a number of issues that may limit their use. Typical antipsychotics can often cause significant sedation and extrapyramidal symptoms, which may diminish their behavioral benefits.[98] Particular care should be exercised when treating patients with DLB with neuroleptic agents owing to their marked sensitivity to the adverse effects associated with these medications.[5] Recent concerns have centered on a meta-analysis that revealed a small but statistically significant increase in the risk of overall mortality among elderly dementia patients treated with atypical antipsychotic agents.[104] These findings prompted the US Food and Drug Administration to issue a "black box" warning covering all available atypical antipsychotic medications, which highlighted this risk and emphasized that these medications are not formally approved for the treatment of behavioral disorders in patients with dementia.[105] Although this warning was not extended to the typical antipsychotic drugs, subsequent analyses have found that the increased mortality rates associated with the use of these drugs in elderly subjects may be even greater than those seen with atypical antipsychotic agents.[106] Given the relative small effect size and uncertain etiology for the increased mortality rates uncovered in these studies, the judicious use of antipsychotic medications may still be warranted in a subset of patients with behavioral symptoms of appropriate severity that have not improved despite other interventions.

Summary

Neuropsychiatric symptoms are a significant source of increased morbidity, caregiver stress and cost of care in dementia. Frequently reported behavioral syndromes include aggression, depression, apathy, motor hyperactivity and psychosis. Individual symptoms correlate with specific patterns of regional cerebral dysfunction and degenerative changes. Distinctive patterns of psychopathology are seen in different dementing disorders and may be related to the anatomical localization of the degenerative changes characteristic of each disease. Pharmacological and non-pharmacological treatment interventions may help to reduce the frequency, severity and impact of these symptoms for both the patient and the caregiver.

Acknowledgements

Preparation of this chapter has been supported by the National Institute on Aging (P50 AG 16570), the Alzheimer's Disease Research Centers of California and the Sidell–Kagan Foundation.

Disclosures: Drs. Teng and Marshall have nothing to disclose. Dr. Cummings has provided consultation to the following pharmaceutical companies: Avanir, AstraZeneca, Eisai, EnVivo, Forest, Janssen, Lilly, Lundbeck, Merz, Myriad, Neurochem, Novartis, Ono, Pfizer, Sanofi-Aventis, Sepracor, and Takeda.

References

1. Lyketsos CG, Steinberg M, Tschanz JT *et al.* Mental and behavioral disturbances in dementia: findings from the Cache County Study on Memory in Aging. *American Journal of Psychiatry* 2000;**157**(5):708–14.

2. Mega MS, Cummings JL, Fiorello T, Gornbein J. The spectrum of behavioral changes in Alzheimer's disease. *Neurology* 1996;**46**(1):130–5.

3. Liu W, Miller BL, Kramer JH *et al.* Behavioral disorders in the frontal and temporal variants of frontotemporal dementia. *Neurology* 2004;**62**(5):742–8.

4. Neary D, Snowden JS, Gustafson L *et al.* Frontotemporal lobar degeneration: a consensus on clinical diagnostic criteria. *Neurology* 1998;**51**(6):1546–54.

5. McKeith IG, Dickson DW, Lowe J *et al.* Diagnosis and management of dementia with Lewy bodies: third report of the DLB Consortium. *Neurology* 2005; **65**(12):1863–72.

6. McKhann G, Drachman D, Folstein M *et al.* Clinical diagnosis of Alzheimer's disease: report of the NINCDS–ADRDA Work Group under the auspices of Department of Health and Human Services Task Force on Alzheimer's Disease. *Neurology* 1984;**34**(7):939–44.

7. Roman GC, Tatemichi TK, Erkinjuntti T *et al.* Vascular dementia: diagnostic criteria for research studies. Report of the NINDS–AIREN International Workshop. *Neurology* 1993;**43**(2):250–60.

8. Hwang TJ, Masterman DL, Ortiz F, Fairbanks LA, Cummings JL. Mild cognitive impairment is associated with characteristic neuropsychiatric symptoms. *Alzheimer Disease and Associated Disorders* 2004; **18**(1):17–21.

9. Aarsland D, Cummings JL, Larsen JP. Neuropsychiatric differences between Parkinson's disease with dementia and Alzheimer's disease. *International Journal of Geriatric Psychiatry* 2001; **16**(2):184–91.

10. Litvan I, Mega MS, Cummings JL, Fairbanks L. Neuropsychiatric aspects of progressive supranuclear palsy. *Neurology* 1996;**47**(5):1184–9.

11. Litvan I, Cummings JL, Mega M. Neuropsychiatric features of corticobasal degeneration. *Journal of Neurology, Neurosurgery and Psychiatry* 1998; **65**(5):717–21.

12. Deimling GT, Bass DM. Symptoms of mental impairment among elderly adults and their effects on family caregivers. *Journal of Gerontology* 1986; **41**(6):778–84.

13. Yaffe K, Fox P, Newcomer R *et al.* Patient and caregiver characteristics and nursing home placement in patients with dementia. *Journal of the American Medical Association* 2002; **287**(16):2090–7.

14. Beeri MS, Werner P, Davidson M, Noy S. The cost of behavioral and psychological symptoms of dementia (BPSD) in community dwelling Alzheimer's disease patients. *International Journal of Geriatric Psychiatry* 2002;**17**(5):403–8.

15. Coen RF, Swanwick GR, O'Boyle CA, Coakley D. Behaviour disturbance and other predictors of carer burden in Alzheimer's disease. *International Journal of Geriatric Psychiatry* 1997;**12**(3):331–6.

16. Mourik JC, Rosso SM, Niermeijer MF, Duivenvoorden HJ, van Swieten JC, Tibben A. Frontotemporal dementia: behavioral symptoms and caregiver distress. *Dementia Geriatric Cognitive Disorders* 2004;**18**(3–4): 299–306.

17. Marin DB, Green CR, Schmeidler J *et al.* Noncognitive disturbances in Alzheimer's disease: frequency, longitudinal course, and relationship to cognitive symptoms. *Journal of the American Geriatrics Society* 1997;**45**(11):1331–8.

18. Tractenberg RE, Weiner MF, Cummings JL, Patterson MB, Thal LJ. Independence of changes in behavior from cognition and function in community-dwelling persons with Alzheimer's disease: a factor analytic approach. *Journal of Neuropsychiatry and Clinical Neurosciences* 2005;**17**(1):51–60.

19. Levy ML, Cummings JL, Fairbanks LA *et al.* Longitudinal assessment of symptoms of depression, agitation, and psychosis in 181 patients with Alzheimer's disease. *American Journal of Psychiatry* 1996;**153**(11):1438–43.

20. Hirono N, Mori E, Ishii K *et al.* Frontal lobe hypometabolism and depression in Alzheimer's disease. *Neurology* 1998;**50**(2):380–3.

21. Tekin S, Mega MS, Masterman DM *et al.* Orbitofrontal and anterior cingulate cortex neurofibrillary tangle burden is associated with agitation in Alzheimer disease. *Annals of Neurology* 2001;**49**(3):355–61.

22. Hamilton M. A rating scale for depression. *Journal of Neurology, Neurosurgery and Psychiatry* 1960;**23**:56–62.

23. Cohen-Mansfield J. Agitated behaviors in the elderly. II. Preliminary results in the cognitively

deteriorated. *Journal of the American Geriatric Society* 1986;**34**(10):722–7.

24. Alexopoulos GS, Abrams RC, Young RC, Shamoian CA. Cornell Scale for Depression in Dementia. *Biological Psychiatry* 1988;**23**(3):271–84.

25. Robert PH, Clairet S, Benoit M *et al.* The Apathy Inventory: assessment of apathy and awareness in Alzheimer's disease, Parkinson's disease, and mild cognitive impairment. *International Journal of Geriatric Psychiatry* 2002;**17**:1099–105.

26. Reisberg B, Borenstein J, Salob SP *et al.* Behavioral symptoms in Alzheimer's disease phenomenology and treatment. *Journal of Clinical Psychiatry* 1987; **48**(Suppl):9–15.

27. Cummings JL, Mega M, Gray K *et al.* The Neuropsychiatric Inventory: comprehensive assessment of psychopathology in dementia. *Neurology* 1994;**44**(12):2308–14.

28. Cummings JL. The Neuropsychiatric Inventory: assessing psychopathology in dementia patients. *Neurology* 1997;**48**(Suppl 6):S10–16.

29. Mack JL, Patterson MB, Tariot PN. Behavior Rating Scale for Dementia: development of test scales and presentation of data for 555 individuals with Alzheimer's disease. *Journal of Geriatric Psychiatry and Neurology* 1999;**12**(4):211–23.

30. McShane RH. What are the syndromes of behavioral and psychological symptoms of dementia? *International Psychogeriatrics* 2000;**12**(Suppl 1):147.

31. Burns A, Folstein S, Brandt J, Folstein M. Clinical assessment of irritability, aggression, and apathy in Huntington and Alzheimer disease. *Journal of Nervous and Mental Disease* 1990;**178**(1):20–6.

32. Hirono N, Mori E, Tanimukai S *et al.* Distinctive neurobehavioral features among neurodegenerative dementias. *Journal of Neuropsychiatry and Clinical Neurosciences* 1999;**11**(4):498–503.

33. Aarsland D, Litvan I, Larsen JP. Neuropsychiatric symptoms of patients with progressive supranuclear palsy and Parkinson's disease. *Journal of Neuropsychiatry and Clinical Neurosciences* 2001;**13**(1):42–9.

34. Kuhn DR, Greiner D, Arseneau L. Addressing hypersexuality in Alzheimer's disease. *Journal of Gerontological Nursing* 1998;**24**(4):44–50.

35. Mendez MF, Chen AK, Shapira JS, Miller BL. Acquired sociopathy and frontotemporal dementia. *Dementia and Geriatric Cognitive Disorders* 2005; **20**(2–3):99–104.

36. Senanarong V, Cummings JL, Fairbanks L *et al.* Agitation in Alzheimer's disease is a manifestation of frontal lobe dysfunction. *Dementia and Geriatric Cognitive Disorders* 2004;**17**(1–2):14–20.

37. Sultzer DL, Mahler ME, Mandelkern MA *et al.* The relationship between psychiatric symptoms and

regional cortical metabolism in Alzheimer's disease. *Journal of Neuropsychiatry and Clinical Neurosciences* 1995;**7**(4):476–84.

38. Hirono N, Mega MS, Dinov ID, Mishkin F, Cummings JL. Left frontotemporal hypoperfusion is associated with aggression in patients with dementia. *Archives of Neurology* 2000;**57**(6):861–6.

39. Franceschi M, Anchisi D, Pelati O *et al.* Glucose metabolism and serotonin receptors in the frontotemporal lobe degeneration. *Annals of Neurology* 2005;**57**(2):216–25.

40. Mendez MF, McMurtray A, Chen AK *et al.* Functional neuroimaging and presenting psychiatric features in frontotemporal dementia. *Journal of Neurology, Neurosurgery and Psychiatry* 2006;**77**(1):4–7.

41. Chemerinski E, Petracca G, Sabe L, Kremer J, Starkstein SE. The specificity of depressive symptoms in patients with Alzheimer's disease. *American Journal of Psychiatry* 2001;**158**(1):68–72.

42. Lyketsos CG, Lee HB. Diagnosis and treatment of depression in Alzheimer's disease. A practical update for the clinician. *Dementia and Geriatric Cognitive Disorders* 2004;**17**(1–2):55–64.

43. Katz IR. Diagnosis and treatment of depression in patients with Alzheimer's disease and other dementias. *Journal of Clinical Psychiatry* 1998; **59**(Suppl 9):38–44.

44. Olin JT, Schneider LS, Katz IR *et al.* Provisional diagnostic criteria for depression of Alzheimer disease. *American Journal of Geriatric Psychiatry* 2002; **10**(2):125–8.

45. Ferretti L, McCurry SM, Logsdon R, Gibbons L, Teri L. Anxiety and Alzheimer's disease. *Journal of Geriatric Psychiatry and Neurology* 2001;**14**(1):52–8.

46. Reisberg B, Auer SR, Monteiro I, Boksay I, Sclan SG. Behavioral disturbances of dementia: an overview of phenomenology and methodologic concerns. *International Psychogeriatrics* 1996;**8**(Suppl 2):169–80; discussion 181–2.

47. Fuh JL, Liu CK, Mega MS, Wang SJ, Cummings JL. Behavioral disorders and caregivers' reaction in Taiwanese patients with Alzheimer's disease. *International Psychogeriatrics* 2001;**13**(1):121–8.

48. Zubenko GS. Clinicopathologic and neurochemical correlates of major depression and psychosis in primary dementia. *International Psychogeriatrics* 1996; **8**(Suppl 3):219–23; discussion 269–72.

49. Starkstein SE, Petracca G, Chemerinski E, Kremer J. Syndromic validity of apathy in Alzheimer's disease. *American Journal of Psychiatry* 2001; **158**(6):872–7.

50. Landes AM, Sperry SD, Strauss ME, Geldmacher DS. Apathy in Alzheimer's disease. *Journal of the American Geriatric Society* 2001;**49**(12):1700–7.

51. Craig AH, Cummings JL, Fairbanks L *et al.* Cerebral blood flow correlates of apathy in Alzheimer disease. *Archives of Neurology* 1996;**53**(11):1116–20.

52. Benoit M, Koulibaly PM, Migneco O *et al.* Brain perfusion in Alzheimer's disease with and without apathy: a SPECT study with statistical parametric mapping analysis. *Psychiatry Research* 2002;**114**(2):103–11.

53. McMurtray AM, Chen AK, Shapira JS *et al.* Variations in regional SPECT hypoperfusion and clinical features in frontotemporal dementia. *Neurology* 2006;**66**:517–22.

54. Benoit M, Clairet S, Koulibaly PM, Darcourt J, Robert PH. Brain perfusion correlates of the apathy inventory dimensions of Alzheimer's disease. *International Journal of Geriatric Psychiatry* 2004;**19**(9):864–9.

55. Marshall GA, Fairbanks LA, Tekin S, Vinters HV, Cummings JL. Neuropathologic correlates of apathy in Alzheimer's disease. *Dementia and Geriatric Cognitive Disorders* 2006;**21**(3):144–7.

56. Algase DL. Wandering in dementia. *Annual Review of Nursing Research* 1999;**17**:185–217.

57. Nyatsanza S, Shetty T, Gregory C *et al.* A study of stereotypic behaviours in Alzheimer's disease and frontal and temporal variant frontotemporal dementia. *Journal of Neurology, Neurosurgery, and Psychiatry* 2003;**74**(10):1398–402.

58. Rolland Y, Payoux P, Lauwers-Cances V *et al.* A SPECT study of wandering behavior in Alzheimer's disease. *International Journal of Geriatric Psychiatry* 2005;**20**(9):816–20.

59. Simard M, van Reekum R, Cohen T. A review of the cognitive and behavioral symptoms in dementia with Lewy bodies. *Journal of Neuropsychiatry and Clinical Neurosciences* 2000;**12**(4):425–50.

60. Sultzer DL. Psychosis and antipsychotic medications in Alzheimer's disease: clinical management and research perspectives. *Dementia and Geriatric Cognitive Disorders* 2004;**17**(1–2):78–90.

61. Mosimann UP, Rowan EN, Partington CE *et al.* Characteristics of visual hallucinations in Parkinson disease dementia and dementia with Lewy bodies. *American Journal of Geriatric Psychiatry* 2006; **14**(2):153–60.

62. Mega MS, Lee L, Dinov ID *et al.* Cerebral correlates of psychotic symptoms in Alzheimer's disease. *Journal of Neurology, Neurosurgery and Psychiatry* 2000; **69**(2):167–71.

63. Kotrla KJ, Chacko RC, Harper RG, Jhingran S, Doody R. SPECT findings on psychosis in Alzheimer's disease. *American Journal of Psychiatry* 1995; **152**(10):1470–5.

64. Pasquier J, Michel BF, Brenot-Rossi I *et al.* Value of (99m)Tc-ECD SPET for the diagnosis of dementia with Lewy bodies. *European Journal of Nuclear Medicine and Molecular Imaging* 2002;**29**(10):1342–8.

65. O'Brien JT, Firbank MJ, Mosimann UP, Burn DJ, McKeith IG. Change in perfusion, hallucinations and fluctuations in consciousness in dementia with Lewy bodies. *Psychiatry Research* 2005; **139**(2):79–88.

66. Starkstein SE, Vazquez S, Petracca G *et al.* A SPECT study of delusions in Alzheimer's disease. *Neurology* 1994;**44**(11):2055–9.

67. Mentis MJ, Weinstein EA, Horwitz B *et al.* Abnormal brain glucose metabolism in the delusional misidentification syndromes: a positron emission tomography study in Alzheimer disease. *Biological Psychiatry* 1995;**38**(7):438–49.

68. Staff RT, Venneri A, Gemmell HG *et al.* HMPAO SPECT imaging of Alzheimer's disease patients with similar content-specific autobiographic delusion: comparison using statistical parametric mapping. *Journal of Nuclear Medicine* 2000;**41**(9):1451–5.

69. Perry EK, McKeith I, Thompson P *et al.* Topography, extent, and clinical relevance of neurochemical deficits in dementia of Lewy body type, Parkinson's disease, and Alzheimer's disease. *Annals of the New York Academy of Sciences* 1991;**640**:197–202.

70. Zubenko GS, Moossy J, Martinez AJ *et al.* Neuropathologic and neurochemical correlates of psychosis in primary dementia. *Archives of Neurology* 1991;**48**(6):619–24.

71. Forstl H, Burns A, Levy R, Cairns N. Neuropathological correlates of psychotic phenomena in confirmed Alzheimer's disease. *British Journal of Psychiatry* 1994;**165**(2):53–9.

72. Harding AJ, Broe GA, Halliday GM. Visual hallucinations in Lewy body disease relate to Lewy bodies in the temporal lobe. *Brain* 2002;**125**(Pt 2): 391–403.

73. Lyketsos CG, Corazzini K, Steele C. Mania in Alzheimer's disease. *Journal of Neuropsychiatry and Clinical Neurosciences* 1995;**7**(3):350–2.

74. Depp CA, Jeste DV. Bipolar disorder in older adults: a critical review. *Bipolar Disorders* 2004; **6**(5):343–67.

75. Gafoor R, O'Keane V. Three case reports of secondary mania: evidence supporting a right frontotemporal locus. *European Psychiatry* 2003;**18**(1):32–3.

76. Claggett MS. Nutritional factors relevant to Alzheimer's disease. *Journal of the American Dietetic Association* 1989;**89**(3):392–6.

77. Snowden JS, Bathgate D, Varma A *et al.* Distinct behavioural profiles in frontotemporal dementia and semantic dementia. *Journal of Neurology, Neurosurgery, and Psychiatry* 2001;**70**(3):323–32.

78. Bliwise DL. Sleep disorders in Alzheimer's disease and other dementias. *Clinical Cornerstone* 2004; **6**(Suppl 1A):S16–28.

79. Vitiello MV, Prinz PN. Alzheimer's disease. Sleep and sleep/wake patterns. *Clinics in Geriatric Medicine* 1989; 5(2):289–99.

80. Boeve BF, Silber MH, Ferman TJ, Lucas JA, Parisi JE. Association of REM sleep behavior disorder and neurodegenerative disease may reflect an underlying synucleinopathy. *Movement Disorders* 2001;16(4): 622–30.

81. Reisberg B, Franssen E, Sclan SG, Kluger A, Ferris SH. Stage specific incidence of potentially remediable behavioral symptoms in aging and Alzheimer disease. *Bulletin of Clinical Neurosciences* 1989;54:95–112.

82. Sultzer DL, Levin HS, Mahler ME, High WM, Cummings JL. A comparison of psychiatric symptoms in vascular dementia and Alzheimer's disease. *American Journal of Psychiatry* 1993;150(12): 1806–12.

83. Aharon-Peretz J, Kliot D, Tomer R. Behavioral differences between white matter lacunar dementia and Alzheimer's disease: a comparison on the neuropsychiatric inventory. *Dementia and Geriatric Cognitive Disorders* 2000;11(5):294–8.

84. Fuh JL, Wang SJ, Cummings JL. Neuropsychiatric profiles in patients with Alzheimer's disease and vascular dementia. *Journal of Neurology, Neurosurgery and Psychiatry* 2005;76(10):1337–41.

85. Ikeda M, Fukuhara R, Shigenobu K et al. Dementia associated mental and behavioural disturbances in elderly people in the community: findings from the first Nakayama study. *Journal of Neurology, Neurosurgery and Psychiatry* 2004;75(1):146–8.

86. Srikanth S, Nagaraja AV, Ratnavalli E. Neuropsychiatric symptoms in dementia: frequency, relationship to dementia severity and comparison in Alzheimer's disease, vascular dementia and frontotemporal dementia. *Journal of the Neurological Sciences* 2005;236(1–2):43–8.

87. Kales HC, Maixner DF, Mellow AM. Cerebrovascular disease and late-life depression. *American Journal of Geriatric Psychiatry* 2005;13(2):88–98.

88. Gorno-Tempini ML, Dronkers NF, Rankin KP et al. Cognition and anatomy in three variants of primary progressive aphasia. *Annals of Neurology* 2004; 55(3):335–46.

89. Mendez MF, Perryman KM, Miller BL, Cummings JL. Behavioral differences between frontotemporal dementia and Alzheimer's disease: a comparison on the BEHAVE-AD rating scale. *International Psychogeriatrics* 1998;10(2):155–62.

90. Bozeat S, Gregory CA, Ralph MA, Hodges JR. Which neuropsychiatric and behavioural features distinguish frontal and temporal variants of frontotemporal dementia from Alzheimer's disease? *Journal of Neurology, Neurosurgery and Psychiatry* 2000; 69(2):178–86.

91. Marczinski CA, Davidson W, Kertesz A. A longitudinal study of behavior in frontotemporal dementia and primary progressive aphasia. *Cognitive and Behavioral Neurology* 2004;17(4):185–90.

92. Aarsland D, Ballard C, Larsen JP, McKeith I. A comparative study of psychiatric symptoms in dementia with Lewy bodies and Parkinson's disease with and without dementia. *International Journal of Geriatric Psychiatry* 2001;16(5):528–36.

93. Boxer AL, Geschwind MD, Belfor N et al. Patterns of brain atrophy that differentiate corticobasal degeneration syndrome from progressive supranuclear palsy. *Archives of Neurology* 2006;63(1):81–6.

94. Cohen-Mansfield J. Use of patient characteristics to determine nonpharmacologic interventions for behavioral and psychological symptoms of dementia. *International Psychogeriatrics* 2000;12 (Suppl 1): 373–80.

95. Teri L. Combined therapy: a research overview. *International Psychogeriatrics* 2000;12(Suppl 1): 381–6.

96. Cohen-Mansfield J. Nonpharmacologic interventions for inappropriate behaviors in dementia: a review, summary, and critique. *American Journal of Geriatric Psychiatry* 2001;9(4):361–81.

97. Emre M, Aarsland D, Albanese A et al. Rivastigmine for dementia associated with Parkinson's disease. *New England Journal of Medicine* 2004;351(24): 2509–18.

98. Sink KM, Holden KF, Yaffe K. Pharmacological treatment of neuropsychiatric symptoms of dementia: a review of the evidence. *Journal of the American Medical Association* 2005;293(5):596–608.

99. Wynn ZJ, Cummings JL. Cholinesterase inhibitor therapies and neuropsychiatric manifestations of Alzheimer's disease. *Dementia and Geriatric Cognitive Disorders* 2004;17(1–2):100–8.

100. Gauthier S, Wirth Y, Mobius HJ. Effects of memantine on behavioural symptoms in Alzheimer's disease patients: an analysis of the Neuropsychiatric Inventory (NPI) data of two randomised, controlled studies. *International Journal of Geriatric Psychiatry* 2005; 20(5):459–64.

101. Taragano FE, Lyketsos CG, Mangone CA, Allegri RF, Comesana-Diaz E. A double-blind, randomized, fixed-dose trial of fluoxetine vs. amitriptyline in the treatment of major depression complicating Alzheimer's disease. *Psychosomatics* 1997;38(3): 246–52.

102. Katona CL, Hunter BN, Bray J. A double-blind comparison of the efficacy and safety of paroxetine and imipramine in the treatment of depression with dementia. *International Journal of Geriatric Psychiatry* 1998;13(2):100–8.

103. Huey ED, Putnam KT, Grafman J. A systematic review of neurotransmitter deficits and treatments in frontotemporal dementia. *Neurology* 2006; **66**(1):17–22.

104. Schneider LS, Dagerman KS, Insel P. Risk of death with atypical antipsychotic drug treatment for dementia: meta-analysis of randomized placebo-controlled trials. *Journal of the American Medical Association* 2005;**294**(15):1934–43.

105. US Food and Drug Administration. FDA Public Health Advisory: deaths with antipsychotics in elderly patients with behavioral disturbances. Washington, DC: US Food and Drug Administration. http://www.fda.gov/cder/drug/advisory/antipsychotics.htm (accessed March 3, 2006).

106. Wang PS, Schneeweiss S, Avorn J *et al*. Risk of death in elderly users of conventional vs. atypical antipsychotic medications. *New England Journal of Medicine* 2005; **353**(22):2335–41.

Chapter 8

Neuroimaging in dementia

Maria Carmela Tartaglia and Howard Rosen

Introduction

Despite the tremendous technological advancement in medicine, diagnosis of dementia caused by neurodegenerative disease continues to be made almost exclusively based on the clinical interpretation of patients' symptoms, supported by cognitive assessment with neuropsychological testing. Not surprisingly, the accuracy of diagnosis varies with the expertise of the center where a patient is evaluated, and with the rarity of the clinical presentation.[1,2] For unusual clinical presentations, accuracy can be disappointingly low.[3] In addition, diagnosis of neurodegenerative diseases that cause dementia is currently not made until an individual's level of cognitive impairment has already robbed them of their ability to work and perform other functions important for self-esteem and independence, such as driving and management of their finances.

The introduction of computed tomographic (CT) scanning in the 1970s offered the possibility of safe, non-invasive visualization of the human brain in vivo. Since that time, the chief goals for brain imaging in dementia have been quite simple: first, to facilitate early diagnosis by differentiating patients with neurodegenerative disease from normal individuals at the earliest possible time in the illness; and, second, to differentiate various causes of neurodegeneration, such as Alzheimer's disease (AD), frontotemporal dementia (FTD), dementia with Lewy bodies (DLB), corticobasal degeneration (CBD) and progressive supranuclear palsy (PSP), from each other. While early diagnosis offers the best opportunity for preserving function, accurate diagnosis is critical so that treatments can be tailored to the specific disease. The first step toward achieving these goals is the exclusion of non-neurodegenerative diseases mimicking

neurodegenerative dementias. While such entities are not as common as AD,[4] structural imaging with CT or magnetic resonance imaging (MRI) are usually extremely sensitive to them. In contrast, neurodegenerative diseases do not cause gross structural abnormalities that are easily differentiated from normal aging. Therefore, researchers have had to develop more sophisticated approaches to help with the differential diagnosis of degenerative dementias.

Neurodegenerative diseases cause a complex set of changes in the brain, the earliest of which are believed to be metabolic abnormalities that emerge secondary to the accumulation of abnormal proteins within neurons and glial cells. These proteins differ depending upon the neurodegenerative condition; β-amyloid 42 in AD, α-synuclein in DLB, tau or TAR DNA-binding protein (TDP-43) in FTD and prion proteins in Creutzfeldt–Jakob disease (CJD). These abnormal proteins lead to a cascade of changes, including loss of neuronal function with neurotransmitter dysfunction, loss of synapses and ultimately cell death. Ideally, brain-imaging technology should strive to measure the most specific and earliest of these changes, such as the accumulation of disease-specific proteins. While we appear to be at the dawn of an era where this will be possible, most of the imaging research in dementia to date has attempted to quantify structural and functional changes that occur in association with cell dysfunction or cell death. These efforts have been pursued using a variety of imaging technologies. The goal of this chapter is to provide a broad overview of the various methods that have been used to image neurodegenerative disease and to highlight the relative advantages and disadvantages of each. As will be discussed at the end of the chapter, even as we gain the ability to image the most specific abnormalities associated with neurodegeneration, it is unlikely that any single technique will be sufficient for diagnosis, but rather a combination of techniques will be useful for making a diagnosis and possibly for guiding treatment.

The Behavioral Neurology of Dementia, eds. Bruce L. Miller and Bradley F. Boeve. Published by Cambridge University Press.

Regional changes in basic metabolism and structure

Each degenerative disease appears to selectively affect specific regions of the brain; consequently the pattern of regional dysfunction or atrophy is a clue to diagnosis. The earliest studies documenting these changes were conducted with metabolic imaging using radioactive materials, but more recently, increasingly sophisticated analysis of structural imaging has revealed parallel findings in the patterns of tissue loss in dementia, suggesting that these changes can be measured more easily, and at a lower cost than previously estimated.

Glucose metabolism and brain perfusion
Positron emission tomography and single-photon emission computed tomography

Brain imaging with radioactively labeled compounds, usually administered intravenously, has long been a mainstay in the study of neurodegenerative disease. The most commonly used techniques are single-photon emission computed tomography (SPECT) and positron emission tomography (PET). Both SPECT and PET can be used to measure the uptake of a variety of compounds. The most reliable SPECT method has used ^{99m}Tc-labeled hexamethylpropyleneamine oxime (HMPAO), which crosses the blood–brain barrier and is taken up in proportional relationship to blood flow, allowing the tracking of cerebral perfusion. The PET compound most efficiently used in diagnosis is [^{18}F]-fluorodeoxyglucose (FDG), which crosses the blood–brain barrier and is taken up by metabolically active cells, thus providing a measure of brain activity. These techniques provide unique information about brain function that may not be available with structural imaging, and they can show metabolic abnormalities in structurally normal brain.

One of the first techniques to show a specific abnormality in AD was FDG-PET; the parietal and superior/posterior temporal regions show reduced glucose metabolism in those with AD compared with normal older control subjects.[5] Subsequent studies have consistently demonstrated bilateral temporoparietal hypoperfusion or hypometabolism in patients with AD (Fig. 8.1, closed arrows).[6,7] In the late 1990s, studies began to suggest that the earliest of these changes occurred in the medial portion of the parietal cortex, in the posterior cingulate or retrosplenial region (Fig. 8.1, open arrows).[8] Frontal lobe hypoperfusion is often also reported in AD, but usually in

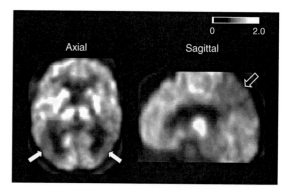

Fig. 8.1. Fluorodeoxyglucose (FDG) positron emission tomography of a patient with Alzheimer's disease showing subtle regional decreases in FDG uptake in the posterior temporal lobes (closed arrows) and the posterior cingulated region (open arrow).

conjunction with temporoparietal abnormalities.[8] These findings suggest that PET and SPECT can be helpful in discriminating patients with clinically diagnosed AD from age-matched controls as well as from patients with vascular dementia (VaD) and FTD.[9] Use of FDG-PET has better sensitivity but lower specificity than SPECT for discriminating AD from normal aging.[10,11] A histopathological study revealed that FDG-PET had a sensitivity of 93% and a specificity of 63% in predicting a pathological diagnosis of AD.[12] This was in contrast to clinical diagnosis of AD, which had a high specificity (100%) but lower sensitivity (75%). Studies with SPECT have a sensitivity of 63% and a specificity of 93% unless combined with clinical diagnosis, where the combination of SPECT evidence of temporoparietal hypoperfusion and clinical diagnosis of AD has a sensitivity of 96% and a specificity of 84%.[13] Thus, regional metabolism studied with PET and SPECT clearly correlates with the presence of neurodegenerative disease; however, these techniques have not yet been perfected to the point where they have the specificity and sensitivity to substitute for a clinical diagnosis.

In recent years, the clinical syndrome of mild cognitive impairment (MCI) has received a great deal of attention as a stage where early diagnosis of AD may be possible. Patients with MCI are at high risk for progression to AD, converting to dementia at a rate of about 12% per year.[14] A number of studies have found that the severity of temporoparietal metabolism as estimated by FDG-PET is helpful in distinguishing patients with a progressive course from those with a non-progressive course.[15–18] Posterior cingulate hypometabolism on SPECT has also been used to predict progression in this setting.[19]

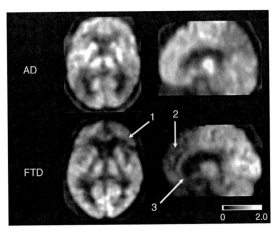

Fig. 8.2. Fluorodeoxyglucose (FDG) positron emission tomography of the same patient as in Fig. 8.1 as well as another patient with frontotemporal dementia (FTD), showing decreased FDG uptake in the lateral (1), medial (2) and orbital (3) portions of the frontal lobe in FTD. AD, Alzheimer's disease.

The observation that AD is associated with metabolic abnormalities in the temporal and parietal regions complements the observation that the non-AD dementias are associated with hypometabolism in different regions, suggesting that PET and SPECT can assist in differential diagnosis. One of the most useful of these observations has been the fact that FTD is associated with hypometabolism in the frontal and anterior temporal regions, which has been demonstrated to separate FTLD from AD (Fig. 8.2).[20,21–24] A recent study of patients with AD and FTD whose diagnoses were ultimately confirmed at autopsy showed that FDG-PET increases diagnostic accuracy beyond clinical features alone.[25] In contrast, DLB is associated with decreased occipitotemporal metabolism compared with AD, consistent with the increased difficulty such patients have with visual processing.[26–28]

In an effort to estimate the overall utility of metabolic imaging in differentiating various forms of dementia, Talbot et al.[29] conducted a large study of SPECT in a group of patients with dementia from a variety of causes including AD, frontotemporal lobar degeneration (FTLD), VaD and DLB, and they identified specific patterns predictive of the clinical diagnosis, including patchy regions of hypometabolism suggestive of VaD, frontal hypometabolism suggestive of FTLD, and temporoparietal metabolism suggestive of AD. These findings were consistent with a study in a group of patients suffering from various dementias who had autopsy confirmation of diagnosis,

which showed that SPECT imaging can be highly accurate in identifying the type of dementia.[30]

Regional brain metabolism studied with PET and SPECT has often been linked with cognitive and behavioral changes in dementia.[31,32] In one of the earliest studies, Haxby et al.[33] used PET to demonstrate that right–left hemisphere metabolic asymmetry in AD correlated with the degree of language versus visuospatial impairment. Subsequently, metabolic imaging has also been used to link metabolism to function in a variety of cognitive and behavioral domains, including memory, which has been linked to hippocampal metabolism;[34] awareness of deficit, which has been linked to right frontal metabolism;[35] and behavioral/emotional variables such as apathy, which is linked to metabolism in the anterior cingulate region.[36]

In summary, metabolic imaging with PET and SPECT helps to differentiate patients with neurodegenerative disease from normal older individuals and to discriminate between various causes of dementia. These techniques are not yet sufficiently accurate to substitute for clinical judgement, but in some cases they can supplement the clinical assessment to improve the accuracy of diagnosis. One such example is the differentiation of FTLD from AD. Additionally, the fact that these measures correlate with the level of behavioral and cognitive impairment suggest that they may be useful surrogate markers in clinical trials of therapeutic agents.[37] For example, improved cerebral metabolism with treatment might predict drug efficacy. This hypothesis has yet to be fully confirmed, but studies have demonstrated preserved or increased glucose metabolism in patients with AD after treatment with cholinesterase inhibitors.[38,39]

Problems with SPECT and particularly PET include expense, lack of availability and the required use of radioactive materials. As detailed below, MRI and CT may be capable of obtaining diagnostically equivalent data using perfusion techniques, and structural imaging with MRI is also yielding similar information about regional brain abnormalities, potentially eliminating the need for PET and SPECT regional metabolic studies.

Regional cerebral perfusion measured with magnetic resonance and computed tomography

Regional cerebral blood volumes can be quantified with MRI by magnetically labeling water molecules in the arteries prior to their entry into the brain and then tracking these molecules as they enter the cerebral tissues, a technique referred to as arterial spin labeling. Using MRI, several investigators have shown reduced cerebral perfusion in AD in the medial and lateral parietal, superior temporal and lateral frontal lobes – the same regions where SPECT and PET demonstrate abnormalities.[40–42] Perfusion MRI in FTD has also demonstrated decreased frontal perfusion and increased parietal perfusion relative to AD, with frontal perfusion deficits in FTD being correlated with deficits in judgement and problem solving.[43] While MR perfusion is less expensive than PET and SPECT, and does not involve exposure to radioactivity, the technique has not yet matured to the point that it is an adequate substitute for PET and SPECT imaging. This is because MR perfusion studies are based on MR imaging approaches such as echo-planar imaging, which are highly susceptible to distortion or loss of signals in the parts of the brain adjacent to air-filled bone.[44,45] Thus, orbital and inferior temporal regions, which are adjacent to air-filled sinuses in the skull, are not yet well imaged with this technique. As methods evolve to avoid these problems, MR perfusion may become a more and more attractive technique in dementia research.

Similarly, CT is now capable of tracking cerebral perfusion using intravenous contrast. Although this has rarely been used to study dementia,[46] CT scanning may offer another relatively inexpensive approach to tracking regional changes occurring in dementia.

Regional tissue content/atrophy

Many of the metabolic abnormalities described with PET and SPECT are visible to the naked eye, which can easily detect that some regions of the brain are drawing less glucose or blood than others. In contrast, because normal aging causes a significant degree of cerebral volume loss, it can be more difficult to appreciate whether certain brain regions are disproportionately atrophied. The ability to acquire increasingly higher resolution images of the brain and the emergence of more powerful techniques for structural image analysis have allowed the routine measurement of atrophy in various brain regions, with findings that are remarkably concordant with metabolic studies.

Regional tissue content with computed tomography

Computed tomography is the most widely used technique for scanning the brain, and creates images using X-rays. Because it was the first technique to provide a detailed image of the brain, it has the longest history of use in dementia. In 1975, the first report appeared highlighting the utility of CT scans in separating dementia cases from possibly reversible causes of cognitive impairment.[47] Although CT can delineate many non-degenerative causes of dementia, most patients with uncomplicated, persistent and progressive memory impairment do not suffer from a non-degenerative condition. In a large study of 513 patients referred to a memory clinic, CT scanning failed to reveal any reversible causes that were not picked up clinically in the 362 patients who were demented.[48]

Early use of CT also included prognostication regarding disease progression. For instance, patients with moderate or severe cerebral atrophy were found to have a worse short-term prognosis than those with questionable or mild atrophy.[49] Although CT scanning is still regularly used for diagnostic assessments and for studies of brain–behavior correlation,[50] its resolution is much lower than that of MRI; consequently, research on most aspects of degenerative dementias has moved away from CT scanning.

Regional tissue content with magnetic resonance imaging

Most modern structural imaging in dementia has used MRI, which acquires brain images with magnetic fields and radiowaves. There are a number of good review articles concerning structural imaging in dementia, particularly in AD.[51–59]

One of the most straightforward approaches to structural image analysis is to measure the volume of specific regions that might be particularly impacted by a disease of interest. Usually, this is accomplished by circling the region on a series of two-dimensional images. In AD, the medial temporal lobes, in particular the hippocampus and entorhinal cortex, are among the earliest sites of pathological involvement.[60] For this reason, many studies have focused on hippocampal volumes and demonstrated decreased volumes in AD compared with age-matched controls.[61–68] Also, volumes in the adjacent entorhinal cortex are reduced in AD,[61,64,67–69] consistent with the fact that this may be the earliest site of neuronal pathology.[60] However, the hippocampus and entorhinal cortex are not unique in showing decreased volume in patients with AD. Other regions include the amygdala,[65] anterior parahippocampal gyrus,[65] corpus callosum[70,71] and the frontal,[72] temporal[64,72] and occipital lobes,[72] indicating that much of the brain shrinks in AD.

In the past, regional volume measurements were limited to selected portions of the medial temporal lobe, or to large lobar structures that are relatively easy to identify. More recently, investigators have begun to measure smaller cortical regions such as the cingulate cortex, which metabolic studies suggest might show reduced posterior volume. This method offers the possibility of bringing volumetric imaging in line with metabolic studies by breaking the cerebral cortex into smaller structures that might show disproportionate volume loss compared with the rest of the brain. A recent study of cingulate volumes in familial AD suggests that this approach is valuable.[73] Jones and colleagues measured four regions of the cingulate cortex, including the rostral and caudal parts of the anterior cingulate, as well as the posterior and retrosplenial cingulate. All areas of the cingulate cortex were reduced in volume in AD compared with controls, although the posterior cingulate cortex was more atrophied than the other segments. Imaging with MRI has also been used to study patients with MCI. Several studies have shown that hippocampal volumes[74] and volumes in other brain regions[75] predict the likelihood of progression, although precise prognostication in an individual is still not achievable.

The utility of regional volume loss in the diagnosis of AD remains unsettled. As is the case with metabolic studies, most imaging studies are performed using clinical diagnosis as the "gold standard," and very few studies have been done in autopsy-confirmed patient groups. In most volumetric studies, there is at least some overlap between patients and controls, so imaging measures correctly identify between 80 and 100% of patients, depending on the study and the region being measured. Given that most of these patients are clearly demented at the time of study, the added value of imaging in this setting is questionable.

All the research described above used cross-sectional approaches. Another approach taken by some investigators has been to look at longitudinal changes. These studies have demonstrated greater atrophy rates in whole brain volume,[76-83] hippocampus,[84-86] entorhinal cortex[85,87] and the temporal area as a whole,[85,88,89] both in AD and in MCI compared with age-matched controls. Some of these studies have demonstrated that rates of atrophy are another feature predicting conversion from MCI to dementia.[86]

Structural imaging has also been studied as a means of differentiating various causes of dementia. This has been studied extensively in FTLD, where early observations documented visible volume loss in the frontal and anterior temporal regions, and subsequent studies have gone on to quantify these changes. The term FTLD serves as the overarching name for a set of disorders with different clinical manifestations, all associated with a predominance of frontal and/or temporal pathology. Structural imaging studies using MRI have demonstrated that the behavioral variant of FTD is associated with reduced frontal lobe volumes compared with controls, while semantic dementia (SD) shows reduced temporal lobe volumes.[90,91] Frontal and temporal volumes in these syndromes are significantly smaller in FTD and SD than in AD. One recent study showed that frontal lobe volumes correctly classified 93% of patients with FTD, but specificity compared with patients with AD was not reported.[92] A recent study demonstrated hippocampal and amygdala atrophy in both AD and FTLD compared with controls.[93] After segregating the different FTLD subtypes into SD and the behavioral variant of FTD, they found smaller hippocampal and amygdala volumes in SD compared with the frontal variant.

While lobar, hippocampal and amygdala volumes are useful in discriminating between dementia etiologies, techniques for analyzing tissue loss in specific subregions of the frontal and temporal lobes have been even more revealing. Many of these findings were facilitated by a technique called voxel-based morphometry (VBM). In contrast to region-of-interest-based techniques, where a specific region is identified and circled in each individual, VBM quantifies regional tissue content by resizing each subject's image to fit into a standardized space, so that a given coordinate in this space should correspond to the same anatomical structure in every subject.[94] The resolution of the technique is on the order of 1–2 cm, so relatively small regions can be related to diagnosis or other conditions of interest without an a-priori hypothesis about their size, shape or location. Thus, the technique allows the analysis of changes across the entire brain in a much shorter time than can be accomplished using manually identified regions of interest.

Studies using VBM in FTLD have revealed that the disorder is associated in general with loss of gray matter in the frontal and temporal lobes, but it is particularly associated with loss in the ventromedial frontal cortex, the posterior orbital frontal regions, the insula bilaterally and the left anterior cingulate cortex.[90] These regions are frontal components of the

105

brain's emotional processing systems,[95] so their involvement in FTLD explains the unique behavioral symptoms seen in that disorder. These findings are consistent with autopsy studies demonstrating progressive changes in these same regions in increasingly advanced cases of FTD,[96] and also with PET and SPECT studies showing similar patterns of metabolic impairment in FTD as in AD.[97] The SD subgroup also showed atrophy in the amygdala, which is a critical component of basic emotional processing.[98] Because VBM looks for relationships with behavior across many regions of the brain, statistical corrections are necessary for the many comparisons in every analysis,[99] potentially limiting the sensitivity of the technique, particularly for single subject analysis.

While most studies examining structural differences across dementia syndromes looked at clinically diagnosed populations, recent studies have extended these findings to autopsy-confirmed patients. A recent study using VBM in a group of 21 patients with pathologically confirmed FTD demonstrated atrophy of the inferior and medial temporal regions as well as the inferior frontal lobes in the FTD group compared with controls.[100] Recently, Rabinovici et al.[101] compared patients with pathologically confirmed FTLD and AD and verified that the medial frontal, orbitofrontal and insular volume changes in FTLD were more severe than in AD, whereas AD was associated with more significant changes in the parietal and occipital regions, as would be expected based on the metabolic studies. In addition, ventral striatal volumes were decreased in FTLD compared with AD.

Structural imaging has also demonstrated significant relationships between local changes in brain volume and cognitive or behavioral changes in dementia. In AD, several studies have found correlations between hippocampal volumes and episodic memory performance, consistent with the long-established role for this structure in memory consolidation.[102] Disproportionate loss of visuospatial function in AD, as indicated by very poor figure copying, has been linked to right lateral temporal tissue loss.[103] Many studies of non-AD dementias, particularly FTLD, have yielded findings that shed light on poorly understood frontal and anterior temporal brain functions. For instance, in the language domain, intensive study of word knowledge in dementia has helped to define the role of the temporal lobes in semantic processing. Picture naming in FTLD, which relies on an intact semantic memory, correlates with tissue content in the temporal lobe,[90,104] and recent studies

have further defined this role by showing a dissociation between naming of living stimuli, which appears to depend on right medial anterior temporal region, and naming of non-living stimuli, which is associated with tissue content in the left posterior middle temporal gyrus.[104] Structural imaging has elucidated important information regarding the role of various brain regions in emotional processing. Right anterior temporal tissue volume in dementia is associated with the ability to identify facial expressions of emotion[105] and with empathy,[106] which explains, in part, the profound insensitivity seen in patients with FTLD, particularly those with right temporal involvement.[107] In addition, other behaviors in FTLD correlate with specific subregions within the frontal and insular cortex. Disinhibition correlates with anterior cingulate atrophy, while apathy correlates with right medial frontal atrophy, which suggests differing roles for these regions in the regulation of goal-directed behavior.[108] Right insular and orbitofrontal tissue loss has been correlated with overeating in FTLD, consistent with the role these structures play in processing food rewards.[109,110] Many of the findings discussed above were identified using VBM, as well as manual identification of regions of interest.

Another technique for structural image analysis is the measurement of cortical thickness. Similar to VBM, cortical thickness mapping examines changes in structure across the entire cerebrum; however, rather than averaging the amount of tissue in a particular volume of space, this technique measures the thickness of cerebral cortex under each segment of the cerebral cortical surface. A recent application of this technique to AD and MCI found decreases in mean cortical thickness in both groups compared with controls, with those with MCI showing an intermediate thickness between normal elderly and AD.[111] The largest degree of thinning in AD and MCI was in the inferior and middle temporal gyri. These results are consistent with autopsy studies in normal aging and AD, showing cortical thinning as a result of cytoarchitectural changes such as neuronal loss, synaptic degeneration and cell shrinkage.[112–114] Cortical thickness measurement has also demonstrated differences between AD and FTLD similar to those identified using VBM.[115]

In summary, structural imaging, particularly with MRI, has advanced impressively since the advent of CT, with increasingly higher resolution images. Although at first glance the main structural change in dementia, atrophy, appears to be more diffuse than

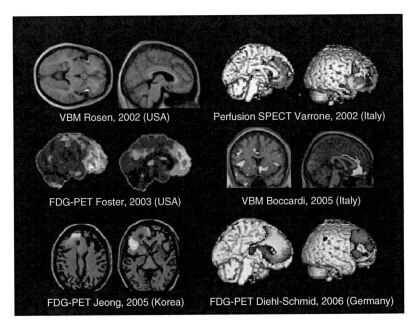

VBM Rosen, 2002 (USA)

Perfusion SPECT Varrone, 2002 (Italy)

FDG-PET Foster, 2003 (USA)

VBM Boccardi, 2005 (Italy)

FDG-PET Jeong, 2005 (Korea)

FDG-PET Diehl-Schmid, 2006 (Germany)

Fig. 8.3. Imaging findings in frontotemporal dementia from various groups. All show a similar pattern of changes affecting the medial and orbital portions of the frontal lobes. VBM, voxel-based morphometry of structural magnetic resonance imaging (USA,[90] Italy[116]); FDG-PET, fluorodeoxyglucose positron emission tomography (USA,[117] Korea,[118] Germany[119]); perfusion SPECT, perfusion single-photon emission computed tomography (Italy[120]).

the metabolic deficits described above, careful attention to specific regions of interest has identified the types of abnormality that would be expected based on the known patterns of pathology in dementia, and that are specific to the cause of neurodegeneration. Emerging techniques for examining changes across the entire brain relatively quickly, such as VBM and cortical thickness mapping, have made it easier to identify these regionally specific patterns of atrophy, and demonstrated patterns of atrophy that are remarkably consistent with the metabolic deficits identified using PET and SPECT scanning. Figure 8.3 illustrates the remarkable overlap in findings between metabolic and structural imaging studies performed by different research groups around the world. As with metabolic imaging, MRI-based measures do not appear to be sensitive or specific enough to substitute for the clinical evaluation. Like metabolic imaging, MRI measures of regional volume clearly correlate with patients' cognitive and behavioral status. The fact that MR scanners are ubiquitous and less expensive to use than PET and SPECT machines makes MRI an attractive alternative to these techniques. Whether the abnormalities seen with structural imaging are more sensitive or less sensitive to disease than metabolic imaging has not yet been determined. One potential disadvantage to MRI that must be considered is that structural changes may evolve more slowly than metabolic changes; consequently, the question of which

might be more useful for following disease progression or treatment effects must be studied before one could be chosen for this purpose.

In addition, while regional reductions in glucose metabolism, perfusion and tissue content have been the focus of the great majority of imaging studies in dementia, alternative techniques for brain imaging have begun to be more commonly applied to dementia, offering opportunities to study different aspects of neurodegenerative disease.

Alternative structural analyses
Diffusion-weighted imaging and diffusion tensor imaging

Diffusion-weighted imaging (DWI) with MRI is based on the analysis of the random motion of water molecules in the brain. In many cases, local cerebral pathology, such as stroke, leads to decreased local diffusion. Probably the most meaningful application of simple DWI in neurodegenerative disease is in CJD, where decreased diffusion in cerebral cortex (called "cortical ribboning"), often with associated decreased diffusion in the basal ganglia, is highly sensitive and specific for the diagnosis of CJD (sensitivity of 91%, specificity of 95%) (Fig. 8.4).[121] Variant CJD is often associated with high signals in the pulvinar region, with a sensitivity of 78% and specificity of 100% in one study.[122]

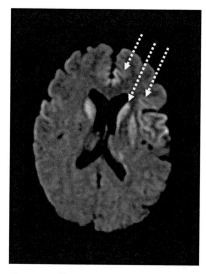

Fig. 8.4. Diffusion-weighted abnormalities (arrows) in the basal ganglia and cortical ribboning in Creutzfeld-Jakob disease. (Image courtesy of Michael Geschwind and Paolo Vitali, UCSF.)

An important variation of DWI is diffusion tensor imaging (DTI). Whereas DWI evaluates diffusion of water in all directions, DTI evaluates diffusion of water separately in each of the three main directions (right/left, front/back, up/down) in the brain. The key to understanding how DTI works lies in the distinction between isotropic and *an*isotropic diffusion. Isotropic diffusion refers to the state when molecules are diffusing equally in all directions. Anisotropic diffusion refers to when molecules are diffusing more in a particular direction than in other directions. This anisotropic diffusion, where there is coherent molecular motion, can also be called "flow." Anisotropic diffusion and isotropic diffusion have different effects on the MR signal, which enables diffusion measurements to be acquired. In certain biological structures, such as muscle or axonal fibers, there is an ordered arrangement that causes the diffusion of water to be significantly greater along the axis of those fibers. In healthy white matter tracts, an extensive number of neuronal axons all traveling in the same direction means that this tissue will have a high degree of anisotropic diffusion in a particular direction.[123–126] Therefore, diffusion measurements can provide information concerning the type of matter present in a given voxel, as well as its orientation, using a parameter called fractional anisotropy. These analyses are often aided by identifying tracts of interest in each individual, a technique sometimes referred to as tractography. Although most of the pathology in neurodegenerative

diseases, particularly in AD, occurs in gray matter, this has secondary effects on white matter. Increasing disorganization in white matter tracts would decrease the anisotropy of diffusion along the tract. Accordingly, altered diffusion has been reported in the temporal lobe white matter, posterior cerebral white matter, and corpus callosum of patients with very mild and moderate AD.[41,127–129] Recently, Zhang et al.[130] identified reduced fractional anisotropy in the portion of the cingulum bundle connecting the hippocampus to the posterior cingulate region in patients with MCI and AD compared with controls. The use of this measure provided improved classification of patients from controls compared with hippocampal volumes alone.[130] White matter tract integrity has also been correlated with measures of episodic memory in AD and MCI.[131]

Diffusion tensor imaging is also being used more to examine differences across dementia subtypes. A recent study found decreased fractional anisotropy in the parietal lobes in DLB compared with AD, consistent with the metabolic studies and with the prominent visuospatial difficulties often seen in these patients.[132] In FTD, decreased fractional anisotropy has been identified in the superior longitudinal fasciculus, which connects frontal and parietal regions, while SD shows decreased fractional anisotropy in the inferior longitudinal fasciculus, connecting temporal with parietal regions. Integrity of the superior longitudinal fasciculus in this study was correlated with a clinical measure of behavior and executive function.[133]

Alternative metabolic and functional approaches

Magnetic resonance spectroscopy

In vivo proton magnetic resonance spectroscopy (^{1}H MRS) with MRI allows non-invasive sampling of brain chemistry by measuring the levels of relatively few specific metabolites, including N-acetyl-aspartate (NAA), choline, creatine, lactate and glutamate. Because NAA is thought to be a marker of neuronal integrity, many studies have focused on NAA content in patients with dementia. Content of NAA is consistently reported as lower in patients with AD compared with cognitively normal elderly subjects, in various portions of the brain[134–138] and in the parietal gray matter and hippocampus.[139,140] A different pattern of NAA loss has been reported in VaD, with the greatest losses in the frontal and parietal cortex but no significant losses in the medial temporal lobe.[141] Thalamic lacunes were associated with greater NAA reductions in the frontal cortex than lacunes located outside the thalamus, which supports the idea that disruption of subcortical–cortical connections may contribute to cognitive dysfunction in VaD. Myoinositol, a marker associated with gliosis, has also been reported as high in patients with AD.[135] Decreased NAA and increased myo-inositol have also been reported in MCI.[142]

A few studies of non-AD dementias have used ^{1}H MRS, including FTD,[143,144] prion diseases,[145] Huntington's disease[146] and acquired immunodeficiency syndrome–dementia complex.[147] In one study comparing patients with AD and FTD, the NAA/creatine ratio was reduced in the posterior cingulate cortex in those with AD and FTD/Pick's disease, but the patients with AD showed a greater decrease posteriorly while the patients with FTD/Pick's disease displayed greater frontal decreases.[148] Proton MRS has also been used, though relatively infrequently, for brain–behavior correlations.

Iron-dependent T$_2$-weighted contrast with magnetic resonance

Iron-dependent T$_2$-weighted contrast has been reported as increased in a number of regions in AD, including the hippocampus, entorhinal cortex, globus pallidus, putamen and caudate.[149–151] Although, the significance of the increased iron is still being investigated, there appears to be increasing reports to suggest that altered iron metabolism or its accumulation is associated with toxicity or cell injury.

Functional activation using magnetic resonance imaging

With the exception of MR perfusion, the MR techniques discussed until now measure structural features of the brain that change very slowly over time in neurodegenerative disease. They are a consequence of microscopic changes in neuronal structure (for instance synaptic and dendritic complexity), which influence neuronal function and so structural changes will correlate with changes in behavior. Since the late 1980s, it has also been possible to study brain activity related to cognitive processing using PET, most commonly using radiolabeled water.[152] This is because increased synaptic activity leads to local increases in blood flow; as a result, blood flow during a task of interest can be compared with blood flow during a comparison task to identify regions selectively involved in the task of interest. This phenomenon can now be studied with functional MRI (fMRI), which has largely supplanted PET scanning for this purpose. Most commonly, this is accomplished by measuring the blood oxygen level-dependent (BOLD) signal, which occurs because the local increases in blood flow associated with synaptic activity are in excess of what is needed to supply metabolic demand; consequently these vessels contain blood that is relatively high in oxygenated hemoglobin, and the corresponding oxidized state of the iron causes local increases in magnetic susceptibility.[153] The ability of MRI to measure indirectly synaptic activity in response to cognitive demands provides an approach that may be the best correlate of cognitive performance and may be a promising technique for following disease progression and treatment response. The tasks can be tailored to examine specific domains of function pertinent to whatever subtype of dementia is being studied.

Brain activation patterns in dementia have shown variable results. The simplest prediction for fMRI studies would be that decreased performance in dementia would be associated with decreased BOLD signal, implying decreased synaptic activity during relevant cognitive tasks. In contrast to this prediction, several studies have shown increased activation in AD, particularly in the early stages of the disease. Saykin et al.[154] assessed semantic processing in mild AD and found that patients activated regions not activated in controls, and found increased activation in regions that were activated in controls. These patients still scored within the normal range for most tasks, suggesting the possibility that increased activation represented a form of compensation. Some studies have shown a combination of decreases and increases in activation in AD. Patients with AD doing a visuospatial processing task showed decreased activation in parietal cortex compared with controls, but increased activation in occipitotemporal cortex.[155] These authors suggested compensation as the basis for some of the altered activation patterns, specifically that parietal dysfunction in mild to moderate AD is compensated by recruitment of the ventral visual pathway for visuospatial processing. Similarly, an fMRI study of memory encoding in AD showed increased frontal activation, but also decreased medial temporal lobe activation.[156] Other studies have demonstrated decreases in medial temporal activation during memory tasks.[157–159]

Similarly, studies of MCI have revealed complex activation patterns. An early study of elderly patients with "isolated memory decline" showed patterns of decreased hippocampal activation similar to AD.[157] Conversely, other studies have shown increased medial temporal activation during a visual-encoding task in patients with MCI whose cognition subsequently worsened,[160] although this same group of investigators showed decreased medial temporal activation in patients with AD.[161] These authors hypothesized that increased activation in medial temporal regions reflects a compensatory response to AD pathology and could serve as a marker for impending clinical decline. Another recent study of individuals with MCI found decreased hippocampal activation, but these subjects were notably more impaired on memory tasks than those with MCI in some other studies, consistent with the idea that compensatory mechanisms eventually fail, resulting in lower levels of activation.[162]

There has been limited use of fMRI in the non-AD dementias. Rombouts et al.[159] studied verbal working memory in early FTD and AD and found decreased activation in frontal and parietal regions in FTD. The FTD group displayed a stronger response in the cerebellum, which was interpreted as a possible compensatory mechanism. A recent study showed increased temporal lobe activation in dementia with Lewy bodies compared with AD on a visual motion-processing task.[163]

Activation patterns seen with fMRI correlate with many clinical features in AD, consistent with the fact that these techniques indirectly evaluate neuronal function. For example, several of the studies described above in AD found that medial temporal activation was correlated with memory performance,[161,162] and some studies have demonstrated correlations between performance and activation in other brain regions during memory-encoding tasks.[164] Recently, a study of emotional processing in AD showed increased amygdala activation during face processing, which was correlated with the severity of irritability and agitation.[165] Small increases in brain activation have been seen after treatment with cholinesterase inhibitors;[166] however, given that both increases and decreases in activation have been seen at all stages of cognitive impairment from MCI to AD, and it is not yet clear what parameters predict increased versus decreased activation for a given cognitive task, the role of fMRI in diagnosis or monitoring of patients with dementia is still unclear.

Resting-state functional magnetic resonance imaging

The metabolic activity during periods when patients are not actively engaged in cognitive processing has proven relevant to dementia. Several regions across the brain, often with related functions, covary in terms of the rise and fall of their BOLD signal during these periods. The networks of regions seen with this type of analysis are referred to as resting-state networks. The network that has received the most attention in AD is the so-called default mode network, which includes the posterior cingulate, inferior parietal, inferolateral temporal, ventral anterior cingulate and hippocampal regions.[167,168] This default mode network shows decreased activity in AD, which is quite consistent with the metabolic and structural data reviewed above highlighting these regions as being affected particularly severely in AD[168,169] and in MCI.[169,170] Other networks have relevance to other dementias. For instance, a "salience" network that includes the dorsal anterior cingulate and orbital frontoinsular regions and tracks with emotional measures may be more relevant to FTD.[171] The precise functions of these networks and the physiological basis of alterations in the functions of these networks have yet to be determined. However, their use for patients with dementia is very attractive because they can be studied in nearly any patient who can have an MRI scan, in contrast to the sometimes complex paradigms used for fMRI activation studies.

Imaging of neurotransmitter systems with positron emission tomography

Metabolic imaging using PET and SPECT allows a level of versatility in imaging that is still unachievable using MRI. This is because the MRI signal is based on intrinsic properties of the brain such as water content and other simple chemical parameters. In contrast, PET and SPECT can image any molecule which can be safely introduced into the body and labeled with a radioactive ion. One approach that takes unique advantage of the capabilities of metabolic imaging is the study of neurotransmitter systems using molecules that bind to neurotransmitter receptors or interact with neurotransmitter systems in other ways. For example, in AD, imaging of the cholinergic system is possible using a variety of agents that interact with acetylcholine receptors and acetylcholinesterase, a key enzyme whose function decreases in AD.[172]

Imaging with one such agent, N-[^{11}C]-methyl-4-piperidyl acetate (MP4A), a radiolabeled acetylcholine analogue, shows reductions in estimated acetylcholinesterase activity in multiple cortical regions, with the greatest reduction in the parietotemporal cortex.[173] This type of imaging could be helpful in guiding therapy, by establishing parameters to predict who would respond best to neurotransmitter manipulation and by following the effects of treatment. In fact, PET imaging has shown significant increases in [^{11}C]-nicotine-binding sites after 3 months of treatment with rivastigmine, and this increase correlates with improvements on attentional tasks at 12 months.[174]

Measurement of cholinergic function has applications beyond the diagnosis of AD. For instance, cognitive deterioration in patients with Parkinson's disease (PD) may be caused by spread of Lewy body pathology outside the substantia nigra, or the development of superimposed AD. In either case, effects on cholinergic function are likely. A recent PET study with MP4A and [^{18}F]-fluorodopa (F-DOPA) evaluated cholinergic and dopaminergic function in PD and with patients with PD with dementia (PDD).[175] While F-DOPA uptake in the striatum was decreased in both groups, cortical MP4A binding was severely decreased in PDD compared with controls, but only moderately decreased in PD. The PDD group had decreased MP4A binding, particularly in the parietal regions. The ability to measure each of these neurotransmitters systems could help to guide treatments specific to each system.

Amyloid imaging with positron emission tomography

All the structural and metabolic imaging techniques discussed above provide relatively non-specific indicators of brain pathology because they do not provide a direct measure of the molecular changes leading to disease. For example, FDG-PET scanning cannot differentiate temporoparietal hypometabolism caused by DLB from that in AD. The recent development of new PET ligands for imaging disease-specific pathology may revolutionize brain imaging in neurodegenerative disease. Specifically, agents that bind in vivo to plaques containing β-amyloid, the hallmark protein that accumulates in AD, are now being evaluated in clinical trials. A number of different compounds are being evaluated for this purpose[176–178] but radiolabeled Pittsburgh compound B [^{11}C]-PIB, is, currently the furthest along in development and

the most widely used. In the first study of the clinical utility of PIB, Klunk et al.[177] demonstrated marked retention of [^{11}C]-PIB in the frontal, parietal, temporal and occipital cortices, as well as the striatum, in patients with AD compared with controls. Because [^{11}C]-PIB labels amyloid plaques that are not normally present in healthy brains, the images in AD usually appear dramatically different from images in healthy controls, allowing easy visual interpretation of PIB images.[179]

Since the first reports on [^{11}C]-PIB, subsequent studies have gone on to show increased PIB retention in patients with MCI,[180] and several reports have examined PIB retention in non-AD dementias.[181–184] A recent study by Rabinovici et al.[181] included seven patients with a clinical diagnosis of AD and 12 with FTLD. All seven in the AD group had increased [^{11}C]-PIB scans by visual inspection, while most (8/12) in the FTLD group and 5/5 controls had no increase in [^{11}C]-PIB retention, consistent with the proposal that non-AD dementia will not usually show increased [^{11}C]-PIB retention. The increased [^{11}C]-PIB retention in the four patients with FTLD may represent AD pathology mimicking the clinical presentation of FTLD, or it may represent coexisting pathology. Use of [^{11}C]-PIB has also been studied in patients with PD, where a complex scenario occurs, with some patients showing cortical [^{11}C]-PIB staining and others showing staining limited to the brainstem.[184]

While amyloid imaging is a promising approach for diagnosis of neurodegenerative disease, this technique should be used cautiously as it gains wider use. The presence of increased PIB retention should not be considered tantamount to a diagnosis of AD. The few studies in non-AD dementias have highlighted the fact that complex results may emerge, and the interpretation of these findings will require much more study. In addition [^{11}C]-PIB studies have demonstrated increased retention in up to 20% of healthy older individuals who are cognitively normal.[185,186] Whether such patients are destined to develop dementia is still an open question. The fact that increased [^{11}C]-PIB retention can occur in cognitively normal individuals is consistent with pathological studies indicating that up to 37% of autopsies in patients who were cognitively normal prior to death show pathology meeting the National Institute on Aging NIA-Reagan criteria for a high or intermediate likelihood of AD.[187] As the review above clearly demonstrates, there are many other techniques to image changes in brain occurring secondary to neurodegenerative

Table 8.1. Summary of various imaging techniques used in dementia, with relative advantages and disadvantages

Method	Typical findings	Advantages	Disadvantages
Standard structural CT	Regional reductions in tissue content (atrophy)	Inexpensive, ubiquitous	Lower resolution than MRI; poor differentiation of white matter versus gray matter changes
Standard structural MRI	Regional reductions in gray matter content (atrophy)	Ubiquitous; many available techniques for analysis; has been used extensively in dementia	Sensitivity to disease and to changes in function versus metabolic imaging not established
Diffusion-weighted imaging	Increased diffusion in CJD	Uniquely sensitive to CJD	Utility in other dementias unclear; sometimes difficult to read; approach to quantitative analysis not yet established
Diffusion tensor imaging	Decreased organization in white matter tracts	Novel approach to white matter assessment; assesses unique aspect of cerebral structure	Relatively little use in dementia thus far; utility in study of dementia not yet established
Perfusion MRI	Regional deficits in brain perfusion	Non-invasive indirect indicator of metabolic function; no radiation exposure	Reliant on artifact-prone imaging sequences; sensitivity versus other techniques not established
Magnetic resonance spectroscopy	Decreased NAA/creatine ratio	Assesses unique aspects of chemical content of the brain	Sensitivity and utility in dementia not clearly established
Functional MRI (active and resting state)	Changes in BOLD signal representing synaptic activity	Capable of tracking cognitive performance on individual tasks	Sensitivity and utility in dementia not clearly established; both increases and decreases have been documented, but meaning in each case unclear
[18F]-Fluorodeoxyglucose PET	Regional changes in glucose metabolism	Long history of findings in dementia; metabolic changes may image dysfunction not detectable in structural imaging	Expensive; exposure to radiation; sensitivity versus other techniques not well established
Neurotransmitter system imaging using PET ligands	Changes in neurotransmitter function	Neurotransmitter function is an important contributor to function; may be relevant to specific symptoms and treatments	Sensitivity for diagnosis not well established; may only be relevant to specific symptoms; may not be suitable for tracking overall disease course
Amyloid imaging using PET	Pathological accumulation of disease-specific proteins (β-amyloid)	Detects disease specific protein; may be most suitable for diagnosis	Sensitivity not yet established; may be positive prior to any disease-related impairment
Perfusion with SPECT (e.g. with [99mTc]-HMPAO)	Regional changes in cerebral perfusion	Long history of use in dementia; SPECT less expensive than PET	SPECT lower resolution than PET; radiation exposure

Notes:
CT, computed tomography; MRI, magnetic resonance imaging; PET, positron emission tomography; SPECT, single-photon emission computed tomography; NAA, N-acetyl-aspartate; BOLD, blood oxygen level-dependent; HMPAO, hexamethylpropyleneamine oxime; CJD, Creutzfeldt–Jakob disease.

disease that are capable of tracking function over varying time intervals, depending on the technique. The likelihood is that techniques for imaging specific molecular pathology, such as use of [11C]-PIB, will be combined with one or more of these other imaging techniques to identify these molecular abnormalities and to quantify their effects in the brain.

Summary

Brain imaging offers a wide variety of approaches for studying the changes in the brain induced by neurodegenerative disease, each with its own advantages and disadvantages (Table 8.1). In addition to the approaches highlighted here, which primarily utilize MRI, PET and SPECT imaging, other approaches for quantifying changes in the brain not discussed here, including electroencephalography and magnetoencephalography, could be considered "imaging" approaches, as they depict regional changes across the brain; these, however, are beyond the scope of this chapter.[188] Despite the availability of methods for imaging many aspects of structure and function, including white matter tract integrity, neurotransmitter function, task-related synaptic activity and chemical content, the bulk of imaging research in dementia is still focused on regional abnormalities in glucose metabolism, perfusion and tissue content. The simple goal of making early and accurate diagnosis solely with imaging has not been achieved for the common degenerative diseases, although DWI has emerged as a critically important diagnostic tool in CJD. In certain contexts, such as differentiation of FTD from AD, imaging can be a valuable addition to the clinical assessment. The arrival of amyloid imaging may herald the emergence of a new era when imaging of the specific metabolic abnormality associated with each degenerative syndrome will vastly improve diagnostic accuracy. However, we must be cautious as we embrace this technology in order to avoid misdiagnosis and to recognize the possibility of multiple metabolic abnormalities accounting for a patient's clinical presentation. The future of brain imaging will likely involve combinations of imaging techniques to identify the presence of a molecular abnormality, to gage its impact on the brain structure and function and to predict and follow the effects of treatment.

References

1. Litvan, I., Y. Agid, N. Sastry et al. What are the obstacles for an accurate clinical diagnosis of Pick's disease? A clinicopathologic study. [See comments.] Neurology, 1997; 49(1): 62–9. [Published erratum appears in Neurology 1997; 49(6): 1755.]

2. Knopman, D. S., B. F. Boeve, J. E. Parisi et al. Antemortem diagnosis of frontotemporal lobar degeneration. Ann Neurol, 2005; 57(4): 480–8.

3. Mendez, M. F., M. Cherrier, K. M. Perryman et al. Frontotemporal dementia versus Alzheimer's disease: Differential cognitive features. Neurology, 1996; 47: 1189–94.

4. Clarfield, A. M. The decreasing prevalence of reversible dementias: an updated meta-analysis. Arch Intern Med, 2003; 163(18): 2219–29.

5. Rapoport, S. I. Positron emission tomography in normal aging and Alzheimer's disease. Gerontology, 1986; 32(Suppl 1): 6–13.

6. Mielke, R. and W. D. Heiss. Positron emission tomography for diagnosis of Alzheimer's disease and vascular dementia. J Neural Transm Suppl, 1998; 53: 237–50.

7. Silverman, D. H., G. W. Small and M. E. Phelps. Clinical value of neuroimaging in the diagnosis of dementia. Sensitivity and specificity of regional cerebral metabolic and other parameters for early identification of Alzheimer's disease. Clin Positron Imaging, 1999; 2(3): 119–30.

8. Minoshima, S., B. Giordani, S. Berent et al. Metabolic reduction in the posterior cingulate cortex in very early Alzheimer's disease. Ann Neurol, 1997; 42(1): 85–94.

9. Devous, M. D. Functional brain imaging in the dementias: role in early detection, differential diagnosis, and longitudinal studies. Eur J Nucl Med Mol Imaging, 2002; 29(12): 1685–96.

10. Hoffman, J. M., M. W. Hanson, K. A. Welsh et al. Interpretation variability of [18]FDG-positron emission tomography studies in dementia. Invest Radiol, 1996; 31(6): 316–22.

11. van Heertum, R. L. and R. S. Tikofsky. Positron emission tomography and single-photon emission computed tomography brain imaging in the evaluation of dementia. Semin Nucl Med, 2003; 33(1): 77–85.

12. Hoffman, J. M., K. A. Welsh-Bohmer, M. Hanson et al. FDG PET imaging in patients with pathologically verified dementia. J Nucl Med, 2000; 41(11): 1920–8.

13. Jagust, W., R. Thisted, M. D. Devous St. et al. SPECT perfusion imaging in the diagnosis of Alzheimer's disease: a clinical–pathologic study. Neurology, 2001; 56(7): 950–6.

14. Petersen, R. C., R. Doody, A. Kurz et al. Current concepts in mild cognitive impairment. Arch Neurol, 2001; 58(12): 1985–92.

15. Mosconi, L. Brain glucose metabolism in the early and specific diagnosis of Alzheimer's disease. FDG-PET studies in MCI and AD. Eur J Nucl Med Mol Imaging, 2005; 32(4): 486–510.

16. Anchisi, D., B. Borroni, M. Franceschi et al. Heterogeneity of brain glucose metabolism in mild cognitive impairment and clinical progression to Alzheimer disease. Arch Neurol, 2005; 62(11): 1728–33.

17. Drzezga, A., T. Grimmer, M. Riemenschneider et al. Prediction of individual clinical outcome in MCI by means of genetic assessment and (18)F-FDG PET. J Nucl Med, 2005; 46(10): 1625–32.

18. Chetelat, G., F. Eustache, F. Viader et al. FDG-PET measurement is more accurate than neuropsychological assessments to predict global cognitive deterioration in patients with mild cognitive impairment. Neurocase, 2005; 11(1): 14–25.

19. Johnson, K. A., E. K. Moran, J. A. Becker et al. Single photon emission computed tomography perfusion differences in mild cognitive impairment. J Neurol Neurosurg Psychiatry, 2007; 78(3): 240–7.

20. Jagust, W. J., B. R. Reed, J. P. Seab et al. Clinical-physiologic correlates of Alzheimer's disease and frontal lobe dementia. Am J Physiol Imaging, 1989; 4: 89–96.

21. Miller, B. L., J. L. Cummings, J. Villanueva-Meyer et al. Frontal lobe degeneration: clinical, neuropsychological, and SPECT characteristics. Neurology, 1991; 41(9): 1374–82.

22. Salmon, E., B. Sadzot, P. Maquet *et al.* Differential diagnosis of Alzheimer's disease with PET. *J Nucl Med*, 1994; **35**(3): 391–8.

23. Frisoni, G. B., G. Pizzolato, C. Geroldi *et al.* Dementia of the frontal type: neuropsychological and [99Tc]-HM-PAO SPECT features. *J Geriatr Psychiatry Neurol*, 1995; **8**: 42–8.

24. Edwards-Lee, T., B. L. Miller, D. F. Benson *et al.* The temporal variant of frontotemporal dementia. *Brain*, 1997; **120**(Pt 6): 1027–40.

25. Foster, N. L., J. L. Heidebrink, C. M. Clark *et al.* FDG-PET improves accuracy in distinguishing frontotemporal dementia and Alzheimer's disease. *Brain*, 2007; **130**(Pt 10): 2616–35.

26. Albin, R. L., S. Minoshima, C. J. D'Amato *et al.* Fluoro-deoxyglucose positron emission tomography in diffuse Lewy body disease. *Neurology*, 1996; **47**(2): 462–6.

27. Lobotesis, K., J. D. Fenwick, A. Phipps *et al.* Occipital hypoperfusion on SPECT in dementia with Lewy bodies but not AD. *Neurology*, 2001; **56**(5): 643–9.

28. Gilman, S., R. A. Koeppe, R. Little *et al.* Differentiation of Alzheimer's disease from dementia with Lewy bodies utilizing positron emission tomography with [^{18}F] fluorodeoxyglucose and neuropsychological testing. *Exp Neurol*, 2005; **191**(Suppl 1): S95–103.

29. Talbot, P. R., J. J. Lloyd, J. S. Snowden *et al.* A clinical role for ^{99m}Tc-HMPAO SPECT in the investigation of dementia? *J Neurol Neurosurg Psychiatry*, 1998; **64**(3): 306–13.

30. Read, S. L., B. L. Miller, I. Mena *et al.* SPECT in dementia: clinical and pathological correlation. *J Am Geriatr Soc*, 1995; **43**(11): 1243–7.

31. de Leon, M. J., S. H. Ferris, A. E. George *et al.* Positron emission tomographic studies of aging and Alzheimer disease. *Am J Neuroradiol*, 1983; **4**(3): 568–71.

32. Teipel, S. J., M. Ewers, O. Dietrich *et al.* [Reliability of multicenter magnetic resonance imaging: results of a phantom test and in vivo measurements by the German Dementia Competence Network.] *Nervenarzt*, 2006; **77** (9): 1086–95.

33. Haxby, J. V., R. Duara, C. L. Grady *et al.* Relations between neuropsychological and cerebral metabolic asymmetries in early Alzheimer's disease. *J Cereb Blood Flow Metab*, 1985; **5**: 193–200.

34. Mosconi, L., S. de Santi, J. Li *et al.* Hippocampal hypometabolism predicts cognitive decline from normal aging. *Neurobiol Aging*, 2008; **29**(5): 676–92.

35. Salmon, E., D. Perani, K. Herholz *et al.* Neural correlates of anosognosia for cognitive impairment in Alzheimer's disease. *Hum Brain Mapp*, 2006; **27**(7): 588–97.

36. Benoit, M., P. M. Koulibaly, O. Migneco *et al.* Brain perfusion in Alzheimer's disease with and without apathy: a SPECT study with statistical parametric mapping analysis. *Psychiatry Res*, 2002; **114**(2): 103–11.

37. Mueller, S. G., M. W. Weiner, L. J. Thal *et al.* Ways toward an early diagnosis in Alzheimer's disease: the Alzheimer's Disease Neuroimaging Initiative (ADNI). *Alzheimers Dement*, 2005; **1**(1): 55–66.

38. Stefanova, E., A. Wall, O. Almkvist *et al.* Longitudinal PET evaluation of cerebral glucose metabolism in rivastigmine treated patients with mild Alzheimer's disease. *J Neural Transm*, 2006; **113**(2): 205–18.

39. Teipel, S. J., A. Drzezga, P. Bartenstein *et al.* Effects of donepezil on cortical metabolic response to activation during (18)FDG-PET in Alzheimer's disease: a double-blind cross-over trial. *Psychopharmacology (Berl)*, 2006; **187**(1): 86–94.

40. Sandson, T. A., M. O'Connor, R. A. Sperling *et al.* Noninvasive perfusion MRI in Alzheimer's disease: a preliminary report. *Neurology*, 1996; **47**(5): 1339–42.

41. Bozzao, A., R. Floris, M. E. Baviera *et al.* Diffusion and perfusion MR imaging in cases of Alzheimer's disease: correlations with cortical atrophy and lesion load. *Am J Neuroradiol*, 2001; **22**(6): 1030–6.

42. Johnson, N. A., G. H. Jahng, M. W. Weiner *et al.* Pattern of cerebral hypoperfusion in Alzheimer disease and mild cognitive impairment measured with arterial spin-labeling MR imaging: initial experience. *Radiology*, 2005; **234**(3): 851–9.

43. Du, A. T., G. H. Jahng, S. Hayasaka *et al.* Hypoperfusion in frontotemporal dementia and Alzheimer disease by arterial spin labeling MRI. *Neurology*, 2006; **67**(7): 1215–20.

44. Ojemann, J. G., E. Akbudak, A. Z. Snyder *et al.* Anatomic localization and quantitative analysis of gradient refocused echo-planar fMRI susceptibility artifacts. *Neuroimage*, 1997; **6**(3): 156–67.

45. Gorno-Tempini, M. L., C. Hutton, O. Josephs *et al.* Echo time dependence of BOLD contrast and susceptibility artifacts. *Neuroimage*, 2002; **15**(1): 136–42.

46. Zimny, A., M. Sasiadek, J. Leszek *et al.* Does perfusion CT enable differentiating Alzheimer's disease from vascular dementia and mixed dementia? A preliminary report. *J Neurol Sci*, 2007; **257**(1–2): 114–20.

47. Fox, J. H. and M. S. Huckman. Computerized tomography: a recent advance in evaluating senile dementia. *Geriatrics*, 1975; **30**(11): 97–100.

48. Farina, E., S. Pomati and C. Mariani. Observations on dementias with possibly reversible symptoms. *Aging (Milan)*, 1999; **11**(5): 323–8.

49. Fox, J. H., J. L. Topel and M. S. Huckman. Use of computerized tomography in senile dementia. *J Neurol Neurosurg Psychiatry*, 1975; **38**(10): 948–53.

50. Lavenu, I., F. Pasquier, F. Lebert *et al.* Explicit memory in frontotemporal dementia: the role of medial temporal atrophy. *Dement Geriatr Cogn Disord*, 1998; **9**(2): 99–102.

51. Anstey, K. J. and J. J. Maller. The role of volumetric MRI in understanding mild cognitive impairment and similar classifications. *Aging Ment Health*, 2003; **7**(4): 238–50.

52. Atiya, M., B. T. Hyman, M. S. Albert *et al.* Structural magnetic resonance imaging in established and prodromal Alzheimer disease: a review. *Alzheimer Dis Assoc Disord*, 2003; **17**(3): 177–95.

53. Chetelat, G. and J. C. Baron. Early diagnosis of Alzheimer's disease: contribution of structural neuroimaging. *Neuroimage*, 2003; **18**(2): 525–41.

54. Good, C. D. Dementia and ageing. *Br Med Bull*, 2003; **65**: 159–68.

55. Petrella, J. R., R. E. Coleman and P. M. Doraiswamy. Neuroimaging and early diagnosis of Alzheimer disease: a look to the future. *Radiology*, 2003; **226**(2): 315–36.

56. Small, S. A. Imaging Alzheimer's disease. *Curr Neurol Neurosci Rep*, 2003; **3**(5): 385–92.

57. Norfray, J. F. and J. M. Provenzale. Alzheimer's disease: neuropathologic findings and recent advances in imaging. *Am J Roentgenol*, 2004; **182**(1): 3–13.

58. Kantarci, K. Magnetic resonance markers for early diagnosis and progression of Alzheimer's disease. *Expert Rev Neurother*, 2005; **5**(5): 663–70.

59. Ramani, A., J. H. Jensen and J. A. Helpern. Quantitative MR imaging in Alzheimer disease. *Radiology*, 2006; **241**(1): 26–44.

60. Braak, H. and E. Braak. Neuropathological staging of Alzheimer-related changes. *Acta Neuropathol*, 1991; **82**(4): 239–59.

61. Bobinski, M., J. Wegiel, H. M. Wisniewski *et al.* Atrophy of hippocampal formation subdivisions correlates with stage and duration of Alzheimer disease. *Dementia*, 1995; **6**(4): 205–10.

62. Fox, N. C., P. A. Freeborough and M. N. Rossor. Visualisation and quantification of rates of atrophy in Alzheimer's disease. *Lancet*, 1996; **348**(9020): 94–7.

63. Jack, C. R., Jr., R. C. Petersen, Y. C. Xu *et al.* Medial temporal atrophy on MRI in normal aging and very mild Alzheimer's disease. *Neurology*, 1997; **49**(3): 786–94.

64. Juottonen, K., M. P. Laakso, R. Insausti *et al.* Volumes of the entorhinal and perirhinal cortices in Alzheimer's disease. *Neurobiol Aging*, 1998; **19**(1): 15–22.

65. Krasuski, J. S., G. E. Alexander, B. Horwitz *et al.* Volumes of medial temporal lobe structures in patients with Alzheimer's disease and mild cognitive impairment (and in healthy controls). *Biol Psychiatry*, 1998; **43**(1): 60–8.

66. Csernansky, J. G., L. Wang, S. Joshi *et al.* Early DAT is distinguished from aging by high-dimensional mapping of the hippocampus. Dementia of the Alzheimer type. *Neurology*, 2000; **55**(11): 1636–43.

67. Du, A. T., N. Schuff, D. Amend *et al.* Magnetic resonance imaging of the entorhinal cortex and hippocampus in mild cognitive impairment and Alzheimer's disease. *J Neurol Neurosurg Psychiatry*, 2001; **71**(4): 441–7.

68. Killiany, R. J., B. T. Hyman, T. Gomez-Isla *et al.* MRI measures of entorhinal cortex vs hippocampus in preclinical AD. *Neurology*, 2002; **58**(8): 1188–96.

69. Bobinski, M., M. J. de Leon, A. Convit *et al.* MRI of entorhinal cortex in mild Alzheimer's disease. *Lancet*, 1999; **353**(9146): 38–40.

70. Hampel, H., S. J. Teipel, G. E. Alexander *et al.* Corpus callosum atrophy is a possible indicator of region- and cell type-specific neuronal degeneration in Alzheimer disease: a magnetic resonance imaging analysis. *Arch Neurol*, 1998; **55**(2): 193–8.

71. Teipel, S. J., W. Bayer, G. E. Alexander *et al.* Progression of corpus callosum atrophy in Alzheimer disease. *Arch Neurol*, 2002; **59**(2): 243–8.

72. Rusinek, H., M. J. de Leon, A. E. George *et al.* Alzheimer disease: measuring loss of cerebral gray matter with MR imaging. *Radiology*, 1991; **178**(1): 109–14.

73. Jones, B. F., J. Barnes, H. B. Uylings *et al.* Differential regional atrophy of the cingulate gyrus in Alzheimer disease: a volumetric MRI study. *Cereb Cortex*, 2006; **16**(12): 1701–8.

74. Jack, C. R., Jr., R. C. Petersen, Y. C. Xu *et al.* Prediction of AD with MRI-based hippocampal volume in mild cognitive impairment. *Neurology*, 1999; **52**(7): 1397–403.

75. Killiany, R. J., T. Gomez-Isla, M. Moss *et al.* Use of structural magnetic resonance imaging to predict who will get Alzheimer's disease. *Ann Neurol*, 2000; **47**(4): 430–9.

76. Fox, N. C., E. K. Warrington, P. A. Freeborough *et al.* Presymptomatic hippocampal atrophy in Alzheimer's disease. A longitudinal MRI study. *Brain*, 1996; **119**(Pt 6): 2001–7.

77. Fox, N. C., E. K. Warrington, P. A. Freeborough *et al.* Presymptomatic hippocampal atrophy in Alzheimer's disease. *Brain*, 1996; **119**: 2001–7.

78. Fox, N. C., R. I. Scahill, W. R. Crum *et al.* Correlation between rates of brain atrophy and cognitive decline in AD. *Neurology*, 1999; **52**(8): 1687–9.

79. Fox, N. C., S. Cousens, R. Scahill *et al.* Using serial registered brain magnetic resonance imaging to measure disease progression in Alzheimer disease: power calculations and estimates of sample size to detect treatment effects. *Arch Neurol*, 2000; **57**(3): 339–44.

80. Fox, N. C., W. R. Crum, R. I. Scahill *et al.* Imaging of onset and progression of Alzheimer's disease with voxel-compression mapping of serial magnetic resonance images. *Lancet*, 2001; **358**(9277): 201–5.

115

81. Chan, D., N. C. Fox, R. Jenkins *et al.* Rates of global and regional cerebral atrophy in AD and frontotemporal dementia. *Neurology*, 2001; **57**(10): 1756–63.

82. Chan, D., J. C. Janssen, J. L. Whitwell *et al.* Change in rates of cerebral atrophy over time in early-onset Alzheimer's disease: longitudinal MRI study. *Lancet*, 2003; **362**(9390): 1121–2.

83. Thompson, P. M., K. M. Hayashi, G. de Zubicaray *et al.* Dynamics of gray matter loss in Alzheimer's disease. *J Neurosci*, 2003; **23**(3): 994–1005.

84. Jack, C. R., Jr., R. C. Petersen, Y. Xu *et al.* Rate of medial temporal lobe atrophy in typical aging and Alzheimer's disease. *Neurology*, 1998; **51**(4): 993–9.

85. Schott, J. M., N. C. Fox, C. Frost *et al.* Assessing the onset of structural change in familial Alzheimer's disease. *Ann Neurol*, 2003; **53**(2): 181–8.

86. Jack, C. R., Jr., R. C. Petersen, Y. Xu *et al.* Rates of hippocampal atrophy correlate with change in clinical status in aging and AD. *Neurology*, 2000; **55**(4): 484–9.

87. Du, A. T., N. Schuff, X. P. Zhu *et al.* Atrophy rates of entorhinal cortex in AD and normal aging. *Neurology*, 2003; **60**(3): 481–6.

88. Wang, D., J. B. Chalk, S. E. Rose *et al.* MR image-based measurement of rates of change in volumes of brain structures. Part II: application to a study of Alzheimer's disease and normal aging. *Magn Reson Imaging*, 2002; **20**(1): 41–8.

89. Rusinek, H., S. de Santi, D. Frid *et al.* Regional brain atrophy rate predicts future cognitive decline: 6-year longitudinal MR imaging study of normal aging. *Radiology*, 2003; **229**(3): 691–6.

90. Rosen, H. J., M. L. Gorno-Tempini, W. P. Goldman *et al.* Patterns of brain atrophy in frontotemporal dementia and semantic dementia. *Neurology*, 2002; **58**(2): 198–208.

91. Liu, W., B. L. Miller, J. H. Kramer *et al.* Behavioral disorders in the frontal and temporal variants of frontotemporal dementia. *Neurology*, 2004; **62**(5): 742–8.

92. Fukui, T. and A. Kertesz. Volumetric study of lobar atrophy in Pick complex and Alzheimer's disease. *J Neurol Sci*, 2000; **174**(2): 111–21.

93. Barnes, J., J. L. Whitwell, C. Frost *et al.* Measurements of the amygdala and hippocampus in pathologically confirmed Alzheimer disease and frontotemporal lobar degeneration. *Arch Neurol*, 2006; **63**(10): 1434–9.

94. Ashburner, J. and K. J. Friston. Voxel-based morphometry: the methods. *Neuroimage*, 2000; **11**(Pt 1): 805–21.

95. Phillips, M. L., W. C. Drevets, S. L. Rauch *et al.* Neurobiology of emotion perception. I: The neural basis of normal emotion perception. *Biol Psychiatry*, 2003; **54**(5): 504–14.

96. Kril, J. J. and G. M. Halliday. Clinicopathological staging of frontotemporal dementia severity: correlation with regional atrophy. *Dement Geriatr Cogn Disord*, 2004; **17**(4): 311–15.

97. Ibach, B., S. Poljansky, J. Marienhagen *et al.* Contrasting metabolic impairment in frontotemporal degeneration and early onset Alzheimer's disease. *Neuroimage*, 2004; **23**(2): 739–43.

98. Tranel, D. and H. Damasio. Neuroanatomical correlates of electrodermal skin conductance responses. *Psychophysiology*, 1994; **31**(5): 427–38.

99. Friston, K. J., A. Holmes, J. B. Poline *et al.* Detecting activations in PET and fMRI: levels of inference and power. *Neuroimage*, 1996; **4**(Pt 1): 223–35.

100. Whitwell, J. L., K. A. Josephs, M. N. Rossor *et al.* Magnetic resonance imaging signatures of tissue pathology in frontotemporal dementia. *Arch Neurol*, 2005; **62**(9): 1402–8.

101. Rabinovici, G. D., S. C. Allison, M. L. Gorno-Tempini *et al.* Voxel-based morphometry in autopsy-proven frontotemporal lobar degeneration and Alzheimer's disease. In *58th Annual Meeting of the American Academy of Neurology*, San Diego, CA, 2006.

102. Cahn, D. A., E. V. Sullivan, P. K. Shear *et al.* Structural MRI correlates of recognition memory in Alzheimer's disease. *J Int Neuropsychol Soc*, 1998; **4**(2): 106–14.

103. Boxer, A. L., J. H. Kramer, A.-T. Du *et al.* Focal right inferotemporal atrophy in AD with disproportionate visual constructive impairment. *Neurology*, 2003; **61**: 1485–91.

104. Brambati, S. M., D. Myers, A. Wilson *et al.* The anatomy of category-specific object naming in neurodegenerative diseases. *J Cogn Neurosci*, 2006; **18**(10): 1644–53.

105. Rosen, H. J., M. R. Wilson, G. F. Schauer *et al.* Neuroanatomical correlates of impaired recognition of emotion in dementia. *Neuropsychologia*, 2006; **44**(3): 365–73.

106. Rankin, K. P., M. L. Gorno-Tempini, S. C. Allison *et al.* Structural anatomy of empathy in neurodegenerative disease. *Brain*, 2006; **129**(Pt 11): 2945–56.

107. Gorno-Tempini, M. L., K. P. Rankin, J. D. Woolley *et al.* Cognitive and behavioral profile in a case of right anterior temporal lobe neurodegeneration. *Cortex*, 2004; **40**(4–5): 631–44.

108. Rosen, H. J., S. C. Allison, G. F. Schauer *et al.* Neuroanatomical correlates of behavioural disorders in dementia. *Brain*, 2005; **128**(Pt 11): 2612–15.

109. Woolley, J. D., M. L. Gorno-Tempini, W. W. Seeley *et al.* Binge eating is associated with right orbitofrontal-insular-striatal atrophy in frontotemporal dementia. *Neurology*, 2007; **69**(14): 1424–33.

110. Rolls, E. T. The orbitofrontal cortex and reward. *Cereb Cortex*, 2000; **10**(3): 284–94.

111. Singh, V., H. Chertkow, J. P. Lerch *et al.* Spatial patterns of cortical thinning in mild cognitive impairment and Alzheimer's disease. *Brain*, 2006; **129**(Pt 11): 2885–93.

112. Henderson, G., B. E. Tomlinson and P. H. Gibson. Cell counts in human cerebral cortex in normal adults throughout life using an image analysing computer. *J Neurol Sci*, 1980; **46**(1): 113–36.

113. Davies, C. A., D. M. Mann, P. Q. Sumpter *et al.* A quantitative morphometric analysis of the neuronal and synaptic content of the frontal and temporal cortex in patients with Alzheimer's disease. *J Neurol Sci*, 1987; **78**(2): 151–64.

114. Regeur, L. Increasing loss of brain tissue with increasing dementia: a stereological study of post-mortem brains from elderly females. *Eur J Neurol*, 2000; **7**(1): 47–54.

115. Du, A. T., N. Schuff, J. H. Kramer *et al.* Different regional patterns of cortical thinning in Alzheimer's disease and frontotemporal dementia. *Brain*, 2007; **130**(Pt 4): 1159–66.

116. Boccardi, M., F. Sabattoli, M. P. Lasko *et al.* Frontotemporal dementia as a neural system disease. *Neurobiol Aging*, 2005; **26**(1): 37–44.

117. Foster, N. L. Validating FDG-PET as a biomarker for frontotemporal dementia. *Exp Neurol*, 2003; **184**(Suppl 1): S2–8.

118. Jeong, Y., S. S. Cho, J. M. Park *et al.* 18F-FDG PET findings in frontotemporal dementia: an SPM analysis of 29 patients. *J Nucl Med*, 2005; **46**(2): 233–9.

119. Diehl-Schmid, J., T. Grimmer, A. Drzezga *et al.* Decline of cerebral glucose metabolism in frontotemporal dementia: a longitudinal ^{18}F-FDG-PET-study. *Neurobiol Aging*, 2006; **28**(1): 42–50.

120. Varrone, A., S. Pappatà, C. Caraco *et al.* (2002). Voxel-based comparison of rCBF SPET images in frontotemporal dementia and Alzheimer's disease highlights the involvement of different cortical networks. *Eur J Nucl Med Mol Imaging*, 2002; **29**(11): 1447–54.

121. Young, G. S., M. D. Geschwind, N. J. Fischbein *et al.* Diffusion-weighted and fluid-attenuated inversion recovery imaging in Creutzfeldt–Jakob disease: high sensitivity and specificity for diagnosis. *Am J Neuroradiol*, 2005; **26**(6): 1551–62.

122. Zeidler, M., R. J. Sellar, D. A. Collie *et al.* The pulvinar sign on magnetic resonance imaging in variant Creutzfeldt–Jakob disease. *Lancet*, 2000; **355**(9213): 1412–18.

123. Moseley, M., Y. Cohen, J. Kucharczyk *et al.* Diffusion-weighted MR imaging of anisotropic water diffusion in cat central nervous system. *Radiology*, 1990; **176**(2): 439–45.

124. Beaulieu, C. and P. S. Allen. Determinants of anisotropic water diffusion in nerves. *Magn Reson Med*, 1994; **31**(4): 394–400.

125. Henkelman, R. M., G. J. Stanisz, J. K. Kim *et al.* Anisotropy of NMR properties of tissues. *Magn Reson Med*, 1994; **32**(5): 592–601.

126. Basser, P. J., J. Mattiello and D. LeBihan. Estimation of the effective self-diffusion tensor from the NMR spin echo. *J Magn Reson Series B*, 1994; **103**(3): 247–54.

127. Hanyu, H., H. Sakurai, T. Iwamoto *et al.* Diffusion-weighted MR imaging of the hippocampus and temporal white matter in Alzheimer's disease. *J Neurol Sci*, 1998; **156**(2): 195–200.

128. Sandson, T. A., O. Felician, R. R. Edelman *et al.* Diffusion-weighted magnetic resonance imaging in Alzheimer's disease. *Dement Geriatr Cogn Disord*, 1999; **10**(2): 166–71.

129. Bozzali, M., M. Franceschi, A. Falini *et al.* Quantification of tissue damage in AD using diffusion tensor and magnetization transfer MRI. *Neurology*, 2001; **57**(6): 1135–7.

130. Zhang, Y., N. Schuff, G. H. Jahng *et al.* Diffusion tensor imaging of cingulum fibers in mild cognitive impairment and Alzheimer disease. *Neurology*, 2007; **68**(1): 13–19.

131. Huang, J. and A. P. Auchus. Diffusion tensor imaging of normal appearing white matter and its correlation with cognitive functioning in mild cognitive impairment and Alzheimer's disease. *Ann N Y Acad Sci*, 2007; **1097**: 259–64.

132. Firbank, M. J., A. M. Blamire, M. S. Krishnan *et al.* Diffusion tensor imaging in dementia with Lewy bodies and Alzheimer's disease. *Psychiatry Res*, 2007; **155**(2): 135–45.

133. Borroni, B., S. M. Brambati, C. Agosti *et al.* Evidence of white matter changes on diffusion tensor imaging in frontotemporal dementia. *Arch Neurol*, 2007; **64**(2): 246–51.

134. Klunk, W. E., K. Panchalingam, J. Moossy *et al.* N-Acetyl-L-aspartate and other amino acid metabolites in Alzheimer's disease brain: a preliminary proton nuclear magnetic resonance study. *Neurology*, 1992; **42**(8): 1578–85.

135. Miller, B. L., R. A. Moats, T. Shonk *et al.* Alzheimer disease: depiction of increased cerebral myo-inositol with proton MR spectroscopy. *Radiology*, 1993; **187**(2): 433–7.

136. Schuff, N., D. L. Amend, D. J. Meyerhoff *et al.* Alzheimer disease: quantitative H-1 MR spectroscopic imaging of frontoparietal brain. *Radiology*, 1998; **207**(1): 91–102.

137. Kantarci, K., C. R. Jack, Jr., Y. C. Xu *et al.* Regional metabolic patterns in mild cognitive impairment and

117

Alzheimer's disease: A ^{1}H MRS study. *Neurology*, 2000; **55**(2): 210–17.

138. Jessen, F., W. Block, F. Traber *et al.* Proton MR spectroscopy detects a relative decrease of *N*-acetylaspartate in the medial temporal lobe of patients with AD. *Neurology*, 2000; **55**(5): 684–8.

139. Huang, W., G. E. Alexander, L. Chang *et al.* Brain metabolite concentration and dementia severity in Alzheimer's disease: a (1)H MRS study. *Neurology*, 2001; **57**(4): 626–32.

140. Schuff, N., A. A. Capizzano, A. T. Du *et al.* Selective reduction of *N*-acetylaspartate in medial temporal and parietal lobes in AD. *Neurology*, 2002; **58**(6): 928–35.

141. Schuff, N., A. A. Capizzano, A. T. Du *et al.* Different patterns of *N*-acetylaspartate loss in subcortical ischemic vascular dementia and AD. *Neurology*, 2003; **61**(3): 358–64.

142. Franczak, M., R. W. Prost, P. G. Antuono *et al.* Proton magnetic resonance spectroscopy of the hippocampus in patients with mild cognitive impairment: a pilot study. *J Comput Assist Tomogr*, 2007; **31**(5): 666–70.

143. Coulthard, E., M. Firbank, P. English *et al.* Proton magnetic resonance spectroscopy in frontotemporal dementia. *J Neurol*, 2006; **253**(7): 861–8.

144. Garrard, P., J. M. Schott, D. G. MacManus *et al.* Posterior cingulate neurometabolite profiles and clinical phenotype in frontotemporal dementia. *Cogn Behav Neurol*, 2006; **19**(4): 185–9.

145. Macfarlane, R. G., S. J. Wroe, J. Collinge *et al.* Neuroimaging findings in human prion disease. *J Neurol Neurosurg Psychiatry*, 2007; **78**(7): 664–70.

146. Gomez-Anson, B., M. Alegret, E. Munoz *et al.* Decreased frontal choline and neuropsychological performance in preclinical Huntington disease. *Neurology*, 2007; **68**(12): 906–10.

147. Schifitto, G., B. A. Navia, C. T. Yiannoutsos *et al.* Memantine and HIV-associated cognitive impairment: a neuropsychological and proton magnetic resonance spectroscopy study. *AIDS*, 2007; **21**(14): 1877–86.

148. Mihara, M., N. Hattori, K. Abe *et al.* Magnetic resonance spectroscopic study of Alzheimer's disease and frontotemporal dementia/Pick complex. *Neuroreport*, 2006; **17**(4): 413–16.

149. Bartzokis, G., D. Sultzer, J. Cummings *et al.* In vivo evaluation of brain iron in Alzheimer disease using magnetic resonance imaging. *Arch Gen Psychiatry*, 2000; **57**(1): 47–53.

150. Haacke, E. M., N. Y. Cheng, M. J. House *et al.* Imaging iron stores in the brain using magnetic resonance imaging. *Magn Reson Imaging*, 2005; **23**(1): 1–25.

151. Schenck, J. F., E. A. Zimmerman, Z. Li *et al.* High-field magnetic resonance imaging of brain iron in Alzheimer disease. *Top Magn Reson Imaging*, 2006; **17**(1): 41–50.

152. Petersen, S. E., P. T. Fox, M. I. Posner *et al.* Positron emission tomographic studies of the processing of single words. *J Cogn Neurosci*, 1989; **1**: 153–70.

153. Logothetis, N. K. MR imaging in the non-human primate: studies of function and of dynamic connectivity. *Curr Opin Neurobiol*, 2003; **13**(5): 630–42.

154. Saykin, A. J., L. A. Flashman, S. A. Frutiger *et al.* Neuroanatomic substrates of semantic memory impairment in Alzheimer's disease: patterns of functional MRI activation. *J Int Neuropsychol Soc*, 1999; **5**(5): 377–92.

155. Prvulovic, D., D. Hubl, A. T. Sack *et al.* Functional imaging of visuospatial processing in Alzheimer's disease. *Neuroimage*, 2002; **17**(3): 1403–14.

156. Gron, G., D. Bittner, B. Schmitz *et al.* Subjective memory complaints: objective neural markers in patients with Alzheimer's disease and major depressive disorder. *Ann Neurol*, 2002; **51**(4): 491–8.

157. Small, S. A., G. M. Perera, R. DeLaPaz *et al.* Differential regional dysfunction of the hippocampal formation among elderly with memory decline and Alzheimer's disease. *Ann Neurol*, 1999; **45**(4): 466–72.

158. Kato, T., D. Knopman and H. Liu. Dissociation of regional activation in mild AD during visual encoding: a functional MRI study. *Neurology*, 2001; **57**(5): 812–16.

159. Rombouts, S. A., J. C. van Swieten, Y. A. Pijnenburg *et al.* Loss of frontal fMRI activation in early frontotemporal dementia compared to early AD. *Neurology*, 2003; **60**(12): 1904–8.

160. Dickerson, B. C., D. H. Salat, J. F. Bates *et al.* Medial temporal lobe function and structure in mild cognitive impairment. *Ann Neurol*, 2004; **56**(1): 27–35.

161. Dickerson, B. C., D. H. Salat, D. N. Greve *et al.* Increased hippocampal activation in mild cognitive impairment compared to normal aging and AD. *Neurology*, 2005; **65**(3): 404–11.

162. Petrella, J. R., L. Wang, S. Krishnan *et al.* Cortical deactivation in mild cognitive impairment: high-field-strength functional MR imaging. *Radiology*, 2007; **245**(1): 224–35.

163. Sauer, J., D. H. ffytche, C. Ballard *et al.* Differences between Alzheimer's disease and dementia with Lewy bodies: an fMRI study of task-related brain activity. *Brain*, 2006; **129**(Pt 7): 1780–8.

164. Diamond, E. L., S. Miller, B. C. Dickerson *et al.* Relationship of fMRI activation to clinical trial memory measures in Alzheimer disease. *Neurology*, 2007; **69**(13): 1331–41.

165. Wright, C. I., B. C. Dickerson, E. Feczko *et al.* A functional magnetic resonance imaging study of amygdala responses to human faces in aging and mild Alzheimer's disease. *Biol Psychiatry*, 2007; **62**(12): 1388–95.

166. Shanks, M. F., W. J. McGeown, K. E. Forbes-McKay *et al.* Regional brain activity after prolonged cholinergic enhancement in early Alzheimer's disease. *Magn Reson Imaging*, 2007; **25**(6): 848–59.

167. Greicius, M. D., B. Krasnow, A. L. Reiss *et al.* Functional connectivity in the resting brain: a network analysis of the default mode hypothesis. *Proc Natl Acad Sci USA*, 2003; **100**(1): 253–8.

168. Greicius, M. D., G. Srivastava, A. L. Reiss *et al.* Default-mode network activity distinguishes Alzheimer's disease from healthy aging: evidence from functional MRI. *Proc Natl Acad Sci USA*, 2004; **101**(13): 4637–42.

169. Rombouts, S. A., F. Barkhof, R. Goekoop *et al.* Altered resting state networks in mild cognitive impairment and mild Alzheimer's disease: an fMRI study. *Hum Brain Mapp*, 2005; **26**(4): 231–9.

170. Sorg, C., V. Riedl, M. Muhlau *et al.* Selective changes of resting-state networks in individuals at risk for Alzheimer's disease. *Proc Natl Acad Sci USA*, 2007; **104**(47): 18760–5.

171. Seeley, W. W., V. Menon, A. F. Schatzberg *et al.* Dissociable intrinsic connectivity networks for salience processing and executive control. *J Neurosci*, 2007; **27**(9): 2349–56.

172. Kikuchi, T., T. Okamura, K. Fukushi *et al.* Cerebral acetylcholinesterase imaging: development of the radioprobes. *Curr Top Med Chem*, 2007; **7**(18): 1790–9.

173. Iyo, M., H. Namba, K. Fukushi *et al.* Measurement of acetylcholinesterase by positron emission tomography in the brains of healthy controls and patients with Alzheimer's disease. *Lancet*, 1997; **349**: 1805–9.

174. Kadir, A., T. Darreh-Shori, O. Almkvist *et al.* Changes in brain ^{11}C-nicotine binding sites in patients with mild Alzheimer's disease following rivastigmine treatment as assessed by PET. *Psychopharmacology (Berl)*, 2007; **191**(4): 1005–14.

175. Hilker, R., A. V. Thomas, J. C. Klein *et al.* Dementia in Parkinson disease: functional imaging of cholinergic and dopaminergic pathways. *Neurology*, 2005; **65**(11): 1716–22.

176. Verhoeff, N. P., A. A. Wilson, S. Takeshita *et al.* In-vivo imaging of Alzheimer disease beta-amyloid with ^{11}C]SB-13 PET. *Am J Geriatr Psychiatry*, 2004; **12**(6): 584–95.

177. Klunk, W. E., H. Engler, A. Nordberg *et al.* Imaging brain amyloid in Alzheimer's disease with Pittsburgh Compound-B. *Ann Neurol*, 2004; **55**(3): 306–19.

178. Small, G. W., V. Kepe, L. M. Ercoli *et al.* PET of brain amyloid and tau in mild cognitive impairment. *N Engl J Med*, 2006; **355**(25): 2652–63.

179. Ng, S., V. L. Villemagne, S. Berlangieri *et al.* Visual assessment versus quantitative assessment of ^{11}C-PIB PET and ^{18}F-FDG PET for detection of Alzheimer's disease. *J Nucl Med*, 2007; **48**(4): 547–52.

180. Kemppainen, N. M., S. Aalto, I. A. Wilson *et al.* PET amyloid ligand ^{11}C]PIB uptake is increased in mild cognitive impairment. *Neurology*, 2007; **68**(19): 1603–6.

181. Rabinovici, G. D., A. J. Furst, J. P. O'Neil *et al.* ^{11}C-PIB PET imaging in Alzheimer disease and frontotemporal lobar degeneration. *Neurology*, 2007; **68**(15): 1205–12.

182. Engler, H., A. Forsberg, O. Almkvist *et al.* Two-year follow-up of amyloid deposition in patients with Alzheimer's disease. *Brain*, 2006; **129**(Pt 11): 2856–66.

183. Boxer, A. L., G. D. Rabinovici, V. Kepe *et al.* Amyloid imaging in distinguishing atypical prion disease from Alzheimer disease. *Neurology*, 2007; **69**(3): 283–90.

184. Maetzler, W., M. Reimold, I. Liepelt *et al.* [(11)C]PIB binding in Parkinson's disease dementia. *Neuroimage*, 2008; **39**(3): 1027–33.

185. Mintun, M. A., G. N. Larossa, Y. I. Sheline *et al.* [11]C]PIB in a nondemented population: potential antecedent marker of Alzheimer disease. *Neurology*, 2006; **67**(3): 446–52.

186. Pike, K. E., G. Savage, V. L. Villemagne *et al.* Beta-amyloid imaging and memory in non-demented individuals: evidence for preclinical Alzheimer's disease. *Brain*, 2007; **130**(Pt 11): 2837–44.

187. Bennett, D. A., J. A. Schneider, Z. Arvanitakis *et al.* Neuropathology of older persons without cognitive impairment from two community-based studies. *Neurology*, 2006; **66**(12): 1837–44.

188. Rossini, P. M., S. Rossi, C. Babiloni *et al.* Clinical neurophysiology of aging brain: from normal aging to neurodegeneration. *Prog Neurobiol*, 2007; **83**(6): 375–400.

Chapter 9

Epidemiology and risk factors

Kristine Yaffe and Deborah E. Barnes

Introduction

As prior chapters have discussed, dementia is a neurodegenerative syndrome that encompasses many different specific diseases. Alzheimer's disease (AD) is the most common cause of dementia, accounting for approximately 70% of dementia cases; vascular dementia (VaD) accounts for another 10–20%. To date, most epidemiologic research on dementia has examined prevalence, incidence and risk factors for either all-cause dementia or for AD. Therefore, in this chapter, we also will discuss primarily what is known about the epidemiology of all-cause dementia and AD, with reference to other specific dementias when data are available.

The impending public health crisis of dementia

Prevalence

The prevalence of all-cause dementia, as well as AD and VaD, increases with age. For AD alone, prevalence may be as high as 10% in adults over the age of 65 years and nearly 50% in adults over 85 (Evans *et al.*, 1989). In 2000, there were approximately 4.5 million people in the USA with AD. It is estimated that this number will nearly triple to 13.2 million by 2050 (Hebert *et al.*, 2003) (Fig. 9.1). This increase in the prevalence of AD over the next 50 years will primarily reflect increased life expectancy and the aging of adults who were born during the "baby boom" after World War II (1946–1964), who will make up an increasingly large proportion of our population.

Incidence

The incidence of all-cause dementia, as well as AD and VaD, rises exponentially with age, with an approximate doubling in incidence every 5 years (Jorm and Jolley, 1998). A meta-analysis found that the overall incidence of new moderate-severity dementia cases in the USA is approximately 2.4, 5.0, 10.5, 17.7 and 27.5 per 1000 person-years for the age groups 65–69, 70–74, 75–79, 80–84 and 85–89 years, respectively (Fig. 9.2). For AD, the age-specific incidence rates are 1.6, 3.5, 7.8, 14.8 and 26.0, respectively. Incidence rates are two to three times higher if mild-severity cases are included.

Costs

In 1991, it was estimated that the total lifetime cost of caring for a patient with AD was US$174 000 (Ernst and Hay, 1994). Nationally, this reflected direct and indirect costs of $67.3 billion. Given increases in the prevalence of AD as well as inflation, current direct and indirect costs of caring for persons with AD are at least $100 billion (Alzheimer's Association, 2005). These costs are expected to rise dramatically over the next 50 years as the prevalence of disease rises and would be even higher if other forms of dementia were included.

The direct costs of caring for those with AD and dementia include nursing home or paid healthcare, especially in the later stages of the disease. However, most people with AD live at home, and much of their care is provided informally by family and friends (Rice *et al.*, 1993). The indirect costs of dementia include lost productivity, absenteeism and worker-replacement costs for these caregivers.

The potential for prevention

Given the dramatic increases that are expected in both the prevalence and costs of AD and other dementias, it is critical to identify factors that are associated with increased disease risk and to develop successful prevention and treatment strategies. Because AD and most dementias occur most commonly in very old age, interventions that delay the onset of disease have the potential to reduce prevalence dramatically

The Behavioral Neurology of Dementia, eds. Bruce L. Miller and Bradley F. Boeve. Published by Cambridge University Press. © Cambridge University Press 2009.

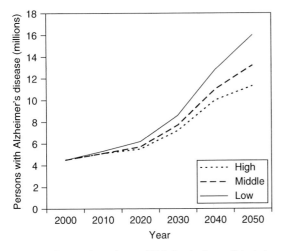

Fig. 9.1. Projected prevalence of Alzheimer's disease (Adapted from Hebert *et al.* (2003). Alzheimer disease in the US population: prevalence estimates using the 2000 census. *Arch Neurol* **60**(8): 1119–22, with permission. Copyright © 2003 American Medical Association. All rights reserved.)

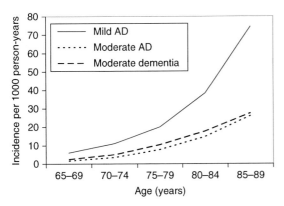

Fig. 9.2. Age-specific incidence rates for dementia and Alzheimer's disease (AD) in the USA. (Adapted from Jorm and Jolley (1998). The incidence of dementia: a meta-analysis. *Neurology* **51**(3): 728–33, with permission.)

over time. One study estimated that delaying the mean onset of AD by 5 years would reduce the expected prevalence by more than 1 million cases after 10 years and more than 4 million cases after 50 years (Brookmeyer *et al.*, 1998) (Fig. 9.3).

Risk factors for dementia

Gender

There is no difference between women and men in the age-specific incidence of all-cause dementia. However, this may reflect a difference in the types of dementia

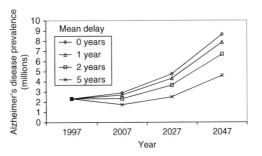

Fig. 9.3. Potential impact of interventions to delay onset of Alzheimer's disease. (Adapted from Brookmeyer *et al.* (1998). Projections of Alzheimer's disease in the United States and the public health impact of delaying disease onset. *Am J Public Health* **88**(9): 1337–42, with permission.)

that they tend to develop. Two meta-analyses have found that women are more likely to develop AD than men, especially in very old age (odds ratio [OR], 1.56; 95% confidence interval [CI], 1.16–2.10) (Gao *et al.*, 1998; Jorm and Jolley, 1998). This association persists even after taking into consideration the greater longevity of women. In addition, there is evidence that men are at increased risk of VaD, especially at younger ages (Jorm and Jolley, 1998). It is possible that these gender differences reflect differences in the risk factors that women and men are typically exposed to (e.g. greater cardiovascular disease in men leading to increased risk of VaD; lower educational or physical activity levels in women leading to increased risk of AD). However, several large studies have found no differences between women and men in the incidence of AD and VaD (Rocca *et al.*, 1998; Hebert *et al.*, 2001), and it remains controversial whether observed gender differences reflect true differences in underlying disease etiology or are the result of measurement bias or uncontrolled confounding.

Race/ethnicity

Several studies performed in the USA have found that the incidence of dementia and AD are approximately two times higher in African-Americans and Hispanics than whites (Folstein *et al.*, 1991; Tang *et al.*, 2001). Interestingly, one study has found that the prevalence of dementia among Nigerians in Africa is substantially lower than among African-Americans in the USA (Hendrie *et al.*, 1995), even after accounting for age and survival differences. Internationally, the prevalences of dementia and AD appear to be lower in Asian countries than in the USA (Japan, China and

India) (Jorm and Jolley, 1998; Manly et al., 1999). In addition, dementia prevalence among Japanese men in Japan is lower than among Japanese-American men living in Hawaii (White et al., 1996). Taken together, these studies suggest that ethnic differences may largely result from environmental, rather than purely genetic, factors. Additional research is needed to determine why these ethnic differences exist and to develop interventions that target those at highest risk.

Education

There is considerable evidence that older adults with greater education are less likely to develop AD and dementia (Breteler et al., 1992; Stern et al., 1994). One highly cited study analyzed writing samples from nuns when they were 22 years old and found that sisters with high idea density and grammatical complexity early in life were less likely to develop AD later in life (Snowdon et al., 1996). This may reflect, in part, a measurement bias, in which older adults with more education or higher intelligence perform better on cognitive tests, making AD and dementia more difficult to detect. However, there is growing evidence that education may be associated with greater cognitive or neuronal reserves, which may protect against or minimize the impact of neurodegenerative disorders (Stern, 2002). Studies in mice have found that being raised in an "enriched" environment – which includes larger cages with more mice and access to colorful tunnels, toys and running wheels – is associated with enhanced neurogenesis in areas of the brain involved in learning and memory as well as reduced cerebral deposition of β-amyloid, which is a pathological hallmark of AD (van Praag et al., 1999; Lazarov et al., 2005).

Cardiovascular factors

Traditionally, AD has been viewed as a neurodegenerative disorder distinct from VaD. However, autopsy studies have suggested that many patients with clinical AD also have evidence of vascular pathology. In one study, subjects who had both brain infarcts and AD pathology at autopsy were more likely to have exhibited the clinical symptoms of AD during their lifetimes, suggesting that cerebrovascular disease may influence both the presence and the severity of clinical AD (Snowdon et al., 1997). There also is growing evidence that risk factors for cardiovascular disease, such as diabetes mellitus, hypertension and high plasma homocysteine, are associated with increased risk of dementia. Research related to each

of these risk factors, as well as the effects of combined cardiovascular risk factors, is described in more detail in the following sections.

Diabetes mellitus

Population-based, longitudinal studies have consistently found that older adults with diabetes experienced approximately a two-fold increase in dementia risk (Areosa and Grimley, 2002). When specific dementia subtypes are examined, diabetes is associated more strongly with VaD than AD (Hassing et al., 2002; MacKnight et al., 2002). For example, in the Canadian Study of Health and Aging, a prospective, population-based study of more than 5000 older adults, subjects with diabetes experienced double the risk of VaD (relative risk [RR], 2.0; 95% CI, 1.2–3.6) but no significant increase in the risk of AD (RR, 1.3; 95% CI, 0.8–2.0) (MacKnight et al., 2002). Studies also have found that older women with impaired fasting glucose, which is a prediabetic condition, experience a two-fold increase in the risk of significant cognitive decline (Yaffe et al., 2004a). Additional studies are needed to determine whether optimal glycemic control or other treatments in people with diabetes may lower their risk of developing dementia.

Hypertension

A recent systematic review has concluded that hypertension in midlife, especially if not treated effectively, is associated with poor cognitive function and an increased risk of dementia and AD in late life (Qiu et al., 2005). In the Honolulu-Asia Aging Study, which was a longitudinal study of approximately 3700 older Japanese-American men, the risk of dementia was almost tripled in men who had systolic blood pressure ≥ 160 mmHg during midlife that was not treated with antihypertensive medication (OR, 2.8; 95% CI, 1.1–7.2) (Launer et al., 2000). In late life, both very high systolic blood pressure and very low diastolic blood pressure have been associated with increased risk of dementia and AD (Qiu et al., 2005). It has been proposed that high blood pressure may lead to dementia by increasing the risk of ischemia and stroke, whereas low blood pressure in late life may lead to dementia by increasing the risk of cerebral hypoperfusion and hypoxia. As described in more detail in the section below on antihypertensive medications, there is some evidence from randomized, controlled trials that treatment of hypertension may reduce the risk of dementia, although the data are far from conclusive and additional studies are needed.

Homocysteine

Elevated concentrations of plasma total homocysteine are an indicator of inadequate folate and vitamin B_{12} status and have been linked to a variety of poor vascular outcomes, including increased risk of stroke, carotid atherosclerosis, coronary artery disease and death from cardiovascular causes (Malouf et al., 2003). In addition, there is some evidence that high homocysteine concentrations may be associated with increased risk of dementia (Ellinson et al., 2004). In the Framingham Study, in which more than 1000 older adults were followed for a median of 8 years, elevated plasma total homocysteine levels were associated with increased risk of both all-cause dementia and AD, even after adjustment for plasma levels of folate and other B vitamins (for dementia: RR, 1.4 per 1 standard deviation [SD] increase, 95% CI, 1.1–1.9; for AD, RR, 1.8 per 1 SD increase, 95% CI, 1.3–2.5); in contrast, low folate and vitamin B levels were not associated with dementia risk in this study (Seshadri et al., 2002). In the Washington Heights–Inwood Columbia Aging Project, which included 679 older adults followed for about 5 years, the association between high homocysteine concentrations and AD risk was modest and not statistically significant (HR, 1.4; 95% CI, 0.8–2.4) (Luchsinger et al., 2004). These studies have raised hope that dietary supplementation with folic acid and/or vitamin B_{12} may lower dementia risk in older adults. However, a small number of randomized controlled trials conducted to date suggest that folic acid supplementation, with or without vitamin B_{12}, appears to have little or no effect on cognitive outcomes in either healthy older adults or those with cognitive impairment (Malouf et al., 2003).

Multiple cardiovascular risk factors

Several studies have evaluated the effects of multiple or composite cardiovascular risk factors on risk of dementia. Among members of a large health-maintenance organization, subjects who had diabetes, hypertension, high cholesterol or were smokers at midlife were more likely to develop dementia later in life, and the effects of each factor were approximately additive (Whitmer et al., 2005). Similarly, the "metabolic syndrome," which is a clustering of disorders that include abdominal obesity, hypertriglyceridemia, low levels of high density lipoprotein, hypertension and/or hyperglycemia, has been associated with increased risk of cognitive impairment and cognitive decline, especially in subjects with high levels of inflammation (Yaffe et al., 2004b). One study also found that both diabetes and hypertension were associated with greater cognitive decline in middle-aged adults (Knopman et al., 2001).

Radiologically identifiable risk factors

Several studies also have found that older adults with evidence of cerebrovascular disease on magnetic resonance imaging (MRI) studies are at increased risk of developing dementia, even if these did not result in clinically recognized events such as strokes or transient ischemic attacks. In the Rotterdam Scan Study, which is a prospective, population-based study of risk factors for cognitive decline and dementia in the Netherlands, subjects who had silent brain infarcts on cerebral MRI scans at baseline were more than twice as likely to develop dementia during follow-up (HR, 2.26; 95% CI, 1.09–4.70) (Vermeer et al., 2003). Furthermore, those subjects who experienced new infarcts during follow-up exhibited a faster rate of cognitive decline. Similarly, in the Cardiovascular Health Cognition Study, which included cerebral MRIs from more than 3600 older adults, imaging findings that were associated with increased risk of dementia included larger ventricles, white matter disease and large infarcts (Kuller et al., 2003).

Behavioral/lifestyle factors

Mental activity

There is growing evidence that mental activity may protect against cognitive decline and dementia. Several prospective, observational studies have found that older adults who engage in mentally stimulating activities, such as reading or playing games, are less likely to develop dementia and AD (Scarmeas et al., 2001; Wilson et al., 2002a,b; Verghese et al., 2003). In a biracial community study of older adults in Chicago, a 1 point increase in cognitive activity score was associated with a 64% reduction in the risk of developing AD (OR, 0.36; 95% CI, 0.2–0.6) (Wilson et al., 2002a). It has been hypothesized that mental activity may help older adults to build or maintain a mental reserve that may delay the onset of overt dementia symptoms (Stern, 2002).

A large, randomized controlled trial examined the effects of cognitive training for memory, reasoning or speed of mental processing in older adults and found that cognitive training resulted in marked and sustained improvements in the specific areas trained (Ball et al., 2002). However, cognitive training did not generalize across domains and did not affect everyday functioning; its long-term impact on dementia incidence is not known. Additional trials of other forms of mental activity are needed.

Physical activity

Several lines of evidence also suggest that physical activity may protect against cognitive decline and dementia in older adults. A meta-analysis of randomized, controlled trials found that sedentary older adults who were randomized to exercise interventions experienced short-term improvements in cognitive function relative to controls (0.48 per 1 SD versus 0.16 per 1 SD; $p < 0.05$) (Colcombe and Kramer, 2003). In addition, several prospective, observational studies have found that older adults who exercise are less likely to experience cognitive decline and dementia (Abbott et al., 2004; Weuve et al., 2004). In a study of almost 6000 older women, those in the highest quartile of blocks walked per week were 34% less likely to experience substantial cognitive decline compared with those in the lowest quartile (OR, 0.66; 95% CI, 0.54–0.82), after adjustment for age, education, smoking and health and functional status (Yaffe et al., 2001).

It has been hypothesized that physical activity could reduce the risk of dementia and AD through a vascular mechanism, since it is well established that physical activity reduces the risk of certain vascular diseases and vascular risk factors (e.g. coronary heart disease, hypertension, stroke) (US Department of Health and Human Services, 1996). In addition, studies in mice have found that mice who are raised with a running wheel experience enhanced neurogenesis and reduced β-amyloid deposition that is similar in magnitude to that seen in those raised in a fully "enriched" environment (van Praag et al., 1999; Adlard et al., 2005).

Alcohol

Several studies have found that light-to-moderate drinkers have a 30–50% reduction in the risk of cognitive decline, AD and VaD compared with non-drinkers (Ruitenberg et al., 2002; Mukamal et al., 2003; Stampfer et al., 2005), although the definition of light-to-moderate drinking has varied substantially between the studies (from < 1 drink/day to 1–3 drinks/day). As with studies of the association between alcohol consumption and cardiovascular disease, there is some evidence of a U-shape relationship, in which high alcohol consumption does not appear to be protective.

Smoking

Although several early case–control studies found that smokers had a reduced risk of AD, this may have been explained by participation or survival bias (e.g. cases who were smokers may have been less likely to participate in the study or more likely to die early in the course of their disease). More recent population-based, prospective studies have found that the incidence of AD is approximately doubled in older adults who are current smokers (Almeida et al., 2002).

Dietary factors

Laboratory studies have suggested that oxidative stress may contribute to the pathogenesis of AD (Behl, 2005), leading to the hypothesis that high dietary intake of antioxidants – either through food or supplements – might lower disease risk. In the Rotterdam study, consumption of foods high in vitamins E and C was associated with reduced risk of AD, particularly in current smokers (Engelhart et al., 2002). In the Canadian Study of Health and Aging, subjects who reported use of either multivitamins or combined E and C supplements were approximately 50% less likely to experience significant cognitive decline over 5 years of follow-up (Maxwell et al., 2005). However, several other large, prospective, observational studies have found no association between vitamin intake (either through diet or supplements) and dementia risk (e.g. Washington Heights–Inwood Columbia Aging Project, Honolulu-Asia Aging Study). Furthermore, although one randomized, controlled trial found that subjects with AD experienced slower disease progression when taking vitamin E compared with those taking placebo (Sano et al., 1997), a more recent trial found no evidence that vitamin E slowed progression to dementia in subjects with mild cognitive impairment (Petersen et al., 2005). Therefore, it remains unclear whether the observed associations between antioxidant use and dementia are real or reflect uncontrolled confounding or other biases.

Results from large, prospective, population-based studies of fish and omega-3 polyunsaturated fatty acid (PUFA) consumption also have been mixed (Lim et al., 2006). In the Rotterdam Study, greater fish consumption at baseline was associated with reduced risk of dementia (RR, 0.4; 95% CI, 0.2–0.9) and AD (RR, 0.3; 95% CI, 0.1–0.9) over the first 2 years of follow-up (Kalmijn et al., 1997), whereas consumption of omega-3 PUFAs was not associated with either dementia (RR, 1.07; 95% CI, 0.94–1.22) or AD (RR, 1.07; 95% CI, 0.91–1.25) over a longer follow-up period of 6 years (Grant, 2003). Similarly, in the Chicago Health and Aging Project, a community-based study of more than 6000 older adults, fish consumption was associated with slower rate of cognitive decline whereas omega-3 PUFA consumption was not (Morris *et al.*, 2005). Two large randomized controlled trials are underway to determine whether dietary supplementation with omega-3 PUFAs has beneficial effects on cognitive outcomes; both are scheduled to be completed in 2007 (Lim *et al.*, 2006).

Psychosocial factors

Depression

Depression is associated with poor cognitive test performance (Christensen *et al.*, 1997) and occurs in 30–50% of dementia patients (Lyketsos *et al.*, 2002; Starkstein *et al.*, 2005). Several longitudinal studies have found that older people with depressive symptoms have an increased risk of cognitive decline and dementia (Geerlings *et al.*, 2000; Wilson *et al.*, 2002c), while others have found that depressive symptoms appear to coincide with (Dufouil *et al.*, 1996) or follow (Chen *et al.*, 1999) dementia onset rather than precede it. In the Study of Osteoporotic Fractures, a longitudinal study of almost 6000 older women, those with high depressive symptoms at baseline were significantly more likely to experience cognitive decline over 4 years (adjusted OR, 2.1; 95% CI, 1.4–3.1), and there was evidence of increased risk of dementia, although this was of borderline statistical significance (adjusted OR, 2.3; 95% CI, 0.9–5.9) (Yaffe *et al.*, 1999). A meta-analysis has concluded that the risk of dementia is approximately doubled in older adults with a history of depression (Jorm, 2001).

Several hypotheses have been proposed to explain the association between depression and dementia (Jorm, 2001): depression may be an early symptom or prodrome for dementia in some older adults; it may bring forward the clinical symptoms of disease, leading to earlier diagnosis; or it may be a reaction to early cognitive deficits in some cases. Depression also may lead directly to hippocampal damage through an elevation in cortisol (Brown *et al.*, 2004). Several studies have found that cognitive function improves in older adults following treatment of depressive symptoms (Butters *et al.*, 2000; Doraiswamy *et al.*, 2003), while others suggest that these improvements may be a result of practice effects (Nebes *et al.*, 2003). Additional research is needed to determine whether treatment of depressive symptoms may reduce the risk of dementia.

Social engagement

Several studies have found that older adults with limited social networks or low levels of social activities are more likely to develop dementia (Fratiglioni *et al.*, 2004). In a study of more than 1200 older people living in the Kungsholmen district of Stockholm, Sweden, subjects who had poor or limited social networks experienced a 60% increase in the risk of developing dementia (RR, 1.6; 95% CI, 1.2–2.1), after adjustment for age, sex, education, baseline cognitive score and depression (Fratiglioni *et al.* 2000). Similarly, in a longitudinal study of more than 1700 older people living in northern Manhattan, New York, those who had engaged in social activities during the past month at baseline were less likely to develop dementia during follow-up (RR, 0.85; 95% CI, 0.77–0.94) (Scarmeas *et al.*, 2001). The social activities examined included visiting with friends or relatives; going out to movies, restaurants, clubs or centers; doing voluntary community work; and going to a church or synagogue. Fratiglioni *et al.* (2004) have proposed that social, mental and physical activities might reduce the risk of dementia by acting through similar mechanisms, which could include increasing cognitive reserve, reducing vascular disease and/or reducing stress and the glucocorticoid cascade. However, a recent analysis in the Honolulu-Asia Aging Study found that the association between low social engagement and risk of dementia was restricted to those subjects who experienced a decline in social engagement from midlife to late life (HR, 1.87; 95% CI, 1.12–3.13), suggesting that low social engagement in late life might also reflect prodromal dementia (Saczynski *et al.*, 2006).

Other factors

Head trauma

After age and family history, head injury with loss of consciousness was one of the earliest factors to be associated with increased risk of dementia and AD (Heyman *et al.*, 1984). The EURODEM pooled reanalysis of data from early case–control studies found that a history of head injury was associated with almost double the risk of AD (OR, 1.8; 95% CI, 1.3–2.7) (Brayne, 1991). However, more recent longitudinal studies, including the Rotterdam Study and the Canadian Study of Health and Aging, have found no significant association between head injury and risk of AD or dementia (Mehta *et al.*, 1999; Lindsay *et al.*, 2002). It is biologically plausible that head injury could lead to the development of β-amyloid-containing diffuse neocortical plaques, which have been observed in some boxers with dementia pugilistica. However,

125

findings from observational studies are inconsistent, and it is unclear whether head injury represents a true risk factor for AD or dementia.

Medications for prevention

Based on the epidemiologic findings described in the preceding sections, several randomized, controlled trials have been performed to investigate the use of various strategies to prevent or delay onset of dementia. In most of these studies, dementia was a secondary outcome, and power to detect an association was sometimes limited. However, these trials reflect the best evidence available of the potential of these interventions to prevent dementia.

Antihypertensive medications

Several large-scale randomized controlled trials have examined the possibility that treatment of hypertension in older adults might prevent cognitive decline and dementia, with mixed results (Qiu et al., 2005). The Systolic Hypertension in the Elderly Program (SHEP) found that treatment of isolated systolic hypertension with thiazide diuretics significantly reduced the risk of stroke and cardiovascular events but not of cognitive impairment or dementia (SHEP Cooperative Research Group, 1991), although there was some evidence that differential drop-out rates in the placebo and treatment groups might have obscured a potential beneficial effect on cognition (Di Bari et al., 2001). In contrast, the trial of Systolic Hypertension in Europe (Syst-Eur) found that patients with isolated systolic hypertension who received active treatment (which included the calcium channel blocker nitrendipine followed by the angiotensin-converting enzyme [ACE] inhibitor enalapril, hydrochlorothiazide or both) versus placebo experienced a 50% reduction in the incidence of dementia (Forette et al., 1998). A third trial examined the impact of the ACE inhibitor perindopril (with or without the diuretic inadapmide) in subjects with a history of stroke or transient ischemic attack and found that subjects in the active treatment group experience a reduced risk of dementia with recurrent stroke but not of overall dementia (Tzourio et al., 2003). Additional trials are needed to clarify which antihypertensive treatments, if any, may protect against cognitive decline and dementia, and whether specific patient populations should be targeted.

Statins

Evidence from in vivo, in vitro and observational studies has suggested that statins might protect against dementia and AD (Rea et al., 2005). However, a recent randomized, controlled trial of statins in more than 20 000 adults aged 40–80 years with coronary disease, occlusive arterial disease or diabetes found that, although statins were associated with important reductions in mortality and cardiovascular disease outcomes, no differences between the treatment and placebo groups were observed for the outcomes of cognitive impairment or dementia (Heart Protection Study Collaborative Group, 2002). A recent systematic review identified four randomized, controlled trials of at least 6 months' duration, and none reported finding a positive effect of statins on cognition in non-demented older people (Xiong et al., 2005).

Non-steroidal anti-inflammatory drugs

Several observational studies have found that older adults who used non-steroidal anti-inflammatory drugs (NSAIDs) had a reduced risk of dementia (McGeer et al., 1996; Szekely et al., 2004). In addition, there is considerable evidence that AD is associated with inflammatory and immune changes in the brain, including acute phase proteins and activated microglial cells in and around amyloid plaques and complement proteins around tangles (Aisen and Davis, 1994). However, randomized, controlled trials have found that NSAIDs do not appear to prevent AD in healthy older people or to slow progression of disease in those with AD (Aisen et al., 2003). Furthermore, several selective cyclooxygenase-2 inhibitors, which are types of NSAID, have recently been withdrawn from the market owing to increased risk of cardiovascular events.

Hormone therapy

A large number of both biological and observational studies had suggested that hormone-replacement therapy might protect against cognitive decline and dementia in postmenopausal women (Yaffe, 2001). However, several recent randomized controlled trials have found that, contrary to expectations, hormone-replacement therapy has adverse effects on cognitive outcomes. The Heart and Estrogen/progestin Replacement Study (HERS) found that older women with coronary disease who were treated with conjugated estrogen plus progestin performed more poorly than the placebo group on a verbal fluency test at follow-up (Grady et al., 2002). Furthermore, the Women's

Health Initiative Memory Study (WHIMS) found that older women treated with conjugated estrogen, either alone or in combination with progestin, were twice as likely as those treated with placebo to develop dementia or mild cognitive impairment (Shumaker *et al.*, 2003, 2004). Another trial found that estrogen was not an effective therapy in patients with AD who had had a hysterectomy (Mulnard *et al.*, 2000).

Taken together, these studies suggest that conjugated estrogen should not be prescribed either to prevent or to treat AD or dementia. However, it remains possible that different formulations or doses of estrogens may be beneficial, or at least not harmful. A recent randomized controlled trial of raloxifene, a selective estrogen-reuptake modulator (SERM), found that women taking the higher dose (120 mg/day) were 33% less likely to develop mild cognitive impairment (RR, 0.67; 95% CI, 0.46–0.98) and had slightly, but not statistically significantly, lower risks of AD (RR, 0.52; 95% CI, 0.22–1.21) (Yaffe *et al.*, 2005).

Vitamin E

A recent three-arm, double-blind, placebo-controlled trial compared the effects of vitamin E, donepezil and placebo on progression to dementia in subjects with mild cognitive impairment (Petersen *et al.*, 2005). Over 3 years of follow-up, there were no significant differences between the placebo and vitamin E groups (HR, 1.02; 95% CI, 0.74–1.41). In the donepezil group, the risk of progression to dementia was lower at months 6 and 12 but did not differ significantly from placebo at the end of the study (HR, 0.80; 95% CI, 0.57–1.13). Furthermore, several trials have found that vitamin E supplementation may increase risk of cardiovascular outcomes (Alpha-Tocopherol Beta Carotene Cancer Prevention Study Group, 1994; Waters *et al.*, 2002).

Summary

Several large, prospective, observational studies have identified a variety of factors that may prevent or delay onset of dementia and AD. These include cardiovascular risk factors (diabetes, hypertension, high plasma homocysteine, high cholesterol), behavioral risk factors (lack of exercise, lack of mental stimulation, no alcohol consumption, smoking, diet) and psychosocial risk factors (depressive symptoms, lack of social engagement). To date, randomized, controlled trials of most pharmacologic interventions have yielded disappointing results, although antihypertensive medications and newer formulations of

estrogens appear to hold some potential. Additional randomized controlled trials are needed to determine whether other interventions, especially those that target cardiovascular, behavioral and psychosocial risk factors, may result in reduced prevalence and incidence of dementia and AD over the next 50 years. In the future, drugs that target amyloid deposition and removal also should be evaluated for their primary prevention potential.

References

Abbott, R. D., L. R. White, G. W. Ross *et al.* (2004). Walking and dementia in physically capable elderly men. *JAMA* **292**(12): 1447–53.

Adlard, P. A., V. M. Perreau, V. Pop and C. W. Cotman (2005). Voluntary exercise decreases amyloid load in a transgenic model of Alzheimer's disease. *J Neurosci* **25**(17): 4217–21.

Aisen, P. S. and K. L. Davis (1994). Inflammatory mechanisms in Alzheimer's disease: implications for therapy. *Am J Psychiatry* **151**(8): 1105–13.

Aisen, P. S., K. A. Schafer, M. Grundman *et al.* (2003). Effects of rofecoxib or naproxen vs placebo on Alzheimer disease progression: a randomized controlled trial. *JAMA* **289**(21): 2819–26.

Almeida, O. P., G. K. Hulse, D. Lawrence and L. Flicker (2002). Smoking as a risk factor for Alzheimer's disease: contrasting evidence from a systematic review of case-control and cohort studies. *Addiction* **97**(1): 15–28.

The Alpha-Tocopherol Beta Carotene Cancer Prevention Study Group (1994). The effect of vitamin E and beta carotene on the incidence of lung cancer and other cancers in male smokers. *N Engl J Med* **330**(15): 1029–35.

Alzheimer's Association website (2005). Statistics about Alzheimer's Disease: http://www.alz.org/AboutAD/statistics.asp#8.

Areosa, S. A. and E. V. Grimley (2002). Effect of the treatment of type II diabetes mellitus on the development of cognitive impairment and dementia. *Cochrane Database Syst Rev* (4): CD003804.

Ball, K., D. B. Berch, K. F. Helmers *et al.* (2002). Effects of cognitive training interventions with older adults: a randomized controlled trial. *JAMA* **288**(18): 2271–81.

Behl, C. (2005). Oxidative stress in Alzheimer's disease: implications for prevention and therapy. *Subcell Biochem* **38**: 65–78.

Brayne, C. (1991). The EURODEM collaborative re-analysis of case-control studies of Alzheimer's disease: implications for public health. *Int J Epidemiol* **20**(Suppl 2): S68–71.

Breteler, M. M., J. J. Claus, C. M. van Duijn, L. J. Launer and A. Hofman (1992). Epidemiology of Alzheimer's disease. *Epidemiol Rev* **14**: 59–82.

Brookmeyer, R., S. Gray and C. Kawas (1998). Projections of Alzheimer's disease in the United States and the public health impact of delaying disease onset. *Am J Public Health* **88**(9): 1337–42.

Brown, E. S., F. P. Varghese and B. S. McEwen (2004). Association of depression with medical illness: does cortisol play a role? *Biol Psychiatry* **55**(1): 1–9.

Butters, M. A., J. T. Becker, R. D. Nebes *et al.* (2000). Changes in cognitive functioning following treatment of late-life depression. *Am J Psychiatry* **157**(12): 1949–54.

Chen, P., M. Ganguli, B. H. Mulsant and S. T. DeKosky (1999). The temporal relationship between depressive symptoms and dementia: a community-based prospective study. *Arch Gen Psychiatry* **56**(3): 261–6.

Christensen, H., K. Griffiths, A. Mackinnon and P. Jacomb (1997). A quantitative review of cognitive deficits in depression and Alzheimer-type dementia. *J Int Neuropsychol Soc* **3**(6): 631–51.

Colcombe, S. and A. F. Kramer (2003). Fitness effects on the cognitive function of older adults: a meta-analytic study. *Psychol Sci* **14**(2): 125–30.

Di Bari, M., M. Pahor, L. V. Franse *et al.* (2001). Dementia and disability outcomes in large hypertension trials: lessons learned from the systolic hypertension in the elderly program (SHEP) trial. *Am J Epidemiol* **153**(1): 72–8.

Doraiswamy, P. M., K. R. Krishnan, T. Oxman *et al.* (2003). Does antidepressant therapy improve cognition in elderly depressed patients? *J Gerontol A Biol Sci Med Sci* **58**(12): M1137–44.

Dufouil, C., R. Fuhrer, J. F. Dartigues and A. Alperovitch (1996). Longitudinal analysis of the association between depressive symptomatology and cognitive deterioration. *Am J Epidemiol* **144**(7): 634–41.

Ellinson, M., J. Thomas and A. Patterson (2004). A critical evaluation of the relationship between serum vitamin B, folate and total homocysteine with cognitive impairment in the elderly. *J Hum Nutr Diet* **17**(4): 371–83; quiz 385–7.

Engelhart, M. J., M. I. Geerlings, A. Ruitenberg *et al.* (2002). Dietary intake of antioxidants and risk of Alzheimer disease. *JAMA* **287**(24): 3223–9.

Ernst, R. L. and J. W. Hay (1994). The US economic and social costs of Alzheimer's disease revisited. *Am J Public Health* **84**(8): 1261–4.

Evans, D. A., H. H. Funkenstein, M. S. Albert *et al.* (1989). Prevalence of Alzheimer's disease in a community population of older persons. Higher than previously reported. *JAMA* **262**(18): 2551–6.

Folstein, M. F., S. S. Bassett, J. C. Anthony, A. J. Romanoski and G. R. Nestadt (1991). Dementia: case ascertainment in a community survey. *J Gerontol* **46**(4): M132–8.

Forette, F., M. L. Seux, J. A. Staessen *et al.* (1998). Prevention of dementia in randomised double-blind placebo-controlled Systolic Hypertension in Europe (Syst-Eur) trial. *Lancet* **352**(9137): 1347–51.

Fratiglioni, L., H. X. Wang, K. Ericsson, M. Maytan and B. Winblad (2000). Influence of social network on occurrence of dementia: a community-based longitudinal study. *Lancet* **355**(9212): 1315–19.

Fratiglioni, L., S. Paillard-Borg and B. Winblad (2004). An active and socially integrated lifestyle in late life might protect against dementia. *Lancet Neurol* **3**(6): 343–53.

Gao, S., H. C. Hendrie, K. S. Hall and S. Hui (1998). The relationships between age, sex, and the incidence of dementia and Alzheimer disease: a meta-analysis. *Arch Gen Psychiatry* **55**(9): 809–15.

Geerlings, M. I., R. A. Schoevers, A. T. Beekman *et al.* (2000). Depression and risk of cognitive decline and Alzheimer's disease. Results of two prospective community-based studies in the Netherlands. *Br J Psychiatry* **176**: 568–75.

Grady, D., K. Yaffe, M. Kristof *et al.* (2002). Effect of postmenopausal hormone therapy on cognitive function: the Heart and Estrogen/progestin Replacement Study. *Am J Med* **113**(7): 543–8.

Grant, W. B. (2003). Diet and risk of dementia: does fat matter? The Rotterdam Study. *Neurology* **60**(12): 2020–1.

Hassing, L. B., B. Johansson, S. E. Nilsson *et al.* (2002). Diabetes mellitus is a risk factor for vascular dementia, but not for Alzheimer's disease: a population-based study of the oldest old. *Int Psychogeriatr* **14**(3): 239–48.

Heart Protection Study Collaborative Group (2002). MRC/BHF Heart Protection Study of cholesterol lowering with simvastatin in 20 536 high-risk individuals: a randomised placebo-controlled trial. *Lancet* **360**(9326): 7–22.

Hebert, L. E., P. A. Scherr, J. J. McCann, L. A. Beckett and D. A. Evans (2001). Is the risk of developing Alzheimer's disease greater for women than for men? *Am J Epidemiol* **153**(2): 132–6.

Hebert, L. E., P. A. Scherr, J. L. Bienias, D. A. Bennett and D. A. Evans (2003). Alzheimer disease in the US population: prevalence estimates using the 2000 census. *Arch Neurol* **60**(8): 1119–22.

Hendrie, H. C., B. O. Osuntokun, K. S. Hall *et al.* (1995). Prevalence of Alzheimer's disease and dementia in two communities: Nigerian Africans and African Americans. *Am J Psychiatry* **152**(10): 1485–92.

Heyman, A., W. E. Wilkinson, J. A. Stafford *et al.* (1984). Alzheimer's disease: a study of epidemiological aspects. *Ann Neurol* **15**(4): 335–41.

Jorm, A. F. (2001). History of depression as a risk factor for dementia: an updated review. *Aust N Z J Psychiatry* **35**(6): 776–81.

Jorm, A. F. and D. Jolley (1998). The incidence of dementia: a meta-analysis. *Neurology* **51**(3): 728–33.

Kalmijn, S., L. J. Launer, A. Ott *et al.* (1997). Dietary fat intake and the risk of incident dementia in the Rotterdam Study. *Ann Neurol* **42**(5): 776–82.

Knopman, D., L. L. Boland, T. Mosley *et al.* (2001). Cardiovascular risk factors and cognitive decline in middle-aged adults. *Neurology* 56(1): 42–8.

Kuller, L. H., O. L. Lopez, A. Newman *et al.* (2003). Risk factors for dementia in the cardiovascular health cognition study. *Neuroepidemiology* 22(1): 13–22.

Launer, L. J., G. W. Ross, H. Petrovitch *et al.* (2000). Midlife blood pressure and dementia: the Honolulu-Asia aging study. *Neurobiol Aging* 21(1): 49–55.

Lazarov, O., J. Robinson, Y. P. Tang *et al.* (2005). Environmental enrichment reduces abeta levels and amyloid deposition in transgenic mice. *Cell* 120(5): 701–13.

Lim, W., J. Gammack, J. Van Niekerk and A. Dangour (2006). Omega 3 fatty acid for the prevention of dementia. *Cochrane Database Syst Rev* (1): CD005379.

Lindsay, J., D. Laurin, R. Verreault *et al.* (2002). Risk factors for Alzheimer's disease: a prospective analysis from the Canadian Study of Health and Aging. *Am J Epidemiol* 156(5): 445–53.

Luchsinger, J. A., M. X. Tang, S. Shea *et al.* (2004). Plasma homocysteine levels and risk of Alzheimer disease. *Neurology* 62(11): 1972–6.

Lyketsos, C. G., O. Lopez, B. Jones *et al.* (2002). Prevalence of neuropsychiatric symptoms in dementia and mild cognitive impairment: results from the cardiovascular health study. *JAMA* 288(12): 1475–83.

MacKnight, C., K. Rockwood, E. Awalt and I. McDowell (2002). Diabetes mellitus and the risk of dementia, Alzheimer's disease and vascular cognitive impairment in the Canadian Study of Health and Aging. *Dement Geriatr Cogn Disord* 14(2): 77–83.

Malouf, M., E. J. Grimley and S. A. Areosa (2003). Folic acid with or without vitamin B12 for cognition and dementia. *Cochrane Database Syst Rev* (4): CD004514.

Manly, J. J., D. M. Jacobs and R. Mayeux (1999). Alzheimer disease among different ethnic and racial groups. In *Alzheimer Disease*, 2nd edn, R. D. Terry, R. Katzman, K. L. Bick and S. S. Sisodia (eds.). New York: Lippincott, Williams & Wilkins, pp. 117–32.

Maxwell, C. J., M. S. Hicks, D. B. Hogan, J. Basran and E. M. Ebly (2005). Supplemental use of antioxidant vitamins and subsequent risk of cognitive decline and dementia. *Dement Geriatr Cogn Disord* 20(1): 45–51.

McGeer, P. L., M. Schulzer and E. G. McGeer (1996). Arthritis and anti-inflammatory agents as possible protective factors for Alzheimer's disease: a review of 17 epidemiologic studies. *Neurology* 47(2): 425–32.

Mehta, K. M., A. Ott, S. Kalmijn *et al.* (1999). Head trauma and risk of dementia and Alzheimer's disease: the Rotterdam Study. *Neurology* 53(9): 1959–62.

Morris, M. C., D. A. Evans, C. C. Tangney, J. L. Bienias and R. S. Wilson (2005). Fish consumption and cognitive decline with age in a large community study. *Arch Neurol* 62(12): 1849–53.

Mukamal, K. J., L. H. Kuller, A. L. Fitzpatrick *et al.* (2003). Prospective study of alcohol consumption and risk of dementia in older adults. *JAMA* 289(11): 1405–13.

Mulnard, R. A., C. W. Cotman, C. Kawas *et al.* (2000). Estrogen replacement therapy for treatment of mild to moderate Alzheimer disease: a randomized controlled trial. Alzheimer's Disease Cooperative Study. *JAMA* 283(8): 1007–15.

Nebes, R. D., B. G. Pollock, P. R. Houck *et al.* (2003). Persistence of cognitive impairment in geriatric patients following antidepressant treatment: a randomized, double-blind clinical trial with nortriptyline and paroxetine. *J Psychiatr Res* 37(2): 99–108.

Petersen, R. C., R. G. Thomas, M. Grundman *et al.* (2005). Vitamin E and donepezil for the treatment of mild cognitive impairment. *N Engl J Med* 352(23): 2379–88.

Qiu, C., B. Winblad and L. Fratiglioni (2005). The age-dependent relation of blood pressure to cognitive function and dementia. *Lancet Neurol* 4(8): 487–99.

Rea, T. D., J. C. Breitner, B. M. Psaty *et al.* (2005). Statin use and the risk of incident dementia: the Cardiovascular Health Study. *Arch Neurol* 62(7): 1047–51.

Rice, D. P., P. J. Fox, W. Max *et al.* (1993). The economic burden of Alzheimer's disease care. *Health Aff (Millwood)* 12(2): 164–76.

Rocca, W. A., R. H. Cha, S. C. Waring and E. Kokmen (1998). Incidence of dementia and Alzheimer's disease: a reanalysis of data from Rochester, Minnesota, 1975–1984. *Am J Epidemiol* 148(1): 51–62.

Ruitenberg, A., J. C. van Swieten, J. C. Witteman *et al.* (2002). Alcohol consumption and risk of dementia: the Rotterdam Study. *Lancet* 359(9303): 281–6.

Saczynski, J. S., L. A. Pfeifer, K. Masaki *et al.* (2006). The effect of social engagement on incident dementia: the Honolulu-Asia Aging Study. *Am J Epidemiol* 163(5): 433–40.

Sano, M., C. Ernesto, R. G. Thomas *et al.* (1997). A controlled trial of selegiline, alpha-tocopherol, or both as treatment for Alzheimer's disease. The Alzheimer's Disease Cooperative Study. *N Engl J Med* 336(17): 1216–22.

Scarmeas, N., G. Levy, M. X. Tang, J. Manly and Y. Stern (2001). Influence of leisure activity on the incidence of Alzheimer's disease. *Neurology* 57(12): 2236–42.

Seshadri, S., A. Beiser, J. Selhub *et al.* (2002). Plasma homocysteine as a risk factor for dementia and Alzheimer's disease. *N Engl J Med* 346(7): 476–83.

SHEP Cooperative Research Group (1991). Prevention of stroke by antihypertensive drug treatment in older persons with isolated systolic hypertension. Final results of the Systolic Hypertension in the Elderly Program (SHEP). *JAMA* 265(24): 3255–64.

Shumaker, S. A., C. Legault, S. R. Rapp *et al.* (2003). Estrogen plus progestin and the incidence of dementia and mild cognitive impairment in postmenopausal

129

women: the Women's Health Initiative Memory Study: a randomized controlled trial. *JAMA* **289**(20): 2651–62.

Shumaker, S. A., C. Legault, L. Kuller *et al.* (2004). Conjugated equine estrogens and incidence of probable dementia and mild cognitive impairment in postmenopausal women: Women's Health Initiative Memory Study. *JAMA* **291**(24): 2947–58.

Snowdon, D. A., S. J. Kemper, J. A. Mortimer *et al.* (1996). Linguistic ability in early life and cognitive function and Alzheimer's disease in late life. Findings from the Nun Study. *JAMA* **275**(7): 528–32.

Snowdon, D. A., L. H. Greiner, J. A. Mortimer *et al.* (1997). Brain infarction and the clinical expression of Alzheimer disease. The Nun Study. *JAMA* **277**(10): 813–7.

Stampfer, M. J., J. H. Kang, J. Chen, R. Cherry and F. Grodstein (2005). Effects of moderate alcohol consumption on cognitive function in women. *N Engl J Med* **352**(3): 245–53.

Starkstein, S. E., R. Jorge, R. Mizrahi and R. G. Robinson (2005). The construct of minor and major depression in Alzheimer's disease. *Am J Psychiatry* **162**(11): 2086–93.

Stern, Y. (2002). What is cognitive reserve? Theory and research application of the reserve concept. *J Int Neuropsychol Soc* **8**(3): 448–60.

Stern, Y., B. Gurland, T. K. Tatemichi *et al.* (1994). Influence of education and occupation on the incidence of Alzheimer's disease. *JAMA* **271**(13): 1004–10.

Szekely, C. A., J. E. Thorne, P. P. Zandi *et al.* (2004). Nonsteroidal anti-inflammatory drugs for the prevention of Alzheimer's disease: a systematic review. *Neuroepidemiology* **23**(4): 159–69.

Tang, M. X., P. Cross, H. Andrews, D. *et al.* (2001). Incidence of AD in African-Americans, Caribbean Hispanics, and Caucasians in northern Manhattan. *Neurology* **56**(1): 49–56.

Tzourio, C., C. Anderson, N. Chapman *et al.* (2003). Effects of blood pressure lowering with perindopril and indapamide therapy on dementia and cognitive decline in patients with cerebrovascular disease. *Arch Intern Med* **163**(9): 1069–75.

US Department of Health and Human Services (1996). *Physical Activity and Health: A report of the Surgeon General.* Atlanta, GA: US Department of Health and Human Services, Centers for Disease Control and Prevention, National Center for Chronic Disease Prevention and Health Promotion.

van Praag, H., B. R. Christie, T. J. Sejnowski and F. H. Gage (1999). Running enhances neurogenesis, learning, and long-term potentiation in mice. *Proc Natl Acad Sci USA* **96**(23): 13427–31.

Verghese, J., R. B. Lipton, M. J. Katz *et al.* (2003). Leisure activities and the risk of dementia in the elderly. *N Engl J Med* **348**(25): 2508–16.

Vermeer, S. E., N. D. Prins, T. den Heijer *et al.* (2003). Silent brain infarcts and the risk of dementia and cognitive decline. *N Engl J Med* **348**(13): 1215–22.

Waters, D. D., E. L. Alderman, J. Hsia *et al.* (2002). Effects of hormone replacement therapy and antioxidant vitamin supplements on coronary atherosclerosis in postmenopausal women: a randomized controlled trial. *JAMA* **288**(19): 2432–40.

Weuve, J., J. H. Kang, J. E. Manson *et al.* (2004). Physical activity, including walking, and cognitive function in older women. *JAMA* **292**(12): 1454–61.

White, L., H. Petrovitch, G. W. Ross *et al.* (1996). Prevalence of dementia in older Japanese-American men in Hawaii: the Honolulu-Asia Aging Study. *JAMA* **276**(12): 955–60.

Whitmer, R. A., S. Sidney, J. Selby, S. C. Johnston and K. Yaffe (2005). Midlife cardiovascular risk factors and risk of dementia in late life. *Neurology* **64**(2): 277–81.

Wilson, R. S., D. A. Bennett, J. L. Bienias *et al.* (2002a). Cognitive activity and incident AD in a population-based sample of older persons. *Neurology* **59**(12): 1910–4.

Wilson, R. S., C. F. Mendes De Leon, L. L. Barnes *et al.* (2002b). Participation in cognitively stimulating activities and risk of incident Alzheimer disease. *JAMA* **287**(6): 742–8.

Wilson, R. S., L. L. Barnes, C. F. Mendes de Leon *et al.* (2002c). Depressive symptoms, cognitive decline, and risk of AD in older persons. *Neurology* **59**(3): 364–70.

Xiong, G. L., A. Benson and P. M. Doraiswamy (2005). Statins and cognition: what can we learn from existing randomized trials? *CNS Spectr* **10**(11): 867–74.

Yaffe, K. (2001). Estrogens, selective estrogen receptor modulators, and dementia: what is the evidence? *Ann N Y Acad Sci* **949**: 215–22.

Yaffe, K., T. Blackwell, R. Gore *et al.* (1999). Depressive symptoms and cognitive decline in nondemented elderly women: a prospective study. *Arch Gen Psychiatry* **56**(5): 425–30.

Yaffe, K., D. Barnes, M. Nevitt, L. Y. Lui and K. Covinsky (2001). A prospective study of physical activity and cognitive decline in elderly women: women who walk. *Arch Intern Med* **161**(14): 1703–8.

Yaffe, K., T. Blackwell, A. M. Kanaya *et al.* (2004a). Diabetes, impaired fasting glucose, and development of cognitive impairment in older women. *Neurology* **63**(4): 658–63.

Yaffe, K., A. Kanaya, K. Lindquist *et al.* (2004b). The metabolic syndrome, inflammation, and risk of cognitive decline. *JAMA* **292**(18): 2237–42.

Yaffe, K., K. Krueger, S. R. Cummings *et al.* (2005). Effect of raloxifene on prevention of dementia and cognitive impairment in older women: the Multiple Outcomes of Raloxifene Evaluation (MORE) randomized trial. *Am J Psychiatry* **162**(4): 683–90.

Chapter 10

Animal models of dementia

Erik D. Roberson and Aimee W. Kao

Recent decades have witnessed major advances in diagnosing neurodegenerative diseases such as Alzheimer's disease (AD) and frontotemporal dementia (FTD), together with a wealth of new information about their clinical course and natural history. However, patients and physicians alike have been frustrated by the lack of available treatments. Solving this problem will require both a better understanding of the molecular mechanisms underlying these diseases and systems for screening the efficacy and safety of new therapeutics. There are several strategies for addressing these issues: studies of human patients themselves and human autopsy tissues, studies of animal models of disease, and more reductionist (cell culture or in vitro) models of disease. In this chapter, we will focus on animal models of neurodegenerative diseases, summarizing their relative advantages and disadvantages, highlighting some of the most important and widely studied models available, and reviewing a few important lessons that have emerged from animal model studies in recent years.

There is no question that studies of affected patients are the "gold standard" for understanding a human disease. As such, animal model studies depend fully on such human research. For example, human genetic studies has identified the mutations that have been used to generate most animal models of disease. Obviously, though, there are advantages to using animal models, and it is useful to consider them explicitly, as they help to clarify both the power and the limitations of animal models.

Ability to study early stages of the disease.
Therapies are most likely to be effective when delivered early in the disease, before irreversible cell death or other changes occur, making it critical to understand the pathophysiology underlying initial stages. Until we have sensitive biomarkers for early disease and the resources to screen large

populations, few such "preclinical" patients are likely to be available for research. Even then, it is difficult to carry out the more interventional studies (e.g. biopsy) necessary to fully characterize a disease in such patients; most neuropathological studies are conducted on postmortem brains with end-stage disease. And true experiments that involve manipulating part of the system to determine its effect are rarely likely to pass ethical tests.

Ability to distinguish mediators from indicators.
Imaging and neuropathological studies reveal many of the lesions that characterize various forms of dementia. Some of these findings are undoubtedly causative and drugs that prevent them could be effective therapies. Others, however, might be compensatory responses and blocking them could even be counterproductive. Of course, yet others may simply be indicators of disease with no causal effects on the pathogenic processes. Distinguishing between these possibilities requires experimental manipulations (either preventing or stimulating the effect in question) that are not possible in patients.

Control over genetic background. It is clear that the onset and/or severity of neurodegenerative diseases is controlled by a variety of genes, many of which have not yet even been identified. In a human population, variability from genetic diversity reduces the power of studies. Animal model studies can be conducted on inbred genetic backgrounds, minimizing genetic variability and increasing statistical power. It is worth noting, though, that variability is also seen even in genetically identical mice, indicating that epigenetic and/or environmental factors also have a strong influence on neurodegenerative pathophysiology.

Ability to perform unbiased screens. Animal models enable both genetic and pharmacological

The Behavioral Neurology of Dementia, eds. Bruce L. Miller and Bradley F. Boeve. Published by Cambridge University Press. © Cambridge University Press 2009.

screening, with the attendant power to detect novel and unexpected interactions. Such studies are not possible in patients, where treatment trials are necessarily limited to agents with a reasonable expectation of efficacy.

Of course, the power of animal models depends on how good the models are. The validity of animal models is often assessed with three questions. First, is the disease model generated in a manner similar to that believed to cause disease in humans? Most available models of dementia utilize transgenes with mutations that cause familial forms of the disease in humans, and so pass this test fairly well. Second, does the phenotype of the disease model look like the real disease? Most animal models have cognitive abnormalities and pathological lesions similar to those that characterize human dementing diseases, although in many cases only a partial "phenocopy" of the disease is present. Finally, do observations in the animal model predict similar observations in the human condition – in particular, are treatments identified in a model effective in patients? Here the jury is still out, and those working in this area are eagerly awaiting the results of clinical trials on therapeutic strategies originally identified in animal models, such as β-amyloid (Aβ) immunotherapy.

Vertebrate models

The mainstay of most animal model work for neurodegenerative diseases has been the transgenic mouse. Rodent models have several advantages for such studies. First, there is considerable anatomic conservation of the brain structures involved. Because neurodegenerative diseases are characterized by a high degree of regional specificity, this is an important consideration, potentially enabling the modeling of selective vulnerability. Second, there is a high degree of genetic conservation between mice and humans; it is estimated that 99% of human genes are present in mice and the vast majority are syntenic, or in the same chromosomal arrangement (Tecott, 2003). Third, there are powerful methods for analyzing rodent behavior that enable detection of phenotypes relating to clinical dementia syndromes, including tests of learning and memory, motor impairment and social dysfunction (Crawley, 2000).

The main disadvantage of rodent models is the time and expense involved. Most of the phenotypes are age dependent, so the mice that are used in many studies must be aged for several months or years.

Beyond the fact that this slows the pace of mouse model research, it also creates great expense for housing and husbandry; a large laboratory easily spends tens of thousands of dollars per month just on animal housing costs.

Mouse models of Alzheimer's disease
Human amyloid precursor protein models

The first animal models of AD were transgenic mice with neuronal expression of human amyloid precursor protein (hAPP) carrying familial AD mutations (Games et al., 1995; McGowan et al., 2006). Commonly studied lines include PDAPP and related J20 mice (Games et al., 1995; Mucke et al., 2000), Tg2576 mice (Hsiao et al., 1996), APP23 mice (Sturchler-Pierrat et al., 1997) and TgCRND8 mice (Chishti et al., 2001). In large part, these lines remain the mainstays for AD research using animal models, including both studies dissecting underlying pathophysiological mechanisms and preclinical testing of new treatments.

All hAPP mice have age-dependent amyloid plaque deposition and memory deficits (Kobayashi and Chen, 2005; McGowan et al., 2006). However, not all aspects of AD are modeled. Neurofibrillary tangles (NFT) do not form, although reducing endogenous tau in these mice does preclude most of the Aβ-induced deficits (Roberson et al., 2007). Neuron loss is also not a prominent feature (Irizarry et al., 1997a,b; Takeuchi et al., 2000). The use of hAPP mice as an AD model has been criticized by some because of the lack of NFT pathology and neuron loss. However, they do seem to be good models of AD-related synaptic loss and dendritic simplification (Mucke et al., 2000; Buttini et al., 2002; Lanz et al., 2003; Chin et al., 2004; Moolman et al., 2004; Wu et al., 2004; Spires et al., 2005). These mice are best considered as an animal model of Aβ-induced neuronal dysfunction, a phenomenon that may precede Aβ-induced neurodegeneration and contribute to cognitive impairment (Selkoe, 2002; Palop et al., 2006).

While the relative contributions of neuronal dysfunction and neuron loss to AD-related cognitive deficits await further study, it is worth noting that hAPP mice have already contributed to the development of many of the AD therapies now in clinical trials (Roberson and Mucke, 2006). For example, the plaque-clearing effects of Aβ immunization were initially identified in hAPP mice (Schenk et al., 1999), and vaccination appears to have a similar effect on amyloid deposits in human subjects (Nicoll et al., 2003, 2006).

These mice have also helped to elucidate the pathogenic role of Aβ oligomers. Although their abundant amyloid plaques were the aspect of the phenotype that attracted the most initial attention, it later became clear that the memory deficits in these mice did not correlate well with the plaque load (Holcomb et al., 1998; Westerman et al., 2002; Palop et al., 2003; Kobayashi and Chen, 2005; Lesné et al., 2006). Rather, the deficits in these mice seem to be linked to synaptic dysfunction caused by soluble oligomers of Aβ (Walsh et al., 2002; Cleary et al., 2005; Lesné et al., 2006).

Presenilin models
Mutations affecting APP are not the only genetic causes of AD, and other mutations have also been used to create animal models. Mutations in the gene *PS1*, which encodes presenilin 1, are the most common cause of autosomal dominant AD (Cruts and Rademakers, 2008). Mutant *PS1* transgenic mice have high levels of Aβ42 (the 42-residue form of Aβ) but do not form plaques and have no striking learning and memory deficits (Duff et al., 1996; Janus et al., 2000). However, crossing these *PS1* transgenics with hAPP mice (producing what are called PSAPP mice) causes hAPP/Aβ-induced deficits to appear at earlier ages and with greater severity (Borchelt et al., 1997; Holcomb et al., 1998). This is consistent with the fact that many mutations altering presenilin increase the production of the more pathogenic Aβ42 peptides (Borchelt et al., 1996; Scheuner et al., 1996).

Increasing Aβ production is not the only effect of mutant presenilin, however. There is increasing attention paid to loss-of-function effects of these mutations (Shen and Kelleher, 2007). For example, presenilin loss of function leads to increased calcium release from intracellular stores (Leissring et al., 2000; LaFerla, 2002; Kasri et al., 2006; Tu et al., 2006) and also stimulates tau phosphorylation (Baki et al., 2004). Conditional presenilin knockout mice (presenilin deficiency during development is lethal) have abnormal tau phosphorylation, neurodegeneration and deficits in synaptic plasticity and learning and memory impairments (Saura et al., 2004). Because these mice do not have increased Aβ levels, their abnormalities support the idea that presenilin loss of function may contribute to AD pathogenesis (Shen and Kelleher, 2007).

Apolipoprotein E models
While apolipoprotein E (ApoE) is not a genetic cause per se of AD, it is by far the strongest genetic risk factor for the disease (Farrer et al., 1997; Raber et al., 2004; Bertram et al., 2007). There are three isoforms of *ApoE*: ApoE2, ApoE3 and ApoE4. These are encoded by three alleles, ε2, ε3 and ε4. Roughly half of all those with sporadic AD have at least one ε4 allele (Saunders et al., 1993). Several different ApoE-based animal models of AD have been developed.

Most of the ApoE in normal brain is produced by glia, but neurons produce ApoE after injury (Xu et al., 2006). Transgenic mice expressing ApoE from a neuron-specific promoter exhibit learning and memory deficits in females (Raber et al., 1998, 2000). The gender dependence of this effect is interesting because ApoE4 is a stronger risk factor for AD in women than in men (Payami et al., 1996). The basis of the differential gender effect in mice may relate to the fact that ApoE4 decreases androgen receptor levels; because females have lower levels of circulating androgens, they would be more sensitive to this effect (Raber et al., 2002; Raber, 2004). Mouse models also indicate that neuronal ApoE4 lacks the neuroprotective effects that are seen with neuronal production of ApoE3 (Buttini et al., 1999).

Human ε4 has also been "knocked-in" to the mouse *ApoE* locus, retaining the endogenous sequences that regulate the formation of ApoE. These mice have abnormalities in synaptic plasticity (Trommer et al., 2004). Pathogenic proteolysis also alters ApoE in neurons (Huang et al., 2001), and mice with just this truncated form of ApoE4 develop neurodegeneration and behavioral deficits (Harris et al., 2003).

Combination models
In addition to the PSAPP combination model mentioned above, other multiply transgenic models have been described. First, both human ε3 and human ε4 transgenics have been crossed with hAPP mice, helping to explore interactions between Aβ and ApoE. Presence of ApoE4 dramatically increases amyloid plaque distribution relative to that seen with ApoE3 (Holtzman et al., 2000; Buttini et al., 2002). Interestingly, even before plaque deposition begins, ApoE4/hAPP mice have more synaptic and behavioral deficits than ApoE3/hAPP mice (Raber et al., 2000; Buttini et al., 2002), suggesting that ApoE isoforms may have differential effects on Aβ oligomers, in addition to the plaques.

Mutations in the human tau gene cause FTD, but not AD, so models with these transgenes are discussed in more detail below. However, many of these mutant tau transgenes have been introduced in combination

133

with other AD-related transgenes in attempts to improve the modeling of the neurofibrillary pathology seen in AD. Such models include the TAPP line (a cross between the Tg2576 hAPP line and the JNPL3 tau transgenic; Lewis *et al.*, 2001) and the 3×Tg line, which contains human *APP* and *PS1* with familial AD mutations and human tau with an FTD mutation (Oddo *et al.*, 2003). These lines have revealed that Aβ can stimulate tau phosphorylation and accumulation, but that tau overexpression does not strongly affect Aβ deposits (Lewis *et al.*, 2001; Oddo *et al.*, 2004).

Finally, although synuclein pathology is often thought of mostly in the context of parkinsonian dementias, there is important clinical and pathological overlap between these disorders and AD (Perl *et al.*, 1998). Doubly transgenic hAPP/α-synuclein lines revealed that Aβ stimulates synuclein accumulation (Masliah *et al.*, 2001). Both memory deficits and motor abnormalities were worse in the bigenic mice than in the singly transgenic parental lines (Masliah *et al.*, 2001).

Mouse models of frontotemporal dementia

The first genetic mutations discovered to cause FTD in humans were in the tau gene on chromosome 17 (Hutton *et al.*, 1998; Poorkaj *et al.*, 1998; Spillantini *et al.*, 1998; Clark *et al.*, 1998), and mutant tau transgenic mice have remained the primary animal model of FTD. One of the first such models was the JNPL3 line, which produces human tau with the P301L mutation (Lewis *et al.*, 2000). These mice develop progressive motor deficits, neurofibrillary tau aggregates and neurodegeneration. More recently, a line called rTg4510 was developed, which also produces the P301L tau mutant, but from a transgene that can be turned off by feeding the animal doxycycline (Santa-Cruz *et al.*, 2005). These mice also have behavioral deficits and neurofibrillary tau pathology, but when the transgene is turned off, the two phenomena dissociate; learning and memory impairments resolve, while tau aggregation continues (SantaCruz *et al.*, 2005). This suggests that soluble forms of mutant tau contribute to neuronal dysfunction in these mice.

The pathology of FTD reveals involvement of several different glia types (reviewed in Roberson, 2006), and animal models have extended our understanding of the role of both microglia and astrocytes in FTD. Studies with a P301S mutant line further supported the idea that mutant tau causes synaptic loss and neuronal

dysfunction even before tau aggregates appear and neuron loss occurs (Yoshiyama *et al.*, 2007). In these mice, tau-induced microglial activation appears to be an early step in pathogenesis (Yoshiyama *et al.*, 2007). Cell type-specific promoters have also been used to express mutant human tau in astrocytes (Forman *et al.*, 2005). These mice also develop neuronal dysfunction before tau aggregation, apparently as a result of impaired astrocytic glutamate uptake from decreased expression of the glutamate transporter GLT-1 (Dabir *et al.*, 2006).

The rapid pace of new discoveries in FTD, including roles for progranulin, TAR DNA-binding protein 43 (TDP-43), valosin-containing protein and charged multivesicular body protein 2B, raises hopes and expectations for the future (Watts *et al.*, 2004; Skibinski *et al.*, 2005; Baker *et al.*, 2006; Cruts *et al.*, 2006; Neumann *et al.*, 2006). Animal models based on these molecules are likely to contribute significantly to our understanding of different subtypes of FTD. In addition, most of the behavioral assessment of FTD models to date has focused on learning and memory, as these tests are well established from research on AD models. Growing interest in social function and dysfunction in rodents has produced new behavioral methods that should enable investigations into how and why FTD targets social domains.

Invertebrate models

In this section, we will summarize the potential advantages of invertebrates in the study of human neurodegenerative disease, review what has been learned from existing models of AD and FTD in flies and worms, and finally discuss key questions left in the field and the role that invertebrates may play in answering them.

Advantages and limitations of using invertebrates to study neurodegenerative disease

Invertebrates such as the fruit fly *Drosophila melanogaster* and the microscopic worm *Caenorhabditis elegans* represent compelling alternative model systems in which to study human diseases. Their compact lifespan (averaging 25–30 days in flies and 15–20 days in worms) allow for the observation of biological processes from fertilization through development and aging to death. Surprising to many, flies and worms exhibit stereotyped behaviors, including directed searching and foraging and conditional learning and memory, albeit in much simpler forms than vertebrates. In fact, Nobel prize-winning scientist Sydney Brenner in 1973 hand-picked the nematode *C. elegans* as a model organism in which to apply recently developed genetic techniques to study the nervous system. These and the additional powerful tools developed for genetic manipulation of worms and flies represent the greatest advantage of these systems in the study of neurodegenerative disease.

Compared with the 10 billion neurons of the average *Homo sapiens* brain, the fruit fly and worm have approximately 50 000 and 300 neurons, respectively. Their nervous systems are not only much simpler than that of humans, or even rodents, but they are better characterized and understood. In fact, in *C. elegans*, every neuron and its synaptic connections have been mapped. Because of the thin cuticle lining its body, the worm nervous system has the additional advantage of being transparent to light microscopic viewing. *Drosophila* neurodegeneration likewise can conveniently be reflected in eye organization. Invertebrate neurons express many of the same molecules of the mammalian brain. Most of the basic building blocks of the vertebrate nervous system are present, including ion channels, synaptic proteins and neurons with small molecule, amino acid and neuroactive peptide neurotransmitters (such as dopamine, gamma-aminobutyric acid and insulin) (Bargmann, 1998; Yoshihara *et al.*, 2001). Although the complex behaviors and emotions that make us human and are so tragically lost in neurodegenerative diseases cannot be recapitulated in such simple model systems, invertebrates do exhibit stereotyped outputs from their nervous systems, some of which can be measured, including foraging, feeding, hibernation, reproduction, defecation and simple learning. In some cases, these functions can be perturbed by human disease proteins, resulting in the deficit of a function that is both homologous and commensurate to what is seen in humans. For example, when mutant human α-synuclein is expressed in *Drosophila* neurons, the flies show age-dependent loss of dopaminergic neurons, develop intraneuronal inclusions containing α-synuclein and exhibit dysfunctional movement all reminiscent of Parkinson's disease (Feany and Bender, 2000).

Another advantage of invertebrates relates to the ease and rapidity by which genetic manipulation can be carried out. Transgenic worms and flies can be developed in a few weeks instead of the months–years required to produce a transgenic mouse. Once introduced, the phenotype of a transgene can be observed across a much shorter lifespan, and since there are fewer redundant genes in fly and worm genomes, knock-out phenotypes are less likely to be masked. In fact, the entire *Drosophila* and *C. elegans* genomes have been sequenced (The *C. elegans* Sequencing Consortium, 1998; Adams *et al.*, 2000). This allows for easy comparison between functionally or structurally similar genes in different species. When a disease gene is identified in humans, one can identify orthologs in worms or flies with just a few keystrokes. Whole genome comparisons have already shown that there is a high degree of conservation of genes and metabolic pathways between these organisms and humans (Rubin *et al.*, 2000). In fact, of 289 genes implicated in human disease, 61% appear to have orthologs in *Drosophila* (Rubin *et al.*, 2000). Included in this list are multiple genes mutated in neurological disease, including genes for APP and presenilin (AD), Notch (CADASIL), tau (FTD) and parkin (juvenile Parkinson's disease). Whether these gene products play the same role in invertebrates as in mammals and whether they can serve as disease models is in many cases yet to be determined. However, the initial results are promising (see below).

A final advantage of invertebrate systems relates to the number of techniques to study organisms, cells and molecules in vivo. For example, real-time microscopy can be used to follow the in vivo subcellular localization of proteins labeled with fluorescent protein probes. A powerful technique for single-gene silencing in *C. elegans* is RNA interference (RNAi) (Fire *et al.*, 1998). The principle of RNAi as a genetic tool is to silence an endogenous gene using a short anti-sense RNA (called a short interfering RNA, or siRNA) that hybridizes to the mRNA in question, thus targeting that mRNA for degradation or translation arrest. In *C. elegans*, RNAi can be easily achieved by feeding the worm bacteria that produce the siRNA. For example, if one wished to study the function of the *C. elegans* amyloid precursor protein, APL-1, worms could be fed bacteria that have been engineered to produce *apl-1* siRNA. After eating this bacteria, the siRNA would hybridize with endogenous *apl-1* mRNA in the worm cells and inhibit its expression. Such easy genetic manipulation is not yet readily available in vertebrate model systems, which generally require a viral vector to introduce the siRNA into cells.

The question still remains: does invertebrate biology reflect that of mammals with enough fidelity that they can be effective disease models? After all, dementia is characterized by a breakdown in the

135

higher functions and abilities that make us human. Indeed, the complex phenotypes and regional specificity of neurodegenerative diseases cannot be recapitulated in invertebrates. Nonetheless, at their simplest, dementias are diseases of neuronal dysfunction and death, and it is precisely by studying these basic processes that greater understanding of disease can be achieved. Science is riddled with examples of basic research in simple organisms that ultimately have profound and previously unforeseen practical and disease applications in humans. One of the most recent examples is that of the study of apoptosis or programmed cell death. The basic mechanisms of programmed cell death or apoptosis are not only conserved in invertebrates, but their biology and function was pioneered in *C. elegans*, for which the Nobel prize was awarded in 2001 (Marx, 2002). This basic research, which was pioneered in *C. elegans*, has profoundly influenced human research in fields as varied as development, aging, tumor biology and immunology.

Invertebrate models of Alzheimer's disease and frontotemporal dementia

Both the *Drosophila* and the *C. elegans* genomes contain genes that are related to hAPP. In the fly, the protein product is known as APPL (APP-like protein) and in the worm as APL-1 (Rosen *et al.*, 1989; Daigle and Li, 1993). Compared with hAPP, fly APPL and worm APL-1 have similar extracellular E1 and E2 domains, and a highly conserved cytoplasmic C domain. However, these related proteins do not encode the Aβ domain of hAPP and, therefore, produce neither toxic protein fragments nor disease in their hosts. When hAPP is transgenically produced in a *Drosophila* that has had its own APPL deleted, it can ameliorate a subtle behavioral deficit in light-responsive movement (Luo *et al.*, 1992). This suggests that the two proteins have similar functions.

The function of APP has been a focus of intense research. Work in both cell culture and invertebrate models have shed light on this topic. Based on work in *Drosophila*, proposed APP functions include involvement in synapse generation (Torroja *et al.*, 1999a), fast axonal transport (Torroja *et al.*, 1999b) and postdevelopmental neurite arborization (Leyssen *et al.*, 2005). An emerging theme, that of toxic proteins first attacking distal neurites, is supported by the finding that overproduction of APP in *Drosophila* results in accumulation of organelles in distal axons

as well as increased neuronal cell death. This has led to the hypothesis that increased local concentrations of Aβ promote cell death (Gunawardena and Goldstein, 2001). Certainly work in *C. elegans* supports the claim that Aβ production has endogenous toxicity. When Aβ42 is expressed in worm muscle, microarray comparisons of gene expression show that heat shock proteins and genes involved in apoptosis are upregulated (Link *et al.*, 2003).

A major risk factor for development of neurodegenerative diseases is advanced age, yet the causal factors behind this link have been elusive. The field of aging research grew out of the observation that single gene mutations in *C. elegans* could double the lifespan of the organism (Kenyon *et al.*, 1993). With an average lifespan of 2 weeks, the worm is thus an ideal organism to study the relationship between disease and aging. In fact, a recent report suggests that aging can influence the development of diseases of protein aggregation in two ways. Using a model of AD in which Aβ42 is expressed in worm muscle, scientists have shown that the process of aging inhibits both a cell's ability to degrade toxic low-molecular-weight Aβ42 aggregates and the ability to detoxify these aggregates through the formation of larger, non-toxic inclusions, which may be analogous to AD plaques and tangles (Cohen *et al.*, 2006).

Along with neuron loss, the formation of amyloid plaques and NFTs are the cornerstone to a pathological diagnosis of AD and this is one disease characteristic in which invertebrate models have so far fallen short. The situation is different in *Drosophila* and *C. elegans* models of tauopathies. In both animals, production of wild-type or mutant human tau causes accumulation of insoluble aggregates (Wittmann *et al.*, 2001; Kraemer *et al.*, 2003), which in some cases were flame shaped and enriched for hyperphosphorylated tau (Jackson *et al.*, 2002), just as in human disease. Acetylcholine neurons were preferentially affected by overproduced tau (Wittmann *et al.*, 2001). Tau inclusions correlated with, but followed rather than preceded, neuronal degeneration (Jackson *et al.*, 2002), adding further support to the now more generally accepted idea that inclusions are a consequence of but not causative for neurodegenerative disease (Arrasate *et al.*, 2004).

Work in *Drosophila* has further expanded our understanding of the pathogenic mechanism of tau by identifying tau-interacting proteins that may contribute to hyperphosphorylation. Using the same *Drosophila* model of tauopathy, scientists have shown that phosphorylation of tau by the serine/threonine kinase PAR-1 acts as a trigger of sorts for cell death, suggesting a central role for this kinase in tau-related neurodegeneration (Nishimura *et al.*, 2004). In an example of an invertebrate being used for functional validation of findings in mice, Karsten *et al.* (2006) identified puromycin-sensitive aminopeptidase (PSA) as being upregulated in regions of mouse brain resistant to neurodegeneration after overproduction of mutant tau. They then used *Drosophila* to show that loss of PSA exacerbated tau-induced neurodegeneration, while overproduction of PSA ameliorated it (Karsten *et al.*, 2006). These discoveries could translate into potential therapies for several tau-related diseases.

The therapeutic potential of invertebrate model systems

Discoveries of the basic mechanisms of neurodegenerative diseases are but one avenue in which invertebrates can contribute to the development of treatments for AD and FTD. The complexity and phenotypic variability of human disease coupled with ethical considerations have also limited the use of human subjects in the development and testing of disease therapies. Although testing in mice is a necessary step in ultimately bringing therapies to the bedside, drug screening in vertebrates requires large numbers of animals and the subsequent costs of handling and upkeep can be prohibitive. Given their small size, ease of handling and rapid rate of reproduction, invertebrate disease models have no such limitations. Consequently, these model systems represent a major opportunity to screen not only conventional drug therapies but also the hundreds of thousands of small molecules that are being rapidly generated in the hope of finding novel treatments. This type of work is ongoing and will likely yield benefits for human disease not only in neurodegeneration but in other fields of medicine as well.

Summary

The study of neurodegenerative disease using animal models has already had a profound impact on our understanding of disease mechanisms and is poised to contribute to breakthroughs in developing disease treatments. One lesson to be gained from these many model systems is that no single model is ideal in all situations. One transgenic animal model may more closely recapitulate human disease and be useful for studying disease progress and pathogenesis but

be impractical for unbiased genetic screening of disease-modifying molecules. Likewise, another may be more suited for the rapid screening of potential therapies but lack the correct regional vulnerability pattern when expressed in the brain. In order to generate meaningful scientific insight from animal models, it is vital that they be used judiciously, in the correct context and with the goal of answering clearly delineated questions. Only then will the knowledge gained from these animal models be useful in ultimately treating and preventing neurodegenerative disease.

References

Adams, M. D., Celniker S. E., Holt R. A. *et al.* 2000. The genome sequence of *Drosophila melanogaster*. *Science* **287**, 2185–2195.

Arrasate, M., Mitra S., Schweitzer E. S., Segal M. R., Finkbeiner S. 2004. Inclusion body formation reduces levels of mutant huntingtin and the risk of neuronal death. *Nature* **431**, 805–810.

Baker, M., Mackenzie I. R., Pickering-Brown S. M. *et al.* 2006. Mutations in progranulin cause tau-negative frontotemporal dementia linked to chromosome 17. *Nature* **442**, 916–919.

Baki, L., Shioi J., Wen P. *et al.* 2004. PS1 activates PI3K thus inhibiting GSK-3 activity and tau overphosphorylation: effects of FAD mutations. *EMBO J.* **23**, 2586–2596.

Bargmann, C. I. 1998. Neurobiology of the *Caenorhabditis elegans* genome. *Science* **282**, 2028–2033.

Bertram, L., McQueen M. B., Mullin K., Blacker D., Tanzi R. E. 2007. Systematic meta-analyses of Alzheimer disease genetic association studies: the AlzGene database. *Nat. Genet.* **39**, 17–23.

Borchelt, D. R., Thinakaran G., Eckman C. B. *et al.* 1996. Familial Alzheimer's disease-linked presenilin 1 variants elevate Aβ1–42/1–40 ratio in vitro and in vivo. *Neuron* **17**, 1005–1013.

Borchelt, D. R., Ratovitski T., Van Lare J. *et al.* 1997. Accelerated amyloid deposition in the brains of transgenic mice coexpressing mutant presenilin 1 and amyloid precursor proteins. *Neuron* **19**, 939–945.

Brenner, S. 1973. The genetics of behaviour. *Br. Med. Bull.* **29**, 269–271.

Buttini, M., Orth M., Bellosta S. *et al.* 1999. Expression of human apolipoprotein E3 or E4 in the brains of *Apoe$^{-/-}$* mice: isoform-specific effects on neurodegeneration. *J. Neurosci.* **19**, 4867–4880.

Buttini, M., Yu G.-Q., Shockley K. *et al.* 2002. Modulation of Alzheimer-like synaptic and cholinergic deficits in transgenic mice by human apolipoprotein E depends on isoform, aging, and overexpression of amyloid β peptides but not on plaque formation. *J. Neurosci.* **22**, 10539–10548.

137

Chin, J., Palop J. J., Yu G.-Q. *et al.* 2004. Fyn kinase modulates synaptotoxicity, but not aberrant sprouting, in human amyloid precursor protein transgenic mice. *J. Neurosci.* **24**, 4692–4697.

Chishti, M. A., Yang D. S., Janus C. *et al.* 2001. Early-onset amyloid deposition and cognitive deficits in transgenic mice expressing a double mutant form of amyloid precursor protein 695. *J. Biol. Chem.* **276**, 21562–21570.

Clark, L. N., Poorkaj P., Wszolek Z. *et al.* 1998. Pathogenic implications of mutations in the tau gene in pallido-ponto-nigral degeneration and related neurodegenerative disorders linked to chromosome 17. *Proc. Natl. Acad. Sci. USA* **95**, 13103-13107.

Cleary, J. P., Walsh D. M., Hofmeister J. J. *et al.* 2005. Natural oligomers of the amyloid-β protein specifically disrupt cognitive function. *Nat. Neurosci.* **8**, 79–84.

Cohen, E., Bieschke J., Perciavalle R. M., Kelly J. W., Dillin A. 2006. Opposing activities protect against age-onset proteotoxicity. *Science* **313**, 1604–1610.

Crawley, J. N. 2000. *What's Wrong with my Mouse?: Behavioral Phenotyping of Transgenic and Knockout Mice.* New York: Wiley-Liss.

Cruts M., Rademakers R. 2008. *Alzheimer Disease and Frontotemporal Dementia Mutation Database.* http://www.molgen.ua.ac.be/ADMutations/default.cfm. (accessed October 2008).

Cruts, M., Gijselinck I., van der Zee J. *et al.* 2006. Null mutations in progranulin cause ubiquitin-positive frontotemporal dementia linked to chromosome 17q21. *Nature* **442**, 920–924.

Dabir, D. V., Robinson M. B., Swanson E. *et al.* 2006. Impaired glutamate transport in a mouse model of tau pathology in astrocytes. *J. Neurosci.* **26**, 644–654.

Daigle, I., Li C. 1993. apl-1, a *Caenorhabditis elegans* gene encoding a protein related to the human β-amyloid protein precursor. *Proc. Natl. Acad. Sci. USA* **90**, 12045–12049.

Duff, K., Eckman C., Zehr C. *et al.* 1996. Increased amyloid-β42(43) in brains of mice expressing mutant presenilin 1. *Nature* **383**, 710–713.

Farrer, L. A., Cupples L. A., Haines J. L. *et al.* 1997. Effects of age, sex, and ethnicity on the association between apolipoprotein E genotype and Alzheimer disease. A meta-analysis. *JAMA* **278**, 1349–1356.

Feany, M. B., Bender W. W. 2000. A *Drosophila* model of Parkinson's disease. *Nature* **404**, 394–398.

Fire, A., Xu S., Montgomery M. K. *et al.* 1998. Potent and specific genetic interference by double-stranded RNA in *Caenorhabditis elegans. Nature* **391**, 806–811.

Forman, M. S., Lal D., Zhang B. *et al.* 2005. Transgenic mouse model of tau pathology in astrocytes leading to nervous system degeneration. *J. Neurosci.* **25**, 3539–3550.

Games, D., Adams D., Alessandrini R. *et al.* 1995. Alzheimer-type neuropathology in transgenic mice overexpressing V717F β-amyloid precursor protein. *Nature* **373**, 523–527.

Gunawardena, S., Goldstein L. S. B. 2001. Disruption of axonal transport and neuronal viability by amyloid precursor protein mutations in Drosophila. *Neuron* **32**, 389–401.

Harris, F., Brecht W. J., Xu Q. *et al.* 2003. Carboxyl-terminal-truncated apolipoprotein E4 causes Alzheimer's disease-like neurodegeneration and behavioral deficits in transgenic mice. *Proc. Natl. Acad. Sci. USA* **100**, 10966–10971.

Holcomb, L., Gordon M. N., McGowan E. *et al.* 1998. Accelerated Alzheimer-type phenotype in transgenic mice carrying both mutant amyloid precursor protein and presenilin 1 transgenes. *Nat. Med.* **4**, 97–100.

Holtzman, D. M., Bales K. R., Tenkova T. *et al.* 2000. Apolipoprotein E isoform-dependent amyloid deposition and neuritic degeneration in a mouse model of Alzheimer's disease. *Proc. Natl. Acad. Sci. USA* **97**, 2892–2897.

Hsiao, K., Chapman P., Nilsen S. *et al.* 1996. Correlative memory deficits, Aβ elevation, and amyloid plaques in transgenic mice. *Science* **274**, 99–102.

Huang, Y., Liu X. Q., Wyss-Coray T. *et al.* 2001. Apolipoprotein E fragments present in Alzheimer's disease brains induce neurofibrillary tangle-like intracellular inclusions in neurons. *Proc. Natl. Acad. Sci. USA* **98**, 8838–8843.

Hutton, M., Lendon C. L., Rizzu P. *et al.* 1998. Association of missense and 5′-splice-site mutations in tau with the inherited dementia FTDP-17. *Nature* **393**, 702–705.

Irizarry, M. C., McNamara M., Fedorchak K., Hsiao K., Hyman B. T. 1997a. APP$_{Sw}$ transgenic mice develop age-related Aβ deposits and neuropil abnormalities, but no neuronal loss in CA1. *J. Neuropathol. Exp. Neurol.* **56**, 965–973.

Irizarry, M. C., Soriano F., McNamara M. *et al.* 1997b. Aβ deposition is associated with neuropil changes, but not with overt neuronal loss in the human amyloid precursor protein V717F (PDAPP) transgenic mouse. *J. Neurosci.* **17**, 7053–7059.

Jackson, G. R., Wiedau-Pazos M., Sang T. K. *et al.* 2002. Human wild-type tau interacts with wingless pathway components and produces neurofibrillary pathology in Drosophila. *Neuron* **34**, 509–519.

Janus, C., D'Amelio S., Amitay O. *et al.* 2000. Spatial learning in transgenic mice expressing human presenilin 1 (PS1) transgenes. *Neurobiol. Aging* **21**, 541–549.

Karsten, S. L., Sang T. K., Gehman L. T. *et al.* 2006. A genomic screen for modifiers of tauopathy identifies puromycin-sensitive aminopeptidase as an inhibitor of tau-induced neurodegeneration. *Neuron* **51**, 549–560.

Kasri, N. N., Kocks S. L., Verbert L. *et al.* 2006. Up-regulation of inositol 1,4,5-trisphosphate receptor

138

type 1 is responsible for a decreased endoplasmic-reticulum Ca^{2+} content in presenilin double knock-out cells. *Cell Calcium* **40**, 41–51.

Kenyon, C., Chang J., Gensch E., Rudner A., Tabtiang R. 1993. A *C. elegans* mutant that lives twice as long as wild type. *Nature* **366**, 461–464.

Kobayashi, D. T., Chen K. S. 2005. Behavioral phenotypes of amyloid-based genetically modified mouse models of Alzheimer's disease. *Genes Brain Behav.* **4**, 173–196.

Kraemer, B. C., Zhang B., Leverenz J. B. *et al.* 2003. Neurodegeneration and defective neurotransmission in a *Caenorhabditis elegans* model of tauopathy. *Proc. Natl. Acad. Sci. USA* **100**, 9980–9985.

LaFerla, F. M. 2002. Calcium dyshomeostasis and intracellular signalling in Alzheimer's disease. *Nat. Rev. Neurosci.* **3**, 862–872.

Lanz, T. A., Carter D. B., Merchant K. M. 2003. Dendritic spine loss in the hippocampus of young PDAPP and Tg2576 mice and its prevention by the ApoE2 genotype. *Neurobiol. Dis.* **13**, 246–253.

Leissring, M. A., Akbari Y., Fanger C. M. *et al.* 2000. Capacitative calcium entry deficits and elevated luminal calcium content in mutant presenilin-1 knockin mice. *J. Cell Biol.* **149**, 793–798.

Lesné, S., Koh, M. T., Kotilinek L., Kayed R. *et al.* 2006. A specific amyloid-β protein assembly in the brain impairs memory. *Nature* **440**, 352–357.

Lewis, J., McGowan E., Rockwood J. *et al.* 2000. Neurofibrillary tangles, amyotrophy and progressive motor disturbance in mice expressing mutant (P301L) tau protein. *Nat. Genet.* **25**, 402–405.

Lewis, J., Dickson D. W., Lin W. L. *et al.* 2001. Enhanced neurofibrillary degeneration in transgenic mice expressing mutant tau and APP. *Science* **293**, 1487–1491.

Leyssen, M., Ayaz D., Hébert S. S. *et al.* 2005. Amyloid precursor protein promotes post-developmental neurite arborization in the Drosophila brain. *EMBO J.* **24**, 2944–2955.

Link, C. D., Taft A., Kapulkin V. *et al.* 2003. Gene expression analysis in a transgenic *Caenorhabditis elegans* Alzheimer's disease model. *Neurobiol. Aging* **24**, 397–413.

Luo, L., Tully T., White K. 1992. Human amyloid precursor protein ameliorates behavioral deficit of flies deleted for *Appl* gene. *Neuron* **9**, 595–605.

Marx, J. 2002. Nobel Prize in Physiology or Medicine. Tiny worm takes a star turn. *Science* **298**, 526.

Masliah, E., Rockenstein E., Veinbergs I. *et al.* 2001. β-Amyloid peptides enhance α-synuclein accumulation and neuronal deficits in a transgenic mouse model linking Alzheimer's disease and Parkinson's disease. *Proc. Natl. Acad. Sci. USA* **98**, 12245–12250.

McGowan, E., Eriksen J., Hutton M. 2006. A decade of modeling Alzheimer's disease in transgenic mice. *Trends Genet.* **22**, 281–289.

Moolman, D. L., Vitolo O. V., Vonsattel J. P., Shelanski M. L. 2004. Dendrite and dendritic spine alterations in Alzheimer models. *J. Neurocytol.* **33**, 377–387.

Mucke, L., Masliah E., Yu G.-Q. *et al.* 2000. High-level neuronal expression of $A\beta_{1-42}$ in wild-type human amyloid protein precursor transgenic mice: synaptotoxicity without plaque formation. *J. Neurosci.* **20**, 4050–4058.

Neumann, M., Sampathu D. M., Kwong L. K. *et al.* 2006. Ubiquitinated TDP-43 in frontotemporal lobar degeneration and amyotrophic lateral sclerosis. *Science* **314**, 130–133.

Nicoll, J. A., Wilkinson D., Holmes C. *et al.* 2003. Neuropathology of human Alzheimer disease after immunization with amyloid-beta peptide: a case report. *Nat. Med.* **9**, 448–452.

Nicoll, J. A., Barton E., Boche D. *et al.* 2006. Aβ species removal after $A\beta_{42}$ immunization. *J. Neuropathol. Exp. Neurol.* **65**, 1040–1048.

Nishimura, I., Yang Y., Lu B. 2004. PAR-1 kinase plays an initiator role in a temporally ordered phosphorylation process that confers tau toxicity in Drosophila. *Cell* **116**, 671–682.

Oddo, S., Caccamo A., Shepherd J. D. *et al.* 2003. Triple-transgenic model of Alzheimer's disease with plaques and tangles: intracellular Aβ and synaptic dysfunction. *Neuron* **39**, 409–421.

Oddo, S., Billings L., Kesslak J. P., Cribbs D. H., LaFerla F. M. 2004. Aβ immunotherapy leads to clearance of early, but not late, hyperphosphorylated tau aggregates via the proteasome. *Neuron* **43**, 321–332.

Palop, J. J., Jones B., Kekonius L. *et al.* 2003. Neuronal depletion of calcium-dependent proteins in the dentate gyrus is tightly linked to Alzheimer's disease-related cognitive deficits. *Proc. Natl. Acad. Sci. USA* **100**, 9572–9577.

Palop, J. J., Chin J., Mucke L. 2006. A network dysfunction perspective on neurodegenerative diseases. *Nature* **443**, 768–773.

Payami, H., Zareparsi S., Montee K. R. *et al.* 1996. Gender difference in apolipoprotein E-associated risk for familial Alzheimer disease: a possible clue to the higher incidence of Alzheimer disease in women. *Am. J. Hum. Genet.* **58**, 803–811.

Perl, D. P., Olanow C. W., Calne D. 1998. Alzheimer's disease and Parkinson's disease: distinct entities or extremes of a spectrum of neurodegeneration? *Ann. Neurol.* **44**, S19–31.

Poorkaj, P., Bird T. D., Wijsman E. *et al.* 1998. Tau is a candidate gene for chromosome 17 frontotemporal dementia. *Ann. Neurol.* **43**, 815–825.

Raber, J. 2004. Androgens, apoE, and Alzheimer's disease. *Sci. Aging Knowl. Environ.* **11**, re2.

139

Raber, J., Wong D., Buttini M. *et al.* 1998. Isoform-specific effects of human apolipoprotein E on brain function revealed in *ApoE* knockout mice: increased susceptibility of females. *Proc. Natl. Acad. Sci. USA* **95**, 10914–10919.

Raber, J., Wong D., Yu G.-Q. *et al.* 2000. Alzheimer's disease: apolipoprotein E and cognitive performance. *Nature* **404**, 352–354.

Raber, J., LeFevour A., Buttini M., Mucke L. 2002. Androgens protect against apolipoprotein E4-induced cognitive deficits. *J. Neurosci.* **22**, 5204–5209.

Raber, J., Huang Y., Ashford J. W. 2004. ApoE genotype accounts for the vast majority of AD risk and AD pathology. *Neurobiol. Aging* **25**, 641–650.

Roberson, E. D. 2006. Frontotemporal dementia. *Curr. Neurol. Neurosci. Rep.* **6**, 481–489.

Roberson, E. D., Mucke L. 2006. 100 years and counting: prospects for defeating Alzheimer's disease. *Science* **314**, 781–784.

Roberson, E. D., Scearce-Levie K., Palop J. J. *et al.* 2007. Reducing endogenous tau ameliorates Aβ-induced deficits in an Alzheimer's disease mouse model. *Science* **316**, 750–754.

Rosen, D. R., Martin-Morris L., Luo L. Q., White K. 1989. A Drosophila gene encoding a protein resembling the human β-amyloid protein precursor. *Proc. Natl. Acad. Sci. USA* **86**, 2478–2482.

Rubin, G. M., Yandell M. D., Wortman J. R. *et al.* 2000. Comparative genomics of the eukaryotes. *Science* **287**, 2204–2215.

SantaCruz, K., Lewis J., Spires T. *et al.* 2005. Tau suppression in a neurodegenerative mouse model improves memory function. *Science* **309**, 476–481.

Saunders, A. M., Strittmatter W. J., Schmechel D. *et al.* 1993. Association of apolipoprotein E allele ε4 with late-onset familial and sporadic Alzheimer's disease. *Neurology* **43**, 1467–1472.

Saura, C. A., Choi S. Y., Beglopoulos V. *et al.* 2004. Loss of presenilin function causes impairments of memory and synaptic plasticity followed by age-dependent neurodegeneration. *Neuron* **42**, 23–36.

Schenk, D., Barbour R., Dunn W. *et al.* 1999. Immunization with amyloid-β attenuates Alzheimer-disease-like pathology in the PDAPP mouse. *Nature* **400**, 173–177.

Scheuner, D., Eckman C., Jensen M. *et al.* 1996. Secreted amyloid β-protein similar to that in the senile plaques of Alzheimer's disease is increased in vivo by the presenilin 1 and 2 and APP mutations linked to familial Alzheimer's disease. *Nat. Med.* **2**, 864–870.

Selkoe, D. J. 2002. Alzheimer's disease is a synaptic failure. *Science* **298**, 789–791.

Shen, J., Kelleher R. J., III 2007. The presenilin hypothesis of Alzheimer's disease: evidence for a loss-of-function pathogenic mechanism. *Proc. Natl. Acad. Sci. USA* **104**, 403–409.

Skibinski, G., Parkinson N. J., Brown J. M. *et al.* 2005. Mutations in the endosomal ESCRTIII-complex subunit CHMP2B in frontotemporal dementia. *Nat. Genet.* **37**, 806–808.

Spillantini, M. G., Murrell J. R., Goedert M. *et al.* 1998. Mutation in the tau gene in familial multiple system tauopathy with presenile dementia. *Proc. Natl. Acad. Sci. USA* **95**, 7737–7741.

Spires, T. L., Meyer-Luehmann M., Stern E. A. *et al.* 2005. Dendritic spine abnormalities in amyloid precursor protein transgenic mice demonstrated by gene transfer and intravital multiphoton microscopy. *J. Neurosci.* **25**, 7278–7287.

Sturchler-Pierrat, C., Abramowski D., Duke M. *et al.* 1997. Two amyloid precursor protein transgenic mouse models with Alzheimer disease-like pathology. *Proc. Natl. Acad. Sci. USA* **94**, 13287–13292.

Takeuchi, A., Irizarry M. C., Duff K. *et al.* 2000. Age-related amyloid β deposition in transgenic mice overexpressing both Alzheimer mutant presenilin 1 and amyloid beta precursor protein Swedish mutant is not associated with global neuronal loss. *Am. J. Pathol.* **157**, 331–339.

Tecott, L. H. 2003. The genes and brains of mice and men. *Am. J. Psychiatry* **160**, 646–656.

The *C. elegans* Sequencing Consortium. 1998. Genome sequence of the nematode *C. elegans*: a platform for investigating biology. *Science* **282**, 2012–2018.

Torroja, L., Packard M., Gorczyca M., White K., Budnik V. 1999a. The Drosophila β-amyloid precursor protein homolog promotes synapse differentiation at the neuromuscular junction. *J. Neurosci.* **19**, 7793–7803.

Torroja, L., Chu H., Kotovsky I., White K. 1999b. Neuronal overexpression of APPL, the *Drosophila* homologue of the amyloid precursor protein (APP), disrupts axonal transport. *Curr. Biol.* **9**, 489–492.

Trommer, B. L., Shah C., Yun S. H. *et al.* 2004. ApoE isoform affects LTP in human targeted replacement mice. *Neuroreport* **15**, 2655–2658.

Tu, H., Nelson O., Bezprozvanny A. *et al.* 2006. Presenilins form ER Ca^{2+} leak channels, a function disrupted by familial Alzheimer's disease-linked mutations. *Cell* **126**, 981–993.

Walsh, D. M., Klyubin I., Fadeeva J. V. *et al.* 2002. Naturally secreted oligomers of amyloid β protein potently inhibit hippocampal long-term potentiation in vivo. *Nature* **416**, 535–539.

Watts, G. D., Wymer J., Kovach M. J. *et al.* 2004. Inclusion body myopathy associated with Paget disease of bone and frontotemporal dementia is caused by mutant valosin-containing protein. *Nat. Genet.* **36**, 377–381.

Westerman, M. A., Cooper-Blacketer D., Mariash A. *et al.* 2002. The relationship between Aβ and memory in the Tg2576 mouse model of Alzheimer's disease. *J. Neurosci.* **22**, 1858–1867.

140

Wittmann, C. W., Wszolek M. F., Shulman J. M. *et al.* 2001. Tauopathy in Drosophila: neurodegeneration without neurofibrillary tangles. *Science* **293**, 711–714.

Wu, C. C., Chawla F., Games D. *et al.* 2004. Selective vulnerability of dentate granule cells prior to amyloid deposition in PDAPP mice: digital morphometric analyses. *Proc. Natl. Acad. Sci. USA* **101**, 7141–7146.

Xu, Q., Bernardo A., Walker D. *et al.* 2006. Profile and regulation of apolipoprotein E (ApoE) expression in the CNS in mice with targeting of green fluorescent protein gene to the ApoE locus. *J. Neurosci.* **26**, 4985–4994.

Yoshihara, M., Ensminger A. W., Littleton J. T. 2001. Neurobiology and the Drosophila genome. *Funct. Integr. Genomics* **1**, 235–240.

Yoshiyama, Y., Higuchi M., Zhang B. *et al.* 2007. Synapse loss and microglial activation precede tangles in a P301S tauopathy mouse model. *Neuron* **53**, 337–351.

Neuropathology of dementia

Marcelo N. Macedo, Eun-Joo Kim and William W. Seeley

Introduction

Age-related neurodegenerative diseases represent an increasing public health crisis. In the USA, individuals 85 years of age or older are the fastest growing segment of society, projected to exceed 10 million citizens before 2050.[1] The risk of developing Alzheimer's disease (AD) doubles every five years after age 65,[2] suggesting that the prevalence of dementia will escalate dramatically in the next 40 years.

Major advances in neuroimaging, genetics, molecular biology and neuropathology have begun to refine our understanding of the dementias, providing hope for new therapies. Structural and functional imaging studies now map dementia-related regional and network-level dysfunction in unprecedented detail, and transgenic animals provide testable disease models, bringing new insights into dementia pathogenesis. Genetic studies have identified numerous disease-causing mutations and provide a foothold for understanding the molecular pathology of dementia. Conversely, careful separation of patients with dementia into pathologically homogeneous groupings has accelerated the search for new causative mutations. Accurate prediction of pathology will become even more critical when molecule-specific treatments emerge.

With new discoveries and shifts in opinion, diagnostic frameworks for dementia have evolved rapidly. Formal clinical and pathological diagnostic research criteria for the dementias continue to be revised, with the goal of optimizing clinical–pathological correlations. However, even among patients seen at dementia referral centers, clinical and pathological diagnoses remain discordant in a significant minority of patients.[3,4] Necessarily, neuropathology remains the gold standard for dementia diagnosis.

This chapter reviews the neuropathology of dementia from the behavioral neurologist's point of view, relating commonly encountered clinical syndromes to histopathological disease signatures seen at autopsy. Each disorder features a characteristic pattern of early neuronal and regional vulnerability, with resulting neurological first symptoms. In turn, each disorder shows a typical progression of regional degeneration with associated downstream symptoms and histopathologic hallmarks that reflect specific disease genes and proteins. Nonetheless, overlap and uncertainty continue to complicate the task at the bedside and at the microscope, and we highlight these ambiguities throughout the chapter. Whenever possible, we emphasize the distinction between clinical and pathological terms, seeking to maintain clarity and underscore lingering challenges in clinical–pathological correlation.

Selective vulnerability

Selective vulnerability provides a unifying framework in neurodegenerative disease. Patients decline because aberrant, misfolded proteins disrupt homeostasis within specific neurons found in specific brain regions that participate in large-scale distributed neural networks to support cognition, behavior and movement. Each dementia illustrates these principles in a different way, as highlighted in Table 11.1. In the clinic, the behavioral neurologist relies on selective vulnerability; without it, each disorder would present with global deficits early on, making differential diagnosis even more precarious.

For the neuroscientist studying dementia, limited information is available about how selective vulnerability works. Why do neurons that die early in one disease persist through end stages of another? These natural experiments may harbor critical information about the mechanisms that undermine – or protect – neuronal populations. Furthermore, successful dementia treatments may require better models of how disease proteins interact with disease-susceptible neurons and networks.

Table 11.1. Selective vulnerability in neurodegenerative dementia

Disease/syndrome	Early symptom(s)	Early network/region	Early neuron	Proteins	Genes[a]
Alzheimer's disease	Episodic memory loss	Medial temporal–posterior cingulate–precuneus	Entorhinal cortex layer II pyramidal neurons	Aβ42, Tau	APP, PS1, PS2
Frontotemporal lobar degeneration					
Frontotemporal dementia, behavioral variant	Apathy, disinhibition, loss of self- and other-awareness	Anterior cingulate–frontoinsula cortex	Von Economo neurons	Tau = TDP-43	MAPT, PGRN
Semantic dementia	Anomia, loss of word meaning, emotional detachment	Temporal pole–amygdala–frontoinsula	Unknown	TDP-43 ≫ Tau	MAPT, PGRN
Progressive non-fluent aphasia	Non-fluent aphasia motor speech impairment	Dominant perisylvian and dorsal insular cortex	Unknown	Tau > TDP-43	MAPT, PGRN
Motor neuron disease	Motor weakness, spasticity	Primary motor cortex and spinal cord anterior horn	Upper and lower motor neurons	Ubiquitin, TDP-43	SOD1, TDP-43[b]
Corticobasal degeneration	Assymetric akinesia-rigidity, dystonia, apraxia, and executive, behavioral or motor speech impairment	Medial posterior frontal, dorsal frontoparietal	Unknown	Tau ≫ TDP-43	MAPT, PGRN
Progressive supranuclear palsy	Falls, executive dysfunction	Dentate nucleus, dorsal midbrain, subthalamic nucleus	Unknown	Tau	MAPT
Dementia with Lewy bodies	REM sleep-behavior disorder, arousal fluctuations, visual hallucinations, parkinsonism	Descending/ascending brainstem projection streams	Long-range brainstem projection neurons	α-Synuclein	SNCA, LRRK-2
Multiple system atrophy (MSA)					
MSA-P	Autonomic insufficiency, parkinsonism	Brainstem–spinal cord (IMLCC) sympathetic control, nigrostriatal circuit	Preganglionic sympathetic neurons, nigral dopaminergic and putaminal MSP neurons	α-Synuclein	
MSA-C	Autonomic insufficiency, ataxia	Brainstem–spinal cord (IMLCC) sympathetic control, cerebellar pathways	Preganglionic sympathetic neurons, olivopontine and cerebellar Purkinje neurons	α-Synuclein	
Huntington's disease	Chorea, depression, executive dysfunction	Dorsal frontal–striatal–thalamic circuit	Caudate MSP neurons	Huntingtin	IT15

Notes:

IMLCC, intermediolateral cell column; MSP, medium spiny projection; TDP-43, TAR DNA-binding protein; Aβ42, β-amyloid 42 residue form.

[a]Only the most common associations with autosomal dominant inheritance are listed.

[b]SOD1 mutations (superoxide dismutase) are associated with ubiquitin-positive, TDP-43-negative intraneuronal inclusions.[153]

The dementias

To constrain the scope of this chapter, we focus on the degenerative dementia syndromes commonly encountered by the dementia specialist. Across these conditions, shared underlying histopathological features include, to varying degrees, the presence of reactive gliosis, microvacuolation and synapse loss, followed by neuronal drop-out, more extensive gliosis and loss of cortical architecture.[5,6] These changes are accompanied by cortical and subcortical volume loss, which can be appreciated grossly at autopsy or in vivo with high-resolution magnetic resonance imaging (MRI). Distributed patterns of regional atrophy may reflect a tendency of neurodegenerative diseases to target specific functional networks of interconnected brain regions.[7] Culprit neurons, vulnerable within these networks, have been identified for some diseases but not others. In the following sections, we touch briefly on the clinical, neuronal and regional features of each disease, en route to a more detailed discussion of the signature underlying histopathologies.

Alzheimer's disease

Alzheimer's disease (AD) accounts for more than half of all patients with dementia[8] and remains the best characterized disease in its class. The overall US prevalence of AD is estimated at 4.5 million, translating to roughly 1600 per 100 000, with an incidence of 14 per 1000 person-years after age 65.[1,9] Early symptoms most often involve anterograde episodic memory impairment, which reflects hierarchical pathology within the medial temporal lobe.[5,10,11] Layer II entorhinal cortex pyramidal neurons are strikingly affected, isolating the hippocampus from a vital input source.[12] Perhaps because of the anatomic and functional connectivity of medial temporal with posterior cingulo-parietotemporal structures, evidence for dysfunction within parietal association cortex is seen even in presymptomatic individuals genetically at risk for AD.[13] Particularly in patients with early-onset AD, first symptoms may also emphasize language,[14,15] visuospatial,[15] primary or secondary visual[15,16] or even frontal-executive deficits.[17] Prominent, early social–emotional or motor system complaints should raise suspicion for an alternative diagnosis.

The typical AD brain shows hippocampal atrophy, with diffuse and relatively symmetric volume loss in parietal, temporal and frontal association cortices. This pattern is more pronounced in posterior than anterior brain regions. Primary motor and sensory cortices may be conspicuously spared, even into advanced clinical dementia.[18] The neuropathological hallmarks of AD are shown in Fig. 11.1. Despite advances in AD molecular pathophysiology, neuritic plaques and neurofibrillary tangles (NFTs) remain the diagnostic hallmarks of the disease 100 years after their first description.[19] The neuritic plaques are complex spherical structures composed of extracellular deposits of β-amyloid peptide Aβ42, which forms a central core. The remainder of the sphere is composed of a halo of dystrophic neurites, with interspersed Aβ42 peptide. Small numbers of reactive astrocytes and activated microglia complete the neuritic plaque complex. Diffuse plaques, in contrast, lack a dense core and radially oriented dystrophic neurites, and are less reliable in distinguishing patients with dementia from healthy aged individuals.[20] The NFTs are insoluble intracellular aggregates of abnormally hyperphosphorylated microtubule-associated protein tau.[21] Both neuritic plaques and NFTs are easy to detect with silver stains, such as Bielschowsky or Gallyas, or by immunohistochemistry using antibodies to Aβ (neuritic plaques) or hyperphosphorylated tau (NFTs). While neuritic plaques tend to be evenly distributed across the neocortex, with less specific laminar distributions, NFTs target mesial temporal structures, especially layers II and IV, possibly explaining why NFT distribution better corresponds with clinical impairment than the pattern and number of neuritic plaques.[22,23] Granulovacuolar degeneration, neuronal loss, amyloid deposition in the subarachnoid and cerebral arteries (amyloid angiopathy), Hirano bodies and glial reactions are additional AD histological features not routinely used to diagnose or stage disease.[24–27]

Several published research criteria compete for a role in AD pathological diagnosis. The Consortium to Establish a Registry for Alzheimer's disease (CERAD) criteria use semiquantitative neuritic plaque frequency adjusted for age and the presence of dementia.[28] Braak and Braak defined six stages of NFT pathology[29] in which AD progresses from transentorhinal (stage I) and entorhinal (stage II) regions in early disease to limbic areas (stages III, IV), the neocortical sensory association and prefrontal regions (stage V), and finally primary sensory and motor fields (stage VI). In 1997, the National Institute on Aging and the Ronald and Nancy Reagan Institute of the Alzheimer's Association proposed the NIA–Reagan criteria, which combined the modified CERAD criteria with Braak staging methods and required clinical dementia to

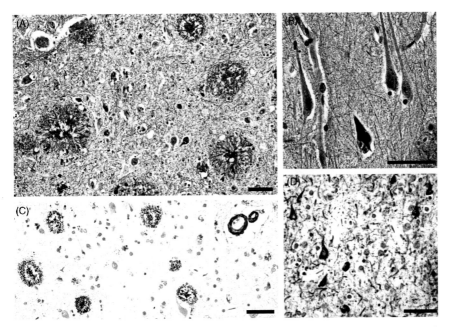

Fig. 11.1. Alzheimer's disease. (A) Neuritic plaques (NPs) and neuron loss in entorhinal cortex. The NPs show dense cores and radially oriented dystrophic neurites. (B) A typical neurofibrillary tangle in CA1. Bielschowsky silver stain. (C) Beta-amyloid immunohistochemistry demonstrates frequent plaques in posterior cingulate cortex, accompanied by cerebral amyloid angiopathy (inset). Hematoxylin counterstain. (D) Immunohistochemical stains for hyperphosphorylated tau show aggregation in neurofibrillary tangles and cortical dystrophic neurites. (CP-13 antibody, courtesy of Dr. Peter Davies.) Hematoxylin counterstain. Scale bars = 50 μm.

make a final "high likelihood" AD pathological diagnosis.[30] Despite all of these efforts, AD heterogeneity continues to challenge existing frameworks. Patients with symptoms before age 65, for example, show a significantly greater frontoparietal neuritic plaque and NFT burden and synapse loss compared with older patients with AD.[31,32] Similar neuroimaging findings, using both functional and structural approaches, have been reported.[33,34]

Prevailing theories of AD pathogenesis emphasize the overproduction and accumulation of neurotoxic Aβ42 and other oligomeric forms of soluble Aβ. These toxic species are derived from abnormal processing of amyloid precursor protein (APP) and, according to this amyloid cascade hypothesis, cause direct neuronal degeneration.[35] Other disease models emphasize tau. The production and accumulation of hyperphosphorylated tau protein has been hypothesized to cause microtubule dysfunction, compromising axonal transport and leading to synaptic loss and ultimately retrograde degeneration.[36] Molecular genetic studies of familial AD have revealed autosomal dominant inheritance patterns in individuals with early-onset AD,[37] in association with three genes: *APP* on chromosome 21, *PS1* (presenilin 1)

on chromosome 14, and *PS2* (presenilin 2) on chromosome 1.[38–40] In part because these mutations directly or indirectly increase Aβ production, the amyloid cascade is widely considered the most relevant pathogenic mechanism in AD. However, neuritic plaques are often found in non-demented elderly brains,[41] and, as mentioned, NFT frequency is more strongly correlated than neuritic plaque frequency with clinical AD severity. These observations underscore the amount remaining to be learned about the etiology and pathogenesis of AD.

Frontotemporal lobar degeneration

Frontotemporal lobar degeneration (FTLD) is a pathological umbrella term that refers to a group of disorders united by degeneration of the frontal lobes, anterior temporal lobes or both. The term frontotemporal dementia (FTD), in contrast, now most commonly refers to the clinical syndromes that result from FTLD pathology (Fig. 11.2). Symptoms typically begin in the sixth decade of life, and the prevalence of FTD, 15 per 100 000, equals that of AD among dementia patients under age 65 years.[42] The incidence of FTD is 3.3 per 100 000 person-years for ages 50 to 59, also equal to that of AD.[43]

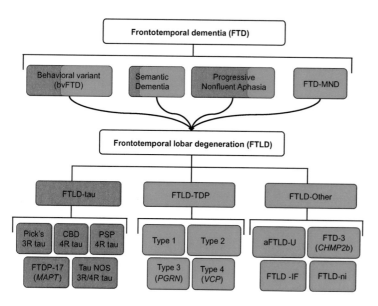

Fig. 11.2. Classification and pathological correlates of the frontotemporal dementias. Colored boxes illustrate the approximate proportion of patients with each syndrome who are found to have FTLD-tau (orange) vs. FTLD-TDP (blue) vs. other FTLD pathology (green). Strong genetic associations with each subtype, if known, are shown in parentheses. MND, motor neuron disease; CBD, corticobasal degeneration; PSP, progressive supranuclear palsy; FTDP-17, frontotemporal dementia with parkinsonism linked to chromosome 17; PGRN, progranulin; VCP, valosin-containing protein; aFTLD-U, atypical FTLD with ubiquitin-positive inclusions; FTD-3, FTD linked to chromosome 3 mutations in the charged multivesicular body protein 2b (CHMP2b); FTLD-IF, FTLD with neuronal intermediate filament inclusions; FTLD-ni, FTLD with no inclusions.

Research criteria for FTD have specified three major clinical subtypes: a behavioral variant (bvFTD), semantic dementia (SD) and progressive non-fluent aphasia (PNFA).[44] Each subtype features a distinctive set of early deficits, relating to focal neurodegeneration within vulnerable cortical regions (Fig. 11.3). The behavioral variant, sometimes referred to as frontal variant FTD or simply FTD, is the most common of the three subtypes and begins with prominent changes in social cognition, emotion and behavior. Typical early symptoms include apathy, disinhibition, repetitive and compulsive behaviors, and a failing ability to represent the self and others, manifesting as shallow insight and lack of empathy. In parallel, patients develop early focal degeneration of the pre- and subgenual anterior cingulate cortex and frontal insula, as well as the rostromedial frontal cortex (reviewed by M. L. Schroeter et al.[45]). Based on neuroimaging[46,47] and pathologic[48] studies of very mild bvFTD, these paralimbic regions may represent the sites of earliest injury. Semantic dementia, also referred to as temporal variant FTD, presents with progressive loss of meaning for words, objects and emotions as a result of focal degeneration of the temporal poles and amygdalae.[49,50] Affected patients with greater left-sided atrophy first develop naming and comprehension deficits, accompanied by fluent, empty spontaneous speech. Right-hemisphere predominant SD, in contrast, manifests as early emotional detachment and failure to comprehend the feelings of others, followed by face recognition difficulties.[44,51,52]

Left- and right-hemisphere symptoms then appear in all patients as the illness encroaches on whichever temporal pole was less affected at onset. The third FTD subtype, PNFA, is defined by non-fluent speech with agrammatism, phonemic paraphasias and anomia, often with speech apraxia, reflecting dominant inferior frontal, perisylvian and dorsal insular degeneration.[14] Motor neuron disease (MND) may co-occur with bvFTD-like symptoms or, less commonly, with SD or PNFA,[53] and the term FTD-MND has been applied to each of these scenarios. Most commonly, FTD-MND affects lower motor neurons to the bulbar and upper limb musculature.

The gross FTLD pathology pattern depends more on the clinical syndrome than on the underlying histopathology (Figure 11.3). Atrophy is almost always more prominent anteriorly but distributes unevenly in frontal vs. temporal lobes and right vs. left hemispheres. Affected regions show cortical thinning, blurring of the gray-white junction, and ex vacuo ventricular enlargement. The anterior corpus callosum, basal ganglia and substantia nigra may also show prominent atrophy.[54] At the microscopic level, the field now recognizes two major FTLD histopathological subcategories, based on the associated intracellular inclusion proteins: tau-positive FTLD (FTLD-tau) and TDP-43-positive FTLD (FTLD-TDP).[55] Additional subtypes are recognized but account for only a small minority of patients (Figure 11.2).

FTLD-tau encompasses Pick's disease, corticobasal degeneration (CBD), progressive supranuclear

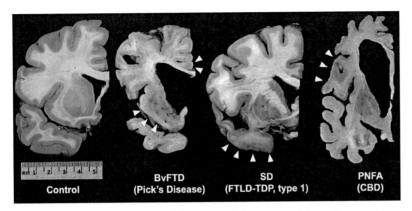

Fig. 11.3. Contrasting regional vulnerability patterns in frontotemporal dementia. Coronal slabs near the temporal pole demonstrate regions of early and severe degeneration (arrowheads) in the three major FTD syndromes. BvFTD targets orbital frontoinsular and medial frontal structures, SD the inferior temporal pole (and frontoinsula). In PNFA, there is prominent dorsal and lateral frontal atrophy, including Broca's area (arrowheads). Underlying histopathologies for the cases shown are listed in parentheses. PNFA photograph courtesy Dr. Ian Mackenzie.

palsy (PSP), and frontotemporal dementia with parkinsonism linked to chromosome 17 (FTDP-17). These heterogeneous disorders feature filamentous tau deposits in neurons and glia as their most salient histopathological hallmark.[56] Tau has six isoforms in the adult brain, generated through alternative splicing of exons 2, 3, and, 10. Exon 10 encodes the fourth repeated sequence, resulting in three 3-repeat (3R) and three 4-repeat (4R) isoforms. Pick's disease is usually a 3R-tauopathy. FTDP-17 may include 3R, 4R or a mix of 3R and 4R isoforms. In the majority of CBD and PSP cases, the 4R isoform predominates.[54] Additional tauopathies have been described that do not fall cleanly into one of the major FTLD-tau subtypes.[57]

The pathological hallmark of Pick's disease is the Pick body, a round, circumscribed, argyrophilic neuronal cytoplasmic inclusion (Figure 11.4). Pick cells, swollen, achromatic 'ballooned' neurons, further support the diagnosis.[58] Pick bodies stain positively with Bielschowsky but not Gallyas silver staining,[59] and they are easy to detect among hippocampal dentate gyrus granule cells due to the high neuronal density of this region. Pick body detection in superficial layers of affected cortex is less reliable, and the relationship between these inclusions and the overall degenerative process remains uncertain. Pick bodies may also be found in amygdala, basal ganglia, and brainstem monoaminergic nuclei.[58] Most Pick bodies stain positively with hyperphosphorylated tau protein immunohistochemistry. Other tau-immunoreactive findings, such as less well circumscribed neuronal

cytoplasmic and glial inclusions of various morphologies, including gray and white matter coils, threads, and so-called ramified astrocytes (Figure 4) are also variably detected in Pick's disease.[60] FTDP-17 was initially reported by Wilhelmsen et al.[61] as a single FTD family linked to chromosome 17q21-22 and Hutton et al.[62] identified the culprit gene, *MAPT*, four years later. Now numerous families have been described that share FTD clinical features, parkinsonism, amyotrophy, tau pathology, and mutations in *MAPT*,[63-65] cultivating the notion that FTLD-tau subtypes belong to a common family.

FTLD-TDP, perhaps the most common FTLD subcategory,[66] features ubiquitinated TDP-43 immunoreactive neuronal inclusions, also easy to visualize in dentate granule cells and affected cortex (Figure 5). Four major FTLD-TDP subtypes, based on the subcellular localization and laminar distribution of pathology, have been described.[67,68] While FTLD-TDP subtyping remains a matter of active study, it seems clear that some patients feature TDP-43 inclusions nearly confined to long, swollen dystrophic neurites, whereas others show neuritic and perikaryal inclusions that vary in size, shape, and compactness. In familial FTLD-TDP due to mutations in progranulin *(PGRN)* and in some patients with sporadic disease, cigar-shaped or lentiform intranuclear neuronal inclusions[69] can be found in affected cortical and limbic regions. When these various pathomorphologies co-occur with upper or lower motor neuron loss, the term FTLD-MND is applied.[70] Importantly, mutations in the gene

147

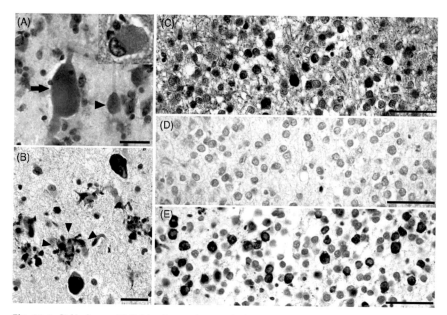

Fig. 11.4. Pick's disease. (A) Pick bodies are circumscribed, neuronal cytoplasmic inclusions detectable with hematoxylin and eosin stains (inset), whereas Pick cells are ballooned, achromatic neurons. A ballooned von Economo neuron (arrow) in anterior cingulate cortex is shown with a neighboring pyramidal neuron (arrowhead). Cresyl violet. (B) In this patient with behavioral variant frontotemporal dementia, tau immunohistochemistry reveals frequent cortical Pick bodies and associated glial pathology, including glial threads and ramified astrocytes (arrowheads). (C–E) Pick bodies are easily detected in dentate granule cells with the Bielschowsky silver stain (C) and tau immunohistochemistry (E, CP-13 antibody), but not the Gallyas silver stain (D). Scale bars, 25 μm (A,B) and 50 μm (C–E).

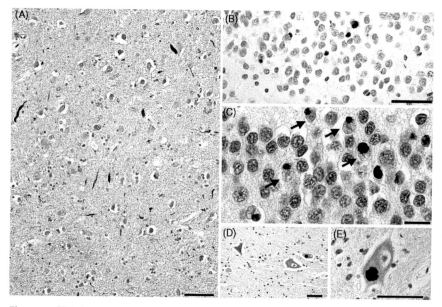

Fig. 11.5. FTLD-TDP. (A) FTLD-TDP often shows scattered TDP-43-immunoreactive pathology, including neuritic profiles as seen in the inferior temporal pole of this patient with semantic dementia (FTLD-TDP, type 1 (68)). (B) Rounded, neuronal cytoplasmic inclusions are also commonly seen in dentate gyrus (shown) or other affected regions. Ubiquitin immunohistochemistry, hematoxylin counterstain. (C) Neurons containing TDP-43 cytoplasmic inclusions (arrows) lack normal nuclear TDP-43 immunoreactivity (seen here in adjacent dentate granule cells without inclusions). TDP-43 immunohistochemistry, hematoxylin counterstain. (D, E) TDP-43-immunoreactive inclusions are also found in hippocampus, frontal cortex, and motor neurons from patients with ALS and FTLD-MND (shown). Scale bars indicate 50 microns.

encoding TDP-43 (*TARDBP*) cause amyotrophic lateral sclerosis, affirming the pathogenic role of TDP-43 and the link between FTD and MND.[71]

When FTLD pathology is neither tau nor TDP-43 immunoreactive, it is described according to the relevant inclusion protein, if known, or using other descriptive terminology. For example, FTLD with neuronal intermediate filament inclusions is now referred to as FTLD-intermediate filament (FTLD-IF). This illness features inclusions that stain positively with neurofilament antibodies, ubiquitin, and α-internexin but negatively for tau, α- synuclein, and TDP-43.[72–75] Alpha-internexin may be the most sensitive marker for these inclusions,[74] but the precise role of this protein in FTLD-IF pathogenesis remains uncertain. The term dementia lacking distinctive histopathology (DLDH, now referred to as FTLD-no inclusions, or FTLD-ni) played an important role in identifying autopsied patients with non-Pick's, non-AD dementia,[76] but most patients previously given this label were later found to have had FTLD-TDP.[77] Other important subtypes within the non-tau, non-TDP category include atypical FTLD with ubiquitin positive inclusions (aFTLD-U) and FTD-3, which results from mutations in *CHMP-2b* and shows ubiquitinated inclusions containing no known disease protein.[78–80]

Important clues to the FTLD pathogenesis puzzle have been amassed in the past four years. In 2006, chromosome 17q21 mutations in *PGRN* were identified as a major cause of familial tau-negative FTLD, and the pathology in these patients was later confirmed to be FTLD-TDP.[81–83] Despite the close relationship between FTLD-TDP and FTLD-MND, *PGRN* mutations rarely underlie familial FTLD-MND,[84] for which causative genes remain unknown. Progranulin is a growth factor involved in cell proliferation and repair, and most mutations described to date result in haploinsufficiency.[85] Consequently, progranulin replacement strategies for patients with familial FTLD-U represent an exciting frontier in FTD treatment.

No histopathological staging system has been adopted for FTLD research, in part owing to the anatomical and pathological heterogeneity of the disorder. Using gross anatomical observations, however, Broe and colleagues[48] proposed an FTLD morphological staging scheme, suggesting that degeneration begins in dorsomedial and orbital-insular frontal cortices and hippocampus (Stage 1); spreads to other anterior frontal regions, temporal poles, and basal ganglia (Stage 2); undercuts white matter, leading to lateral ventricular dilatation and callosal thinning (Stage 3); and finally produces severe diffuse atrophy throughout the anterior brain, encroaching on posterior temporal and parietal regions (Stage 4). Within the sites of early FTLD atrophy, no population of selectively vulnerable neurons had been identified until 2006, when von Economo neurons (VENs) were shown to undergo early, selective dropout in FTLD but not AD.[86] VENs are large, bipolar projection neurons found only in anterior cingulate and frontoinsular cortex (Figure 6). Though the connectivity and functions of these cells remain to be elucidated, VEN-containing regions form the core of the FTLD anatomic injury pattern,[45] may represent the sites of earliest injury,[47,48] and show robust functional connectivity in the healthy human brain.[87] Intriguingly, VENs have been identified only in great apes, humans, cetaceans and elephants: large-brained mammals that may share social-emotional functions lost in FTD.[88,89] Further investigations are needed to define the basic biology of these cells and the circuits to which they contribute.

Imperfect correlations persist between FTD clinical syndromes, on the one hand, and FTLD pathological subtypes, on the other. Nonetheless, recent studies have clarified the most common associations. BvFTD remains the most challenging prediction problem, with roughly equal numbers resulting from FTLD-tau and FTLD-TDP.[4,90] SD usually reflects FTLD-TDP, though a significant minority may have underlying Pick's disease or even AD pathology.[90–92] PNFA is most often a tauopathy,[91,93] CBD or PSP, and commonly clinical PNFA evolves into a corticobasal or PSP-like syndrome after an initial period of isolated language and motor speech impairment.[94] Clinical FTD with MND is almost always due to FTLD-MND, with TDP-43 immunoreactive inclusions in affected cortex and motor neurons. These relationships are illustrated in Figure 11.2.

The dementia–movement disorder tauopathies: corticobasal degeneration and progressive supranuclear palsy

Corticobasal degeneration (CBD) is an under-recognized neurodegenerative illness with a prevalence of 5–7 per 100 000, and an incidence of 0.6–0.9 per 100 000 per year, though these estimates may more accurately reflect the numbers presenting to movement

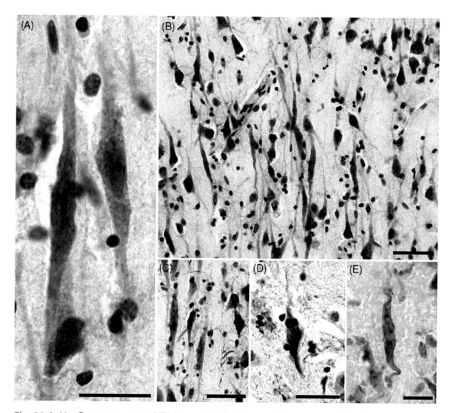

Fig. 11.6. Von Economo neurons (VENs): an early cellular target in frontotemporal lobe degeneration (FTLD). (A,B) Normal anterior cingulate cortex VENs in a neurologically unaffected control. The VENs are large projection neurons with a bipolar dendritic architecture (A) that form clusters near small arterioles (B, center). Cresyl violet. (C) In Alzheimer's disease, VENs show no selective vulnerability, do not form tangles and maintain normal clustering and morphology despite local neurofibrillary pathology. CP-13 antibody, cresyl violet counterstain. (D) In Pick's disease, VENs are severely depleted, and surviving neurons often show dense hyperphosphorylated tau protein accumulation. CP-13 antibody, hematoxylin counterstain. (E) In FTLD-TDP, VENs may exhibit abnormal twisting and kinking of proximal dendrites and neuronal cytoplasmic inclusions (not shown). Cresyl violet. Scale bars, 25 μm (A,E) and 50 μm (B–D).

disorders specialists.[95] Men and women are equally affected,[96] with a mean age of onset in the early sixties,[97,98] and the disease is usually sporadic. We now recognize that CBD can accompany the PNFA syndrome, as just described, or a movement disorder with salient cognitive–behavioral manifestations. The classical movement disorder features progressive, asymmetric, akinetic-rigid parkinsonism; dystonia; myoclonus; and cortical signs, such as limb apraxia, visuospatial dysfunction, alien limb phenomena or cortical sensory disturbance. All are related to medial frontoparietal and striatopallidal degeneration. Regardless of the most function-limiting aspect of the CBD syndrome, cognitive impairment is common and often involves executive functions, verbal fluency, praxis, visual construction or hemispatial attention.[99] Patients with early, debilitating dystonia and parkinsonism are difficult to assess for cognitive impairment, possibly undermining prior attempts to document dementia in the illness.[100–102]

At autopsy, patients with CBD exhibit frontal, parietal and insular atrophy with sparing involvement of temporal and occipital cortex (see Fig. 11.2). Although profound asymmetry may be more common in CBD than other disorders, a symmetric pattern is also seen in some patients. Pre- and postcentral gyri are affected, consistent with the cortical motor and sensory signs seen in CBD antemortem. Nigral depigmentation can be prominent, but otherwise the brainstem is grossly unremarkable. Microscopically, tau-immunoreactive astrocytic plaques are considered by some to be the most specific histopathologic marker (Fig. 11.7). These annular clusters of short astrocytic processes are found in both affected neocortex and affected striatum; they may be difficult to identify in some patients with CBD, and, to complicate matters, can

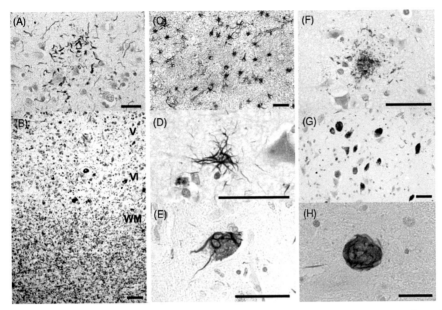

Fig. 11.7. Overlapping tau pathology in corticobasal degeneration (CBD) and progressive supranuclear palsy (PSP). In CBD, tau pathology takes the form of astrocytic plaques (A, Gallyas silver stain) and dense glial thread and coil pathology that fills the white matter (B, CP-13 antibody). Subcortical white matter tauopathy is accompanied by exuberant subcortical reactive astrocytosis (C, antibody to glial fibrillary acidic protein). Thorny astrocytes (D) and coiled tangles (E) may be seen in both CBD and PSP (Gallyas silver stain), while tufted astrocytes (F, CP-13 antibody) are more characteristic of PSP. Conspicuous globose tangles in the midbrain make the PSP diagnosis (G,H, Gallyas). Scale bars, 25 μm (A,H) and 50 μm (B–G).

be seen sparsely populating the cortex in PSP.[103] Dense white matter involvement with tau-positive glial threads and small round oligodendroglial inclusions referred to as coiled bodies, however, are nearly universal in CBD and distinguish it from Pick's disease and PSP. Thorny astrocytes, ballooned neurons (also seen in Pick's disease), and tau-positive neuronal cytoplasmic inclusions called coiled tangles or pretangles may also be seen in affected cortex.[60]

Progressive supranuclear palsy (PSP) is a cognitive–behavioral–movement disorder, also typically sporadic, that affects both men and women and has a mean onset in the sixth decade.[104] The crude and age-adjusted prevalences of PSP are 6.5 and 5 per 100 000, respectively.[105] Early symptoms include axial rigidity with gait instability, often leading to recurrent, dramatic injurious falls facilitated by frontally mediated apathy, mental rigidity, executive dysfunction and poor judgement. An oculomotor disorder soon accompanies the syndrome and worsens falling, especially when patients travel downward on slopes or stairways while impulsively bypassing the precaution of handrails. Square wave jerks are followed by slowed saccades, vertical greater than horizontal, before a full-blown supranuclear gaze palsy (also worse for

vertical gaze) emerges. Pseudobulbar palsy, featuring dysarthria, dysphagia and emotional incontinence, may also occur in later stages. The cognitive executive syndrome is usually not late. Indeed, early onset cognitive–behavioral dysfunction (at least two of apathy, impairment in abstract reasoning, decreased verbal fluency, utilization or imitation behavior, or frontal release signs) provides supportive evidence for PSP according to published research criteria.[104]

At autopsy, PSP cortical atrophy, if present, is usually subtle and frontal. In contrast, diencephalic, dorsal midbrain and cerebellar dentate atrophy is prominent enough to be seen grossly. Globus pallidus, subthalamic nucleus, superior colliculus and superior cerebellar peduncle (carrying dentate nucleus efferents) are particularly affected.[106] On microscopic examination, rounded or globe-shaped NFTs, referred to as globose tangles (Fig. 11.7), are distributed throughout affected brainstem nuclei and are considered diagnostic of PSP in the absence of extensive AD-type (flame-shaped) cortical NFTs and neuritic plaques. In PSP, tau immunohistochemistry demonstrates both glial and neuronal inclusions. Glial cells featuring tau-positive and argyrophilic inclusions, referred to as tufted astrocytes, are more common in PSP than in

151

CBD, though they can be seen in both (Fig. 11.7).[107] Thorny astrocytes, also seen in CBD, are seen in PSP-affected cortex, highlighting the close pathomorphological kinship of these related tauopathies.

The clinical[108] and pathological[60] overlap between PSP and CBD highlights an emerging and important nosological problem with how we conceptualize neurodegenerative diseases. Patients with the clinical PSP syndrome may have pathological features more consistent with CBD and vice versa, even among family members with an identical tau mutation.[109] Both CBD and PSP are associated with 4R isoform tauopathy and the H1 tau haplotype, further supporting their close affiliation.[110] Even so, why two diseases with such extensive pathophysiological overlap so often manifest with divergent clinical presentations remains an important problem to be solved.[111,112]

The dementia–movement disorder synucleinopathies

Dementia with Lewy bodies

Dementia with Lewy bodies (DLB) is the second overall cause of dementia after AD, accounting for 15–25% of cases in published autopsy series.[113–115] It typically occurs in later life, with a mean onset of 75 years of age.[116] The dementia involves prominent attentional deficits, executive dysfunction and visuospatial impairment. According to the revised DLB clinical consensus guidelines, fluctuating cognition, recurrent visual hallucinations and parkinsonism remain the core clinical diagnostic features.[117] Thus, with dementia as a required feature, any two of three core features warrant a probable DLB diagnosis, while one of two core features suffice for possible DLB. The criteria also include three suggestive features, REM sleep-behavior disorder, severe neuroleptic sensitivity and low dopamine transporter uptake in basal ganglia demonstrated by imaging (single-photon emission computed tomography or positron emission tomography). Any of these with at least one core feature suffice for probable DLB; possible DLB is assigned to patients with dementia who lack core features but have at least one suggestive feature. Repeated falls, syncope and autonomic dysfunction (e.g. orthostatic hypotension, urinary incontinence), delusions and visual misperceptions and distortions are also commonly associated with the illness.

The brain in DLB may appear surprisingly normal or show minimal frontal or parietal atrophy on gross examination.[118] A depigmented substantia nigra and

locus coeruleus are often seen in the brainstem. Disruption of these and other ascending brainstem monoaminergic streams may account for the mismatch between widespread cognitive impairment and mild gross atrophy. The diagnostic histological hallmark is the Lewy body (LB), a rounded intracytoplasmic inclusion containing α-synuclein. Two LB subtypes, brainstem and cortical, have been described based on morphological features and regional distribution. Brainstem LBs feature the classical LB morphology that predominates in Parkinson's disease, with an eosinophilic central core and a paler peripheral halo easily detected with hematoxylin and eosin (H&E) stain (Fig. 11.8). The substantia nigra, cholinergic pedunculopontine tegmental nucleus, serotonergic raphe nucleus and noradrenergic locus ceruleus are frequently affected, producing characteristic DLB clinical features that arise only in late stages of other dementias, if they arise at all. Compared with brainstem LBs, cortical LBs have an irregular shape without a central eosinophilic core and peripheral halo. Therefore, ubiquitin or (preferably) α-synuclein immunohistochemistry (Fig. 11.8) is required for the detection of cortical LBs. In cerebral cortex, LBs are usually seen in deep cortical layers (V, VI) and found most abundantly in cingulate gyrus, entorhinal cortex and amygdala, as well as temporal and insular cortices.[119,120] Frontal, parietal and occipital cortex, however, can be less affected and cerebellum is typically spared.[121,122] Lewy neurites, almost always coexisting with LBs, are another characteristic DLB marker (Fig. 11.8). These aggregated α-synuclein deposits are seen prominently in the CA2 region of the hippocampus, and may also be detected in brainstem and cortex.[123–125]

The regional distribution of LBs in DLB has been categorized into the following types: brainstem predominant, limbic (transitional), and diffuse neocortical.[113] Patients with isolated brainstem involvement raise the possibility that DLB is, at its core, a disease of the brainstem nuclei that support cortical arousal and attention, autonomic control and movement. The transition into limbic cortex may herald more prominent amnesia and psychosis, whereas cortical LBs may relate to advancing, global dementia. Lewy-related pathology can be graded, as suggested by the most recent report of the DLB consortium, according to the abundance of LBs and Lewy neurites, though the relationship between α-synuclein burden and clinical severity remains uncertain.

Depending on the series, as many as 80% of brains from patients with DLB show concomitant AD

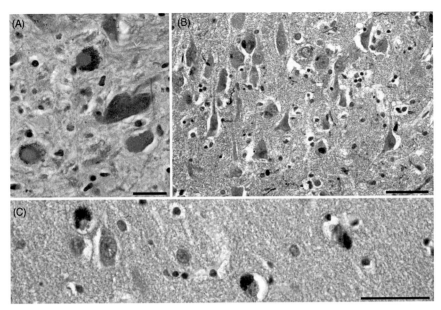

Fig. 11.8. Dementia with Lewy bodies. (A) Classical brainstem Lewy bodies in the substantia nigra. Hematoxylin and eosin stain. (B) Lewy neurites in hippocampal CA2. (C) Cortical Lewy bodies in posterior cingulate cortex. Alpha-synuclein antibody, hematoxylin counterstain. Scale bars, 25 μm (A) and 50 μm (B,C).

pathology, variably consisting of widespread neocortical neuritic plaques and NFTs that are insufficient to fulfill diagnostic criteria for AD.[126] The degree of coexisting AD pathology is strongly associated with the clinical DLB phenotype and, consequently, DLB clinical diagnostic accuracy. That is, patients are more likely to be correctly diagnosed with DLB during life if they have a high burden of DLB pathology in the relative absence of AD-related histopathological changes.[127–129] Further deepening the diagnostic quagmire, no pathological hallmark distinguishes DLB from Parkinson's disease apart from the extent and distribution of LB pathology, but even these features show significant overlap in clinically distinct cohorts. The prevailing notion is that α-synuclein pathophysiology creates a spectrum of clinical disorders; what drives the diversity of this spectrum remains an important area for future research.

Multiple system atrophy

Multiple system atrophy (MSA) is a sporadic neurodegenerative disease characterized by a variable combination of parkinsonism, cerebellar ataxia, autonomic insufficiency and corticospinal tract dysfunction. The prevalence of MSA is 4.4 per 100 000, with an annual incidence of 3 per 100 000 among persons over 50 years of age.[130,131] There is an equal distribution among males and females, with a mean onset early in the sixth decade.[132] A 1998 consensus conference proposed two clinical MSA types: MSA-P for patients with predominant parkinsonism and MSA-C for those with predominant cerebellar ataxia.[133] Almost all patients with MSA develop autonomic symptoms, including orthostatic hypotension, sexual dysfunction and urinary incontinence. Cognitive deficits may be subtle or late appearing and usually involve frontal-executive impairment, with deficits in attentional set-shifting, spatial working memory and verbal memory all reported.[134–136]

At autopsy, patients with MSA show varying degrees of gross atrophy of the cerebellum, pons, medulla and the posterolateral putamen. Nigral depigmentation and putaminal discoloration are frequent, especially in patients with MSA-P. Neuronal loss in MSA is prominent and may be cell specific (Table 11.1) despite the observation that MSA α-synuclein accumulation occurs predominantly within oligodendroglia.[137,138] According to MSA diagnostic consensus criteria, definite neuropathological MSA requires a characteristic density and distribution of glial cytoplasmic inclusions.[133] These eosinophilic, α-synuclein-positive, flame- or sickle-shaped inclusions in oligodendroglia are widely distributed in white matter, basal ganglia (especially putamen), substantia nigra, pontine nuclei, medulla and cerebellum.[139–142] Similar inclusions may also be found in neuronal cytoplasm and nuclei, and glial nuclei; these are referred to as neuronal cytoplasmic inclusions, neuronal nuclear inclusions and glial nuclear inclusions, respectively. All of these inclusions have been reported to be α-synuclein immunoreactive[143] In addition, selective neuronal loss and iron pigment accumulation and gliosis in basal ganglia, substantia nigra, pons and cerebellum are increasingly recognized.

Since the first α-synuclein gene mutation was identified in autosomal dominant Parkinson's disease,[144] α-synuclein has been considered the protein responsible for this class of neurodegenerative disorders, often referred to as "synucleinopathies." United by α-synuclein-immunoreactive inclusions, the synucleinopathies include Parkinson's disease, Parkinson's disease with dementia (PDD), DLB and MSA. Although the etiology of MSA remains unknown and the disease is rarely familial,[145,146] the neuropathology of the disease suggests a strong molecular link between MSA and the other synucleinopathies. Insights from research into DLB, MSA, Parkinson's disease and PDD may complement and inform each other as the field moves forward.

Huntington's disease

Huntington's disease (HD) is an autosomal dominant inherited disorder that presents with motor, cognitive and psychiatric symptoms. In the USA, the prevalence of HD is estimated at 5–7 per 100 000.[147] It typically manifests in the fourth or fifth decade and equally affects men and women. Chorea is the most prominent motor feature, accompanied by dystonia early in the course. As the disease progresses, rigidity, bradykinesia and akinesia unfold.[148] Cognitive impairments develop early, including executive dysfunction, memory impairment and visuospatial deficits.[149] About 50% of those with HD present with psychiatric symptoms, such as depression, anxiety and compulsivity, which may precede motor impairment by years or perhaps even decades, though it can be difficult to disentangle the psychological threat of HD from its primary neuropsychiatric consequences and a chaotic family environment.[150,151]

Gross examination in HD reveals prominent atrophy of the frontal lobe, caudate nucleus, putamen and globus pallidus. Bilateral caudate atrophy represents the most characteristic feature and occurs from tail, to body, to head with a dorsal worse than ventral distribution.[152] Ventricles are enlarged, whereas cerebellum, brainstem and spinal cord are less affected. Microscopically, HD shows neuronal loss and astrocytosis in neostriatum and pallidum, with the medium-sized, spiny projection neurons most vulnerable while large aspiny interneurons are relatively spared.[153] Cerebral cortex and hippocampus show mild to moderate degenerative changes, which may account, in part, for HD cognitive and behavioral impairments, though frontostriatal circuit damage, via the caudate, may play a more primary role in producing these features. Vonsattel et al.[154] established a grading system (0–4) based on gross and histological findings of the striatum, ranging from grade 0 (no specific neuropathological abnormalities) to grade 4 (severe striatal atrophy, neuronal loss and astrocytosis).

Huntington's disease results from a mutation in the IT15 gene on chromosome 4p63, resulting in an unstable trinucleotide (CAG) expansion that alters huntingtin protein encoding.[155] Normally, CAG repeats number 10–35, but in HD repeat length exceeds 39, leading to a polyglutamine strand of variable length at the N-terminus. Repeat number correlates with a younger age of symptom onset and an earlier age at death.[156,157] The function of huntingtin remains poorly understood, but it is widely expressed in humans. How abnormal huntingtin in HD produces neuropathological abnormalities remains unclear, but mutant huntingtin might not only have a toxic gain of function derived from polyglutamine aggregation but may also disturb the neuroprotective function of wild-type huntingtin.[158] Targeted neuronal injury may also relate to alterations in neighboring neuronal or glial support.[159]

Summary

Postmortem neuropathological examination remains the definitive method for identifying neurodegenerative disease. Since the mid 1990s molecular pathology and genetics have pushed forward our understanding of dementia pathogenesis, offering the prospect of new treatments. Disease protein immunohistochemistry has become the essential component of dementia neuropathological evaluation, usurping the role of classical cell-staining methods. Recent clinicopathological correlation studies highlight the difficulty of accurately predicting pathology at the bedside, but growing attention to clinical and imaging biomarkers fuels hope for improved antemortem diagnosis. The behavioral neurologist must strive for this goal, as diagnostic accuracy will impact the success of molecule-specific treatments, including those already in clinical trials for AD. However, a comprehensive view of the dementias—and possibly effective therapies—will require more integrative models that address not only the aberrant proteins of each disease but also how those proteins interact with genetic, epigenetic and environmental factors to erode disease-susceptible neurons, brain regions and distributed functional networks.

Acknowledgements

We thank Drs. Stephen DeArmond and Bruce Miller for helpful comments and Dr. DeArmond for assistance with photomicrography. Finally, we thank our patients and their families for contributing to dementia research.

References

1. Hebert LE, Scherr PA, Bienias JL, Bennett DA, Evans DA. Alzheimer disease in the US population: prevalence estimates using the 2000 census. *Arch Neurol* 2003;**60**(8):1119–22.

2. Bachman DL, Wolf PA, Linn RT *et al.* Incidence of dementia and probable Alzheimer's disease in a general population: the Framingham Study. *Neurology* 1993;**43**(3 Pt 1):515–19.

3. Knopman DS, Boeve BF, Parisi JE *et al.* Antemortem diagnosis of frontotemporal lobar degeneration. *Ann Neurol* 2005;**57**(4):480–8.

4. Forman MS, Farmer J, Johnson JK *et al.* Frontotemporal dementia: clinicopathological correlations. *Ann Neurol* 2006;**59**(6):952–62.

5. Brun A, Gustafson L. Limbic lobe involvement in presenile dementia. *Arch Psychiatr Nervenkr* 1978;**226**(2):79–93.

6. Brun A, Liu X, Erikson C. Synapse loss and gliosis in the molecular layer of the cerebral cortex in Alzheimer's disease and in frontal lobe degeneration. *Neurodegeneration* 1995;**4**(2):171–7.

7. Mesulam MM. Large-scale neurocognitive networks and distributed processing for attention, language, and memory. *Ann Neurol* 1990;**28**(5):597–613.

8. Ritchie K, Lovestone S. The dementias. *Lancet* 2002;**360**(9347):1759–66.

9. Kukull WA, Higdon R, Bowen JD *et al.* Dementia and Alzheimer disease incidence: a prospective cohort study. *Arch Neurol* 2002;**59**(11):1737–46.

10. Braak H, Braak E. Staging of Alzheimer's disease-related neurofibrillary changes. *Neurobiol Aging* 1995;**16**(3):271–284.

11. Hyman BT, Damasio AR. Hierarchical vulnerability of the entorhinal cortex and the hippocampal formation to Alzheimer neuropathological changes: a semiquantitative study. *Neurology* 1990;**40**:403.

12. Hyman BT, Damasio AR, Van Hoesen GW, Barnes CL. Alzheimer's disease: cell-specific pathology isolates the hippocampal formation. *Science* 1984;**298**:83–95.

13. Reiman EM, Caselli RJ, Yun LS, Chen K *et al.* Preclinical evidence of Alzheimer's disease in persons homozygous for the epsilon 4 allele for apolipoprotein E. *N Engl J Med* 1996;**334**(12):752–8.

14. Gorno-Tempini ML, Dronkers NF, Rankin KP *et al.* Cognition and anatomy in three variants of primary progressive aphasia. *Ann Neurol* 2004;**55**(3):335–46.

15. Galton CJ, Patterson K, Xuereb JH, Hodges JR. Atypical and typical presentations of Alzheimer's disease: a clinical, neuropsychological, neuroimaging and pathological study of 13 cases. *Brain* 2000;**123** Pt 3:484–98.

16. Zakzanis KK, Boulos MI. Posterior cortical atrophy. *Neurologist* 2001;**7**(6):341–9.

17. Johnson J, Head E, Kim R *et al.* Clinical and pathological evidence for a frontal variant of Alzheimer disease. *Arch Neurol* 1999;**56**(10):1233–9.

18. Brun A, Gustafson L. Distribution of cerebral degeneration in Alzheimer's disease. A clinico-pathological study. *Arch Psychiatr Nervenkr* 1976;**223**(1):15–33.

19. Alzheimer A. Uber einen eigenartigen, schweren Erkrankungsprozess der Hirnrinde. *Neurol Zbl* 1906;**25**:1134.

20. Dickson DW. The pathogenesis of senile plaques. *J Neuropathol Exp Neurol* 1997;**56**(4):321–39.

21. Goedert M. Tau protein and the neurofibrillary pathology of Alzheimer's disease. *Trends Neurosci* 1993;**16**(11):460–5.

22. Arnold SE, Hyman BT, Flory J, Damasio AR, Van Hoesen GW. The topographical and neuroanatomical distribution of neurofibrillary tangles and neuritic plaques in the cerebral cortex of patients in Alzheimer's disease. *Cerebral Cortex* 1991;**1**(1):103–16.

23. Arriagada PV, Growdon JH, Hedley-Whyte ET, Hyman BT. Neurofibrillary tangles but not senile plaques parallel duration and severity of Alzheimer's disease. *Neurology* 1992;**42**(3 Pt 1):631–9.

24. Ball MJ. Neuronal loss, neurofibrillary tangles and granulovacuolar degeneration in the hippocampus with ageing and dementia. *A quantitative study. Acta Neuropathol (Berl)* 1977;**37**(2):111–8.

25. Vinters HV. Cerebral amyloid angiopathy. *A critical review. Stroke* 1987;**18**(2):311–24.

26. Gibson PH, Tomlinson BE. Numbers of Hirano bodies in the hippocampus of normal and demented people with Alzheimer's disease. *J Neurol Sci* 1977;**33**(1–2):199–206.

155

27. Itagaki S, McGeer PL, Akiyama H, Zhu S, Selkoe D. Relationship of microglia and astrocytes to amyloid deposits of Alzheimer disease. *J Neuroimmunol* 1989;**24** (3):173–82.

28. Mirra S, Heyman A, McKeel D *et al.* The consortium to establish a registry for Alzheimer's disease (CERAD). Part II. Standardization of the neuropathologic assessment of Alzheimer's disease. *Neurology* 1991; **41**(4):479–486.

29. Braak H, Braak E. Neuropathological stageing of Alzheimer-related changes. *Acta Neuropathol* 1991; **82**(4):239–59.

30. Hyman BT, Trojanowski JQ. Consensus recommendations for the postmortem diagnosis of Alzheimer disease from the National Institute on Aging and the Reagan Institute Working Group on diagnostic criteria for the neuropathological assessment of Alzheimer disease. *J Neuropathol Exp Neurol* 1997; **56**(10):1095–7.

31. Bigio EH, Hynan LS, Sontag E, Satumtira S, White CL. Synapse loss is greater in presenile than senile onset Alzheimer disease: implications for the cognitive reserve hypothesis. *Neuropathol Appl Neurobiol* 2002;**28** (3):218–27.

32. Marshall GA, Fairbanks LA, Tekin S, Vinters HV, Cummings JL. Early-onset Alzheimer's disease is associated with greater pathologic burden. *J Geriatr Psychiatry Neurol* 2007;**20**(1):29–33.

33. Kim EJ, Cho SS, Jeong Y *et al.* Glucose metabolism in early onset versus late onset Alzheimer's disease: an SPM analysis of 120 patients. *Brain* 2005;**128** (Pt 8):1790–801.

34. Frisoni GB, Pievani M, Testa C *et al.* The topography of grey matter involvement in early and late onset Alzheimer's disease. *Brain* 2007;**130**(Pt 3):720–30.

35. Hardy JA, Higgins GA. Alzheimer's disease: the amyloid cascade hypothesis. *Science* 1992;**256**(5054):184–5.

36. Goedert M, Spillantini MG, Cairns NJ, Crowther RA. Tau proteins of Alzheimer paired helical filaments: abnormal phosphorylation of all six brain isoforms. *Neuron* 1992;**8**(1):159–68.

37. Farrer LA, Myers RH, Cupples LA *et al.* Transmission and age-at-onset patterns in familial Alzheimer's disease: evidence for heterogeneity. *Neurology* 1990;**40** (3 Pt 1):395–403.

38. St George-Hyslop PH, Tanzi RE, Polinsky RJ. The Genetic Defect Causing Familial Alzheimer's Disease Maps on Chromosome 21. *Science* 1987;**235**:885–90.

39. Schellenberg GD, Bird TD, Wijsman EM *et al.* Genetic linkage evidence for a familial Alzheimer's disease locus on chromosome 14. *Science* 1992;**258**:68–671.

40. Levy-Lahad E, Wasco W, Poorkaj P *et al.* Candidate gene for the chromosome 1 familial Alzheimer's disease locus. *Science* 1995;**269**(5226):973–7.

41. Schmitt FA, Davis DG, Wekstein DR *et al.* "Preclinical" AD revisited: neuropathology of cognitively normal older adults. *Neurology* 2000;**55**(3):370–6.

42. Ratnavalli E, Brayne C, Dawson K, Hodges JR. The prevalence of frontotemporal dementia. *Neurology* 2002;**58**(11):1615–21.

43. Knopman DS, Petersen RC, Edland SD, Cha RH, Rocca WA. The incidence of frontotemporal lobar degeneration in Rochester, Minnesota, 1990 through 1994. *Neurology* 2004;**62**(3):506–8.

44. Neary D, Snowden JS, Gustafson L *et al.* Frontotemporal lobar degeneration: a consensus on clinical diagnostic criteria. *Neurology* 1998;**51**(6): 1546–54.

45. Schroeter ML, Raczka K, Neumann J, von Cramon DY. Neural networks in frontotemporal dementia: a meta-analysis. *Neurobiol Aging* 2006;**29**(3):418–26.

46. Seeley WW, Crawford R, Rascovsky K *et al.* Frontal paralimbic network atrophy in very mild behavioral variant frontotemporal dementia. *Arch Neurol* 2008;**65**(2):249–55.

47. Perry RJ, Graham A, Williams G *et al.* Patterns of frontal lobe atrophy in frontotemporal dementia: a volumetric MRI study. *Dement Geriatr Cogn Disord* 2006;**22**(4):278–87.

48. Broe M, Hodges JR, Schofield E *et al.* Staging disease severity in pathologically confirmed cases of fronto temporal dementia. *Neurology* 2003;**60**(6):1005–11.

49. Hodges JR, Patterson K, Oxbury S, Funnell E. Semantic dementia. Progressive fluent aphasia with temporal lobe atrophy. *Brain* 1992;**115** (Pt 6):1783–806.

50. Snowden J. *Semantic dementia.* 2nd edition ed. New York: Oxford University Press; 2000.

51. Seeley WW, Bauer AM, Miller BL *et al.* The natural history of temporal variant frontotemporal dementia. *Neurology* 2005;**64**(8):1384–90.

52. Thompson SA, Patterson K, Hodges JR. Left/right asymmetry of atrophy in semantic dementia: behavioral–cognitive implications. *Neurology* 2003;**61**(9):1196–203.

53. Neary D, Snowden JS, Mann DM *et al.* Frontal lobe dementia and motor neuron disease. *J Neurol Neurosurg Psychiatry* 1990;**53**(1):23–32.

54. Munoz DG, Dickson DW, Bergeron C *et al.* The neuropathology and biochemistry of frontotemporal dementia. *Ann Neurol* 2003;**54**(Suppl 5):S24–8.

55. Mackenzie IR, Neumann M, Bigio EH *et al.* Nomenclature for neuropathologic subtypes of frontotemporal lobar degeneration: consensus recommendations. *Acta Neuropathol* 2009;**117**(1):15–8.

56. Forman MS, Lee VM, Trojanowski JQ. New insights into genetic and molecular mechanisms of brain degeneration in tauopathies. *J Chem Neuroanat* 2000;**20** (3–4):225–44.

57. Bigio EH, Lipton AM, Yen SH *et al.* Frontal lobe dementia with novel tauopathy: sporadic multiple system tauopathy with dementia. *J Neuropathol Exp Neurol* 2001;**60**(4):328–41.

58. Dickson DW. Pick's disease: a modern approach. *Brain Pathol* 1998;**8**(2):339–54.

59. Probst A, Tolnay M, Langui D, Goedert M, Spillantini MG. Pick's disease: hyperphosphorylated tau protein segregates to the somatoaxonal compartment. *Acta Neuropathol (Berl)* 1996;**92**(6):588–96.

60. Feany MB, Mattiace LA, Dickson DW. Neuropathologic overlap of progressive supranuclear palsy, Pick's disease and corticobasal degeneration. *J Neuropathol Exp Neurol* 1996;**55**(1):53–67.

61. Wilhelmsen K, Lynch T, Pavlou E *et al.* Localization of disinhibition–dementia–parkinsonism–amyotrophy complex to 17q21-22. *Am J Hum Genet* 1994;**6**:1159–65.

62. Hutton M, Lendon CL, Rizzu P *et al.* Association of missense and 5'-splice-site mutations in tau with the inherited dementia FTDP-17. *Nature* 1998;**393** (6686):702–5.

63. Foster NL, Wilhelmsen K, Sima AA *et al.* Frontotemporal dementia and parkinsonism linked to chromosome 17: a consensus conference. Conference Participants. *Annals of Neurology* 1997;**41**(6):706–15.

64. Bird TD, Wijsman EM, Nochlin D *et al.* Chromosome 17 and hereditary dementia: linkage studies in three non-Alzheimer families and kindreds with late-onset FAD. *Neurology* 1997;**48**(4):949–54.

65. Heutink P, Stevens M, Rizzu P *et al.* Hereditary frontotemporal dementia is linked to chromosome 17q21-q22: a genetic and clinicopathological study of three Dutch families. *Ann Neurol* 1997;**41**(2):150–9.

66. Lipton AM, White CL, 3rd, Bigio EH. Frontotemporal lobar degeneration with motor neuron disease-type inclusions predominates in 76 cases of frontotemporal degeneration. *Acta Neuropathol (Berl)* 2004;**108** (5):379–85.

67. Mackenzie IR, Baborie A, Pickering-Brown S *et al.* Heterogeneity of ubiquitin pathology in frontotemporal lobar degeneration: classification and relation to clinical phenotype. *Acta Neuropathol* 2006;**112**(5):539–49.

68. Sampathu DM, Neumann M, Kwong LK *et al.* Pathological heterogeneity of frontotemporal lobar degeneration with ubiquitin-positive inclusions delineated by ubiquitin immunohistochemistry and novel monoclonal antibodies. *Am J Pathol* 2006; **169**(4):1343–52.

69. Mackenzie IR, Baker M, Pickering-Brown S *et al.* The neuropathology of frontotemporal lobar degeneration caused by mutations in the progranulin gene. *Brain* 2006;**129**(Pt 11):3081–90.

70. Jackson M, Lennox G, Lowe J. Motor neurone disease–inclusion dementia. *Neurodegeneration* 1996; **5**(4):339–50.

71. Sreedharan J, Blair IP, Tripathi VB *et al.* TDP-43 mutations in familial and sporadic amyotrophic lateral sclerosis. *Science* 2008;**319**(5870):1668–72.

72. Cairns NJ, Grossman M, Arnold SE *et al.* Clinical and neuropathologic variation in neuronal intermediate filament inclusion disease. *Neurology* 2004;**63**(8): 1376–84.

73. Neumann M, Sampathu DM, Kwong LK *et al.* Ubiquitinated TDP-43 in frontotemporal lobar degeneration and amyotrophic lateral sclerosis. *Science* 2006;**314**(5796):130–3.

74. Cairns NJ, Zhukareva V, Uryu K *et al.* alpha-internexin is present in the pathological inclusions of neuronal intermediate filament inclusion disease. *Am J Pathol* 2004;**164**(6):2153–61.

75. Josephs KA, Uchikado H, McComb RD *et al.* Extending the clinicopathological spectrum of neurofilament inclusion disease. *Acta Neuropathol (Berl)* 2005;**109** (4):427–32.

76. Knopman DS, Mastri AR, Frey WHd *et al.* Dementia lacking distinctive histologic features: a common non-Alzheimer degenerative dementia. *Neurology* 1990;**40**(2):251–6.

77. Josephs KA, Jones AG, Dickson DW. Hippocampal sclerosis and ubiquitin-positive inclusions in dementia lacking distinctive histopathology. *Dement Geriatr Cogn Disord* 2004;**17**(4):342–5.

78. Holm IE, Englund E, Mackenzie IR *et al.* A reassessment of the neuropathology of frontotemporal dementia linked to chromosome 3. *J Neuropathol Exp Neurol* 2007;**66**(10):884–91.

79. Mackenzie IR, Foti D, Woulfe J, Hurwitz TA. Atypical frontotemporal lobar degeneration with ubiquitin-positive, TDP-43-negative neuronal inclusions. *Brain* 2008;**131**(Pt 5):1282–93.

80. Josephs KA, Lin WL, Ahmed Z *et al.* Frontotemporal lobar degeneration with ubiquitin-positive, but TDP-43-negative inclusions. *Acta Neuropathol* 2008;**116**(2):159–67.

81. Baker M, Mackenzie IR, Pickering-Brown SM *et al.* Mutations in progranulin cause tau-negative frontotemporal dementia linked to chromosome 17. *Nature* 2006;**442**:916–19.

82. Cruts M, Gijselinck I, van der Zee J *et al.* Null mutations in progranulin cause ubiquitin-positive frontotemporal dementia linked to chromosome 17q21. *Nature* 2006;**442**:920–4.

83. Mukherjee O, Pastor P, Cairns NJ *et al.* HDDD2 is a familial frontotemporal lobar degeneration with ubiquitin-positive, tau-negative inclusions caused by a missense mutation in the signal peptide of progranulin. *Ann Neurol* 2006;**60**(3):314–22.

84. Schymick JC, Yang Y, Andersen PM *et al.* Progranulin mutations and amyotrophic lateral sclerosis or

amyotrophic lateral sclerosis-frontotemporal dementia phenotypes. *J Neurol Neurosurg Psychiatry* 2007;**78**(7):754–6.

85. Gass J, Cannon A, Mackenzie IR *et al.* Mutations in progranulin are a major cause of ubiquitin-positive frontotemporal lobar degeneration. *Hum Mol Genet* 2006;**15**(20):2988–3001.

86. Seeley WW, Carlin DA, Allman JM *et al.* Early frontotemporal dementia targets neurons unique to apes and humans. *Ann Neurol* 2006;**60**(6):660–7.

87. Seeley WW, Menon V, Schatzberg AF *et al.* Dissociable intrinsic connectivity networks for salience processing and executive control. *J Neurosci* 2007;**27**(9):2349–56.

88. Hof PR, Van Der Gucht E. Structure of the cerebral cortex of the humpback whale, Megaptera novaeangliae (Cetacea, Mysticeti, Balaenopteridae). Anat Rec A Discov Mol Cell Evol Biol 2006.

89. Hakeem AY, Sherwood CC, Bonar CJ *et al.* Von Economo neurons in the elephant brain. *Anat Rec (Hoboken)* 2009;**292**(2):242–8.

90. Hodges JR, Davies RR, Xuereb JH *et al.* Clinicopathological correlates in frontotemporal dementia. *Ann Neurol* 2004;**56**(3):399–406.

91. Knibb JA, Xuereb JH, Patterson K, Hodges JR. Clinical and pathological characterization of progressive aphasia. *Ann Neurol* 2006;**59**(1):156–65.

92. Davies RR, Hodges JR, Kril JJ *et al.* The pathological basis of semantic dementia. *Brain* 2005;**128**(Pt 9): 1984–95.

93. Josephs KA, Duffy JR, Strand EA *et al.* Clinicopathological and imaging correlates of progressive aphasia and apraxia of speech. *Brain* 2006;**129**(Pt 6):1385–98.

94. Gorno-Tempini ML, Murray RC, Rankin KP *et al.* Clinical, cognitive and anatomical evolution from nonfluent progressive aphasia to corticobasal syndrome: a case report. *Neurocase* 2004;**10**(6):426–36.

95. Mahapatra RK, Edwards MJ, Schott JM, Bhatia KP. Corticobasal degeneration. *Lancet Neurol* 2004;**3**(12):736–43.

96. Rinne JO, Lee MS, Thompson PD, Marsden CD. Corticobasal degeneration. A clinical study of 36 cases. *Brain* 1994;**117** (Pt 5):1183–96.

97. Wenning GK, Litvan I, Jankovic J *et al.* Natural history and survival of 14 patients with corticobasal degeneration confirmed at postmortem examination. *J Neurol Neurosurg Psychiatry* 1998;**64**(2):184–9.

98. Riley DE, Lang AE. Clinical diagnostic criteria. *Adv Neurol* 2000;**82**:29–34.

99. Graham NL, Bak TH, Hodges JR. Corticobasal degeneration as a cognitive disorder. *Mov Disord* 2003;**18**(11):1224–32.

100. Kompoliti K, Goetz CG, Boeve BF *et al.* Clinical presentation and pharmacological therapy in corticobasal degeneration. *Arch Neurol* 1998;**55**(7):957–61.

101. Grimes DA, Lang AE, Bergeron CB. Dementia as the most common presentation of cortical-basal ganglionic degeneration. *Neurology* 1999;**53**(9): 1969–74.

102. Murray R, Neumann M, Forman MS *et al.* Cognitive and motor assessment in autopsy-proven corticobasal degeneration. *Neurology* 2007;**68**(16):1274–83.

103. Feany MB, Dickson DW. Widespread cytoskeletal pathology characterizes corticobasal degeneration. *Am J Pathol* 1995;**146**(6):1388–96.

104. Litvan I, Agid Y, Calne D *et al.* Clinical research criteria for the diagnosis of progressive supranuclear palsy (Steele-Richardson-Olszewski syndrome): report of the NINDS-SPSP international workshop. *Neurology* 1996;**47**(1):1–9.

105. Nath U, Ben-Shlomo Y, Thomson RG *et al.* The prevalence of progressive supranuclear palsy (Steele-Richardson-Olszewski syndrome) in the UK. *Brain* 2001;**124**(Pt 7):1438–49.

106. Lantos PL. The neuropathology of progressive supranuclear palsy. *J Neural Transm Suppl* 1994;**42**:137–52.

107. Komori T, Arai N, Oda M *et al.* Astrocytic plaques and tufts of abnormal fibers do not coexist in corticobasal degeneration and progressive supranuclear palsy. *Acta Neuropathol (Berl)* 1998;**96**(4):401–8.

108. Pillon B, Blin J, Vidailhet M *et al.* The neuropsychological pattern of corticobasal degeneration: comparison with progressive supranuclear palsy and Alzheimer's disease. *Neurology* 1995;**45**(8):1477–83.

109. Spillantini MG, Goedert M. Tau mutations in familial frontotemporal dementia. *Brain* 2000;**123**(Pt 5):857–9.

110. Houlden H, Baker M, Morris HR *et al.* Corticobasal degeneration and progressive supranuclear palsy share a common tau haplotype. *Neurology* 2001;**56**(12):1702–6.

111. Lang AE, Bergeron, C. Corticobasal degeneration and PSP: the same disease? *Mov Disord* 2002;**17**:1404–5.

112. Nasreddine ZS, Loginov M, Clark LN *et al.* From genotype to phenotype: a clinical pathological, and biochemical investigation of frontotemporal dementia and parkinsonism (FTDP-17) caused by the P301L tau mutation. *Ann Neurol* 1999;**45**(6):704–15.

113. McKeith I, Galasko D, Kosaka K *et al.* Consensus guidlines for the clinical and pathologic diagnosis of dementia with Lewy Bodies. *Neurology* 1996;**47**:1113–24.

114. Holmes C, Cairns N, Lantos P, Mann A. Validity of current clinical criteria for Alzheimer's disease,

vascular dementia, and dementia with Lewy bodies. *Br J Psychiatry* 1999;**174**:45–51.

115. Lim A, Tsuang D, Kukull W *et al*. Clinico-neuropathological correlation of Alzheimer's disease in a community-based case series. *J Am Geriatr Soc* 1999;**47**(5):564–9.

116. Ransmayr G. Dementia with Lewy bodies: prevalence, clinical spectrum and natural history. *J Neural Transm Suppl* 2000(60):303–14.

117. McKeith IG, Dickson DW, Lowe J *et al*. Diagnosis and management of dementia with Lewy bodies: third report of the DLB Consortium. *Neurology* 2005;**65**(12):1863–72.

118. Double KL, Halliday GM, McRitchie DA *et al*. Regional brain atrophy in idiopathic parkinson's disease and diffuse Lewy body disease. *Dementia* 1996;**7**(6):304–13.

119. Perry RH, Irving D, Blessed G, Fairbairn A, Perry EK. Senile dementia of Lewy body type. A clinically and neuropathologically distinct form of Lewy body dementia in the elderly. *J Neurol Sci* 1990;**95**:119–139.

120. Rezaie P, Cairns NJ, Chadwick A, Lantos PL. Lewy bodies are located preferentially in limbic areas in diffuse Lewy body disease. *Neurosci Lett* 1996;**212**(2):111–4.

121. Gomez-Tortosa E, Newell K, Irizarry MC *et al*. Clinical and quantitative pathologic correlates of dementia with Lewy bodies. *Neurology* 1999;**53**(6):1284–91.

122. Giasson B, M-Y Lee, V, Trojanowski, JQ. *Parkinson's disease, dementia with lewy bodies, multiple system atrophy and the spectrum of disease with alpha synuclein inclusions*. 2nd edn. New York: Cambridge University Press; 2004.

123. Dickson DW, Ruan D, Crystal H *et al*. Hippocampal degeneration differentiates diffuse Lewy body disease (DLBD) from Alzheimer's disease: light and electron microscopic immunocytochemistry of CA2-3 neurites specific to DLBD. *Neurology* 1991;**41**(9):1402–9.

124. Dickson D, Schmidt M, Lee V *et al*. Immunoreactivity profile of hippocampal Ca2/3 neurites in diffuse Lewy body disease. *Acta Neuropathologica* 1994;**87**:269–276.

125. Spillantini MG, Crowther RA, Jakes R, Hasegawa M, Goedert M. alpha-Synuclein in filamentous inclusions of Lewy bodies from Parkinson's disease and dementia with lewy bodies. *Proc Natl Acad Sci USA* 1998;**95**(11):6469–73.

126. Kosaka K. Diffuse Lewy body disease. *Neuropathology* 2000;**20**(Suppl):S73–8.

127. Merdes AR, Hansen LA, Jeste DV *et al*. Influence of Alzheimer pathology on clinical diagnostic accuracy in dementia with Lewy bodies. *Neurology* 2003;**60**(10):1586–90.

128. Del Ser T, Hachinski V, Merskey H, Munoz DG. Clinical and pathologic features of two groups of

patients with dementia with Lewy bodies: effect of coexisting Alzheimer-type lesion load. *Alzheimer Dis Assoc Disord* 2001;**15**(1):31–44.

129. Lopez OL, Becker JT, Kaufer DI *et al*. Research evaluation and prospective diagnosis of dementia with Lewy bodies. *Arch Neurol* 2002;**59**(1):43–6.

130. Schrag A, Ben-Shlomo Y, Quinn NP. Prevalence of progressive supranuclear palsy and multiple system atrophy: a cross-sectional study. *Lancet* 1999;**354**(9192):1771–5.

131. Wenning GK, Colosimo C, Geser F, Poewe W. Multiple system atrophy. *Lancet Neurol* 2004;**3**(2):93–103.

132. Wenning GK, Tison F, Ben Shlomo Y, Daniel SE, Quinn NP. Multiple system atrophy: a review of 203 pathologically proven cases. *Mov Disord* 1997;**12**(2):133–47.

133. Gilman S, Low PA, Quinn N *et al*. Consensus statement on the diagnosis of multiple system atrophy. *J Neurol Sci* 1999;**163**(1):94–8.

134. Robbins TW, James M, Owen AM *et al*. Cognitive deficits in progressive supranuclear palsy, Parkinson's disease, and multiple system atrophy in tests sensitive to frontal lobe dysfunction. *J Neurol Neurosurg Psychiatry* 1994;**57**(1):79–88.

135. Meco G, Gasparini M, Doricchi F. Attentional functions in multiple system atrophy and Parkinson's disease. *J Neurol Neurosurg Psychiatry* 1996;**60**(4):393–8.

136. Burk K, Daum I, Rub U. Cognitive function in multiple system atrophy of the cerebellar type. *Mov Disord* 2006;**21**(6):772–6.

137. Sato K, Kaji R, Matsumoto S, Goto S. Cell type-specific neuronal loss in the putamen of patients with multiple system atrophy. *Mov Disord* 2007;**22**(5):738–42.

138. Wenning GK, Tison F, Elliott L, Quinn NP, Daniel SE. Olivopontocerebellar pathology in multiple system atrophy. *Mov Disord* 1996;**11**(2):157–62.

139. Gai WP, Power JH, Blumbergs PC, Blessing WW. Multiple-system atrophy: a new alpha-synuclein disease? *Lancet* 1998;**352**(9127):547–8.

140. Tu PH, Galvin JE, Baba M, Giasson B *et al*. Glial cytoplasmic inclusions in white matter oligodendrocytes of multiple system atrophy brains contain insoluble alpha-synuclein. *Ann Neurol* 1998;**44**(3):415–22.

141. Lantos PL. The definition of multiple system atrophy: a review of recent developments. *J Neuropathol Exp Neurol* 1998;**57**(12):1099–111.

142. Duda JE, Giasson BI, Gur TL *et al*. Immunohistochemical and biochemical studies demonstrate a distinct profile of alpha-synuclein permutations in multiple system atrophy. *J Neuropathol Exp Neurol* 2000;**59**(9):830–41.

143. Lin WL, DeLucia MW, Dickson DW. Alpha-synuclein immunoreactivity in neuronal nuclear inclusions and neurites in multiple system atrophy. *Neurosci Lett* 2004;**354**(2):99–102.

144. Polymeropoulos M, Lavedan C, Leroy E *et al.* Mutation in the alpha-synuclein gene identified in families with Parkinson's diseae. *Science* 1997;**276**:2045–8.

145. Soma H, Yabe I, Takei A *et al.* Heredity in multiple system atrophy. *J Neurol Sci* 2006;**240**(1–2):107–10.

146. Hara K, Momose Y, Tokiguchi S *et al.* Multiplex families with multiple system atrophy. *Arch Neurol* 2007;**64**(4):545–51.

147. Folstein S. *Huntington's Disease: A Disorder of Families.* Baltimore: Johns Hopkins University Press; 1989.

148. Feigin A, Kieburtz K, Bordwell K *et al.* Functional decline in Huntington's disease. *Mov Disord* 1995; **10**(2):211–4.

149. Zakzanis KK. The subcortical dementia of Huntington's disease. *J Clin Exp Neuropsychol* 1998; **20**(4):565–78.

150. Mendez MF. Huntington's disease: update and review of neuropsychiatric aspects. *Int J Psychiatry Med* 1994;**24**(3):189–208.

151. Berrios GE, Wagle AC, Markova IS *et al.* Psychiatric symptoms in neurologically asymptomatic Huntington's disease gene carriers: a comparison with gene negative at risk subjects. *Acta Psychiatr Scand* 2002;**105**(3):224–30.

152. Vonsattel JP, DiFiglia M. Huntington disease. *J Neuropathol Exp Neurol* 1998;**57**(5):369–84.

153. Graveland GA, Williams RS, DiFiglia M. Evidence for degenerative and regenerative changes in neostriatal spiny neurons in Huntington's disease. *Science* 1985;**227**(4688):770–3.

154. Vonsattel J-P, Myers RH, Stevens TJ *et al.* Neuropathological classification of Huntington's disease. *J Neuropath Exp Neurology* 1985;**44**:559–77.

155. The Huntington's Disease Collaborative Research Group. A novel gene containing a trinucleotide repeat that is expanded and unstable on Huntington's disease chromosomes. *Cell* 1993;**72**:971–83.

156. Brandt J, Bylsma FW, Gross R *et al.* Trinucleotide repeat length and clinical progression in Huntington's disease. *Neurology* 1996;**46**(2):527–31.

157. Persichetti F, Srinidhi J, Kanaley L *et al.* Huntington's disease CAG trinucleotide repeats in pathologically confirmed post-mortem brains. *Neurobiol Dis* 1994;**1**(3):159–66.

158. Busch A, Engemann S, Lurz R *et al.* Mutant huntingtin promotes the fibrillogenesis of wild-type huntingtin: a potential mechanism for loss of huntingtin function in Huntington's disease. *J Biol Chem* 2003;**278** (42):41452–61.

159. Zuccato C, Liber D, Ramos C *et al.* Progressive loss of BDNF in a mouse model of Huntington's disease and rescue by BDNF delivery. *Pharmacol Res* 2005;**52** (2):133–9.

160. Mackenzie IR, Bigio EH, Ince PG *et al.* Pathological TDP-43 distinguishes sporadic amyotrophic lateral sclerosis from amyotrophic lateral sclerosis with SOD1 mutations. *Ann Neurol* 2007;**61**(5):427–34.

Cognitive impairment, not demented

Cerebrovascular contributions to amnestic mild cognitive impairment

Charles DeCarli, Adriane Votaw Mayda and Christine Wu Nordahl

Introduction

Advancing age is often accompanied by complaints of impaired memory[1] and reduced performance on a variety of cognitive tasks, particularly tasks that measure memory.[2] Careful cross-sectional examination of cognitive function among community-dwelling elderly, however, reveals a spectrum of cognitive performance from normal to dementia, including impairments in a variety of cognitive domains in the absence of a clinically defined dementia.[3,4] Gradual decline in cognitive ability is a characteristic of longitudinal studies of the elderly, consistent with the aging and mental decline hypothesis, but with substantial individual heterogeneity that suggests much of the age-related differences in memory performance may reflect an admixture of incipient dementia within older populations.[5] The possibility that incipient dementia is prevalent amongst the elderly is further supported by neuropathological studies that reveal evidence of Alzheimer's disease (AD) years before clinical symptoms are evident.[6,7] Although less common, AD pathology can also be found in individuals with no detectable symptoms.[6,8] Finally, AD pathology is often present in individuals with memory impairment who are not demented.[7] Clinical studies of elderly individuals with memory impairment also reveal a rapid rate of conversion to AD, reaching as high as 15% per year. This evidence suggests that significant memory impairment, short of dementia and often denoted as mild cognitive impairment (MCI) in the elderly may be a transition phase between the normal aging process and AD.[9,10]

The concept of MCI has been repeatedly revised since its original description in the 1980s in recognition of the heterogeneity of this syndrome.[11] More recent taxonomies [11] have broadened the definition of MCI to include memory and non-memory deficits while further separating these two conditions into isolated conditions or conditions associated with impairments in additional cognitive domains. These various subtypes are postulated to coincide with separate pathologic entities.[11] For example, isolated amnesia is believed to specific for AD pathology.[7,11] The amnestic MCI (aMCI) subtype has the strongest evidence as a valid prodrome of AD,[7,9–11] has been successfully used as a stratification variable in clinical trials[12] and is associated with increased cerebral amyloid in imaging studies.[13] Interestingly, review of the raw data from one currently published amyloid imaging study suggests a bimodal distribution of amyloid accumulation, with approximately one-half the subjects having amyloid accumulation in the normal range and the other half having accumulation values consistent with AD pathology.[13] This chapter reviews a potential second cause for aMCI: cerebrovascular disease (CVD). In order to begin this discussion, however, we first review the various recognized components of human memory.

Human memory systems: a brief review

Memory is the process by which information is received, encoded, stored and retrieved. Milner et al.[14] have further defined memory as explicit (declarative) and implicit (non-declarative). Explicit memory is denoted as memory of people, places and things. Implicit memory is denoted as memory of reflexive or motor skills. Clinically relevant memory impairment such as aMCI involves deficits in explicit memory.[9] Explicit memory can be further subdivided into semantic memory (memory of facts) and episodic memory (memory of recent events).[15] Episodic memory is the form of explicit memory most affected with aMCI.[9] Successful explicit memory function is believed to involve a number of separate processes, which includes encoding, storage and retrieval.

The Behavioral Neurology of Dementia, eds. Bruce L. Miller and Bradley F. Boeve. Published by Cambridge University Press. © Cambridge University Press 2009.

Encoding is the function by which cerebral resources are directed through the use of attentional mechanisms to the processing of information. Memory encoding is believed to be a function of working memory processes that have specific anatomic localization within frontal, parietal and temporal cortices.[16] Results from neuroimaging studies show that the dorsolateral prefrontal cortex (DLPFC) implements processes critical for organizing items in working memory [17] and that DLPFC connections to the hippocampus are important for long-term memory storage.[18] Conversely, the hippocampus is believed to be responsible for memory consolidation,[19] although the exact role of the hippocampus in memory post-consolidation remains controversial.[20–22] Even from this brief review, it is evident the impairments in episodic memory may result from injury to either frontal systems or the hippocampus. In the next section, we briefly review the substantial evidence favoring hippocampal injury by AD in individuals with aMCI.

Hippocampal injury in Alzheimer's disease

There is overwhelming evidence that the pathological processes of AD begins in the hippocampus and associated allocortical areas[23–25] and that the AD process may begin years before clinical symptoms are evident.[6,26] Clinically, this pathological process is associated with a slowly progressive amnestic syndrome.[7,9,27,28] In addition magnetic resonance imaging (MRI) evidence of hippocampal injury (as manifest by the presence of atrophy) is significantly associated with the extent of memory performance and strongly predictive of future progression to AD dementia.[29–32] Moreover, hippocampal volume is associated with the extent of AD pathology in older individuals and those with AD.[33,34]

It is clear, therefore, from even this most cursory review, that AD pathology affects allocortical structures early in the disease, causing hippocampal injury, and can produce the episodic memory impairment characteristic of AD. In these circumstances, it is evident that aMCI is a common prodrome to AD (Fig. 12.1).[7]

While AD pathology is recognized as common to advancing age, less emphasis has been placed on the equally common prevalence of CVD. This is despite evidence that the lifetime risk for CVD is similar to that of AD among women and higher than AD for men.[35] In the next section, we review the impact of CVD on cognition and its potential role in aMCI.

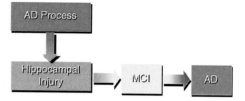

Fig. 12.1. Mild cognitive impairment in early Alzheimer's disease.

Cerebrovascular disease and cognition
The spectrum of vascular brain changes

Before discussing the impact of CVD on cognition, we should first define what we mean by CVD. Stroke or symptoms of transient brain ischemia have long been viewed as the hallmark expression of CVD. Multiple studies conclusively show that the two most significant risk factors for stroke, advancing age and hypertension, are also the most common risk factors for cardiovascular and peripheral vascular disease, suggesting that these disorders share a common mechanism of vascular injury.[36–41] The advent of neuroimaging, however, has shown that a considerable number of cerebral infarcts are clinically silent and share the same risk factors as clinically apparent stroke.[42–47] In addition, the hallmark observations of Hachinski and colleagues relating abnormalities of cerebral white matter to cerebrovascular risk factors (CVRFs)[48–52] have been confirmed and extended.[53–61] The fact that white matter hyperintensities (WMH) significantly predict future stroke[62,63] and mortality[64] lends further support to the notion that WMH are part of a spectrum of vascular-related brain injury.[59,61] Repeated studies showing significant associations between CVRFs and accelerated cerebral atrophy suggest that atrophy may also be part of the spectrum of vascular-related brain injury.[65–68]

Cerebrovascular risk factors can give rise to a spectrum of asymptomatic brain injury. These various forms of brain injury also affect behavior in a variety of ways, further expanding the clinical relevance of CVRFs and the potential interaction between asymptomatic CVD and AD. In the next section, we review evidence supporting the relation between CVRFs, asymptomatic brain injury and cognition.

Impact of cerebrovascular risk factors on cognition in community-dwelling normal individuals

A number of epidemiological studies show strong associations between elevations in middle life blood pressure and the prevalence of later life cognitive impairment and dementia.[69-73] The mechanisms by which CVRFs lead to cognitive impairment remain unclear, but a number of cross-sectional epidemiological studies as well as longitudinal prospective studies suggest that CVRF-related brain changes are associated with these cognitive changes.

Large epidemiological studies, while sometimes limited in the extent of cognitive testing available, consistently show moderate associations between brain atrophy or WMH volumes and diminished cognitive impairment.[74-79] A few smaller, cross-sectional studies consistently suggest deficits in tests of attention and mental processing, although impairments in memory and general intelligence are also seen.[80,83] A number of these studies also show a threshold effect where extensive amounts of WMH are necessary before cognitive impairments are seen.[80-82]

Two studies from the Cardiovascular Health Study have examined the relation between cognitive impairment and clinically silent cerebral infarction.[84,85] While Price et al.[84] focused primarily on the neurological manifestations of silent cerebral infarcts, they did note a significant increase in the number of individuals with a history of memory loss amongst those with silent cerebral infarction. Longstreth et al.[85] examined cognitive function in more detail and noted a significant association between silent cerebral infarctions and diminished performances on the modified Mini-Mental State Examination (MMSE) and the Digit-Symbol Substitution Test (DSS).[85] These findings are remarkably similar to their previously reported effect of WMH on cognition.[75] Findings from these studies have been confirmed in another large population-based study.[86,87]

Unfortunately, these studies did not examine the impact of lifetime cerebrovascular risk on brain structure and cognition. Results from the NHLBI Twin Study, however, confirm the suspected link between CVRFs, brain injury and decline in cognitive performance over time.[58] Lifetime patterns of systolic blood pressure were significantly associated with differences in brain atrophy, WMH volume and 10-year changes in MMSE and DSS scores.[58] Importantly, however, even after correcting for age, education, baseline cognitive performance and incident CVD, there were strongly significant associations between WMH volume, DSS, Benton Visual Retention Test (BVRT) and a Verbal Fluency Test (VFT). Significant associations between brain volume and 10-year differences in MMSE, DSS and VFT were also found.

These results suggest that the cognitive changes associated with elevations in midlife blood pressure may be mediated by the brain injury induced by prolonged elevations of blood pressure (and possibly other CVRFs). A follow-up study of the same subjects explored the pattern of cognitive changes in association with midlife blood pressure patterns more carefully.[67] Cognitive tests selected for this study fell into the two broad functional categories of memory and psychomotor speed. Subjects with combined brain atrophy and WMH were significantly older and had a higher prevalence of CVRFs[67] and performed more poorly on all tests of psychomotor speed even after correcting for age, educational achievement and incident CVD, whereas group differences on memory tests were small. These results confirm the concept that the cognitive changes associated with CVRFs generally impact frontal executive functioning.[67]

Longitudinal studies offer the advantage of examining lifetime CVRF influences on brain–behavior relations. Unfortunately, these studies have generally focused on older individuals,[58,67] while epidemiological studies show that the impact of CVRFs – especially diabetes and hypertension – may occur at a considerably younger age.[88] Seshadri et al.[68] examined the relation between stroke risk factors, brain volume and cognition in a younger group of individuals with an average age of 62 years. Age-corrected differences in brain volume were significantly and positively associated with performance on tests of attention and executive function (e.g. Trails A and B), new learning (e.g. Paired Associates) and visuospatial function (e.g. delayed visual reproduction and Hooper Visual Organization Test), but not with performance on tests of verbal memory or naming. While these results are consistent with those of Swan et al.,[67] they suggest that the impact of CVRFs on brain structure and function may begin shortly after midlife. A follow-up study examining the impact of WMH on the same cohort had similar findings.[89]

In summary, subtle cognitive deficits in community-dwelling essentially normal individuals are associated with CVRFs and appear to be mediated by CVRF-related brain injury. This process begins relatively early in life, as cognitive impairment and brain injury are present to some degree even in individuals 60 years of age or younger. Frontal lobe-mediated cognitive domains of attention, concentration and psychomotor speed are most affected in subjects free of dementia or stroke.[89] Evidence of frontal lobe dysfunction is supported by positron emission tomography (PET) imaging, which finds reduced metabolism in association with vascular-related brain injury, particularly WMH,[80,90] as well as significant associations between frontal lobe metabolism, memory impairment and future cognitive decline in patients with dementia and WMH.[91,92]

These separate lines of evidence coalesce to create a body of evidence that vascular brain injury results in frontal lobe dysfunction and cognitive impairments assumed to relate to frontal lobe function. Given that episodic memory performance involves coordination between DLPFC-mediated working memory and hippocampus-mediated consolidation, it would not be surprising to find associations between vascular disease and aMCI. In the next section, we describe data from our laboratory giving evidence for the existence of a vascular form of aMCI.

Evidence for vascular amnestic mild cognitive impairment

Elderly individuals commonly have WMH and these have been associated with increased risk for MCI.[93,94] Nordahl et al.[95] used WMH as a marker for small-vessel CVD severity to identify and contrast two groups of subjects with aMCI. In this study, the authors proposed that WMH related to small-vessel CVD might play a role in the episodic memory impairment characteristic of aMCI. The authors predicted that WMH might compromise executive control processes that are critical for working memory, which, in turn, may lead to episodic memory deficits

and a diagnosis of aMCI. As discussed above, this theory is based on the preposition that impairments in consolidation and retrieval could occur if information cannot be actively maintained and manipulated at an immediate or short-term level. Therefore, whereas hippocampal dysfunction may be associated with isolated episodic memory impairments, small-vessel CVD may lead to a distinct pattern of deficits that includes both episodic memory impairment and deficits in executive control processes.

To test their hypothesis, the authors examined a group of individuals who were clinically diagnosed with aMCI and used MRI to stratify the subjects into two subgroups: group 1 contained those with severe WMH without hippocampal atrophy (MCI-WMH) and group 2 those with severe hippocampal atrophy without extensive WMH (MCI-HA), as shown in Figure 12.2. Cognitive performance for each of these groups was compared with a group of age-matched control subjects. Importantly, these specific subgroups of aMCI subjects were selected to isolate the different mechanisms by which WMH and hippocampal atrophy may lead to episodic memory impairment in MCI. Although CVD and AD pathology often co-occur, the nature of the interaction is unclear and complex to study owing to the difficulty of disentangling the two in standard clinical samples. Consequently, a highly selected sample was studied in order to investigate the separate roles that each type of brain lesion may play in producing memory impairment.

The study was divided into two parts. First, the authors compared performance of aMCI patients and

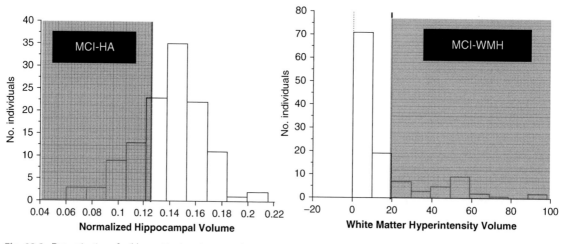

Fig. 12.2. Determination of mild cognitive impairment with severe white matter hyperintensities without hippocampal atrophy (MCI-WMH) and with severe hippocampal atrophy without extensive white matter hyperintensities (MCI-HA).

controls on the neuropsychological tests that were used to diagnose aMCI according to standard criteria.[9] This explored whether standard neuropsychological tests used widely in clinical practice would differ between the two MCI groups. Second, the authors compared the performance of these subjects on a battery of behavioral tasks used widely in the cognitive neuroscience literature. This second series of tasks was designed to explore the different cognitive mechanisms that underlie memory loss in aMCI. The battery included an episodic memory task, two working memory tasks and a version of the Continuous Performance Test (CPT) (see Nordahl et al. [2005][95] for complete details). The authors predicted that both groups of MCI participants would show deficits on the episodic memory task, but that the MCI-WMH group would show additional impairments on the working memory tasks and on the CPT consistent with the hypothesized deficits in frontal function associated with WMH.

Results showed that – by design – individuals in the MCI-HA group had significantly smaller hippocampi than those in the MCI-WMH group but those in this MCI-WMH group did not differ from healthy controls with regard to hippocampal volume. Conversely, the MCI-WMH group had significantly higher WMH volumes than the MCI-HA group, which also did not differ from control volumes. The two MCI groups were equally impaired on all episodic memory tests relative to controls: Wechsler Memory Scale, revised Logical Memory I and II, and Memory Assessment Scale List Learning, Immediate Recall and Delayed Recall.[95] The two MCI groups did not differ from each other or controls on other neuropsychological tasks such as the Digit Span or Boston Naming. There were, however, striking differences in performance on all of the working memory tasks, including the n-back and verbal and spatial variants of the item recognition task, where the MCI-HA group performed similar to normal controls but the MCI-WMH group performed significantly less well. Further testing of executive control using the CPT revealed that MCI-WMH subjects had poorer attention and committed more impulsive errors than the MCI-HA group or normal controls.

This study was designed to test the hypothesis that among individuals diagnosed with aMCI, small-vessel CVD and hippocampal dysfunction give rise to different profiles of cognitive deficits.[95] Results revealed that, although these two groups were virtually indistinguishable on standard neuropsychological tests

administered at the time of diagnosis of MCI, more detailed testing revealed reliable differences between the two subgroups of MCI subjects. Whereas those in the MCI-HA group exhibited relatively specific episodic memory impairment, the MCI-WMH group exhibited deficits on episodic memory, working memory and attentional control tasks. These findings suggest that subjects with MCI-WMH, in contrast to those with MCI-HA, suffered from impaired executive control processes that affect a wide variety of cognitive domains.

Although episodic memory has historically been linked to the hippocampus and surrounding cortices, as noted above, evidence from neuropsychological and neuroimaging studies suggests that the prefrontal cortex plays a critical role in implementing executive control processes that contribute to normal episodic memory functioning.[96] In this study, the MCI-WMH subjects were impaired not only on episodic memory tasks but also on a battery of working memory tasks in both verbal and spatial domains as well as an attentional control task. The authors' interpretation of the data was that episodic memory failure in the MCI-WMH group was secondary to a more general impairment in executive control processes.

Nordahl et al.[95] concluded by hypothesizing that WMH may reflect disruption of the white matter tracts that connect DLPFC with its targets. Disruption of these neural circuits could lead to deficits in executive control processes that impact a wide range of cognitive domains, including episodic memory. The anatomy of this pathological process is unclear, as multiple neural circuits exist that, if disrupted, might lead to the findings described above. For example, lesions affecting connections between the DLPFC and its subcortical targets[97] or lesions affecting the long cortico-cortical connections between prefrontal and posterior parietal cortex[98–100] would be expected to result in impaired working memory and executive control processes.[101–103] Disconnection of the prefrontal, retrosplenial hippocampal circuit may also give rise to the deficits observed.[104,105]

To test the hypothesis of DLPFC dysfunction resulting from WMH, the authors performed a second set of functional MRI (fMRI) experiments on cognitively normal individuals.

White matter hyperintensities and dorsolateral prefrontal activation

In this study, Nordahl et al.[106] used fMRI to examine the relationship between WMH and prefrontal cortex

(PFC) activity in a group of cognitively normal elderly individuals during an episodic retrieval and a verbal working memory task, two tasks in which age-related changes in PFC activity have been observed.[107,108] The WMHs were quantified from structural MRI, and the relationship between global WMH and regional dorsal PFC WMH volume and task-related activity was examined. Two major hypotheses were tested: first that global white matter degeneration would correlate with reduced activation in PFC during each of the memory tasks; and, second, that regional white matter degeneration within dorsal PFC would correlate both with reduced PFC activation as well as with areas that are functionally and anatomically linked to PFC in a task-specific manner. In order to investigate the relationship between WMH volume and PFC activity, Nordahl et al.[106] first identified dorsal and ventral PFC regions of interest based on task-related blood oxygen level dependent (BOLD) activation for each task and then correlated WMH volumes with the magnitude of the activation within these regions. Additional task-related regions of interest were defined in the medial temporal lobes, parietal cortex and cingulate cortex in order to examine the association between dorsal PFC WMH and activity in areas that are functionally related to PFC activity.

Subjects for this study consisted of 15 cognitively normal individuals (4 male/11 female) over the age of 65 years (range, 66–86). Importantly, individuals in this study were not preselected for presence or absence of WMH but were selected on the basis of normal cognitive ability. In this respect, this sample is comparable to samples used in other functional neuroimaging studies of normal aging. The subjects performed the episodic memory and the verbal maintenance task as previously reported.[95]

All subjects performed at a high level of accuracy on the cognitive tasks (generally greater than 80% correct). Total WMH volume was not significantly correlated with memory performance; however, frontal WMH volume was significantly associated with immediate memory recall and there was a trend toward a significant relationship between total WMH and high-load verbal maintenance task. This association between cognitive performance and WMH volumes suggests subtly impaired working memory function even for a group of cognitively normal individuals performing at a very high level of accuracy.

In brief, the results of the fMRI studies revealed a strong relationship between increased global WMH volume and decreased PFC activity during both episodic and working memory performance. Dorsal PFC WMH volume was also strongly correlated with decreased PFC activity as well as with decreased medial temporal and anterior cingulate activity during episodic memory, and posterior parietal and anterior cingulate activity during working memory. Importantly, WMH volume was not correlated with visual cortex activity during a simple visual task, suggesting that non-specific vascular changes associated with WMH did not fundamentally alter the BOLD signal.

These results strongly suggest that WMH disrupt the functional integrity of a widely distributed memory system involving parietal, DLPFC, prefrontal, anterior cingulate and hippocampal regions.[16] Although the exact pathophysiology by which WMH may affect this system requires further research, it is clear that disruption of specific pathways must be involved. As noted above, these might include connections between the DLPFC and its subcortical targets,[97] the long cortico-cortical connections between prefrontal and posterior parietal cortex[98–103] or the prefrontal, retrosplenial, hippocampal circuit.[104,105] Current research is systematically exploring these various pathways using diffusion tensor imaging. We hypothesize that those pathways directly involved in memory system dysfunction by WMH will show reduced fractional anisotropy that is more highly correlated with memory task performance and cognitive activation than regional WMH, indicating the specificity of the identified white matter bundles.

Summary

In this review, we recognize that aMCI is a common expression of early AD pathology.[7] We also note, however, that tests of episodic memory tap a widely distributed neural system involving parietal, frontal, anterior cingulate and medial temporal structures.[16] Cerebrovascular disease, particularly WMH, is common to the aging process. Accumulating evidence suggests that asymptomatic manifestations of CVD can result in clinically relevant memory impairments that may, on occasion, masquerade as aMCI,[95] thereby leading to recognition of two separate mechanisms of disease that can result in aMCI as summarized in Figure 12.3.

More recent research suggests that WMHs affect episodic memory performance through dysfunction of dorsolateral prefrontal systems. Ongoing work seeks to explore both the full impact of WMH on

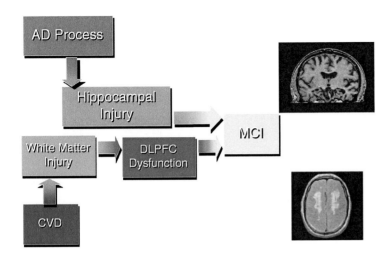

Fig. 12.3. Role of Alzheimer's disease (AD) and cerebrovascular disease (CVD) in mild cognitive impairment (MCI). DLPFC, dorsolateral prefrontal cortex.

age-related working memory impairment as well as identifying specific white matter tracts that may be involved.

An obvious question remains to be asked: to what extent does asymptomatic CVD influence the likelihood of progression from aMCI to dementia? Here the results are mixed. A very early and relatively small study by Wolf et al.[109] suggested a strong additive effect of WMH and atrophy on likelihood of progression from MCI to dementia. This was supported by cross-sectional data showing a multiplicative increase in probability of dementia among community dwelling Latinos having high WMH and small hippocampal volumes.[110] Unfortunately, analysis of a smaller group of MCI subjects did not support these findings.[111] Further work in this area is clearly necessary. It will remain important, however, to understand more fully the specific manner by which asymptomatic CVD may impact brain structure and function to cause cognitive impairment, as most vascular risk factors are treatable and, therefore, this process may be preventable.

References

1. Cutler SJ, Grams AE. Correlates of self-reported everyday memory problems. *J Gerontol Soc Sci* 1988;**43**:S82–S90.

2. La Rue A. *Aging and Neuropsycholgocial Assessment.* New York: Plenum Press, 1992.

3. Robertson D, Rockwood K, Stolee P. The prevalence of cognitive impairment in an elderly Canadian population. *Acta Psychiatr Scand* 1989;**80**:303–309.

4. Graham JE, Rockwood K, Beattie BL, *et al.* Prevalence and severity of cognitive impairment with and without dementia in an elderly population. *Lancet* 1997; **349**:1793–1796.

5. Wilson RS, Beckett LA, Bennett DA, Albert MS, Evans DA. Change in cognitive function in older persons from a community population: relation to age and Alzheimer disease. *Arch Neurol* 1999;**56**:1274–1279.

6. Price JL, Morris JC. Tangles and plaques in nondemented aging and "preclinical" Alzheimer's disease. *Ann Neurol* 1999;**45**:358–368.

7. Morris JC, Storandt M, Miller JP, *et al.* Mild cognitive impairment represents early-stage Alzheimer disease. *Arch Neurol* 2001;**58**:397–405.

8. Bennett DA, Schneider JA, Arvanitakis Z, *et al.* Neuropathology of older persons without cognitive impairment from two community-based studies. *Neurology* 2006;**66**:1837–1844.

9. Petersen RC, Smith GE, Waring SC, *et al.* Mild cognitive impairment: clinical characterization and outcome. *Arch Neurol* 1999;**56**:303–308.

10. Petersen RC, Doody R, Kurz A, *et al.* Current concepts in mild cognitive impairment. *Arch Neurol* 2001;**58**:1985–1992.

11. Petersen RC, Morris JC. Mild cognitive impairment as a clinical entity and treatment target. *Arch Neurol* 2005;**62**:1160–1163; discussion 1167.

12. Petersen RC, Thomas RG, Grundman M, *et al.* Vitamin E and donepezil for the treatment of mild cognitive impairment. *N Engl J Med* 2005;**352**: 2379–2388.

13. Lopresti BJ, Klunk WE, Mathis CA, *et al.* Simplified quantification of Pittsburgh compound B amyloid imaging PET studies: a comparative analysis. *J Nucl Med* 2005;**46**:1959–1972.

14. Milner B, Squire LR, Kandel ER. Cognitive neuroscience and the study of memory. *Neuron* 1998;**20**:445–468.

15. Tulving E. Multiple memory systems and consciousness. *Hum Neurobiol* 1987;**6**:67–80.

16. Baddeley A. Working memory: looking back and looking forward. *Nat Rev Neurosci* 2003;**4**:829–839.

17. Blumenfeld RS, Ranganath C. Dorsolateral prefrontal cortex promotes long-term memory formation through its role in working memory organization. *J Neurosci* 2006;**26**:916–925.

18. Ranganath C. Working memory for visual objects: complementary roles of inferior temporal, medial temporal, and prefrontal cortex. *Neuroscience* 2006;**139**:277–289.

19. Gold JJ, Hopkins RO, Squire LR. Single-item memory, associative memory, and the human hippocampus. *Learn Mem* 2006;**13**:644–649.

20. Squire LR. Memory systems of the brain: a brief history and current perspective. *Neurobiol Learn Mem* 2004;**82**:171–177.

21. Squire LR, Stark CE, Clark RE. The medial temporal lobe. *Annu Rev Neurosci* 2004;**27**:279–306.

22. Moscovitch M, Nadel L, Winocur G, Gilboa A, Rosenbaum RS. The cognitive neuroscience of remote episodic, semantic and spatial memory. *Curr Opin Neurobiol* 2006;**16**:179–190.

23. Braak H, Braak E. Frequency of stages of Alzheimer-related lesions in different age categories. *Neurobiol Aging* 1997;**18**:351–357.

24. Braak H, Braak E. Diagnostic criteria for neuropathologic assessment of Alzheimer's disease. *Neurobiol Aging* 1997;**18**:S85–S88.

25. Braak H, Braak E. Staging of Alzheimer-related cortical destruction. *Int Psychogeriatr* 1997;**9**(Suppl 1): 257–261; discussion 269–272.

26. Morris JC, Price AL. Pathologic correlates of nondemented aging, mild cognitive impairment, and early-stage Alzheimer's disease. *J Mol Neurosci* 2001;**17**:101–118.

27. Petersen RC. Mild cognitive impairment as a diagnostic entity. *J Int Med* 2004;**256**:183–194.

28. Petersen RC, Bennett D. Mild cognitive impairment: is it Alzheimer's disease or not? *J Alzheimers Dis* 2005; **7**:241–245.

29. Grundman M, Jack CR, Jr., Petersen RC, et al. Hippocampal volume is associated with memory but not nonmemory cognitive performance in patients with mild cognitive impairment. *J Mol Neurosci* 2003;**20**:241–248.

30. Jack CR, Jr., Petersen RC, Xu Y, et al. Rates of hippocampal atrophy correlate with change in clinical status in aging and AD. *Neurology* 2000;**55**:484–489.

31. Jack CR, Jr., Petersen RC, Xu YC, et al. Prediction of AD with MRI-based hippocampal volume in mild cognitive impairment. *Neurology* 1999;**52**:1397–1403.

32. DeCarli C, Frisoni GB, Clark CM, et al. Qualitative estimates of medial temporal atrophy as a predictor of progression from mild cognitive impairment to dementia. *Arch Neurol* 2007;**64**:108–115.

33. Bobinski M, de Leon MJ, Wegiel J, et al. The histological validation of post mortem magnetic resonance imaging-determined hippocampal volume in Alzheimer's disease. *Neuroscience* 2000;**95**:721–725.

34. Jack CR, Dickson DW, Parisi JE, et al. Antemortem MRI findings correlate with hippocampal neuropathology in typical aging and dementia. *Neurology* 2002;**58**:750–757.

35. Seshadri S, Beiser A, Kelly-Hayes M, et al. The lifetime risk of stroke: estimates from the Framingham Study. *Stroke* 2006;**37**:345–350.

36. Weber MA. Role of hypertension in coronary artery disease. *Am J Nephrol* 1996;**16**:210–216.

37. Gillum RF. Coronary heart disease, stroke, and hypertension in a US national cohort: the NHANES I Epidemiologic Follow-up Study. National Health and Nutrition Examination Survey. *Ann Epidemiol* 1996;**6**:259–262.

38. Zheng ZJ, Sharrett AR, Chambless LE, et al. Associations of ankle-brachial index with clinical coronary heart disease, stroke and preclinical carotid and popliteal atherosclerosis: the Atherosclerosis Risk in Communities (ARIC) Study. *Atherosclerosis* 1997;**131**:115–125.

39. Papademetriou V, Narayan P, Rubins H, Collins D, Robins S. Influence of risk factors on peripheral and cerebrovascular disease in men with coronary artery disease, low high-density lipoprotein cholesterol levels, and desirable low-density lipoprotein cholesterol levels. HIT Investigators. Department of Veterans Affairs HDL Intervention Trial. *Am Heart J* 1998;**136**:734–740.

40. Cooper R, Cutler J, Desvigne-Nickens P, et al. Trends and disparities in coronary heart disease, stroke, and other cardiovascular diseases in the United States: findings of the national conference on cardiovascular disease prevention. *Circulation* 2000;**102**:3137–3147.

41. Antikainen R, Jousilahti P, Tuomilehto J. Systolic blood pressure, isolated systolic hypertension and risk of coronary heart disease, strokes, cardiovascular disease and all-cause mortality in the middle-aged population. *J Hypertens* 1998;**16**:577–583.

42. Boon A, Lodder J, Heuts-van Raak L, Kessels F. Silent brain infarcts in 755 consecutive patients with a first-ever supratentorial ischemic stroke. Relationship with index-stroke subtype, vascular risk factors, and mortality. *Stroke* 1994;**25**:2384–2390.

43. Brott T, Tomsick T, Feinberg W, et al. Baseline silent cerebral infarction in the Asymptomatic Carotid Atherosclerosis Study. *Stroke* 1994;**25**:1122–1129.

44. Ezekowitz MD, James KE, Nazarian SM, et al. Silent cerebral infarction in patients with nonrheumatic atrial

fibrillation. The Veterans Affairs Stroke Prevention in Nonrheumatic Atrial Fibrillation Investigators. *Circulation* 1995;**92**:2178–2182.

45. Jørgensen HS, Nakayama H, Raaschou HO, Gam J, Olsen TS. Silent infarction in acute stroke patients. Prevalence, localization, risk factors, and clinical significance: the Copenhagen Stroke Study. [See comments.] *Stroke* 1994;**25**:97–104.

46. Kase CS, Wolf PA, Chodosh EH, *et al.* Prevalence of silent stroke in patients presenting with initial stroke: the Framingham Study. *Stroke* 1989;**20**:850–852.

47. Shinkawa A, Ueda K, Kiyohara Y, *et al.* Silent cerebral infarction in a community-based autopsy series in Japan. The Hisayama Study. *Stroke* 1995;**26**:380–385.

48. Steingart A, Lau K, Fox A, *et al.* The significance of white matter lucencies on CT scan in relation to cognitive impairment. *Can J Neurol Sci* 1986;**13**:383–384.

49. Hachinski VC, Potter P, Merskey H. Leuko-araiosis: an ancient term for a new problem. *Can J Neurol Sci* 1986;**13**:533–534.

50. Hachinski VC, Potter P, Merskey H. Leuko-araiosis. *Arch Neurol* 1987;**44**:21–23.

51. Steingart A, Hachinski VC, Lau C, *et al.* Cognitive and neurologic findings in subjects with diffuse white matter lucencies on computed tomographic scan (leuko-araiosis). *Arch Neurol* 1987;**44**:32–35.

52. Steingart A, Hachinski VC, Lau C, *et al.* Cognitive and neurologic findings in demented patients with diffuse white matter lucencies on computed tomographic scan (leuko-araiosis). *Arch Neurol* 1987;**44**:36–39.

53. Yue NC, Arnold AM, Longstreth WT, Jr., *et al.* Sulcal, ventricular, and white matter changes at MR imaging in the aging brain: data from the cardiovascular health study. [See comments.] *Radiology* 1997;**202**:33–39.

54. Ott A, Stolk RP, van Harskamp F *et al.* Diabetes mellitus and the risk of dementia: the Rotterdam Study. [See comments.] *Neurology* 1999;**53**:1937–1942.

55. Manolio TA, Kronmal, RA, Burke GL, *et al.* Magnetic resonance abnormalities and cardiovascular disease in older adults: the Cardiovascular Health Study. *Stroke* 1994;**25**:318–327.

56. Liao D, Cooper L, Cai J, *et al.* Presence and severity of cerebral white matter lesions and hypertension, its treatment, and its control. The ARIC Study. Atherosclerosis Risk in Communities Study. *Stroke* 1996;**27**:2262–2270.

57. Liao D, Cooper L, Cai J, *et al.* The prevalence and severity of white matter lesions, their relationship with age, ethnicity, gender, and cardiovascular disease risk factors: the ARIC Study. *Neuroepidemiology* 1997;**16**:149–162.

58. Swan GE, DeCarli C, Miller BL, *et al.* Association of midlife blood pressure to late-life cognitive decline and brain morphology. *Neurology* 1998;**51**:986–993.

59. DeCarli C, Miller BL, Swan GE, *et al.* Predictors of brain morphology for the men of the NHLBI twin study. *Stroke* 1999;**30**:529–536.

60. Jeerakathil T, Wolf PA, Beiser A, *et al.* Stroke risk profile predicts white matter hyperintensity volume: the Framingham Study. *Stroke* 2004;**35**:1857–1861.

61. Yoshita M, Fletcher E, Harvey D, *et al.* Extent and distribution of white matter hyperintensities in normal aging, MCI, and AD. *Neurology* 2006;**67**:2192–2198.

62. Miyao S, Takano A, Teramoto J, Takahashi A. Leukoaraiosis in relation to prognosis for patients with lacunar infarction. *Stroke* 1992;**23**:1434–1438.

63. Vermeer SE, Hollander M, van Dijk EJ *et al.* Silent brain infarcts and white matter lesions increase stroke risk in the general population: the Rotterdam Scan Study. *Stroke* 2003;**34**:1126–1129.

64. Streifler JY, Eliasziw M, Fox AJ, *et al.* Prognostic importance of leukoaraiosis in patients with ischemic events and carotid artery disease. *Stroke* 1999;**30**:254.

65. Salerno JA, Murphy DG, Horwitz B, *et al.* Brain atrophy in hypertension. A volumetric magnetic resonance imaging study. *Hypertension* 1992;**20**:340–348.

66. Strassburger TL, Lee HC, Daly EM, *et al.* Interactive effects of age and hypertension on volumes of brain structures. *Stroke* 1997;**28**:1410–1417.

67. Swan GE, DeCarli C, Miller BL *et al.* Biobehavioral characteristics of nondemented older adults with subclinical brain atrophy. *Neurology* 2000;**54**: 2108–2114.

68. Seshadri S, Wolf PA, Beiser A, *et al.* Stroke risk profile, brain volume, and cognitive function: the Framingham Offspring Study. *Neurology* 2004;**63**:1591–1599.

69. Elias MF, Wolf PA, D'Agostino RB, Cobb J, White LR. Untreated blodd pressure level is inversely related to cognitive functioning: the Framingham Study. *Am J Epidemiol* 1993;**138**:353–364.

70. Elias MF, D'Agostino RB, Elias PK, Wolf PA. Neuropsychological test performance, cognitive functioning, blood pressure, and age: the Framingham Heart Study. *Exp Aging Res* 1995;**21**:369–391.

71. Elias PK, D'Agostino RB, Elias MF, Wolf PA. Blood pressure, hypertension, and age as risk factors for poor cognitive performance. *Exp Aging Res* 1995; **21**:393–417.

72. Launer LJ, Masaki K, Petrovich H, Foley D, Havlik RJ. The association between mid-life blood pressure levels and late-life cognitive function. The Honolulu-Asia Aging Study. *JAMA* 1995;**274**:1846–1851.

73. Elias MF, Sullivan LM, D'Agostino RB, *et al.* Framingham stroke risk profile and lowered cognitive performance. *Stroke* 2004;**35**:404–409.

74. Longstreth WT, Jr., Arnold AM, Manolio TA, *et al.* Clinical correlates of ventricular and sulcal size on cranial magnetic resonance imaging of 3,301

elderly people. The Cardiovascular Health Study. Collaborative Research Group. *Neuroepidemiology* 2000;**19**:30–42.

75. Longstreth WT, Jr., Manolio TA, Arnold A, *et al.* Clinical correlates of white matter findings on cranial magnetic resonance imaging of 3301 elderly people. The Cardiovascular Health Study. [See comments.] *Stroke* 1996;**27**:1274–1282.

76. Breteler MM. Vascular involvement in cognitive decline and dementia. Epidemiologic evidence from the Rotterdam Study and the Rotterdam Scan Study. *Ann N Y Acad Sci* 2000;**903**:457–465.

77. de Groot JC, de Leeuw FE, Oudkerk M, *et al.* Cerebral white matter lesions and cognitive function: the Rotterdam Scan Study. [See comments.] *Ann Neurol* 2000;**47**:145–151.

78. de Groot JC, de Leeuw FE, Breteler MM. Cognitive correlates of cerebral white matter changes. *J Neur Transm Suppl* 1998;**53**:41–67.

79. Ott A, Stolk RP, Hofman A, *et al.* Association of diabetes mellitus and dementia: the Rotterdam Study. *Diabetologia* 1996;**39**:1392–1397.

80. DeCarli C, Murphy DG, Tranh M, *et al.* The effect of white matter hyperintensity volume on brain structure, cognitive performance, and cerebral metabolism of glucose in 51 healthy adults. *Neurology* 1995;**45**: 2077–2084.

81. Schmidt R, Fazekas F, Koch M, *et al.* Magnetic resonance imaging cerebral abnormalities and neuropsychologic test performance in elderly hypertensive subjects. A case–control study. *Arch Neurol* 1995;**52**:905–910.

82. Boone KB, Miller BL, Lesser IM, *et al.* Cognitive deficits with white-matter lesions in healthy elderly. *Arch Neurol* 1992;**49**:549–554.

83. Breteler MM, van Amerongen NM, van Swieten JC, *et al.* Cognitive correlates of ventricular enlargement and cerebral white matter lesions on MRI: the Rotterdam Study. *Stroke* 1994;**25**:1109–1115.

84. Price TR, Manolio TA, Kronmal RA, *et al.* Silent brain infarction on magnetic resonance imaging and neurological abnormalities in community-dwelling older adults. The Cardiovascular Health Study. CHS Collaborative Research Group. *Stroke* 1997; **28**:1158–1164.

85. Longstreth WT, Jr., Bernick C, Manolio TA, *et al.* Lacunar infarcts defined by magnetic resonance imaging of 3660 elderly people: the Cardiovascular Health Study. *Arch Neurol* 1998;**55**:1217–1225.

86. Vermeer SE, Prins ND, den Heijer T, *et al.* Silent brain infarcts and the risk of dementia and cognitive decline. *N Eng J Med* 2003;**348**:1215–1222.

87. Vermeer SE, Koudstaal PJ, Oudkerk M, Hofman A, Breteler MM. Prevalence and risk factors of silent brain infarcts in the population-based Rotterdam Scan Study. *Stroke* 2002;**33**:21–25.

88. Knopman D, Boland LL, Mosley T, *et al.* Cardiovascular risk factors and cognitive decline in middle-aged adults. *Neurology* 2001;**56**:42–48.

89. Au R, Massaro JM, Wolf PA, *et al.* Association of white matter hyperintensity volume with decreased cognitive functioning: the Framingham Heart Study. *Arch Neurol* 2006;**63**:246–250.

90. Tullberg M, Fletcher E, DeCarli C, *et al.* White matter lesions impair frontal lobe function regardless of their location. *Neurology* 2004;**63**:246–253.

91. Reed BR, Eberling JL, Mungas D, Weiner M, Jagust WJ. Frontal lobe hypometabolism predicts cognitive decline in patients with lacunar infarcts. *Arch Neurol* 2001;**58**:493–497.

92. Reed BR, Eberling JL, Mungas D, Weiner MW, Jagust WJ. Memory failure has different mechanisms in subcortical stroke and Alzheimer's disease. *Ann Neurol* 2000;**48**:275–284.

93. DeCarli C, Miller BL, Swan GE, *et al.* Cerebrovascular and brain morphologic correlates of mild cognitive impairment in the National Heart, Lung, and Blood Institute Twin Study. *Arch Neurol* 2001; **58**:643–647.

94. Lopez OL, Jagust WJ, Dulberg C, *et al.* Risk factors for mild cognitive impairment in the cardiovascular health study cognition study: part 2. *Arch Neurol* 2003; **60**:1394–1399.

95. Nordahl CW, Ranganath C, Yonelinas AP, *et al.* Different mechanisms of episodic memory failure in mild cognitive impairment. *Neuropsychologia* 2005;**43**:1688–1697.

96. Ranganath C, Johnson MK, D'Esposito M. Prefrontal activity associated with working memory and episodic long-term memory. *Neuropsychologia* 2003;**41**: 378–389.

97. Alexander GE, DeLong MR, Strick PL. Parallel organization of functionally segregated circuits linking basal ganglia and cortex. *Annu Rev Neurosci* 1986;**9**:357–381.

98. Cavada C, Goldman-Rakic PS. Posterior parietal cortex in rhesus monkey: II. Evidence for segregated corticocortical networks linking sensory and limbic areas with the frontal lobe. *J Comp Neurol* 1989; **287**:422–445.

99. Cavada C, Goldman-Rakic PS. Posterior parietal cortex in rhesus monkey: I. Parcellation of areas based on distinctive limbic and sensory corticocortical connections. *J Comp Neurol* 1989;**287**:393–421.

100. Selemon LD, Goldman-Rakic PS. Common cortical and subcortical targets of the dorsolateral prefrontal and posterior parietal cortices in the rhesus monkey: evidence for a distributed neural network

subserving spatially guided behavior. *J Neurosci* 1988;**8**:4049–4068.

101. Tekin S, Cummings JL. Frontal-subcortical neuronal circuits and clinical neuropsychiatry: an update. *J Psychosom Res* 2002;**53**:647–654.

102. Cummings JL. Frontal–subcortical circuits and human behavior. *Arch Neurol* 1993;**50**:873–880.

103. Burruss JW, Hurley RA, Taber KH, *et al.* Functional neuroanatomy of the frontal lobe circuits. *Radiology* 2000;**214**:227–230.

104. Petrides M, Pandya DN. Dorsolateral prefrontal cortex: comparative cytoarchitectonic analysis in the human and the macaque brain and corticocortical connection patterns. *Eur J Neurosci* 1999;**11**:1011–1036.

105. Morris R, Pandya DN, Petrides M. Fiber system linking the mid-dorsolateral frontal cortex with the retrosplenial/presubicular region in the rhesus monkey. *J Comp Neurol* 1999;**407**:183–192.

106. Nordahl CW, Ranganath C, Yonelinas AP *et al.* White matter changes compromise prefrontal cortex function in healthy elderly individuals. *J Cogn Neurosci* 2006; **18**:418–429.

107. Grady CL. Functional brain imaging and age-related changes in cognition. *Biol Psychol* 2000;**54**:259–281.

108. Tisserand DJ, Jolles J. On the involvement of prefrontal networks in cognitive ageing. *Cortex* 2003; **39**:1107–1128.

109. Wolf H, Grunwald M, Ecke GM, *et al.* The prognosis of mild cognitive impairment in the elderly. *J Neur Transm Suppl* 1998;**54**:31–50.

110. Wu CC, Mungas D, Petkov CI, *et al.* Brain structure and cognition in a community sample of elderly Latinos. *Neurology* 2002;**59**:383–391.

111. DeCarli C, Mungas D, Harvey D, *et al.* Memory impairment, but not cerebrovascular disease, predicts progression of MCI to dementia. *Neurology* 2004; **63**:220–227.

Chapter 13

Mild cognitive impairment

Brendan J. Kelley and Ronald C. Petersen

Introduction

Most degenerative conditions are characterized by insidious onset and gradually progressive decline. Therefore, the presumption of an early stage in the development of a degenerative disorder in which a person might be "partially symptomatic" is quite plausible. Applied to Alzheimer's disease (AD), the prodromal phase might represent an individual who is slightly forgetful with preservation of other cognitive and functional abilities. Mild cognitive impairment (MCI) refers to the transitional state between normal cognitive changes of aging and the earliest clinical features of dementia. As such, it has become an important topic in clinical practice and research. As initially conceived, MCI referred to memory impairment with preserved non-memory cognitive performance and functional abilities, but more recently, the term has been expanded to include other cognitive domains besides memory. Most literature refers to the amnestic (memory predominant) form of MCI (aMCI), a likely precursor of Alzheimer's disease (AD).[1–3]

In recent years, a tremendous amount of information has been published regarding the early diagnosis of dementia. Consequently, a more general construct of MCI and of specific subtypes of MCI has been adopted as the prodromal phases of various diseases. The general framework of MCI as the incipient phase of a degenerative disease remains an important concept. Research since the mid 1990s on MCI has shown the criteria to be reliable, and the outcomes of patients are known. Some predictors of progression from MCI to AD are known and others are still being evaluated. Neuroimaging studies document a transitional state (between normal and AD) of brain structural and functional features in subjects with MCI, and neuropathological data confirm intermediate pathological findings.

This presumes a benefit to earlier diagnosis of a degenerative disease. Given the overall aging of the world's population,[4] degenerative dementias hold the potential of an impending crisis. A major strategy for averting this disaster involves delaying the onset and/or progression of these diseases. Early diagnosis then becomes paramount in trying to prevent subsequent disability. Most randomized clinical trials so far have been essentially negative, but one trial suggested that donepezil may provide symptomatic benefit for a limited period of time in MCI. We will discuss the implications of MCI for clinical practice and future research.

Historical context

Many investigations of cognitive changes associated with aging have focused on those cognitive changes associated with the extremes of normal aging. Terms such as age-associated memory impairment, aging-associated cognitive decline, benign senescent forgetfulness and late life forgetfulness have been variably used to describe these changes.[5] Age-associated memory impairment (a term popular in the 1980s) refers to people having memory impairment relative to the performance of younger individuals, and it was believed to represent a manifestation of normal aging. Aging-associated cognitive decline expanded this construct to include cognitive domains other than memory, once again referenced to the extremes of normal aging.

By contrast, the MCI construct refers to an abnormal process, with the intent of defining the prodromal stages of a dementing condition. As such, it is fundamentally defined as being different from normal aging (Boxes 13.1 and 13.2).

Epidemiological data on mild cognitive impairment

Since MCI is a relatively recently defined construct, several epidemiological studies had already been

The Behavioral Neurology of Dementia, eds. Bruce L. Miller and Bradley F. Boeve. Published by Cambridge University Press. © Cambridge University Press 2009.

Box 13.1 Worries about memory loss

A 55-year-old lawyer presents for evaluation of her concerns about her memory. Over the past few months, she has been under a great deal of pressure at work and has difficulties remembering the details of her clients' cases. She occasionally misplaces objects at home. Her mother developed AD at age 83, and she confides that this heightens her concerns about her memory. She worries that this may represent the earliest stages of AD.

She scores 30/30 on the Mini-Mental State Examination (MMSE) and her neurologic examination is unremarkable. She seems anxious. Her magnetic resonance scan is normal, including the appearance of the hippocampal structures. Routine laboratory studies are normal. Neuropsychological testing is normal, including very good performance on the learning and delayed recall phases of the Auditory Verbal Learning Test.

Comment
This women represents the "worried well." She is a high-functioning person who has recently been bothered by memory-related symptoms, but she does not have a significant memory problem. Her preserved delayed recall on neuropsychological testing further reassures that she is not suffering a significant memory problem. She can be reassured and followed clinically. Lifestyle modifications aimed at stress management may improve both her anxiety and her overall day-to-day cognitive functioning.

Box 13.2 Progressive memory impairment

A 67-year-old physician is brought to the office by his wife, who expresses concern regarding 3 years of progressive memory impairment. He frequently forgets the details of conversations, misplaces objects at home and repeats questions seeming not to realize they had been answered only minutes before. Within the past year, he has developed difficulty finding words and becomes disoriented in familiar places, including the office building where he has worked for the past 35 years. He retired from his practice 1 year ago, at the urging of his partners. His wife accompanies him when running errands for fear that he will become lost or confused. She turned their finances over to an accountant owing to his inability to continue to manage them himself. His father developed AD at age 75, and his older sister was recently diagnosed with AD at age 78.

He scores 22/30 in the MMSE missing all of the recall items, failing to reproduce the drawing of intersecting pentagons and missing several points on orientation. He becomes confused while trying to subtract serial sevens. His MRI scan shows severe bilateral hippocampal atrophy, accompanied by a moderate degree of global atrophy. Neuropsychological testing documents severe impairment of memory as well as impairment of naming, visuospatial skills and planning/sequencing. Routine laboratory studies are normal.

Comment
This man has dementia, most likely AD. His current cognitive status clearly represents a decline, and this has been progressive in nature. Memory impairment was the first symptom noted, and while it has remained at the core of his complaints, it is now accompanied by impairments in other areas of cognition. These have caused functional impairment. His MRI scan is abnormal, and the hippocampal atrophy is suggestive of AD. His case is included as a counterpoint to the case in Box 13.1 in order to illustrate that many individuals lie between these two extremes. It is these individuals (who are forgetful but not functionally impaired) that are identified as having MCI.

designed and were already underway without having incorporated MCI criteria. There are also several cohort studies that have included these criteria prospectively.[6] Consequently, there is notable variability in the literature with respect to prevalence figures. Table 13.1 shows some of the studies that retrofitted MCI criteria to ongoing longitudinal studies, as well as newer studies utilizing MCI criteria prospectively.

In general, studies of prospectively designed cohorts that employed current MCI criteria have reported prevalence rates of 12–18% among non-demented subjects over age 65 years. As expected, somewhat lower rates are reported when the entire population, including demented subjects, serves as the denominator.[9,10] These figures depend somewhat on the specific subtype of MCI studied and the methods used to implement MCI criteria. For example, using a neuropsychological algorithm to define MCI, prevalence figures are quite variable,[11] likely reflecting the arbitrary nature of the selection of the neuropsychological instruments

Table 13.1. Selected epidemiology/cohort studies of mild cognitive impairment

Reference	Number of participants	Trial type	Diagnosis	Prevalence (%)		
				CIND	AACD	MCI
7	980	P	A		9	3–5
8	2914	R	C	17		5
9	351	P	C	23		12
10	798	P	C			26
11	833	R	A		21	3
6	927	P	C			18
12	806	P	A			5
13	111	P	C			12
14	1704	P	C			16
15	592	P	A			24
16	2768	R	A	9.5		16
17	745	P	C			14

Notes:
CIND, cognitive impairment not demented; AACD, aging-associated cognitive decline; MCI, mild cognitive impairment; P, prospective trials with MCI incorporated into the design; R, retrospective pitting of MCI criteria to an already existing trial; C, clinical diagnosis; A, algorithmic diagnosis.

and cutoff scores. For example, use of a single neuropsychological memory test with one cutoff score to define memory impairment results in an unstable algorithmic definition of MCI.[18] Some studies cited as implying longitudinal instability of the MCI construct in fact demonstrated instability owing to the test–retest variability of the neuropsychological testing that had been used to define MCI, rather than instability of the construct as defined below.[11,18]

Clearly, interpretation of the available epidemiologic data on MCI is complex, with numerous methodological considerations. Overall, the data in Table 13.1 indicate that the prevalence of MCI is probably in the 12–15% range among individuals 65 years and older, with incidence rates in the 1% per year range. These figures are similar to those found in AD.

Clinical characterization and outcomes
Diagnostic criteria and diagnosis

The original criteria for MCI (Table 13.2) were designed to characterize the early stages of an AD-like process, and were thus centered on memory impairment.[3] With subsequent research, it has become apparent that not all subjects with MCI evolve to AD. Therefore, MCI criteria have expanded to include many other types of intermediate cognitive

Table 13.2. Original criteria for mild cognitive impairment

Memory complaint, preferably corroborated by an informant

Memory impairment for age and education

Preserved general cognitive function

Intact activities of daily living

Not demented

impairment that may be precursors to a variety of dementing disorders. An international conference on diagnostic criteria in 2003 expanded the criteria to include other forms of cognitive impairment and helped to translate these findings for primary care practitioners, since these are the individuals most likely to first encounter persons with intermediate degrees of cognitive impairment (Boxes 13.3 and 13.4).[19,20] The main division of MCI is into a amnestic MCI (aMCI) and a non-amestic form (naMCI). Both can then have single or multiple domains. Figure 13.1 shows the diagnostic algorithm currently being used by the National Institute on Aging (NIA) sponsored Alzheimer's Disease Centers program and the Alzheimer's Disease Neuroimaging Initiative to diagnose MCI.[21]

Although the construct of MCI has been expanded, the importance of an accurate clinical history (preferably corroborated by an informant who knows the

Box 13.3 Diagnosing mild cognitive impairment: amnestic subtype

A 64-year-old retired businessman has become increasingly forgetful over the past 2 years. Despite having reduced demands since retirement, he has difficulty keeping track of doctors' appointments and has been disappointed to have forgotten several social events that he wished to attend. His family reports uncharacteristic forgetfulness for the details of conversations and recent events. They are concerned about these recent cognitive changes.

He scores 25/30 on the MMSE, being unable to recall any of the three words and being disoriented to the date. His general neurological examination is normal. He denies symptoms of depression. Mild bilateral hippocampal atrophy is noted on his MRI, but the scan is otherwise normal. His general medical condition is good. Neuropsychological testing identifies mild difficulty learning new material and a prominent deficit in delayed recall of the words on the list from the Auditory Verbal Learning Test and the Logical Memory subtest of the Wechsler Memory Scale III. General intellectual skills, attention, concentration, language and visuospatial functions are preserved.

Comment

This man has aMCI. The insidious onset and gradual progression suggest a degenerative etiology. Although his memory performance is poor, his other cognitive skills remain intact and he does not have a significant functional impairment. Therefore, he does not meet criteria for dementia. His symptoms may represent the earliest clinical manifestations of a degenerative disorder such as AD.

Box 13.4 Diagnosing mild cognitive impairment: non-amnestic subtype

A 70-year-old retired executive presents for evaluation of problems with her driving. She and her passengers have noted difficulties with maintaining and changing lanes as well as with properly orienting her car in parking spaces. Her spouse and several friends have commented that she is much more distractible. Her memory has remained excellent. Additionally, her husband reports that she has become a very "restless" sleeper, frequently flailing her arms and at times seeming to run in her sleep. He recently moved to a separate bed in order to have a more peaceful night's rest. She has inexplicably fallen out of bed on several occasions as well.

She scores 28/30 on the MMSE and is unable to copy intersecting pentagons or to draw a clock face. Her posture is slightly stooped, but neurological examination is otherwise normal. The MRI is unremarkable, demonstrating normal-appearing hippocampal structures. Neuropsychological testing shows normal learning, recall, naming and comprehension. Performance on Part A of the Trail Making Test was slow and she was unable to complete Part B. Her visuospatial skills are quite poor, and attempts to reproduce two- and three-dimensional objects are quite distorted. A polysomnogram demonstrates a REM sleep-behavior disorder.

Comment

She has naMCI-multiple domain, with impairment of attention and concentration as well as visuospatial skills. She has clearly undergone cognitive decline but is not demented. Again, the gradual onset and progressive decline suggest a degenerative course. Her mild extrapyramidal features and REM sleep-behavior disorder, combined with her visuospatial, attentional and executive difficulties, may suggest eventual evolution to dementia with Lewy bodies, but at this time her diagnosis is naMCI.

patient well) has remained of paramount importance. The first criterion for the diagnosis of MCI involves a cognitive concern on the part of the patient or an informant.[22] The physician must then use the combination of history, mental status examination, neuropsychological testing or any other additional information that may be available to determine if the person's cognitive function is normal or compatible with dementia. If it is determined that the patient is neither normal nor demented, and there appears to have been a decline in cognitive function with preservation of most daily activities, the patient can be designated as having MCI. Again, it should be emphasized that clinicians can use various types of information to make this determination and that the corroboration of an informant who knows the individual well is extremely valuable in reaching a conclusion. Fundamentally, the clinical question is whether the person is functioning normally or has already reached the threshold for dementia. Individuals falling somewhere between these two endpoints are designated as having MCI.

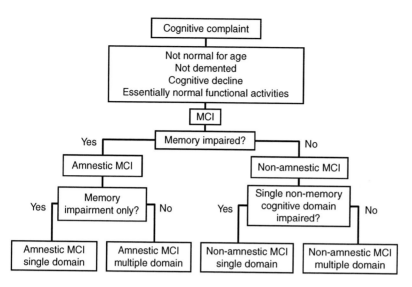

Fig. 13.1. Current diagnostic algorithm for diagnosing and subtyping mild cognitive impairment (MCI). (From Petersen [2004],[19] reprinted by permission.)

Once the diagnosis of MCI is made, the clinician needs to determine whether a memory impairment is present. Screening office memory tests such as a word list with a delayed recall component or more detailed neuropsychological testing can aid in documenting memory functioning. If a memory impairment is present, especially relative to appropriate age and education standards, then the subtype of MCI is aMCI. Neuropsychological testing can aid the clinician in determining whether the person has solely memory (single domain) problems or whether other cognitive domains, such as language, executive function or visuospatial skills, are also impaired (usually to a lesser extent). If memory is impaired with another cognitive domain, then the MCI subtype is aMCI-multiple domain.

Similarly, as indicated in Fig. 13.1, if the patient is determined to be in the MCI category (not normal, not demented) but does not have a significant memory impairment, then the clinician must determine which cognitive domains are impaired. Non-amnestic MCI is subtyped similarly, with single domain (naMCI-single domain) or multiple domain (naMCI-multiple domain). The rationale for this subtyping in clinical practice is to determine the phenotype of the clinical syndrome.

After describing the patient's symptom complex, the clinician determines the etiology of the symptoms. This is done in a similar fashion to making the diagnosis of dementia (Fig. 13.2). In the case of dementia, the clinician determines the subtype of dementia, for example degenerative suggestive of AD or more closely resembling vascular cognitive impairment. This determination is typically done based on the history from the patient and informant, neuroimaging and laboratory testing for other causes of cognitive impairment. After completion of these evaluations, the clinician then classifies the MCI syndrome by likely etiology: degenerative (gradual onset, insidious progression), vascular (abrupt onset, stepwise decline, vascular risk factors, history of strokes, transient ischemic attacks), psychiatric (history of depression, depressed mood or anxiety), or secondary to concomitant medical disorders (e.g. congestive heart failure, diabetes mellitus, systemic cancer). Combining the clinical MCI subtype with the presumed etiology, the clinician can then make a reliable prediction about the outcome of the MCI syndrome, as is shown in Fig. 13.2.

Outcomes

Applying the criteria outlined in Fig. 13.1, patients with aMCI of a presumed degenerative etiology progress to dementia (usually AD) at a rate of 10–15% per year.[3,23] The variability in the literature on this rate of progression reflects, in part, the implementation of the MCI criteria. For example, among the epidemiologic studies discussed above, particularly those that retrofitted neuropsychological criteria to existing databases, rates of progression vary, with some studies reporting lower progression rates.[5,22,24,25] In the large clinical trials studying MCI, progression

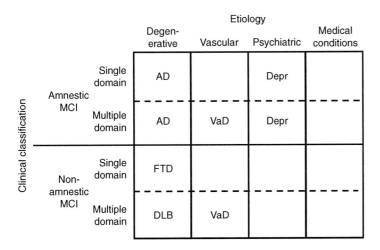

Fig. 13.2. Predicted outcome of mild cognitive impairment (MCI) subtypes according to presumed etiology. FTD, frontotemporal dementia; AD, Alzheimer's disease; VaD, vascular dementia; DLB, dementia with Lewy bodies; Depr, depression. (Adapted from Petersen [2003],[1] reprinted by permission.)

rates varied from 5 to 16% per year.[23] As will be discussed below, there are a number of possible explanations for this variability. Despite this variability in the precise rate of progression reported, all of these progression rates far exceed the population incidence figures for AD of 1–2% per year. In counseling patients, an estimate of 10–12% per year is probably a reasonably accurate prediction.

In a large prospectively designed trial from Germany, MCI subjects diagnosed using the criteria in Figure 13.1 progressed to dementia at rates of 7.2–10.2% per year.[7] Some subjects improved from MCI to normal (approximately 5% per year), but another subset initially improved and subsequently declined, implying instability in clinical course during progression to dementia. The vast majority of dementia cases were believed to represent AD.

Based on the available data from longitudinal studies, it is probably most reasonable to inform patients that individuals meeting criteria for MCI, particularly aMCI of a degenerative etiology, will likely progress to dementia (primarily AD) at a rate of 10% per year. In a typical clinical neurology setting, given that these patients present with a cognitive concern, the progression rate is likely to be in the 10–15% per year range for those meeting the criteria for aMCI. However, in community studies enrolling a more heterogeneous patient population, the rates may be lower, perhaps in the 8–10% per year range. It is also important to inform patients that a small fraction of individuals with MCI will improve and that others may remain clinically stable for many years. Consequently, while MCI (and particularly aMCI) of a presumed degenerative etiology identifies individuals

with an increased risk of developing dementia, the outcome of an individual patient is not absolutely determined by the diagnosis.

Predictors of progression

Identification of factors that may be predictive of which individuals with MCI are more likely to progress to dementia or AD more rapidly than others remains a major area of interest within the field of MCI research. In addition to the obvious benefit in counseling patients and family members, those designing clinical trials of potential therapeutics would like to stratify subjects to maximize the likelihood of progressing to AD over a reasonable period of time. Several potential candidates for predicting progression have emerged: clinical severity, magnetic resonance imaging (MRI) of hippocampal volumes, apolipoprotein E4 (ApoE4) carrier status, biomarkers in cerebrospinal fluid (CSF), positron emission tomography (PET) with [^{18}F]-fluorodeoxyglucose (FDG) and, possibly, PET utilizing a ligand that binds to amyloid or one that binds to both amyloid and tau.

Clinical severity

Individuals having more severe memory impairment are more likely to progress to AD more rapidly than those with less memory impairment. This may account for some of the variability observed in the clinical trials to be discussed below. Also, persons having aMCI-multiple domain subtype will probably progress more rapidly than those having aMCI-single domain. A recent study from the Mayo Clinic reported that individuals with aMCI-multiple domain subtype

177

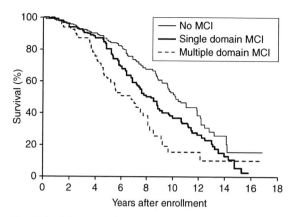

Fig. 13.3. Relative mortality of single domain and multiple domain amnestic mild cognitive impairment (MCI) compared with normal aging. (From Hunderfund *et al.* [2006],[26] reprinted by permission.)

actually had poorer survival than the aMCI-single domain subjects (Fig. 13.3).[26]

Magnetic resonance imaging volumetric studies

A great deal of data exists regarding structural MRI as a predictor of progression from MCI to AD. Hippocampal atrophy (see Ch. 8) has been a prominent and important predictor of subsequent progression from MCI to dementia and AD (Fig. 13.4).[27] More recently, volumetric measurement of entorhinal cortex volume, whole brain volume and ventricular volume have also been shown to be useful.[28] An analysis of a combined measurement of both entorhinal and hippocampal volume reported a small but detectable predictive utility for this combined measurement above and beyond age and cognitive variables.[29] Evaluating the utility of volumetric assessment has been complicated by the variable algorithms used to assess volumes by different investigators, as well as by the populations studied. Although some studies have shown only small added predictive value, the magnitude of this may be greater amongst patients having less readily detectable cognitive impairment. It is hoped that the Alzheimer's Disease Neuroimaging Initiative will address this issue.[21] A recent study suggests that subjective visual assessments of the hippocampal formation may be useful as well.[30]

Apolipoprotein E genotype

Carrier status for the ε4 allele of the *ApoE* gene (giving rise to the ApoE4 isoform) is a recognized risk factor for the development of AD,[31] and this has been documented in numerous studies around the world. Carrier status for ε4 has been demonstrated to be predictive of progression from MCI to AD in several studies of various populations, including the Alzheimer's Disease Cooperative Study (ADCS) MCI Treatment Trial and the Religious Order Study.[32–34] It was also shown to correlate with more rapid progression of hippocampal atrophy as shown by MRI in cognitively normal adults.[35] While this is an important adjunct to the clinical diagnosis of aMCI in predicting progression to AD, it is not recommended for clinical use for several reasons.[36]

Biomarkers in cerebrospinal fluid and plasma

As in AD, biomarkers for MCI are in the early stages of development. There are some indications that the CSF measures of β-amyloid (Aβ) and tau protein may be useful at differentiating subjects with MCI from normal aging[37–39] and that these markers may have utility in predicting progression from MCI to AD.[40,41] A multinational study found that baseline CSF levels of tau phosphorylated at threonine 231, but not total tau protein levels, correlated with cognitive decline and conversion from MCI to AD[42] and with neurofibrillary pathology in AD.[43] A recent study investigated the utility of CSF concentrations of Aβ42 (the 42 residue form of Aβ), total tau (T-tau) and tau phosphorylated at threonine 181 (p-tau) in predicting progression from MCI to AD reported a sensitivity of 95% and specificity of 83% using the combination of elevated T-tau and lowered Aβ42.[44]

The obvious hope is that biochemical markers associated with AD pathology may ultimately provide clinicians insights into which subjects likely have AD pathology at the MCI stage. Biomarkers in CSF continue to be explored in large clinical trials (such as the Alzheimer's Disease Neuroimaging Initiative[21]), but the present data, while intriguing, are insufficient to recommend use of CSF biomarkers in evaluation of MCI. A recent report on the fluctuation of CSF Aβ levels over days may imply that careful design of the conditions under which CSF is collected may make measurement and utility of these biomarkers more robust.[45] Use of plasma Aβ is less well developed, but this or another plasma biomarker may prove useful in the future.[46,47]

Positron emission tomography with [18F]-fluorodeoxyglucose

Some evidence suggests that metabolic changes in the brain may precede structural changes and, therefore, may provide earlier identification of pathological

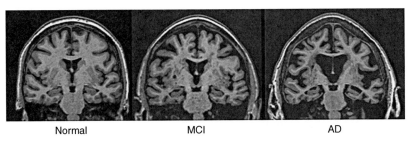

Normal   MCI   AD

Fig. 13.4. Coronal magnetic resonance images showing degrees of hippocampal atrophy in normal, mild cognitive impairment (MCI), and Alzheimer's disease (AD).

processes and thus have prognostic value in the evaluation of individuals having MCI. Studies have investigated FDG-PET as a biological marker in AD, and several report that FDG-PET suggestive of evolving AD among cognitively normal subjects genetically predisposed to develop AD.[48,49] Several studies also indicate that AD patterns of PET at the MCI stage predict progression to AD.[50,51] While intuitive, this technique requires further exploration before it can be recommended for routine clinical use.

Positron emission tomography with ligand binding
The latest imaging techniques attempt in vivo identification of underlying pathology to aid in predicting progression of MCI. Pittsburgh compound B (PiB)[52] binds to amyloid. It can be used as a ligand bound to FDG to image amyloid depositions in the brain. Early studies demonstrated its utility at distinguishing between normal, MCI, and AD subjects. Few longitudinal data are available regarding the outcome of MCI subjects. The limited MCI data available indicate three patterns: PiB retention similar to that of normal subjects, PiB retention mimicking AD subjects, and intermediate patterns. Some subjects with MCI appear to have PiB retention patterns quite similar to that in patients with fully developed AD, while others have no PiB retention, as would be expected in normal subjects. The third group has an intermediate degree of retention, as might be anticipated given the clinical profile of MCI subjects.

The University of California at Los Angeles has developed another ligand-bound FDG tracer, FDDNP (2-(1-(6-[(2-fluoroethyl)(methyl) amino]-2-naphthyl) ethylidene) malononitrile), that labels both amyloid and tau proteins. This would theoretically allow identification of neuritic elements in the brain, including both neuritic plaques and neurofibrillary tangles.[53] While this compound is less specific for AD, it may prove more sensitive at imaging the total pathological

burden. Once again, data are very preliminary and longitudinal studies of both this tracer and PiB will be needed to assess their utility.

Neuropathological correlates
The underlying neuropathological substrate of MCI, particularly aMCI of presumed degenerative etiology, remains an area of active research and debate. Some investigators contend that the neuropathological substrate of AD is already in place and, therefore, we should diagnose these patients as having clinical AD.[54] Along these lines, a study from Washington University reported that AD exists neuropathologically at this point. However, investigators at Washington University do not use MCI as a clinical designation and, as a consequence, likely see only subjects who are more advanced clinically than the MCI state. Therefore, it might be expected that their neuropathological data demonstrate AD.[55] Importantly, this study did not include autopsy data from subjects at the MCI stage or even the Clinical Dementia Rating Scale (CDR) 0.5 stage. Instead, most subjects had progressed clinically to CDR 1. Consequently, these data are perhaps more correctly interpreted as an outcome study rather than a cross-sectional study of subjects with mild degrees of cognitive impairment.

A more recent study from the University of Kentucky concluded that subjects with aMCI had pathological findings similar to those of early AD.[54] These investigators acknowledged that their MCI subjects may have been more clinically advanced than in other studies and that the AD population with which they were compared was in the early clinical stages of AD.

Pathological data in the Religious Order Study demonstrated an intermediate pathology between the neuropathological changes of normal aging and very early AD.[56] These investigators reported that

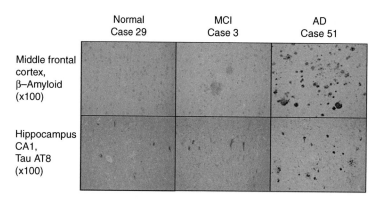

Fig. 13.5. Typical neuropathology in subjects with amnestic mild cognitive impairment (MCI) including neurofibrillary tangles and neuritic amyloid plaque. AD, Alzheimer's disease. (From Petersen *et al.* [2006],[57] reprinted by permission.)

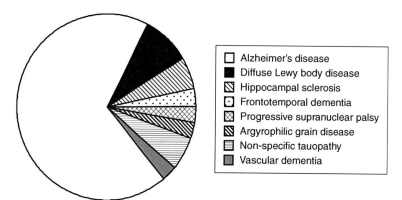

Fig. 13.6. Neuropathological outcome of subjects with history of mild cognitive impairment. (From Petersen [2007],[59] reprinted by permission.)

there is likely a combination of neuropathological findings, including neurodegeneration and vascular pathology, contributing to the clinical picture.

A recent Mayo Clinic study found that subjects who die while their clinical classification was aMCI (using the criteria outlined in Fig. 13.1) had neuropathologic features intermediate between changes of normal aging and AD.[57] Most of these subjects had some degree of medial temporal lobe pathology, usually neurofibrillary tangles, but only sparse diffuse plaques in the neocortex (Fig. 13.5) and had mostly low NIA-Reagan scores for the probability of meeting neuropathology criteria for AD.

A second study from the Mayo Clinic investigated the outcome of subjects with aMCI and, as expected, the vast majority of subjects had progressed to AD. However, as many as 20% had other types of dementing disorders, such as dementia with Lewy bodies, frontotemporal dementia, progressive supranuclear palsy and vascular dementia, although any one of these disorders was quite uncommon (Fig. 13.6).[58]

Therefore, while most of those with aMCI progress to AD, some develop other clinical syndromes.

In summary, the actual pathologic substrate of most aMCI appears to be one of evolving AD. That is, the full AD neuropathologic spectrum is not present at the MCI stage, but many incipient features are evolving (Fig. 13.5).

Clinical trial data in mild cognitive impairment

No treatments approved by the US Food and Drug Administration (FDA) currently exist for MCI. One would not expect an overall treatment indication of MCI anymore than one would expect an overall indication for dementia. However, specific subtypes of MCI might provide potential drug targets. Just as dementia is subdivided into its multiple categories, such as AD, vascular dementia, frontotemporal dementia, one could similarly divide MCI into the various subcategories, shown in Fig. 13.1. To date, most interest

Table 13.3. Clinical trials in mild cognitive impairment

Sponsor	Compound	Number enrolled	Duration (years)	Primary outcome	Progression rate (%)	Result	Reference
ADCS	Donepezil, vitamin E	769	3	AD	16	Partially positive	23
Johnson and Johnson[a]	Galantamine	2048	2	CDR 1	5	Negative	60
Novartis	Rivastigmine	1018	4	AD	5	Negative	61
Merck	Rofecoxib	1457	3–4	AD	5	Negative	62

Notes:
CDR, Clinical Dementia Rating Scale.
[a]Two trials.

has centered on aMCI of a degenerative etiology as a potential drug target, since aMCI likely represents the prodromal stage of AD.

In recent years, five major drug trials of compounds for the treatment of MCI have taken place. These are summarized in Table 13.3. These trials enrolled 4000–5000 subjects worldwide and are now completed. As a whole, they have been disappointing in that none has been notably positive, with one possible exception.[63] There are numerous reasons for this outcome and these will be discussed below.

Alzheimer's Disease Cooperative Study Donepezil and Vitamin E Trials

The ADCS involved 69 centers in the USA and Canada and enrolled 769 subjects with aMCI.[23] Subjects were randomized to three treatment groups: donepezil (10 mg per day), vitamin E (2000 IU per day) or placebo. Subjects in all three groups received a multivitamin. Each subject randomized to one of the three treatment groups was followed with evaluations every 6 months for up to 3 years. The entry criteria included those outlined in Table 13.2 for aMCI and the primary outcome measure was clinical progression to AD. The entry criteria required subjects to have an MMSE of 24 or greater and a score representing an approximate 1.5 to 2 standard deviations below education-adjusted normative values on a modified version of the Wechsler Memory Scale-Revised Logical Memory II subtest. These criteria ensured that the subjects were sufficiently memory impaired to be close to transitioning to AD yet did not meet criteria for dementia.

The study had projected a progression rate of 10–15% per year for the aMCI subjects and was powered to detect a reduction in that rate of 33%. Neither of the two active treatment arms reduced the

risk of progressing to AD over the entire 3 years of the study. However, donepezil reduced the risk of progression to AD for the first 12 months of the study in all subjects and this effect persisted up to 24 months among carriers of ε4. In considering these data, it should be noted that 76% of the 214 conversions from aMCI to AD encountered in the trial were ε4 carriers. Therefore, a treatment effect for donepezil was reported for up to 12–24 months. There was no treatment effect for vitamin E. The secondary measures generally corroborated these primary outcome findings regarding the risk and rate of progression from aMCI to AD.

The aMCI subjects progressed to AD at a rate of 16% per year in this study, quite similar to the design projection. Of the 214 conversions to dementia, 212 were diagnosed with possible or probable AD, indicating that the aMCI criteria were quite specific.

Recommendations based on the outcomes of this trial were somewhat conservative, yet very relevant to patient interactions. The authors concluded that while donepezil could not be generally recommended for the treatment of aMCI, clinicians should discuss the use of this medication with patients on an individual basis. Restated, while there is no FDA-approved treatment for MCI, individualized off-label use of donepezil could be considered for treatment of aMCI based on these data. The second recommendation addressed the question as to whether *APOE* genotyping should be recommended in MCI, with the aim of identifying individuals having a higher likelihood of a clinical progression at an earlier stage in the disease process. In accord with the many consensus panels which have argued against using *APOE* genotyping prior to the diagnostic stage of AD, this study agreed with those recommendations. Here again, while no recommendation is made for genotyping patients with aMCI, the interesting results in this study will

181

lead to further research. Finally, this provided the first demonstration of any intervention's attempt to delay the diagnosis of clinical AD. Prior to this, there had been no clinical trials that had shown ability to delay the onset of clinical AD and as such, this was an important study.

Galantamine

Two studies were undertaken by Johnson and Johnson and coworkers to investigate the impact of their acetylcholinesterase inhibitor, galantamine, on the progression from aMCI to AD.[60] These international studies assessed the rate of progression from aMCI to AD, as measured by progression on the CDR from 0.5 to 1. It is important to note that this study did not use clinical criteria for AD as a conversion point, but rather assessed progression simply by using the CDR. Since it is possible for a subject to progress from aMCI to AD while remaining at the CDR level of 0.5, this design may have resulted in decreased sensitivity. The two trials investigated a total of 2048 subjects, among whom 43% were ε4 carriers. Galantamine did not have a significant effect in either of the trials. A trend in favor of galantamine was present, with 13% on galantamine progressing (versus 18% in the placebo group) in one trial and 17% of the galantamine group progressing (versus 21% of the placebo group) in the second trial. Neither trial reached statistical significance. Scans with MRI were performed on many of the subjects, and there was a suggestion that galantamine may have reduced the rate of whole brain atrophy over the 2-year study period. Despite there being no significant treatment effects in these trials, there was some suggestion of a drug effect, possibly corroborated by MRI volumetric measures.

Rivastigmine

A large study conducted by Novartis investigated its acetylcholinesterase inhibitor rivastigmine.[61] This 3-year study involved 1018 subjects with aMCI and assessed progression from aMCI to AD. This multinational study had many of the same features as the ADCS but encountered difficulties with the implementation of the criteria. The study was conducted in 14 countries using multiple languages and translations of the neuropsychological instruments and enrolled subjects at a milder stage than that in the ADCS trial of donepezil.[64] As a consequence, the lower than expected conversion rate, believed to be related to these operational difficulties, required

extension of the study to 4 years in order to achieve an adequate number of events. Over that time period, 17.3% of subjects taking rivastigmine progressed to AD compared with 21.4% among the placebo group. There was no statistically significant difference between the two groups, but the difference was in the appropriate direction. The study assessed a variety of neuropsychological measures and found no dramatic change in these. Genotyping for ε4 was performed in only a subset of patients, which did not allow this to be included as a stratifying variable in the subsequent analysis. The investigators speculated that the inclusion criteria (which were different from those used in the donepezil trial) as well as the exclusion of patients having symptoms of depression at baseline may have contributed to the lower than expected conversion rate of 5% per year. Despite the lower conversion rate, nearly all subjects who progressed to dementia were diagnosed with AD.

Rofecoxib

A large trial of the cyclooxygenase 2 (COX-2) inhibitor rofecoxib in aMCI subjects was conducted by Merck.[62] This trial enrolled 1457 subjects in a randomized, placebo-controlled, double-blind study assessing the rate of progression from aMCI to AD over 2 years. The progression rate was lower than anticipated, prompting extension of the planned two year study to 3–4 years. This study reported annual conversion rates to AD of 6.4% in the rofecoxib group and 4.5% for the placebo group. This difference achieved statistical significance ($p = 0.011$) in favor of the placebo group. The authors reported that the secondary cognitive measures did not corroborate the primary outcome and consequently tended to dismiss the significance of the finding in favor of placebo. It is uncertain whether this indicates that the COX-2 inhibitor produced a more rapid progression to AD, or whether it was simply spurious. The authors identified several factors that correlated with a greater rate of progression to AD, including lower MMSE score, ε4 carrier status, age, gender and prior use of ginkgo biloba. Including these measures in a multivariate prediction model, the previously noted primary outcome was no longer present. The investigators in this trial modified the memory inclusion criteria to accept a lesser degree of impairment in order to enhance recruitment. It is unclear if this led to a more mildly affected study population or not, but this factor may have contributed to the lower conversion rate.

Trials summary

Taken together, these trials allow some important conclusions. There are several possible factors contributing to the variability in rate of progression from aMCI to AD, including differences in the subject populations recruited, enrollment procedures, the operationalization of the aMCI criteria and the primary outcome measures.[64] As noted above, some international trials were conducted in multiple countries using multiple languages. Translation of the evaluative instruments is one concern, as is the cultural variability as to what constitutes dementia or AD, much less aMCI. It is well known that the clinical judgement of the threshold for AD varies widely among cultures, since the functional requirement for the diagnosis of dementia can be very culture specific. If one extrapolates these difficulties to the clinical context of making the rather subtle diagnosis of aMCI, these cultural differences are likely to be magnified. While it was ambitious for the investigators to undertake these studies in a multinational setting, the logistical difficulties may have hampered the ability to produce reliable results.

Since ε4 carrier status is a strong predictor of progression to AD, variable ε4 carrier rates among the studies are another important factor that likely influenced the outcomes. As noted above, these studies used slightly different implementation procedures for the memory criteria of the aMCI diagnosis. While seemingly innocuous, differing cutoff scores used as inclusion criteria may have had a significant impact on the composition of the study groups. For example, if milder degrees of impairment were utilized in enrollment of the aMCI group, it is quite possible that very mild aMCI and possibly normal subjects (who would have been in the control group of another trial) may have been included in the treatment groups, resulting in a lower than expected conversion rate.

Variability in determination of the primary outcome measure may also have played a role. In addition to cultural differences in the clinical diagnosis of AD, these studies also varied as to how the primary outcome measure was operationalized. One study used the CDR as the outcome, while others used the clinical judgement of the investigators to make the AD diagnosis. Again, since we are studying the subtle phenomenon of the incipient stages of AD, seemingly innocuous differences in implementation criteria may have had a significant impact on outcome measures.

In summary, despite the variability among these studies, several notable factors regarding the construct of aMCI emerge. While the overall progression rate ranged from 5% to 16%, all of these rates were much higher than the population incidence rate for AD of 1–2%. Restated, even the "least successful" trial employing aMCI criteria doubled or tripled the generally reported progression rate of the more generalized population. The ADCS rate of 16% per year far exceeds this general population rate by several-fold. Therefore, while the treatments chosen were essentially ineffective, the study designs documented the utility of using aMCI criteria to enroll an enriched population for evaluating compounds that may have important treatment implications for AD. As treatments for disease modification become available, the aMCI criteria may be an important aid in identifying an appropriate group of individuals to enroll. The ability to identify a group of subjects likely to progress at an accelerated rate would provide an excellent clinical substrate for testing compounds targeting the underlying disease process.

Application to clinical practice

Many clinicians are able to identify patients in their practices who have "partial symptoms" of a dementing disorder, yet are not sufficiently impaired to deserve the label of dementia or AD. Ultimately, the clinical utility of diagnosing these patients as having MCI using the construct discussed here will be determined by its usefulness for these clinicians with respect to patient care. Most literature has investigated the aMCI subtype of a degenerative etiology, likely prodromal to AD. Therefore, this discussion will primarily pertain to that clinical subtype.

A 2001 evidence-based practice parameter from the American Academy of Neurology endorsed the construct of MCI.[65] The authors found that sufficient evidence exists to encourage clinicians to identify and evaluate patients in their practices having clinical features of MCI. These individuals are at increased risk of developing dementia in the future, and should be counseled appropriately. In the future, therapeutic interventions may become available for these patients. A tremendous increase in the extant literature regarding MCI has occurred in the years since publication of the practice parameter. Consequently, the practice parameter will likely be updated in the near future.

As the US demographic evolves to include increasing numbers of older individuals, the number of patients presenting with subtle cognitive concerns will increase, as will the demands, desires and concerns of these individuals. Practicing clinicians will require a diagnostic framework in which to evaluate, classify and ultimately treat these individuals. As the "baby boomers" age into the decades of increased risk for AD, many express growing concern that incipient cognitive difficulties are emerging. Again, if one accepts the premise that individuals pass through a stage of "partial symptoms" en route to developing a degenerative dementia such as AD, then the construct of MCI becomes quite useful in addressing these concerns.

It must be noted that these diagnostic classifications are arbitrary. All would agree that arbitrary distinctions between categories such as MCI and clinically probable AD are artificial when considered in the context of the clinical evolution of AD. Nevertheless, this terminology addresses the need to communicate clearly and effectively with our patients and with each other. The stigma of the diagnostic label of dementia or AD has significant social implications, and the clinical designation of aMCI can be quite useful in characterizing people who do not meet diagnostic criteria for AD or dementia.

How should patients with mild cognitive impairment be counseled?

This is a reasonable question and deserves some attention. It would be appropriate to discuss the evolving nature of the construct of MCI with patients. That is, as research proceeds, there certainly remains discussion in the literature regarding the precise characterization of the diagnostic criteria for MCI. Nevertheless, given a patient who meets the criteria outlined in Figure 13.1 and whose symptoms are felt to be caused by a degenerative process, it would be fair for the clinician to counsel a 10–15% per year risk of progressing to clinically probable AD. To the extent the patient deviates from the criteria, this prediction could be adjusted upward or downward. For example, an ε4 carrier (keeping in mind that testing for *APOE* genotype is not recommended in this clinical situation) having atrophic hippocampal formations on MRI would presumably be at a higher risk of progressing more rapidly. Alternatively, a patient with no family history of dementia, not an ε4 carrier

and having normal medial temporal lobe structures on MRI, it might be predicted that the individual will not progress rapidly. Of course, the regular reassessment, perhaps every 6 months, remains the best adjunct for making this determination.

Counseling patients regarding the implications of this diagnosis is perhaps the most important aspect of diagnosing aMCI at this time. That is, while the patient is cognitively competent, they may wish to begin planning for the future, addressing financial issues, retirement, living arrangements, and so on.

As mentioned above, there are no FDA-approved drugs for MCI. One could certainly discuss use of a cholinesterase inhibitor, and the results from the ADCS trial provide an excellent framework for this discussion. Keeping in mind the modest symptomatic benefit demonstrated in that trial, a highly functioning business person age 66 years wishing to continue to function in the work environment may be inclined towards treatment with donepezil at an earlier stage. Alternatively, a 72-year-old retired person largely engaged in leisure activities may choose to defer treatment until signs of greater impairment evolve. The choice of whether to initiate treatment with a cholinesterase inhibitor is ultimately a personal decision, which must be made after a frank discussion between the clinician and the patient of realistic aims and expectations.

Many physicians recommend lifestyle modification to try to minimize the rate of progression, although definitive data here are limited. Frequently, physicians recommend that patients remain physically active, intellectually engaged, socially active and that they follow a heart-healthy diet.[66,67]

Finally, it is useful and can be quite encouraging to inform patients that MCI is a rapidly evolving topic of investigation and that they should remain in touch with their physician regarding future advancements in this area.

Future directions

Although the construct of MCI has not been adopted by all individuals, it has become useful in both research and clinical practice. It is currently being considered for inclusion in the next revision (5th) of the *Diagnostic and Statistical Manual of Mental Disorders*.[68] As stated above, determination of the utility of the MCI construct will rest with the practicing clinicians.

Continued efforts aim to increase the specificity of outcome prediction for subjects with aMCI. As mentioned, subjects carrying ε4 genotypes and having atrophic hippocampi on MRI will likely progress more rapidly. The FDG-PET markers of progression and CSF biomarkers, such as p-tau and Aβ42, may also provide useful prognostic data. In addition, the newer molecular imaging techniques may provide valuable antemortem insights into the underlying pathology associated with aMCI. Studies investigating PiB and FDDNP are underway. The utility of these measures remains to be seen, but it is likely that some combination of these techniques may prove useful in predicting the outcome of aMCI.

For the practicing clinician, clinical criteria (Fig. 13.1) can be used to identify patients having MCI. Consideration of the suspected etiology will then allow discussion of likely outcomes with the patient (Fig. 13.2). For example, subjects with aMCI of a degenerative etiology will likely progress to AD. However, there is likely to be a second level of utilization of the criteria as well. These clinical considerations, augmented with some combination of the various technological measures mentioned above, may allow for more precision in prognostication. This application of the MCI construct will initially be restricted to research settings, but if the technology proves useful, it may filter into practice at tertiary care centers for the adjudication of difficult cases.

In summary, the construct of MCI serves a useful purpose in sensitizing clinicians to earlier presenting features of dementing disorders. Having been expanded to include non-memory cognitive deficits, MCI can be viewed as a precursor stage to many dementias, and its subtypes may predict specific dementia subtypes. Most literature pertains to the aMCI subtype, which is useful for identifying individuals likely to develop AD in the future. As disease-modifying therapies emerge, the MCI construct may prove useful for identifying subjects early in the course of the disease process in an attempt to treat the disorders before development of significant functional disability. Ultimately, identifying individuals at risk for developing these diseases while still clinically normal may allow for prevention in the future.

References

1. Petersen RC. *Mild Cognitive Impairment: Aging to Alzheimer's Disease.* Oxford: Oxford University Press; 2003.
2. Petersen RC, Doody R, Kurz A *et al.* Current concepts in mild cognitive impairment. *Arch Neurol* 2001; **58**(12):1985–1992.
3. Petersen RC, Smith GE, Waring SC *et al.* Mild cognitive impairment: clinical characterization and outcome. *Arch Neurol* 1999;**56**(3):303–308.
4. Sloane PD, Zimmerman S, Suchindran C *et al.* The public health impact of Alzheimer's disease, 2000–2050: potential implication of treatment advances. *Annu Rev Public Health* 2002;**23**:213–231.
5. Gauthier S, Reisberg B, Zaudig M *et al.* Mild cognitive impairment. *Lancet* 2006;**367**(9518):1262–1270.
6. Lopez OL, Jagust WJ, DeKosky ST *et al.* Prevalence and classification of mild cognitive impairment in the Cardiovascular Health Study Cognition Study: Part 1. *Arch Neurol* 2003;**60**(10):1385–1389.
7. Busse A, Hensel A, Guhne U, Angermeyer MC, Riedel-Heller SG. Mild cognitive impairment: long-term course of four clinical subtypes. *Neurology* 2006; **67**(12):2176–2185.
8. Graham JE, Rockwood K, Beattie BL *et al.* Prevalence and severity of cognitive impairment with and without dementia in an elderly population. *Lancet* 1997;**349** (9068):1793–1796.
9. Unverzagt FW, Gao S, Baiyewu O *et al.* Prevalence of cognitive impairment: data from the Indianapolis Study of Health and Aging. *Neurology* 2001;**57**(9): 1655–1662.
10. Bennett DA, Wilson RS, Schneider JA *et al.* Natural history of mild cognitive impairment in older persons. *Neurology* 2002;**59**(2):198–205.
11. Ritchie K, Artero S, Touchon J. Classification criteria for mild cognitive impairment: a population-based validation study. *Neurology* 2001;**56**(1):37–42.
12. Hanninen T, Hallikainen M, Tuomainen S, Vanhanen M, Soininen H. Prevalence of mild cognitive impairment: a population-based study in elderly subjects. *Acta Neurol Scand* 2002;**106**(3):148–154.
13. Boeve B, McCormick J, Smith G *et al.* Mild cognitive impairment in the oldest old. *Neurology* 2003;**60**(3): 477–480.
14. Petersen R, Roberts R, Knopman D *et al.* Prevalence of mild cognitive impairment in a population-based study. *Neurology* 2007;**68**(Suppl 1):A237.
15. Jungwirth S, Weissgram S, Zehetmayer S, Tragl KH, Fischer P. VITA: subtypes of mild cognitive impairment in a community-based cohort at the age of 75 years. *Int J Geriatr Psychiatry* 2005;**20**(5):452–458.
16. Di Carlo A, Lamassa M, Baldereschi M *et al.* CIND and MCI in the Italian elderly: frequency, vascular risk factors, progression to dementia. *Neurology* 2007; **68**(22):1909–1916.
17. Das SK, Bose P, Biswas A *et al.* An epidemiologic study of mild cognitive impairment in Kolkata, India. *Neurology* 2007;**68**(23):2019–2026.
18. Larrieu S, Letenneur L, Orgogozo JM *et al.* Incidence and outcome of mild cognitive impairment in a

population-based prospective cohort. *Neurology* 2002;**59**(10):1594–1599.

19. Petersen RC. Mild cognitive impairment as a diagnostic entity. *J Intern Med* 2004;**256**(3):183–194.

20. Winblad B, Palmer K, Kivipelto M *et al.* Mild cognitive impairment – beyond controversies, towards a consensus: report of the International Working Group on Mild Cognitive Impairment. *J Intern Med* 2004; **256**(3):240–246.

21. Mueller SG, Weiner MW, Thal LJ *et al.* The Alzheimer's disease neuroimaging initiative. *Neuroimaging Clin N Am* 2005;**15**(4):869–877, xi–xii.

22. Daly E, Zaitchik D, Copeland M *et al.* Predicting conversion to Alzheimer disease using standardized clinical information. *Arch Neurol* 2000;**57**(5):675–680.

23. Petersen RC, Thomas RG, Grundman M *et al.* Vitamin E and donepezil for the treatment of mild cognitive impairment. *N Engl J Med* 2005;**352**(23):2379–2388.

24. Aggarwal NT, Wilson RS, Beck TL, Bienias JL, Bennett DA. Mild cognitive impairment in different functional domains and incident Alzheimer's disease. *J Neurol Neurosurg Psychiatry* 2005;**76**(11):1479–1484.

25. Fischer P, Jungwirth S, Zehetmayer S *et al.* Conversion from subtypes of mild cognitive impairment to Alzheimer dementia. *Neurology* 2007;**68**(4):288–291.

26. Hunderfund AL, Roberts RO, Slusser TC *et al.* Mortality in amnestic mild cognitive impairment: a prospective community study. *Neurology* 2006;**67**(10): 1764–1768.

27. Jack CR, Jr., Petersen RC, Xu YC *et al.* Prediction of AD with MRI-based hippocampal volume in mild cognitive impairment. *Neurology* 1999;**52**(7):1397–1403.

28. Jack CR, Jr., Shiung MM, Weigand SD *et al.* Brain atrophy rates predict subsequent clinical conversion in normal elderly and amnestic MCI. *Neurology* 2005; **65**(8):1227–1231.

29. Devanand DP, Pradhaban G, Liu X *et al.* Hippocampal and entorhinal atrophy in mild cognitive impairment: prediction of Alzheimer disease. *Neurology* 2007; **68**(11):828–836.

30. DeCarli C, Frisoni GB, Clark CM *et al.* Qualitative estimates of medial temporal atrophy as a predictor of progression from mild cognitive impairment to dementia. *Arch Neurol* 2007;**64**(1):108–115.

31. Corder EH, Saunders AM, Strittmatter WJ *et al.* Gene dose of apolipoprotein E type 4 allele and the risk of Alzheimer's disease in late onset families. *Science* 1993; **261**(5123):921–923.

32. Aggarwal NT, Wilson RS, Beck TL *et al.* The apolipoprotein E epsilon4 allele and incident Alzheimer's disease in persons with mild cognitive impairment. *Neurocase* 2005;**11**(1):3–7.

33. Tierney MC, Szalai JP, Snow WG *et al.* A prospective study of the clinical utility of ApoE genotype in the prediction of outcome in patients with memory impairment. *Neurology* 1996;**46**(1):149–154.

34. Petersen RC, Smith GE, Ivnik RJ *et al.* Apolipoprotein E status as a predictor of the development of Alzheimer's disease in memory-impaired individuals. *JAMA* 1995;**273**(16):1274–1278.

35. Jak AJ, Houston WS, Nagel BJ, Corey-Bloom J, Bondi MW. Differential cross-sectional and longitudinal impact of *APOE* genotype on hippocampal volumes in nondemented older adults. *Dement Geriatr Cogn Disord* 2007;**23**(6):282–289.

36. Farrer LA, Cupples LA, Haines JL *et al.* Effects of age, sex, and ethnicity on the association between apolipoprotein E genotype and Alzheimer disease. A meta-analysis. APOE and Alzheimer Disease Meta Analysis Consortium. *JAMA* 1997;**278**(16): 1349–1356.

37. Galasko D, Chang L, Motter R *et al.* High cerebrospinal fluid tau and low amyloid beta42 levels in the clinical diagnosis of Alzheimer disease and relation to apolipoprotein E genotype. *Arch Neurol* 1998; **55**(7):937–945.

38. Galasko D, Clark C, Chang L *et al.* Assessment of CSF levels of tau protein in mildly demented patients with Alzheimer's disease. *Neurology* 1997;**48**(3):632–635.

39. Growdon JH. Biomarkers of Alzheimer disease. *Arch Neurol* 1999;**56**(3):281–3.

40. Sunderland T, Wolozin B, Galasko D *et al.* Longitudinal stability of CSF tau levels in Alzheimer patients. *Biol Psychiatry* 1999;**46**(6):750–755.

41. Stefani A, Martorana A, Bernardini S *et al.* CSF markers in Alzheimer disease patients are not related to the different degree of cognitive impairment. *J Neurol Sci* 2006;**251**(1–2):124–128.

42. Buerger K, Teipel SJ, Zinkowski R *et al.* CSF tau protein phosphorylated at threonine 231 correlates with cognitive decline in MCI subjects. *Neurology* 2002; **59**(4):627–629.

43. Buerger K, Ewers M, Pirttila T *et al.* CSF phosphorylated tau protein correlates with neocortical neurofibrillary pathology in Alzheimer's disease. *Brain* 2006;**129**(Pt 11):3035–3041.

44. Hansson O, Zetterberg H, Buchhave P *et al.* Association between CSF biomarkers and incipient Alzheimer's disease in patients with mild cognitive impairment: a follow-up study. *Lancet Neurol* 2006;**5**(3):228–234.

45. Bateman RJ, Wen G, Morris JC, Holtzman DM. Fluctuations of CSF amyloid-beta levels: implications for a diagnostic and therapeutic biomarker. *Neurology* 2007;**68**(9):666–669.

46. Graff-Radford NR, Crook JE, Lucas J *et al.* Association of low plasma Abeta42/Abeta40 ratios with increased imminent risk for mild cognitive impairment and Alzheimer disease. *Arch Neurol* 2007;**64**(3):354–362.

47. van Oijen M, Hofman A, Soares HD, Koudstaal PJ, Breteler MM. Plasma Abeta(1–40) and Abeta(1–42) and the risk of dementia: a prospective case-cohort study. [See comment.] *Lancet Neurol* 2006;**5**(8):655–660.

48. Small GW, Mazziotta JC, Collins MT *et al.* Apolipoprotein E type 4 allele and cerebral glucose metabolism in relatives at risk for familial Alzheimer disease. *JAMA* 1995;**273**(12):942–947.

49. Reiman EM, Caselli RJ, Yun LS *et al.* Preclinical evidence of Alzheimer's disease in persons homozygous for the epsilon 4 allele for apolipoprotein E. *N Engl J Med* 1996;**334**(12):752–758.

50. Drzezga A, Grimmer T, Riemenschneider M *et al.* Prediction of individual clinical outcome in MCI by means of genetic assessment and (18)F-FDG PET. *J Nucl Med* 2005;**46**(10):1625–1632.

51. Anchisi D, Borroni B, Franceschi M *et al.* Heterogeneity of brain glucose metabolism in mild cognitive impairment and clinical progression to Alzheimer disease. *Arch Neurol* 2005;**62**(11):1728–1733.

52. Klunk WE, Engler H, Nordberg A *et al.* Imaging brain amyloid in Alzheimer's disease with Pittsburgh Compound-B. *Ann Neurol* 2004;**55**(3):306–319.

53. Small GW, Kepe V, Ercoli LM *et al.* PET of brain amyloid and tau in mild cognitive impairment. *N Engl J Med* 2006;**355**(25):2652–2663.

54. Markesbery WR, Schmitt FA, Kryscio RJ *et al.* Neuropathologic substrate of mild cognitive impairment. *Arch Neurol* 2006;**63**(1):38–46.

55. Morris JC, Storandt M, Miller JP *et al.* Mild cognitive impairment represents early-stage Alzheimer disease. *Arch Neurol* 2001;**58**(3):397–405.

56. Bennett DA, Schneider JA, Bienias JL, Evans DA, Wilson RS. Mild cognitive impairment is related to Alzheimer disease pathology and cerebral infarctions. *Neurology* 2005;**64**(5):834–841.

57. Petersen RC, Parisi JE, Dickson DW *et al.* Neuropathologic features of amnestic mild cognitive impairment. *Arch Neurol* 2006;**63**(5):665–672.

58. Jicha GA, Parisi JE, Dickson DW *et al.* Neuropathologic outcome of mild cognitive impairment following progression to clinical dementia. *Arch Neurol* 2006; **63**(5):674–681.

59. Petersen RC. Mild cognitive impairment continuum. *Lifelong Learn Neurol* 2007;**13**(2):15–38.

60. Gold M, Francke S, Nye JS *et al.* Impact of *APOE* genotype on the efficacy of galantamine for the treatment of mild cognitive impairment. *Neurobiol Aging* 2004;**25**(Suppl 2):S521.

61. Feldman HH, Ferris S, Winblad B *et al.* Effect of rivastigmine on delay to diagnosis of Alzheimer's disease from mild cognitive impairment: the InDDEx study. *Lancet Neurol* 2007;**6**(6):501–512.

62. Thal LJ, Ferris SH, Kirby L *et al.* A randomized, double-blind, study of rofecoxib in patients with mild cognitive impairment. *Neuropsychopharmacology* 2005; **30**(6):1204–1215.

63. Petersen RC. Mild cognitive impairment clinical trials. *Nat Rev Drug Discov* 2003;**2**(8):646–653.

64. Petersen RC. MCI treatment trials: failure or not? *Lancet Neurol* 2007;**6**(6):473–475.

65. Petersen RC, Stevens JC, Ganguli M *et al.* Practice parameter: early detection of dementia: mild cognitive impairment (an evidence-based review). Report of the Quality Standards Subcommittee of the American Academy of Neurology. *Neurology* 2001;**56**(9): 1133–1142.

66. Fratiglioni L, Paillard-Borg S, Winblad B. An active and socially integrated lifestyle in late life might protect against dementia. *Lancet Neurol* 2004; **3**(6):343–353.

67. Rovio S, Kareholt I, Helkala EL *et al.* Leisure-time physical activity at midlife and the risk of dementia and Alzheimer's disease. *Lancet Neurol* 2005; **4**(11):705–711.

68. Petersen RC, O'Brien J. Mild cognitive impairment should be considered for DSM-V. *J Geriatr Psychiatry Neurol* 2006;**19**(3):147–154.

Mild cognitive impairment subgroups

Julene K. Johnson

Introduction

Mild cognitive impairment (MCI) is a clinical syndrome that represents a decline of cognitive functioning that is not sufficient to meet criteria for dementia.[1] The cognitive decline is greater than that expected for normal aging but is not sufficient enough to interfere with most activities of daily living. In adults over 65 years of age, cognitive impairment without dementia is two to five times more common than dementia and occurs in approximately 11–27% of the population.[2-7] Most studies suggest that the prevalence of cognitive impairment increases with age. For example, Unverzagt and colleagues[3] reported that 29% of individuals between 65 and 74 years of age and as many as 55% of individuals over age 84 exhibited symptoms of cognitive impairment (without dementia). However, there is considerable variability in prevalence estimates for MCI, in part because of different methods for ascertaining and defining MCI.

Neurodegenerative disorders are proposed to account for the majority of cognitive decline in older adults. Numerous studies suggest that individuals with MCI have an increased risk for converting to dementia, particularly Alzheimer's disease (AD).[8,9] However, the majority of these studies have focused on MCI with predominantly memory impairment. In the studies at the Mayo Clinic, individuals with MCI convert to dementia at approximately 12% per year, compared with healthy older adults, who convert at approximately 1–2% per year.[10] It has also been proposed that most neurodegenerative diseases have an MCI stage; however, the nature of the prodromal stages of non-AD dementias is not yet well known. For example, cognitive decline has been described in preclinical stages of Huntington's disease,[11,12] Parkinson's disease (PD)[13] and sporadic Creutzfeldt–Jakob disease.[14] In addition, mild changes in cognition can also occur in other conditions, such as depression, medical illness and aging.[3,15] One goal is to differentiate mild changes in cognition that are associated with different neurodegenerative diseases or other conditions, and, of course, to differentiate normal from pathological changes of cognition with aging.

The MCI term was popularized by Petersen and colleagues in 1999;[8] however, the term was first used by the New York University group,[16] who defined MCI using the Global Deterioration Scale (GDS),[17] and numerous other terms have been proposed (as discussed below). There is still no consensus about which criteria to use for MCI, and there is considerable debate in the field about the usefulness of various definitions.[15] However, the 1999 criteria proposed by Petersen have been the most widely applied.

It has become increasingly clear that MCI is a heterogeneous clinical syndrome. Some argue that MCI is a transitional stage between healthy aging and dementia.[18] However, others argue that MCI represents early AD.[19,20] Several studies, however, find that some individuals diagnosed with MCI do not progress to dementia, and some even revert to normal.[15,21,22] One goal of MCI research is to differentiate individuals who will decline versus those who remain stable. Heterogeneity is also observed in the clinical presentation. The purpose of this chapter is to discuss MCI in older adults with a particular focus on the recently proposed subgroups of MCI.

Conceptualization of mild cognitive impairment

The concept of MCI developed from the observation that some older adults experience a decline in cognition with age. Reports of cognitive decline in older adults occurred as early as the eighteenth century.[23,24] However, Voijtech A. Kral, a Czech-Canadian neurologist and psychiatrist in Montreal, was one of the first to differentiate types of memory decline in older adults. Kral observed two patterns of memory decline, which he called "benign" and "malignant" senescent forgetfulness in older adults.[25–27] He noticed that some older adults had poor recall of event details but could remember the general information. He also noted that these individuals were aware of the memory difficulty and could usually eventually recall the event. He proposed the term benign senescent forgetfulness because these individuals progressed very slowly. He described a second group of individuals who had poor memory for details and events and did not have insight into their memory deficit. Because these individuals had lower cognitive test scores and decreased survival, he proposed the term malignant senescent forgetfulness to classify these individuals. After 4 years, only 1 of the 20 individuals with the benign form declined, whereas all with the malignant form declined cognitively.[28] Also at this time, Roth et al.[29,30] reported that accumulation of neuritic plaques was related to a decline in cognition and dementia in older adults. Thus, early studies of mild cognitive impairment in older adults documented different profiles of cognitive impairment and linked changes in cognition to neuropathology.

Following these early studies, numerous new clinical terms were proposed to categorize cognitive impairment in older adults (Table 14.1). There was a trend in the 1980s to attribute a slight decline in cognition to a very early stage of dementia (e.g. questionable dementia,[40] minimal dementia,[41] limited dementia).[42] In 1986, the National Institute of Mental Health proposed the term age-associated memory impairment (AAMI) to refer to individuals who scored greater than 1 standard deviation (SD) below *young adults* on tests of memory.[33] This was the first attempt to operationalize a definition of cognitive decline in older adults.

In 1989, the term late-life forgetfulness was proposed to classify individuals who scored 1.5–2.0 SD below age-matched norms on memory tests.[34] Flicker and colleagues[16] identified a group of individuals with MCI as defined by a score of 3 on the GDS.[17] In contrast, age-associated cognitive decline (AACD),[38] age-related cognitive decline (ARCD)[1] and cognitive impairment no dementia (CIND)[1] were developed to classify individuals who exhibit impairment on *any* cognitive domain, including memory. Interestingly, the terms benign senescent forgetfulness, AACD and AAMI are used to characterize cognitive changes associated with normal aging and are not regarded as preclinical stages of neurodegenerative diseases.

Table 14.1. Terms used to label mild cognitive impairment in older adults

	Term	Reference
1962	Benign senescent forgetfulness	27
1962	Malignant senescent forgetfulness	27
1978	Mild cognitive impairment not amounting to dementia	31
1982	Mild cognitive decline (GDS = 3)	17
1982	Questionable dementia (CDR = 0.5)	32
1986	Age-associated memory impairment (AAMI)	33
1989	Late-life forgetfulness (LLF)	34
1991	Possible dementia prodrome (PDP)	35
1991	Mild cognitive impairment (MCI)	16
1992	Mild cognitive impairment	36 (ICD-10)
1993	Mild cognitive disorder	37 (ICD-10)
1994	Age-associated cognitive decline (AACD)	38
1994	Mild cognitive decline	1 (DSM-IV)
1994	Age-related cognitive decline (ARCD)	1
1997	Cognitive impairment no dementia (CIND)	2
1997	Mild cognitive impairment (MCI)	39

Notes:
GDS, Global Deterioration Scale; CDR, Clinical Dementia Rating Scale.

Although used by Flicker and colleagues[16] in 1991 and the World Health Organization[31] in 1978, the term MCI was popularized by Petersen and colleagues in the Mayo Clinic series.[8,10] Following these seminal publications, there was a substantial increase in the number of studies about MCI describing the clinical features, prevalence and outcomes. However, the literature remains challenging to read because different definitions of MCI are used by different groups.[43] In addition, European researchers have focused on AAMI, AACD and normal aging,[15] whereas researchers in the USA have focused on MCI as a prodrome to dementia. Until recently, the majority of studies focused on MCI and memory decline with age. It was not until recently that cognitive decline in non-memory domains was considered.

MCI is generally diagnosed using a combination of clinical judgement, informant report and neuropsychological tests. However, no standard tests or combination of tests are recommended, and different groups use a different combination of tests.

Conceptualization of mild cognitive impairment subgroups

After studying multiple cohorts across the world, it became clear that MCI represented a heterogeneous clinical condition.[7,20,44] One source of heterogeneity involving several studies suggested that individuals with MCI have impairment in non-memory cognitive domains in addition to the disproportionate deficits in memory.[8,45] Furthermore, not all subjects with cognitive decline experience a change in memory.[18,20,46] It was hypothesized that AD could begin with impairment in non-memory cognitive domains.[47] This hypothesis was based, in part, on the observation of atypical presentations of AD that had disproportionate impairment in non-memory cognitive domains such as language, executive function or visuospatial function.[48-50]

In 1999, an international working group convened in Chicago at the *Current Concepts in Mild Cognitive Impairment Conference*[18] and acknowledged that MCI was heterogeneous and proposed MCI subclassifications: (1) MCI (amnestic [aMCI]), (2) MCI (multiple domains slightly impaired – without requiring a memory deficit) and (3) MCI (single, non-memory domain) (Tables 14.2 and 14.3). The working group also proposed that the different subgroups may have different clinical outcomes, with aMCI primarily converting to AD, and non-memory single domain MCI converting to frontotemporal dementia (FTD), dementia with Lewy bodies, primary progressive aphasia (PPA), PD or AD. However, the authors noted that these subgroups were primarily hypothetical, and no conversion data were yet available.

In 2004, another international working group met, this time in Stockholm, to propose consensus diagnostic criteria for MCI.[51] The working group drafted general criteria for MCI: (1) not normal but not demented, (2) cognitive decline (by report and impairment on objective memory tests and/or evidence of decline over time on cognitive tests) and (3) preserved basic activities of daily living. They also discussed the heterogeneity of MCI and included an algorithm for classifying four MCI subgroups: (1) aMCI, (2) aMCI multiple domain, (3) non-amnestic MCI multiple domain, and (4) non-amnestic MCI single domain. A slightly different version of this algorithm was published in the same journal issue by Petersen.[52] Although four subgroups were defined by this algorithm, the multiple domain MCI (with or without memory) is often collapsed into one group

Table 14.2. Original and revised criteria for mild cognitive impairment

	Criteria
Original[8]	1. Memory complaint (noted by individual, informant or physician)
	2. Objective memory impairment on memory test
	3. Preserved general cognitive function
	4. Generally intact activities of daily living
	5. Absence of dementia
Revised[51]	1. Complaint from individual or informant
	2. Change from normal functioning
	3. Decline in any area of cognition
	4. Preserved overall general function but some difficulty in activities of daily living
	5. Absence of dementia

Table 14.3. Proposed conversion diagnoses

Subgroups	Conversion diagnosis
MCI – amnestic	Alzheimer's disease
MCI – single non-memory	Frontotemporal dementia, dementia with Lewy bodies, vascular dementia, primary progressive aphasia, Parkinson's disease, Alzheimer's disease
MCI – multiple domains	Alzheimer's disease, vascular dementia, normal aging

Note:
MCI, mild cognitive impairment.
Adapted from Petersen *et al.* (2001).[18]

(MCI-MCD), yielding three or four subgroups. Neuropsychological testing is generally used to help to determine the specific MCI subgroups, and the cognitive domains of memory, language, executive function and visuospatial skills were recommended to be assessed. However, no specific neuropsychological tests were proposed. The classification of MCI subgroups has not gone without criticism. For example, Rasquin *et al.* (2005)[53] argued that the MCI subgroups have limited clinical relevance.

Clinical heterogeneity in MCI is likely influenced by different underlying etiologies, which contribute to the cognitive decline. As discussed in the introduction, the majority of subjects with MCI are believed to have an underlying neurodegenerative disease. Cognitive decline in the absence of dementia can also occur in other neurodegenerative disorders (e.g. FTD, Huntington's disease) and medical conditions (e.g. depression, schizophrenia). It is not surprising that most neurodegenerative disorders have a preclinical stage, since they often begin insidiously and progress gradually. The majority of research so far has focused on aMCI and risk for AD.

The prevalence of MCI subgroups is not yet well known. In an early study using data from the Cardiovascular Healthy Study, Lopez and colleagues[7] found a higher percentage of subjects with MCI-MCD (16%) compared with aMCI (6%). In the Leipzig Longitudinal Study of the Aged (LEILA 75+), the non-amnestic (single domain) MCI had the highest prevalence rate at 17.4%, followed by aMCI multiple domain at 10.9%. The aMCI single domain had the lowest prevalence rate at 9.3%. In the Vienna-Transdanube-Aging (VITA) study, Jungwirth and colleagues[54] found the highest prevalence rate for non-memory MCI (14.9%), followed by memory impairment + non-amnestic impairment (5.2%) and selective memory impairment (3.7%). The next sections provide further discussion about three subgroups of MCI: aMCI, non-amnestic MCI, and MCI-MCD.

Amnestic mild cognitive impairment (single domain)

The majority of research[50] so far has focused on aMCI. The initial focus of MCI research was on memory decline. According to the 2001 international consensus,[51] aMCI (single domain) is characterized by a relatively selective decline in memory function. Individuals with aMCI present with a subjective memory complaint, preferably corroborated by an informant, have objective impairment on memory tests and are not demented. They commonly perform below the norm for their age on objective measures of verbal or visual episodic memory, such as remembering word lists, stories or pictures.[8,22] Approximately 10–15% of individuals with aMCI convert to dementia per year,[8,55] and 80% convert to dementia over 6 years.[18] Individuals with aMCI commonly convert to clinically diagnosed AD;[8,55,56] however, other neuropathological diagnoses, such as hippocampal sclerosis and argyrophilic grain disease, have been reported[57] and are discussed in more detail below.

Results from several population studies suggest that individuals with aMCI (single domain) are a relatively small group compared with the broader form of MCI.[4,7,21,56,58] In one of the first population-based prevalence estimates of MCI subgroups, the Cardiovascular Healthy Study found that aMCI had a prevalence rate of 6%, while MCI-MCD had a prevalence of 16%.[7]

Non-amnestic mild cognitive impairment (single domain)

Non-memory presentations of MCI have also been proposed,[18,20,47,59] but less is known about the clinical characteristics and outcomes. Although specific non-memory cognitive domains have not been specified, the following summarizes three possible non-memory, single domain MCI presentations: dysexecutive, visuospatial and language.

Dysexecutive

In the original proposal of MCI subgroups, the dysexecutive presentation of MCI was suspected to be a prodrome for FTD.[18] An isolated impairment in executive function has been described in families with known mutations causing FTD prior to the onset of dementia.[60,61] In addition, de Mendonça and colleagues[62] retrospectively described the MCI stage of seven patients with FTD and found both the presence of behavioral change and executive dysfunction prior to the onset of dementia. However, several studies suggest that FTD begins primarily with changes in behavior,[63,64] and executive function is often preserved in the early stages of FTD.[65] Other studies also suggest a combination of behavioral changes and executive dysfunction characterize the first symptoms of FTD.[66] More recently, the term mild behavioral impairment has been proposed to describe late-life changes in behavior that are a possible prodrome for FTD.[67]

Isolated executive dysfunction may also be a prodrome for other neurodegenerative disorders. For example, several studies suggest that isolated executive dysfunction is evident before the onset of dementia in PD.[13,68] In another study, Johnson and colleagues[59] described an individual who died with an isolated executive impairment and found plaque and neurofibrillary tangle neuropathology associated with AD on autopsy. We, therefore, proposed that an isolated executive impairment may represent a dysexecutive presentation of MCI. We are currently following a cohort of individuals who present with isolated impairments on tests of executive function or complain about dysexecutive symptoms (e.g. concentration, multitasking, problem solving) to determine the clinical outcome. Figure 14.1 shows a representative magnetic resonance image (MRI) from one individual diagnosed with dysexecutive MCI in our cohort.

191

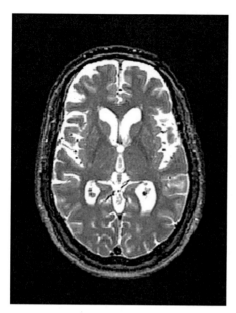

Fig. 14.1. Representative magnetic resonance image of an individual with dysexecutive mild cognitive impairment. Note the prominent atrophy in the frontal and temporal regions and the relative sparing of posterior regions.

Visuospatial

There has been only one study describing a subgroup of MCI with visuospatial defects. Mapstone and colleagues[47] described an individual with MCI who had selective impairment in visuospatial function and a preservation of memory.

Language

A language presentation of MCI has not received much attention apart from the classification of PPA, also called the language variant of frontotemporal dementia. By definition, PPA begins with approximately 2 years of relatively isolated language impairment.[69] A variety of neuropathological conditions can cause PPA, including corticobasal degeneration, Pick's disease, progressive supranuclear palsy, Creutzfeldt–Jakob disease and AD.[70,71] It is not yet clear how PPA will fall within the MCI–language conceptualization.

Mild cognitive impairment multiple cognitive domain

As discussed above, MCI-MCDT (also referred to as md-MCI, "memory plus") is used to classify individuals who have MCI across multiple domains but are not demented. In other words, it is used to classify individuals who do not have a clear disproportionate impairment in one cognitive domain. The term was first proposed in the *Current Concepts in Mild Cognitive Impairment Conference* in 1999.[18] Memory may or may not be included in this classification, which adds to the confusion about this subgroup (see Winblad *et al.*[51]). As discussed above, the prevalence of MCI-MCD appears to be higher than that of aMCI (e.g. prevalence rate of 16% compared with 6% for aMCI in the Cardiovascular Health Study).[7] More than 50% of those with MCI-MCD have memory impairment.[72]

Neuroimaging of subgroups in mild cognitive impairment

Early studies suggested that individuals with MCI had smaller volumes and decreased hypoperfusion of medial temporal cortex.[73] In addition, hippocampal atrophy was found to be a good predictor of conversion from MCI to AD.[74] Therefore, the majority of early imaging studies in MCI focused on the medial temporal lobes and memory. More recently, there are a few studies that examine neuroimaging differences in MCI subgroups. For example, Bell-McGinty and colleagues[75] found that patients with aMCI had volume loss in the left entorhinal cortex and inferior parietal cortex, whereas patients with MCI-MCD had volume loss in the right inferior frontal gyrus, right middle temporal gyrus and bilateral superior temporal gyrus. Another study, by Becker and colleagues,[76] found that subjects with aMCI had significantly greater hippocampal atrophy than controls. In contrast, the subjects with MCI-MCD did not differ from controls in hippocampal volumes. These results suggest that the MCI subgroups may have different neuroimaging profiles. However, additional studies are needed with larger sample sizes.

Clinical outcome for subgroups in mild cognitive impairment

The clinical outcome of MCI subgroups is not yet well understood. Again, the focus has been on studying individuals with aMCI who progress to AD. Only recently have investigators addressed the clinical outcome of MCI subgroups.

Conversion to dementia

In a review of several large longitudinal studies, Petersen and colleagues[18] found that individuals diagnosed with aMCI convert to AD at an annual rate between 6 and 25%, which is substantially higher than conversion to dementia in healthy elderly individuals. In a community-based sample of elderly individuals, subjects classified as having aMCI were approximately four times more likely to progress to AD.[58]

When comparing the different subgroups, there appear to be different risk profiles for converting to dementia. Several studies found that subjects with MCI-MCD have a higher progression rate to dementia than those with aMCI.[53] For example, Alexopoulos and colleagues[77] found that 45% of the individuals with MCI-MCD progressed to dementia after a mean of 3.5 years, compared with 38% of those with single domain non-memory MCI and 25% of those with aMCI In these studies, aMCI had low prognostic value, while MCI-MCD had high prognostic value for conversion to AD. In contrast, Yaffe and colleagues[78] found that individuals with aMCI were more likely to convert to dementia than individuals with single domain, non-memory MCI or MCI-MCD. However, another study did not find a relationship between MCI subgroups and development of dementia.[44] In one study, two-thirds of those patients who progressed to AD had had a prior diagnosis of aMCI.[78] In contrast, 50% of the patients diagnosed with vascular dementia had a prior diagnosis of aMCI, and all patients who converted to a frontal dementia had a prior single non-memory MCI diagnosis. However, several studies point out that some individuals diagnosed with MCI do not progress to dementia, and some even revert to normal.[15,21,22]

Mortality

There have been only a few studies addressing the risk of mortality in subgroups of MCI. In one study, Yaffe and colleagues[78] found that patients with single domain non-memory MCI and MCI-MCD have a greater risk of death than patients with aMCI. After adjusting for baseline score on the Mini-Mental State Examination and demographic, depression, function and medical conditions, the patients with single domain non-memory MCI were more likely to be dead by the time of follow-up.

Neuropathology

Only a small number of individuals have been studied neuropathologically in the MCI stage. Of those, the majority of studies focus on the neuropathology of aMCI. Several early studies reported that individuals with aMCI are likely to meet neuropathological

criteria for AD at autopsy.[19,20,79] However, in a recent study of individuals who died with a diagnosis of aMCI, all 15 had pathological findings involving the medial temporal lobes (mean age, 89 years).[80] Most individuals did not meet the National Institute on Aging–Reagan neuropathological criteria for definite AD, but instead had various transitional stages of AD neuropathology. In addition, there were several comorbid neuropathological diagnoses, including hippocampal sclerosis, argyrophilic grain disease, Lewy bodies and vascular lesions. Jicha and colleagues[57] studied 34 individuals who were originally diagnosed with aMCI and progressed to dementia. In this sample, there was a high percentage of patients diagnosed with argryophilic grain disease, and most subjects had multiple neuropathologic diagnoses.

There are fewer studies describing the neuropathology on single domain, non-memory MCI or MCI-MCD. As described above, we described an individual with isolated executive dysfunction who had plaques and tangles that did not meet criteria for definite AD. However, accumulation of the neurofibrillary tangles and β-amyloid was higher in the midfrontal cortex relative to other cortical regions (i.e. temporal, parietal and occipital cortices), including the hippocampus. Moderate to severe neurofibrillary tangles in the entorhinal cortex and subiculum were seen with relative sparing of area CA1 of the hippocampus. In addition, the posterior cingulate cortex had the highest degree of neurofibrillary degeneration. The predominance of neuropathology in the frontal cortex is similar to the patients we have described with a frontal variant of AD.[48] That is, patients with AD and a disproportionate executive dysfunction also had a greater-than-expected degree of neurofibrillary tangle neuropathology in the frontal cortex. These results suggest that the disproportionate accumulation of neuropathology can be observed early in the disease. Future studies will help to determine the neuropathological diagnoses of the various MCI subgroups.

Conclusions

Mild cognitive impairment is a clinically heterogeneous syndrome characterized by a variety of clinical profiles and underlying etiologies. The concept of MCI has been associated with many different clinical labels, which have contributed to the confusion about the concept. The majority of research about MCI focuses on the amnestic subgroup, which is characterized by a relatively selective decline in memory

193

function. However, it is becoming increasingly recognized that MCI may also involve non-memory cognitive domains.

Mild cognitive impairment is an important clinical syndrome to study because of the risk for conversion to dementia, its functional impairment and the increased risk of death. However, it is important to keep in mind that some individuals diagnosed with MCI do not progress to dementia, and some even revert to normal. The concept of MCI is currently framed as a preclinical stage of AD. However, because most neurodegenerative diseases begin insidiously and gradually progress, it is likely that most neurodegenerative diseases will have an MCI stage once earlier detection is possible. As the window for early detection moves back, it will be possible to identify MCI stages for many other neurodegenerative diseases. Early detection is key because future therapeutic interventions will most likely have maximal effectiveness early in the disease process. It is clear that differential diagnosis is important as MCI stages of different diseases are identified. It is not yet clear if the term MCI will remain as a term to designate a preclinical stage of AD or might be applied to other preclinical diseases.

There is a need to improve the characterization of cognitive impairment in the absence of dementia in both preclinical syndromes and medical conditions, with particular emphasis on non-memory presentations; this will improve our ability to relate the clinical presentation to underlying etiology. Future studies must determine how the MCI stages of different neurodegenerative disorders overlap or differ.

Acknowledgements

The author is supported by NIH R01-AG022538.

References

1. American Psychiatric Association. *Diagnostic and Statistical Manual of Mental Disorders*, 4th edn (DSM-IV). Washington, DC: American Psychiatric Press, 1994.

2. Graham JE, Rockwood K, Beattie BL, *et al.* Prevalence and severity of cognitive impairment with and without dementia in an elderly population. *Lancet* 1997; 349(9068):1793–6.

3. Unverzagt FW, Gao S, Baiyewu O, *et al.* Prevalence of cognitive impairment: data from the Indianapolis Study of Health and Aging. *Neurology* 2001;57(9):1655–62.

4. Schroder J, Kratz B, Pantel J, *et al.* Prevalence of mild cognitive impairment in an elderly community sample. *J Neur Transm Suppl* 1998;54:51–9.

5. Di Carlo A, Baldereschi M, Amaducci L, *et al.* Cognitive impairment without dementia in older people: prevalence, vascular risk factors, impact on disability. The Italian Longitudinal Study on Aging. *J Am Geriatr Soc* 2000;48(7):775–82.

6. Hanninen T, Koivisto K, Reinikainen KJ, *et al.* Prevalence of ageing-associated cognitive decline in an elderly population. *Age Ageing* 1996;25(3):201–5.

7. Lopez OL, Jagust WJ, DeKosky ST, *et al.* Prevalence and classification of mild cognitive impairment in the Cardiovascular Health Study Cognition Study: part 1. *Arch Neurol* 2003;60(10):1385–9.

8. Petersen RC, Smith GE, Waring SC, *et al.* Mild cognitive impairment: clinical characterization and outcome. *Arch Neurol* 1999;56(3):303–8.

9. Morris JC, Storandt M, Miller JP, *et al.* Mild cognitive impairment represents early-stage Alzheimer disease. *Arch Neurol* 2001;58(3):397–405.

10. Petersen RC, Stevens JC, Ganguli M, *et al.* Practice parameter: early detection of dementia: mild cognitive impairment (an evidence-based review). Report of the Quality Standards Subcommittee of the American Academy of Neurology. *Neurology* 2001;56(9):1133–42.

11. Snowden JS, Neary D, Mann DM. Frontotemporal dementia. *Br J Psychiatry* 2002;180:140–3.

12. Ho AK, Sahakian BJ, Brown RG, *et al.* Profile of cognitive progression in early Huntington's disease. *Neurology* 2003;61(12):1702–6.

13. Woods SP, Troster AI. Prodromal frontal/executive dysfunction predicts incident dementia in Parkinson's disease. *J Int Neuropsychol Soc* 2003;9(1):17–24.

14. Zarei M, Nouraei SA, Caine D, Hodges JR, Carpenter RH. Neuropsychological and quantitative oculometric study of a case of sporadic Creutzfeldt–Jakob disease at predementia stage. *J Neurol Neurosurg Psychiatry* 2002;73(1):56–8.

15. Ritchie K, Artero S, Touchon J. Classification criteria for mild cognitive impairment: a population-based validation study. *Neurology* 2001;56(1):37–42.

16. Flicker C, Ferris SH, Reisberg B. Mild cognitive impairment in the elderly: predictors of dementia. *Neurology* 1991;41(7):1006–9.

17. Reisberg B, Ferris SH, de Leon MJ, Crook T. The Global Deterioration Scale for assessment of primary degenerative dementia. *Am J Psychiatry* 1982;139(9):1136–9.

18. Petersen RC, Doody R, Kurz A, *et al.* Current concepts in mild cognitive impairment. *Arch Neurol* 2001; 58(12):1985–92.

19. Morris JC, Storandt M, Miller JP, *et al.* Mild cognitive impairment represents early-stage Alzheimer disease. *Arch Neurol* 2001;58(3):397–405.

20. Lambon Ralph MA, Patterson K, Graham N, *et al.* Homogeneity and heterogeneity in mild cognitive

impairment and Alzheimer's disease: a cross-sectional and longitudinal study of 55 cases. *Brain* 2003;**126** (Pt 11):2350–62.

21. Larrieu S, Letenneur L, Orgogozo JM, *et al.* Incidence and outcome of mild cognitive impairment in a population-based prospective cohort. *Neurology* 2002;**59**(10):1594–9.

22. Collie A, Maruff P. The neuropsychology of preclinical Alzheimer's disease and mild cognitive impairment. *Neurosci Biobehav Rev* 2000;**24**(3):365–74.

23. Schafer D. Gulliver meets Descartes: early modern concepts of age-related memory loss. *J Hist Neurosci* 2003;**12**(1):1–11.

24. Schafer D. No old man ever forgot where he buried his treasure: concepts of cognitive impairment in old age circa 1700. *J Am Geriatr Soc* 2005;**53**(11):2023–7.

25. Kral VA. Neuro-psychiatric observations in an old peoples home; studies of memory dysfunction in senescence. *J Gerontol* 1958;**13**(2):169–76.

26. Kral VA. Senescent memory decline and senile amnestic syndrome. *Am J Psychiatry* 1958;**115**(4):361–2.

27. Kral VA. Senescent forgetfulness: benign and malignant. *Can Med Assoc J* 1962;**86**(6):257–60.

28. Kral VA. Benign senescent forgetfulness. In Katzman R, Terry RD, Bick KL (eds.) *Aging, Vol. 7: Alzheimer's Disease: Senile Dementia and Related Disorders.* New York: Raven Press, 1978, pp. 47–51.

29. Roth M, Tomlinson BE, Blessed G. Correlation between scores for dementia and counts of "senile plaques" in cerebral grey matter of elderly subjects. *Nature* 1966;**209**(18):109–10.

30. Roth M, Tomlinson BE, Blessed G. The relationship between quantitative measures of dementia and of degenerative changes in the cerebral grey matter of elderly subjects. *Proc R Soc Med* 1967;**60**(3):254–60.

31. World Health Organization. *Mental Disorders: Glossary and Guide to Their Classification in Accordance with the Ninth Revision of the International Classification of Diseases.* Geneva: World Health Organization, 1978.

32. Berg L, Hughes CP, Coben LA, *et al.* Mild senile dementia of Alzheimer type: research diagnostic criteria, recruitment, and description of a study population. *J Neurol Neurosurg Psychiatry* 1982;**45**(11):962–8.

33. Crook T, Bartus RT, Ferris SH, *et al.* Age-associated memory impairment: proposed diagnostic criteria and measures of clinical change; report of a National Institute of Mental Health work group. *Dev Neuropsychol* 1986;**2**:261–76.

34. Blackford RLR. Criteria for diagnosing age associated memory impairment: proposed improvements from the field. *Dev Neuropsychol* 1989;**5**:295–306.

35. Heyman A, Fillenbaum GG, Mirra SS. Consortium to Establish a Registry for Alzheimer's Disease (CERAD): clinical, neuropsychological, and neuropathological components. *Aging (Milan)* 1990;**2**(4):415–24.

36. Zaudig M. A new systematic method of measurement and diagnosis of "mild cognitive impairment" and dementia according to ICD-10 and DSM-III-R criteria. *Int Psychogeriatr* 1992;**4**(Suppl 2):203–19.

37. World Health Organization. *The ICD-10 Classification of Mental and Behavioural Disorders: Diagnostic Criteria for Research.* Geneva: World Health Organization, 1993.

38. Levy R. Aging-associated cognitive decline. Working Party of the International Psychogeriatric Association in collaboration with the World Health Organization. *Int Psychogeriatr* 1994;**6**(1):63–8.

39. Petersen RC, Smith GE, Waring SC, *et al.* Aging, memory, and mild cognitive impairment. *Int Psychogeriatr* 1997;**9**(Suppl 1):65–9.

40. Hughes CP, Berg L, Danziger WL, Coben LA, Martin RL. A new clinical scale for the staging of dementia. *Br J Psychiatry* 1982;**140**:566–72.

41. Roth M, Tym E, Mountjoy CQ, *et al.* CAMDEX: a standardised instrument for the diagnosis of mental disorder in the elderly with special reference to the early detection of dementia. *Br J Psychiatry* 1986; **149**:698–709.

42. Gurland BJ, Dean LL, Copeland J, Gurland R, Golden R. Criteria for the diagnosis of dementia in the community elderly. *Gerontologist* 1982;**22**(2):180–6.

43. Ritchie K, Touchon J. Mild cognitive impairment: conceptual basis and current nosological status. *Lancet* 2000;**355**(9199):225–8.

44. Busse A, Bischkopf J, Riedel-Heller SG, Angermeyer MC. Mild cognitive impairment: prevalence and incidence according to different diagnostic criteria. Results of the Leipzig Longitudinal Study of the Aged (LEILA75+). *Br J Psychiatry* 2003;**182**:449–54.

45. Hanninen T, Hallikainen M, Koivisto K, *et al.* Decline of frontal lobe functions in subjects with age-associated memory impairment. *Neurology* 1997;**48**(1):148–53.

46. Ebly EM, Hogan DB, Parhad IM. Cognitive impairment in the nondemented elderly. Results from the Canadian Study of Health and Aging. *Arch Neurol* 1995; **52**(6):612–19.

47. Mapstone M, Steffenella TM, Duffy CJ. A visuospatial variant of mild cognitive impairment: getting lost between aging and AD. *Neurology* 2003;**60**(5):802–8.

48. Johnson JK, Head E, Kim R, Starr A, Cotman CW. Clinical and pathological evidence for a frontal variant of Alzheimer disease. *Arch Neurol* 1999;**56**(10):1233–9.

49. Galton CJ, Patterson K, Xuereb JH, Hodges JR. Atypical and typical presentations of Alzheimer's disease: a clinical, neuropsychological, neuroimaging and pathological study of 13 cases. *Brain* 2000; **123**(Pt 3):484–98.

50. Kanne SM, Balota DA, Storandt M, McKeel DW, Jr., Morris JC. Relating anatomy to function in Alzheimer's disease: neuropsychological profiles predict regional

neuropathology 5 years later. *Neurology* 1998;**50**(4): 979–85.

51. Winblad B, Palmer K, Kivipelto M, *et al.* Mild cognitive impairment: beyond controversies, towards a consensus: report of the International Working Group on Mild Cognitive Impairment. *J Intern Med* 2004;**256** (3):240–6.

52. Petersen RC. Mild cognitive impairment as a diagnostic entity. *J Intern Med* 2004;**256**(3):183–94.

53. Rasquin SM, Lodder J, Visser PJ, Lousberg R, Verhey FR. Predictive accuracy of MCI subtypes for Alzheimer's disease and vascular dementia in subjects with mild cognitive impairment: a 2-year follow-up study. *Dement Geriatr Cogn Disord* 2005;**19**(2–3):113–19.

54. Jungwirth S, Weissgram S, Zehetmayer S, Tragl KH, Fischer P. VITA: subtypes of mild cognitive impairment in a community-based cohort at the age of 75 years. *Int J Geriatr Psychiatry* 2005;**20**(5):452–8.

55. Tierney MC, Szalai JP, Snow WG, *et al.* Prediction of probable Alzheimer's disease in memory-impaired patients: a prospective longitudinal study. *Neurology* 1996;**46**:661–5.

56. Bowen J, Teri L, Kukull W, *et al.* Progression to dementia in patients with isolated memory loss. *Lancet* 1997;**349**:763–5.

57. Jicha GA, Parisi JE, Dickson DW, *et al.* Neuropathologic outcome of mild cognitive impairment following progression to clinical dementia. *Arch Neurol* 2006; **63**(5):674–81.

58. Ganguli M, Dodge HH, Shen C, DeKosky ST. Mild cognitive impairment, amnestic type: an epidemiologic study. *Neurology* 2004;**63**(1):115–21.

59. Johnson JK, Vogt BA, Kim R, Cotman CW, Head E. Isolated executive impairment and associated frontal neuropathology. *Dement Geriatr Cogn Disord* 2004;**17**:360–7.

60. Alberici A, Gobbo C, Panzacchi A, *et al.* Frontotemporal dementia: impact of P301L tau mutation on a healthy carrier. *J Neurol Neurosurg Psychiatry* 2004;**75**(11):1607–10.

61. Geschwind DH, Robidoux J, Alarcon M, *et al.* Dementia and neurodevelopmental predisposition: cognitive dysfunction in presymptomatic subjects precedes dementia by decades in frontotemporal dementia. *Ann Neurol* 2001;**50**(6):741–6.

62. de Mendonça A, Ribeiro F, Guerreiro M, Garcia C. Frontotemporal mild cognitive impairment. *J Alzheimers Dis* 2004;**6**(1):1–9.

63. Passant U, Rosen I, Gustafson L, Englund E. The heterogeneity of frontotemporal dementia with regard to initial symptoms, qEEG and neuropathology. *Int J Geriatr Psychiatry* 2005;**20**(10):983–8.

64. Shinagawa S, Ikeda M, Fukuhara R, Tanabe H. Initial symptoms in frontotemporal dementia and semantic dementia compared with Alzheimer's disease. *Dement Geriatr Cogn Disord* 2006;**21**(2):74–80.

65. Hodges JR, Patterson K, Ward R, *et al.* The differentiation of semantic dementia and frontal lobe dementia (temporal and frontal variants of frontotemporal dementia) from early Alzheimer's disease: a comparative neuropsychological study. *Neuropsychology* 1999;**13**(1):31–40.

66. Lindau M, Almkvist O, Kushi J, *et al.* First symptoms: frontotemporal dementia versus Alzheimer's disease. *Dement Geriatr Cogn Disord* 2000;**11**:286–93.

67. Scholzel-Dorenbos CJ. Mild behavioral impairment: a prodromal stage of frontotemporal lobar degeneration. *J Am Geriatr Soc* 2006;**54**(1):180–1.

68. Janvin CC, Larsen JP, Aarsland D, Hugdahl K. Subtypes of mild cognitive impairment in Parkinson's disease: progression to dementia. *Mov Disord* 2006;**21**(9):1343–9.

69. Mesulam MM. Slowly progressive aphasia without generalized dementia. *Ann Neurol* 1982;**11**(6):592–8.

70. Westbury C, Bub D. Primary progressive aphasia: a review of 112 cases. *Brain Lang* 1997;**60**(3):381–406.

71. Black SE. Focal cortical atrophy syndromes. *Brain Cogn* 1996;**31**(2):188–229.

72. Richards M, Touchon J, Ledesert B, Richie K. Cognitive decline in ageing: are AAMI and AACD distinct entities? *Int J Geriatr Psychiatry* 1999;**14**(7):534–40.

73. Johnson KA, Jones K, Holman BL, *et al.* Preclinical prediction of Alzheimer's disease using SPECT. *Neurology* 1998;**50**(6):1563–71.

74. Jack CR, Jr., Petersen RC, Xu YC, *et al.* Prediction of AD with MRI-based hippocampal volume in mild cognitive impairment. *Neurology* 1999;**52**(7):1397–403.

75. Bell-McGinty S, Lopez OL, Meltzer CC, *et al.* Differential cortical atrophy in subgroups of mild cognitive impairment. *Arch Neurol* 2005;**62**(9):1393–7.

76. Becker JT, Davis SW, Hayashi KM, *et al.* Three-dimensional patterns of hippocampal atrophy in mild cognitive impairment. *Arch Neurol* 2006;**63**(1):97–101.

77. Alexopoulos P, Grimmer T, Perneczky R, Domes G, Kurz A. Progression to dementia in clinical subtypes of mild cognitive impairment. *Dement Geriatr Cogn Disord* 2006;**22**(1):27–34.

78. Yaffe K, Petersen RC, Lindquist K, Kramer J, Miller B. Subtype of mild cognitive impairment and progression to dementia and death. *Dement Geriatr Cogn Disord* 2006;**22**(4):312–19.

79. Berg L, McKeel DW, Jr., Miller JP, *et al.* Clinicopathologic studies in cognitively healthy aging and Alzheimer's disease: relation of histologic markers to dementia severity, age, sex, and apolipoprotein E genotype. *Arch Neurol* 1998;**55**(3):326–35.

80. Petersen RC. Mild cognitive impairment. *Lancet* 2006;**367**(9527):1979.

Chapter 15

Early clinical features of the parkinsonian-related dementias

Bradley F. Boeve

Introduction

Neurologists are confronted with complex patients in whom accurate diagnoses and improvement of symptoms are expected. One useful strategy is to determine if a patient has a constellation of symptoms and findings that fits within a broad category or syndrome, which then narrows the differential diagnosis and allows the clinician to commence a focused work-up. For example, the differential diagnosis and spectrum of available diagnostic studies for a patient with dementia, or a patient with parkinsonism, are rather wide; these are far more restricted in those who have elements of both dementia and parkinsonism. Furthermore, an insidious onset and progressive course suggests a neurodegenerative disease as the likely underlying process. This scenario is relatively common for community neurologists and very common for behavioral neurology and movement disorder specialists at academic centers.

The primary differential diagnosis in a patient with dementia plus parkinsonism who has experienced an insidious onset and progressive course, in probable decreasing prevalence in the population, includes dementia with Lewy bodies (DLB), Parkinson's disease (PD) with dementia (PDD), progressive supranuclear palsy (PSP), corticobasal syndrome (CBS)/corticobasal degeneration (CBD), and frontotemporal dementia (FTD) with parkinsonism linked to chromosome 17 (FTDP-17). One useful exercise in the clinic is to use the interview and examination to explore the following areas of symptomatology: cognitive/neuropsychological, behavioral/neuropsychiatric, motor/extrapyramidal, sleep, autonomic, sensory and other/miscellaneous features. In typical cases, these clinical features permit relatively easy differentiation (Table 15.1).

Several promising therapies that target amyloid in Alzheimer's disease (AD) – recently shown to be efficacious based on laboratory and animal model studies – are being studied in humans, with encouraging initial results. Researches in basic science continue to make advances along similar lines, targeting α-synuclein, tau, progranulin, TAR DNA-bindings protein and other molecules, with 43 (TDP-43), will lead to testable therapies sometime in the future for the non-AD disorders. These therapies will undoubtedly be studied first in patients with fully expressed DLB, PDD, PSP, CBS/CBD, FTDP-17 and so on, and if shown to be beneficial, testing efficacy in patients with milder features of an evolving neurodegenerative disorder will be the next logical step. It is, therefore, critical for clinicians to work with colleagues in other fields and refine existing technologies to allow identification of individuals with very early disease – preferably before any symptoms are manifest.

What do we know about the very early features of the major parkinsonian dementias? For some, such as DLB and PDD, a large body of literature has evolved on early features, but little is known about the very early features of PSP, CBS/CBD and FTDP-17. The primary goal of this chapter is to review the current knowledge of early manifestations of these disorders. Since it is logical to expect that early manifestations may simply reflect milder changes of what is typically seen in the full-blown illness, the clinical features for each disorder will be reviewed in detail, realizing that similar information on some of these disorders is covered in some of the other chapters in this text.

Lewy body disease: dementia with Lewy bodies and Parkinson's disease with dementia

Both DLB and PDD are clinical syndromes associated with underlying Lewy body disease (LBD) pathology. A critical feature in the pathophysiology of DLB and

The Behavioral Neurology of Dementia, eds. Bruce L. Miller and Bradley F. Boeve. Published by Cambridge University Press.
© Cambridge University Press 2009.

Table 15.1. Comparisons between the major parkinsonian-related dementias

	DLB	PDD	PSP	CBS/CBD	FTDP-17
Demographics					
Age of onset (years)	50–90	50–90	50–90	50–80	30–70
Gender predilection	Males	Males	None	None	None
Family history of dementia and/or parkinsonism	Relatively common	Relatively common	Uncommon	Uncommon	Almost always
Proteinopathy	α-Synuclein	α-Synuclein	tau	tau	Progranulin or tau
Typical clinical features					
Cognitive/neuropsychological features	Executive dysfunction, visuospatial dysfunction	Executive dysfunction, visuospatial dysfunction	Executive dysfunction, language dysfunction	Executive dysfunction, language dysfunction, visuospatial dysfunction	Executive dysfunction, language dysfunction
Behavioral/neuropsychiatric features	Visual hallucinations, depression	Visual hallucinations, depression	Apathy without depression, compulsions/obsessions, utilization/imitation behavior	FTD-like features, compulsions/obsessions, depression, apathy	Behavioral disinhibition, loss of empathy/sympathy, compulsions/rituals/stereotypy, hyperorality/dietary changes, apathy without depression
Motor/extrapyramidal features	Bradykinesia, limb rigidity (often symmetric), tremor (often postural more than at rest and symmetric), postural instability, variable Levodopa responsiveness	Bradykinesia, limb rigidity (often asymmetric), tremor (often at rest more than postural and asymmetric), postural instability, positive Levodopa responsiveness	Bradykinesia, axial greater than limb rigidity, postural instability, lack of Levodopa response	Limb bradykinesia, limb apraxia, limb rigidity, myoclonus, alien limb phenomenon, dystonia, postural instability, lack of Levodopa response	Bradykinesia, axial or limb rigidity, limb apraxia, lack of Levodopa response
Sleep disorders	RBD, hypersomnia	RBD, hypersomnia			Poor sleep efficiency/insomnia
Autonomic features	Orthostatic hypotension, erectile dysfunction, constipation, urinary incontinence	Orthostatic hypotension, erectile dysfunction, constipation, urinary incontinence			Multiple autonomic features in one well-studied family
Sensory features	Anosmia	Anosmia, impaired color vision		Cortical sensory loss	
Other features	Fluctuations in cognition or arousal	Fluctuations in motor functioning	Vertical supranuclear gaze palsy, wide-eyed stare with reduced eyeblink frequency, dysphagia, dysarthria, frontal release signs	Supranuclear gaze palsy, dysphagia, dysarthria, frontal release signs, Balint's phenomenon	

Known or suspected early clinical features

Cognitive/neuropsychological features	MCI: any subtype	MCI: any subtype	MCI-SD executive, MCI-SD language (particularly speech apraxia ± PNFA), MCI-MD non-amnestic	MCI-SD executive, MCI-SD language (particularly speech apraxia ± PNFA), MCI-SD visuospatial, MCI-MD non-amnestic	MCI: any subtype
Behavioral/neuropsychiatric features	Visual hallucinations, delusions (false boarder, infidelity, Capgras), depression, anxiety, apathy	Visual hallucinations, delusions (false boarder, infidelity, Capgras), depression, anxiety, apathy	Apathy without depression		Behavioral disinhibition, loss of empathy/ sympathy, compulsions/ rituals/stereotypy, hyperorality/dietary changes, apathy without depression
Motor/extrapyramidal features	Parkinsonism, particularly postural tremor and symmetric rigidity	Parkinsonism, particularly rest tremor and asymmetric rigidity	Parkinsonism, particularly with axial rigidity, postural instability	Monomelic limb apraxia, monomelic limb rigidity	Parkinsonism
Sleep disorders	RBD, hypersomnia	RBD, hypersomnia			Poor sleep efficiency/ insomnia
Autonomic features	Erectile dysfunction, orthostatic hypotension, constipation	Erectile dysfunction, orthostatic hypotension, constipation			Central autonomic dysfunction
Sensory features	Anosmia, impaired color vision	Anosmia, impaired color vision		Monomelic cortical sensory loss	
Other features	Fluctuations	Fluctuations	Vertical supranuclear gaze palsy, wide-eyed stare with reduced eyeblink frequency		

Notes:
DLB, dementia with Lewy bodies; PDD, Parkinson's disease with dementia; PSP, progressive supranuclear palsy; CBS, corticobasal syndrome; CBD, corticobasal degeneration; FTDP-17, frontotemporal dementia with parkinsonism linked to chromosome 17; MCI, mild cognitive impairment; SD, single domain; MD, multiple domain; PNFA, progressive non-fluent aphasia; RBD, REM sleep-behavior disorder.

PDD is the abnormal accumulation of the protein α-synuclein, which is the major constituent of the Lewy bodies and Lewy neurites that define LBD. The primary distinction between the two syndromes on clinical grounds is the temporal association of dementia and parkinsonism: the term PDD is applied when the onset of dementia is at least 1 year after the onset of parkinsonism, and DLB is applied in any other circumstance (dementia onset within 1 year of parkinsonism onset or dementia onset occurring concurrently or anytime before the onset of parkinsonism). While there is considerable overlap between the two disorders, there do appear to be a few important differences in some aspects. They will, therefore, be considered separate clinical syndromes for purposes of this chapter.

These differences may reflect the degree of coexisting neurodegenerative changes, particularly diffuse and neuritic plaques and neurofibrillary tangles, in the brain. This "Alzheimerization" is thought to be a major contributor to the cognitive features in DLB, overshadowing the motor features. Neuropathologic studies indeed show a much greater tendency for coexisting AD-type changes in DLB compared with PDD,[1–3] which likely explains the greater anterograde memory impairment and lack of cuing benefit in subjects with DLB compared with those with PDD.

Diagnostic criteria for dementia with Lewy bodies

The core clinical features for DLB include the presence of dementia plus the following; one feature is necessary for the label of "clinically possible DLB" and two or more features are needed for the diagnosis of "clinically probable DLB":[4]

- recurrent fully formed visual hallucinations
- spontaneous parkinsonism (i.e. not associated with neuroleptic or antiemetic use)
- fluctuations in cognition or arousal
- REM (rapid eye movement) sleep behavior disorder (RBD).

This list should be qualified. Both RBD and neuroleptic sensitivity are considered suggestive features for the diagnosis of DLB.[4] For practical purposes, since few give test doses of haloperidol or chlorpromazine to determine if neuroleptic sensitivity is present (this practice is obviously marginally ethical as well), but RBD is common in DLB, quite specific for DLB (as opposed to AD and FTD) and not overly challenging to assess, the presence of RBD could be considered

a fourth core feature (these features will be elaborated upon below).[5–7]

Typical clinical features of dementia with Lewy bodies

Cognitive/neuropsychological features

Many patients describe the tendency to lose one's train of thought in the middle of a sentence, which some have termed "verbal blocking;" they typically do not have demonstrable dysarthria (other than hypokinesia), apraxia of speech, or aphasia early in the course. Patients and their caregivers often describe forgetfulness for upcoming appointments and social engagements, losing details of recent events and conversations and tendency to repeat questions, yet on office testing these individuals typically perform better than expected on the delayed recall portions of screening mental status examinations. One observation that many clinicians now appreciate is the relative lack of anosagnosia: these patients are typically bothered by their cognitive symptoms and are seeking treatment on how to improve it, whereas patients with AD typically are not overly bothered by their memory impairment or overtly argue with family members that "my memory is fine!" Geographic disorientation can lead to getting lost while driving, or even struggling to locate the bathroom in one's own home. Visuospatial impairment is often easily demonstrated in the office (e.g. intersecting pentagons, Necker cube). Misidentification errors involving people can occur and are particularly upsetting when patients fail to recognize their own spouses or children. Some believe their own reflection in mirrors is someone other than themselves, sometimes leading to conversations or arguments with the perceived individual. Trouble using the telephone, television remote, microwave and household appliances is a common complaint. Bradyphrenia, easy distractibility and difficulties with multitasking and performing sequential tasks are very common.

Impairment in attention/concentration and executive functioning (henceforth these domains will be considered collectively as aspects of "executive functioning") and visuospatial functioning, with relative preservation in confrontation naming and verbal memory, can be considered the prototypical neuropsychological profile of impairment in DLB.[8] In our experience, there can be considerable variability on formal testing even when the tests are performed hours, weeks or months apart. Memory impairment tends to be mild, but it can be severe in some.[9] In mildly affected patients, a discrepancy between a person's functional abilities (poor performance) and his/her findings on neuropsychological testing (good performance) can be striking, sometimes leading the clinician to a strong suspicion of depression, anxiety, stress or other factors as the underlying cause of their cognitive symptoms.

Behavioral/neuropsychiatric features

A defining feature of DLB is the presence of *visual hallucinations*. These hallucinations are often vivid and well-formed false perceptions of insects, animals or people. The hallucinations can be in black and white or in color, and at times they are frightening. Some patients talk to the perceived people or animals, or attempt to shoo them away. Arguments often ensue when family members attempt to convince patients that the images are not actually there. Many patients recognize that the visual experiences are in fact hallucinations and not actually present, and manage to carry out their daily activities relatively undisrupted. Some describe a tendency to blink hard, or look away for a few seconds and then redirect their gaze back, and the image disappears. Others describe them as comical or even consider them as "friends" of sorts. A REM sleep/wakefulness dysregulation has been proposed as a mechanism underlying visual hallucinations, based on polysomnographic monitoring in patients with PD and psychosis, in which the dream imagery of REM sleep may be invading into wakefulness.[10] A similar mechanism has been proposed to underlie hallucinations associated with DLB.[11,12] If further studies substantiate this mechanism, treatments already known to be efficacious in the management of narcolepsy may prove useful in the management of hallucinations, hypersomnolence and similar phenomena associated with DLB.

Visual illusions can also occur in DLB, in which objects are perceived as something different than they actually are. Some typical examples include perceiving chairs, lamps or mailboxes as people or animals. Delusions are also frequent and typically have a paranoid quality, with examples being beliefs that one's belongings have been stolen or that other people are invading or living in the home (i.e. phantom boarder).[13] One particular delusion can evolve around misidentification errors, in which a person believes that his or her spouse has been replaced by an identical-appearing imposter (i.e. Capgras syndrome).[14] Apathy, depression and anxiety are all very common in DLB. Auditory, tactile or olfactory hallucinations are uncommon. Agitation or aggressive behavior tends to occur late in the illness if at all.

Motor/extrapyramidal features

Spontaneous *parkinsonism* (i.e. unrelated to dopamine antagonist exposure) is also a defining characteristic of DLB.[4] Signs and symptoms include masked facies, stooped posture, shuffling gait, bradykinesia, postural instability, difficulty with fine motor skills, sialorrhea and tremor. While some patients have a unilateral or asymmetric rest tremor, with a "pill-rolling" quality that is typical of PD, most have a mild to moderate postural tremor that is often symmetric. Carbidopa/Levodopa can be beneficial for patients with DLB, but the response is more variable than in typical PD. Dopamine agonists are limited by their tendency to exacerbate delusions and hallucinations. Some patients have a several year history of essential/familial tremor or are diagnosed with this entity months or a few years before the cognitive and neuropsychiatric features become more obvious. Myoclonus occurs in some patients, which can complicate differentiation from Creutzfeldt–Jakob disease if progression occurs over a short period of time.

Sleep disorders

REM sleep-behavior disorder is common in DLB.[7,15] Affected patients seem to "act out their dreams," in which they yell, scream, swear, punch, kick, swing, jump out of bed and so on. The dreams often have a chasing or attacking theme, with the patient attempting to protect himself or herself. When the patient is awakened, the description of the dream tends to match the behaviors that had been exhibited. Injuries to patients and their bed partners can occur. The start of RBD often occurs years or even decades before any cognitive or motor symptoms develop (see below), and RBD is intriguing as it tends to occur in certain disorders (such as DLB, PD, PDD and multiple system atrophy) but not others (such as AD, Pick's disease, PSP, CBS/CBD, FTD).[7,16] Dysfunction in brainstem neuronal networks are believed to underlie RBD.[7]

Many patients with DLB also have excessive daytime somnolence, in which they will struggle to stay awake during the day.[17] Other sleep disorders in DLB include insomnia, obstructive sleep apnea, central sleep apnea, restless legs syndrome, and periodic limb movement in sleep.[17]

The importance of recognizing these sleep disorders cannot be overemphasized. We have evaluated hundreds of patients with DLB over the past several years, and we have yet to meet a single patient who does not have one or more primary sleep disorder. Many have three or four sleep disorders and yet none has been diagnosed and treated. All of these sleep disorders are treatable, and maximal improvement in patient symptomatology tends not to happen until all sleep disorders are adequately treated.

Autonomic features

Orthostatic hypotension, impotence, urinary incontinence and constipation are common in DLB.[18,19] The degree of autonomic dysfunction in DLB appears to be intermediate between PD (relatively mild, at least early in the illness) and multiple system atrophy (relatively severe).[20] Lewy bodies have been found in the intermediolateral column of the spinal cord, and in the neurons/plexi of the heart and gut, reflecting the rather widespread nature of Lewy body pathology in the peripheral and central nervous system.[21] In fact, there is now suspicion that the peripheral nervous system may be affected by LBD prior to involvement of the central nervous system (see below).[22]

Sensory features

The ability to recognize odors as part of formal smell testing has not been studied in detail in DLB, but the scant literature so far certainly suggests anosmia is present in a significant proportion of patients.[23]

Other features

Fluctuations are considered a defining feature of DLB;[4] this phenomenon refers to periods of time when cognition and arousal are near normal, contrasting with other periods of more marked confusion or hypersomnolence. This feature is purposely being considered separately since whether fluctuations represent a cognitive issue, a sleep issue, some other process, or a combination of several processes, remains unclear. Although fluctuations have been difficult to operationalize and measure, tools now exist that differentiate fluctuations associated with DLB from those with other disorders.[24–27] However, the methods for measuring fluctuations have not made their way into routine clinical practice.

Diagnostic criteria for Parkinson's disease with dementia

The consensus criteria for the diagnosis of Parkinson's disease with dementia (PDD) were recently published.[28] A hotly debated issue in the development of these criteria was how to determine and operationalize functional impairment due to *cognitive* impairment as opposed to *motor* impairment. It was ultimately decided that the wording below was most fitting, which gives great discretion to the clinician as this point was not operationalized.

The core clinical features for PDD include the following:[28]

1. Diagnosis of PD according to Queen Square Brain Bank criteria
2. A dementia syndrome with insidious onset and slow progression, developing within the context of established PD and diagnosed by history, clinical and mental examination, defined as:
   - impairment in more than one cognitive domain
   - representing a decline from premorbid level
   - deficits severe enough to impair daily life (social, occupational or personal care), independent of the impairment ascribable to motor or autonomic symptoms.

The terms "probable" and "possible" PDD and their associated specific features are detailed in the paper.[28]

Typical clinical features of Parkinson's disease with dementia

Almost all of the material relating to clinical features in DLB applies similarly to PDD, and therefore this information will not be repeated in detail here; those aspects that differ between DLB and PDD are emphasized below.

Cognitive/neuropsychological features

As noted above, the lack of "Alzheimerization" in brains of most patients with PDD likely explains the relative preservation of anterograde memory functioning and benefit from cuing on memory measures in those with PDD compared with those with DLB.[28] Otherwise, the profile of impairment in attention/concentration, executive functioning and visuospatial functioning is similar between PDD and DLB. The symptoms reported by patients are also similar between the two.

Behavioral/neuropsychiatric features

Recurrent and fully formed visual hallucinations, delusions (often with paranoia or phantom boarder themes), apathy, anxiety and depression are all common in PDD.[28] For reasons that are not clear, Capgras syndrome appears to be very rare in PDD.

Motor/extrapyramidal features

The motor features of typical PD–unilateral or asymmetric rest tremor with a "pill-rolling" quality – along with bradykinesia, rigidity, postural instability and Levodopa responsiveness are typically present for several years prior to the onset of dementia.

Sleep disorders

As in DLB, RBD tends to precede the onset of motor, cognitive and neuropsychiatric features of PD and PDD by many years.[12,29] Hypersomnolence is also common in PDD; in fact, the new Consensus Criteria for PDD includes excessive day-time somnolence as a behavioral feature of the disorder.[28] Recent neuropathologic analyses have revealed hypocretin cell loss in the lateral hypothalamus in patients with PD,[30,31] providing a clear mechanism of how hypersomnolence could be a manifestation of LBD pathology. Sleep fragmentation, insomnia, obstructive sleep apnea, central sleep apnea, restless legs syndrome, periodic limb movement disorder and even overt narcolepsy can occur in PD and PDD.[17,32,33]

Autonomic features

The autonomic features in PDD are similar to those in DLB, although the severity of orthostatic hypotension may be greater. Management of this feature can also be very challenging if aggressive dosing of Levodopa is required to minimize parkinsonism.

Sensory features

Anosmia is common in PD and in PDD.

Other features

Fluctuations in PDD have classically been considered in the motor realm, with motor fluctuations being very frequent and challenging to manage. Fluctuations in cognition and arousal clearly occur in PDD but have not been well studied.

Known or suspected early clinical features in Lewy body disease

While there are certainly some differences between patients with DLB and PDD as noted above, it is likely that their early clinical features will be similar and they will, therefore, be considered collectively.

Cognitive/neuropsychological features

This is the only symptom complex where data on both DLB and PDD (at least mild cognitive impairment [MCI] in PD and DLB) exist.[34,35] The concept of MCI is founded on the idea of a transitional state between normal aging and dementia; in other words, one does not evolve from a normal cognitive state on one day to a demented state the next, but rather this likely evolves over months or years. Numerous analyses have supported the concept and utility of the MCI transitional state from normal aging to AD,[36] and there are growing data supporting the same concept from normal aging to MCI to DLB,[34] and from essentially normal cognition in PD to MCI in PD to PDD.[35] Virtually all of the MCI subtypes can evolve into DLB or PDD.

Behavioral/neuropsychiatric features

It is conceivable that visual hallucinations, delusions, depression, anxiety or apathy in the absence of other neurologic features could be early manifestations of LBD. Isolated visual hallucinations may be particularly concerning for evolving LBD.

Motor/extrapyramidal features

Subtle parkinsonism, even when asymptomatic, is an obvious early feature of LBD.

Sleep disorders

The occurrence of RBD in the absence of any coexisting neurologic symptoms is termed "idiopathic RBD." There now exists considerable data suggesting that idiopathic RBD is an early feature of a synucleinopathy in many individuals, often manifesting years or decades prior to the onset of cognitive or motor changes.[7,12,16,37–39] Among the synucleinopathies, since the syndromes of PD, DLB and PDD associated with LBD pathology are far more common than multiple system atrophy, RBD most likely reflects evolving LBD. Recent studies have demonstrated changes on electroencephalography,[40,41] single-photon emission computed tomography (SPECT),[42–44] positron emission tomography (PET),[45] neuropsychological testing,[46] smell testing,[47] color discrimination,[37] cardiac autonomic activity[48] and more subtle abnormalities on measures of autonomic, motor and gait functioning,[37] also suggesting that a more widespread multisystem neurologic disorder is present; these findings are all suggestive of underlying LBD in most subjects with idiopathic RBD.

Hypersomnia has recently been associated with increased risk of PD,[49] and thus also likely PDD and possibly DLB. Whether hypersomnia is a result of intrinsic changes in the brain such as hypocretinergic cell loss,[30,31] or is caused by one or more other primary sleep disorders will need to be investigated in more detail.

Autonomic features

Erectile dysfunction, orthostatic hypotension, urinary incontinence and constipation are common in DLB and PDD, and are likely to reflect LBD pathology in the interomediolateral spinal cord and peripheral autonomic ganglia. Braak and coworkers have recently suggested that LBD pathology begins in the peripheral nervous system and subsequently involves the spinal cord and brain.[22] If true, one would predict that the autonomic features of erectile dysfunction, orthostatic hypotension, urinary incontinence and constipation would precede the cognitive and motor features of PD, PDD and DLB. Ancillary test findings, particularly using cardiac [^{123}I]-meta-iodobenzylguanidine (MIBG) scintigraphy, are also supporting peripheral autonomic nervous system involvement in LBD.[50] Decreased cardiac MIBG uptake has also been found in those with idiopathic RBD.[51]

Sensory features

Dysnosmia/anosmia has clearly been associated with PD. Regardless of whether this is asymptomatic or symptomatic, abnormalities on smell testing may be present early in the course of PD and hence early in PDD; whether dysnosmia occurs early in the course of DLB has not been well studied. The underlying substrate for dysnosmia is thought to reflect the very early involvement of olfactory structures by LBD.[52]

Impaired color vision has also been identified in early PD, and Lewy bodies may be present in the retina in those with DLB.[53]

Alterations on smell and color vision testing have also been shown in subjects with idiopathic RBD.[37]

Other features

Fluctuations in cognition, arousal and motor functioning could theoretically be an early clinical feature in PD, PDD and DLB, but the lack of operationalization of the concept of "fluctuations" and lack of good measurement tools will make this difficult to study. Using one simple and easy-to-use tool, the frequency of fluctuations was high in DLB, low in AD and almost absent in cognitively normal subjects.[27]

Progressive supranuclear palsy

The classic presentation of PSP is the constellation of vertical supranuclear gaze palsy, postural instability and falls, and parkinsonism.

Diagnostic criteria

The features of the classic presentation form the core for the National Institute of Neurological Disorders and Stroke–Society for Progressive Supranuclear Palsy (NINDS-SPSP) clinical criteria;[54] the following features are required for the diagnosis of probable PSP:

1. Core features:
    *   gradually progressive disorder
    *   onset at age 40 or later
    *   vertical supranuclear palsy and prominent postural instability with falls in the first year of disease onset
    *   no evidence of other diseases that could explain the foregoing features, as indicated by mandatory exclusion criteria.
2. Supportive features:
    *   symmetrical akinesia or rigidity, proximal more than distal
    *   abnormal neck posture, especially retrocollis
    *   poor or absence of response of parkinsonism to Levodopa therapy
    *   early dysphagia and dysarthria
    *   early onset of cognitive impairment including at least two of the following: apathy, impairment in abstract thought, decreased verbal fluency, utilization or imitation behavior, or frontal release signs.
3. Exclusion criteria:
    *   recent history of encephalitis
    *   alien limb syndrome, cortical sensory deficits, focal frontal or temporoparietal atrophy
    *   hallucinations or delusions unrelated to dopaminergic therapy
    *   cortical dementia of Alzheimer type
    *   prominent early cerebellar symptoms or prominent early unexplained dysautonomia
    *   severe, asymmetrical parkinsonian signs
    *   neuroradiological evidence of relevant structural abnormalities
    *   Whipple disease, confirmed by polymerase chain reaction.

Typical clinical features

Cognitive/neuropsychological features

It should be emphasized that although PSP is typically considered a "Parkinson-plus syndrome," cognitive and behavioral changes clearly occur in this disorder, which is reflected in the last bullet point of the supportive criteria.

Signs and symptoms of executive dysfunction are most prominent in PSP. Language dysfunction occurs with some frequency as well, particularly apraxia of speech and non-fluent aphasia.[55,56] The concept of "subcortical dementia" has been applied to those with PSP, in which there is slowing of cognitive processing but "cortical" signs such as amnesia and agnosia are infrequent. Letter fluency (i.e. word generation starting with a letter of the alphabet over a specific time period) and cognitive flexibility tend to be particularly impaired.[57–60] Performance on theory of mind tasks has not been well studied.

Behavioral/neuropsychiatric features
Apathy (typically without other features of depression), compulsions/obsessions and utilization/imitation behavior are the most common behavioral and neuropsychiatric features. In fact, some individuals with PSP present as FTD.[61]

Motor/extrapyramidal features
Some of the qualitative features of parkinsonism are diagnostically relevant, particularly *axial greater than appendicular rigidity*; tendency to walk, turn, and sit en bloc; and marked *postural instability* with frequent falls. Retrocollis occurs with some frequency. While some patients may experience a modest benefit with Levodopa therapy, this is typically transient; most patients derive no benefit from this agent.

Sleep disorders
Sleep has only recently been studied in PSP. Both RBD and hypersomnia can occur in PSP[62] but are far less frequent than in PD, PDD and DLB.[7] When RBD does occur in PSP, it tends to begin concurrently with or after the onset of the other neurologic features.[62]

Autonomic features
No autonomic features have been found to be consistently abnormal in PSP.

Sensory features
No sensory features have been consistently abnormal either.

Other features
The *vertical supranuclear gaze palsy* is characteristic of the disorder and is particularly specific for PSP when downgaze is impaired. Pursuits tend to be saccadic in the vertical and horizontal directions of gaze. A wide-eyed stare with reduced eyeblink frequency is also common. Other features include dysphagia, dysarthria (typically spastic ± hypokinetic) and frontal release signs.

Known or suspected early clinical features
Far less is known about the early clinical features in PSP, CBS/CBD and FTDP-17 compared with PDD and DLB. Yet there are obvious features one would suspect to be early in the course.

Cognitive/neuropsychological features
Since executive functioning and, less frequently, language functioning are most likely impaired in PSP, one would predict that MCI-single domain (executive or language) or MCI-multiple domain without amnesia (executive plus language) would be the presenting cognitive syndromes. At the Mayo Clinic Rochester, USA we have encountered patients, who were later proven by autopsy to have PSP, presenting with each of these MCI syndromes, and also one with amnestic MCI. We have also found that among those who present with progressive apraxia of speech and the progressive non-fluent aphasia syndrome almost all those subsequently studied for pathology have had either PSP or CBD pathology.[55,56]

Behavioral/neuropsychiatric features
One can often elicit a history from caregivers that apathy was a prominent early feature of the illness. Obsessions/compulsions can be an early feature as well.[63]

Motor/extrapyramidal features
Parkinsonism with prominent axial rigidity, retrocollis and postural instability with frequent falls would be obvious early motor features, although this has not been studied in great detail.

Other features
Vertical supranuclear gaze palsy and a wide-eyed stare with reduced eyeblink frequency are obvious early ophthalmologic features.

Corticobasal syndrome and corticobasal degeneration
The core clinical features that have been considered characteristic of CBD include progressive asymmetric rigidity and apraxia, with other findings suggesting additional cortical (e.g. alien limb phenomena, cortical sensory loss, myoclonus, mirror movements) and basal ganglionic (e.g. bradykinesia, dystonia, tremor) dysfunction.[64–66] The asymmetry of the findings is key,

and some patients have elements of both rigidity and spasticity in the affected limbs.

Because of the considerable clinicopathologic heterogeneity between those clinically and pathologically diagnosed with CBD,[67,68] some have suggested that the term corticobasal syndrome should be used to describe the constellation of features thought to be most characteristic of CBD.[65]

Diagnostic criteria for CBS

One set of proposed diagnostic criteria for the diagnosis of CBS is shown below.[65]

1. Core features:
   - insidious onset and progressive course
   - no identifiable cause (e.g. tumor, infarct)
   - cortical dysfunction as reflected by at least one of the following:
     - focal or asymmetric ideomotor apraxia
     - alien limb phenomenon
     - cortical sensory loss
     - visual or sensory hemineglect
     - constructional apraxia
     - focal or asymmetric myoclonus
     - apraxia of speech/nonfluent aphasia
   - extrapyramidal dysfunction as reflected by at least one of the following:
     - focal or asymmetric appendicular rigidity lacking prominent and sustained Levodopa response
     - focal or asymmetric appendicular dystonia.
2. Supportive investigations:
   - variable degrees of focal or lateralized cognitive dysfunction, with relative preservation of learning and memory, on neuropsychometric testing
   - focal or asymmetric atrophy on computed tomography or magnetic resonance imaging, typically maximal in parietofrontal cortex
   - focal or asymmetric hypoperfusion on SPECT and hypometabolism on PET, typically maximal in parietofrontal cortex ± basal ganglia ± thalamus

Typical clinical features

Cognitive/neuropsychological features

The cognitive and neuropsychological features of CBS are highly variable: some have no significant cognitive symptoms (other than those related to *apraxia*) nor any impairment on formal neuropsychological testing, while others have a significant dementia syndrome with deficits in many cognitive domains. The cognitive and neuropsychological profiles also depend on the maximally affected cerebral hemisphere and the degree to which the frontal, temporal, parietal and, in some cases, occipital lobes are involved. Yet the fronto-subcortical and parietal neural networks are most consistently affected and, therefore, the domains of executive functioning, language, praxis and visuospatial functioning are most frequently impaired.[59,66,69] As in PSP, apraxia of speech and non-fluent aphasia can occur.[55,56,66,70]

Behavioral/neuropsychiatric features

In one series of patients with CBS, 35% exhibited prominent behavioral/neuropsychiatric features during the course of their illness.[71] Three behavioral syndromes were noted: frontal-lobe syndrome, depression and obsessive–compulsive behavior. These same behavioral syndromes were noted in 22% of 36 patients with pathologically proven CBD, with none experiencing complex visual hallucinations.[72] Thus, FTD-like features, depression and obsessive–compulsive features occur with some frequency in CBS/CBD, but visual hallucinations appear to be very rare.

Motor/extrapyramidal features

The motor and extrapyramidal features in CBS tend to dominate the clinical symptomatology, often causing considerable disability. The features are either unilateral or markedly asymmetric, with *limb bradykinesia*, *apraxia* and *rigidity* being most consistent. More variable degrees of myoclonus, alien limb phenomenon and dystonia can occur. The features tend to be minimally responsive or entirely unresponsive to Levodopa.

Sleep disorders

Sleep has received very little attention in CBS.

Autonomic features

No autonomic features have been found to be consistently abnormal in CBS.

Sensory features

Cortical sensory loss is relatively common in CBS; the resulting pseudoathetosis can add to the alien limb-like features. In very rare instances, a central pain syndrome can evolve that is highly resistant to pharmacotherapy.

Other features

A vertical supranuclear gaze palsy can occur in CBS, as can a wide-eyed stare with reduced eyeblink frequency. Other features include dysphagia, dysarthria (typically spastic ± hypokinetic), postural instability and frontal release signs. Balint's syndrome is relatively uncommon.

Known or suspected early clinical features

Cognitive/neuropsychological features

Since executive functioning, language and visuospatial functioning are the domains most frequently affected in CBS, one would predict that MCI-single domain (executive functioning, language or visuospatial functioning) or MCI-multiple domain without amnesia would be the presenting cognitive syndromes. As noted above, almost all those presenting with apraxia of speech and the progressive non-fluent aphasia syndrome have had either PSP or CBD pathology.[55,56]

Behavioral/neuropsychiatric features

One would predict that one or more of the features reported in the full CBS – FTD-like features, depression, and features of obsessive–compulsive disorder – could be the presenting behavioral/neuropsychiatric manifestations, but so few cases have been well characterized that this remains only speculative.

Motor/extrapyramidal features

Monomelic apraxia or rigidity could certainly be the most common presenting feature in CBS.

Sensory features

Monomelic cortical sensory loss could be the presenting feature in some with CBS. At the Mayo Clinic, several patients we have followed underwent carpal tunnel release surgery for their early complaints of hand paresthesiae (such surgery had no beneficial effect on the paresthesiae in any patient).

Frontotemporal dementia with parkinsonism linked to chromosome 17

The diagnosis of FTDP-17 is applied to those individuals who have both FTD and/or parkinsonism plus linkage to a genetic alteration on chromosome 17 or an identified mutation on chromosome 17. Mutations in either of two genes that are in close proximity to

each other on chromosome 17 have been associated with FTDP-17: genes for microtubule-associated protein tau (*MAPT*)[73] and progranulin (*PGRN*).[74]

Typical clinical features

For those with FTDP-17 associated with mutations in *MAPT* (abbreviated as FTDP-17*MAPT*) (summarized from data and references 75 and 76), the typical age of onset is between 30 and 60, and penetrance appears to be close to 100%. The duration of symptoms from onset to death is typically 3–10 years. Symptomatology usually involves executive dysfunction and altered personality and behavior, with aphasia and parkinsonism evolving in many. Memory impairment occurs less frequently, and visuospatial impairment and limb apraxia are quite rare. Features of motor neuron disease are also infrequent. Tau-positive inclusions in neurons (e.g. neurofibrillary tangles, neuronal threads, Pick bodies) and/or glia (e.g. astrocytic plaques, oligodendroglial coiled bodies) are always present on histologic examination, sometimes accompanied by argyrophilic grains.

For those with FTDP-17 associated with mutations in *PGRN* (abbreviated as FTDP-17*PGRN*) (summarized from data in references 77–86), the typical age of onset is between 45 and 85, and the duration of disease varies from 1 to 13 years. The frequency of mutations in *PGRN* in FTD series is similar to that in *MAPT*.[80] The mode of inheritance follows an autosomal dominant pattern with a high but age-dependent penetrance (90% develop symptoms by age 70).[80] The clinical features have been more variable than in *MAPT* carriers, with not only behavioral and cognitive features commonly present, but also memory impairment, limb apraxia, parkinsonism and visuospatial dysfunction. CBS has also been particularly frequent in the cases reported thus far. No *PGRN* mutation carrier has been reported to date with an amyotrophic lateral sclerosis phenotype. Upon histologic examination, the consistent finding is frontotemporal lobar degeneration (FTLD) with ubiquitin-positive inclusions (FTLD-U); such inclusions are often referred to as "neuronal intranuclear inclusions".[74,78–80,82–86] Immunostaining directed against progranulin stain normal structures and not the ubiquitinated protein that is presumed to be pathogenic; rather, TDP-43 was recently discovered to be the ubiquitinated protein in FTLD-U, FTLD with motor neuron disease and in those with clinical amyotrophic lateral sclerosis.[87]

207

Known or suspected early clinical features

Since mutations in *MAPT* were first reported in 1998, thereby preceding the discovery of mutations in *PGRN* by 8 years, there is far more knowledge about the early clinical features in FTDP-17*MAPT* than FTDP-17*PGRN*. Yet the greater tendency for parietal lobe involvement as well as parkinsonism in FTDP-17 *PGRN* suggests that the very early clinical features may be slightly different between the two proteinopathies.

Cognitive/neuropsychological features

Considering that almost every conceivable cognitive and behavioral syndrome has been associated with mutations in *MAPT* and *PGRN*, one would predict that any of the MCI subtypes could be manifested. Changes on neuropsychological testing (particularly verbal fluency and executive functioning) have been found in asymptomatic *MAPT* mutation carriers, along with changes on brain MRI and PET.[88–90] Impairment in theory-of-mind tasks would certainly be predicted as an early cognitive/neuropsychological feature; there are no published data on this line of research yet, but this is ripe for further study.

Behavioral/neuropsychiatric features

There is a large body of evidence that changes in insight, motivation, social cognition (with resulting disinhibition and loss of empathy/sympathy), sense of morality, food preferences, artistic appreciation and expression, religious affiliation and other behavioral/neuropsychiatric aspects of human existence are affected in FTD.[91–96] Changes on the Neuropsychiatric Inventory (NPI) are also well known in early FTD. There are remarkably few published data on these critical issues in early FTDP-17, and one would predict that changes in behavior may precede the expression of overt cognitive impairment in many individuals with mutations in *MAPT* and *PGRN*. Longitudinal clinical, behavioral/neuropsychiatric and neuroimaging studies in asymptomatic *MAPT* and *PGRN* carriers may provide key insights into the earliest changes in FTD as well as allow elucidation of important brain–behavior relationships.

Motor/extrapyramidal features

Among the mutations in *MAPT*, the N279K mutant is associated with pallido-ponto-nigral degeneration (PPND), and particularly with parkinsonism, and the motor features tend to overshadow the other features among affected relatives. While asymptomatic parkinsonism has not been appreciated in genealogically

at-risk members of a PPND-affected family, myoclonus has.[97] Dystonia is common in this family as well. In most other mutations in *MAPT*, parkinsonism tends to evolve later in the course if at all (an example of longitudinal evolution of parkinsonism in FTDP-17 associated with the *MAPT* mutation leading to S305N is shown by Boeve *et al.*[98]).

Parkinsonism clearly occurs in some affected individuals with *PGRN* mutations, but it is too early to discern if parkinsonism is a prominent early feature associated with specific mutations.

Sleep disorders

The only analyses of sleep published so far in FTDP-17 involved members of the PPND family,[97,99] in which non-REM sleep initiation and maintenance were disrupted in all affected subjects. Severe insomnia was noted in two with the most advanced disorder. Poor sleep efficiency was observed in one subject, who later became symptomatic. Periodic leg movements were increased in three affected subjects. There was no evidence of REM sleep without atonia or RBD, nor any evidence of excessive day-time somnolence. Based on these findings, one could predict that changes in sleep efficiency/maintenance may occur in FTDP-17, but the specificity for this finding in genealogically at-risk individuals remains to be seen. Day-time hypersomnolence and RBD may be very infrequent in the N279K mutant. Additional poly-somnography and multiple sleep latency testing data are needed in other kindreds with *MAPT* mutations to determine the generalizability of these findings. Sleep studies in FTDP-17 associated with *PGRN* mutations have yet to be done.

Autonomic features

Among families with FTDP-17, autonomic functioning has only been studied in the PPND kindred.[97,100] Symptoms included hyperhidrosis, sialorrhea, urinary frequency or incontinence, thermal intolerance, male sexual dysfunction, lacrimation and dryness of the eyes or mouth. None had orthostatic hypotension. Autonomic testing revealed mild to moderate abnormalities in all five affected subjects and minor abnormalities in three asymptomatic at-risk subjects. Findings in affected subjects consisted of preganglionic sudomotor dysfunction in all five, impaired cardiovagal function in three and reduced or absent pupillary near responses in four. Tests of adrenergic function were normal in all subjects. These findings suggest dysfunction in the central autonomic network.

Autonomic studies in FTDP-17 associated with *PGRN* mutations have yet to be done.

Sensory features

Again, only the PPND family has been well studied, and there was no electrophysiologic evidence of peripheral nerve involvement or slowing in central sensory pathways.[101]

Summary

There is clearly more work needed to further characterize the early features of the parkinsonian dementias. A comprehensive approach similar to that of Wszolek and colleagues[101] have performed in the large PPND kindred would be wise in asymptomatic genealogically at-risk individuals with various mutations, particularly if studies are performed longitudinally. The sleep, smell and autonomic changes in evolving LBD likely precede the changes in cognitive and motor functioning. The rarity and difficulties with early diagnosis in PSP and CBS will make characterization of the early features of these disorders challenging.

Acknowledgements

Dr. Boeve is supported by grants P50 AG16574, UO1 AG06786, RO1 AG15866, RO1 AG23195, P50 NS40256, the Alzheimer's Association, and the Robert H. and Clarice Smith and Abigail Van Buren Alzheimer's Disease Research Program of the Mayo Foundation.

References

1. Dickson D. Dementia with Lewy bodies: neuropathology. *J Geriatr Psychiatr Neurol.* 2002;**15**:210–216.

2. Apaydin H, Ahlskog J, Parisi J *et al.* Parkinson's disease neuropathology: later-developing dementia and loss of the Levodopa response. *Arch Neurol.* 2002;**59**:102–112.

3. Tsuboi Y, Dickson D. Dementia with Lewy bodies and Parkinson's disease with dementia: are they different? *Park Relat Disord.* 2005;**11**:S47–S51.

4. McKeith I, Dickson D, Lowe J *et al.* Dementia with Lewy bodies: diagnosis and management: Third report of the DLB Consortium. *Neurology.* 2005;**65**:1863–1872.

5. Knopman D, Boeve B, Petersen R. Essentials of the proper diagnosis of mild cognitive impairment, dementia, and major subtypes of dementia. *Mayo Clin Proc.* 2003;**78**:1290–1308.

6. Boeve B. Dementia with Lewy Bodies. In Petersen R (ed.) *Continuum*, Vol. 10. Minneapolis: American Academy of Neurology, 2004:81–112.

7. Boeve B, Silber M, Saper C *et al.* Pathophysiology of REM sleep behavior disorder and relevance to neurodegenerative disease. *Brain.* 2007;**130**: 2770–2788.

8. Ferman T, Smith G, Boeve B *et al.* Neuropsychological differentiation of dementia with Lewy bodies from normal aging and Alzheimer's disease. *Clin Neuropsychol.* 2006;**20**:623–636.

9. Simard M, van Reekum R, Cohen T. A review of the cognitive and behavioral symptoms in dementia with Lewy bodies. *J Neuropsychiatr Clin Neurosci.* 2000;**12**:425–450.

10. Arnulf I, Bonnet AM, Damier P *et al.* Hallucinations, REM sleep, and Parkinson's disease: a medical hypothesis. *Neurology.* 2000;**55**:281–288.

11. Boeve B, Silber M, Parisi J *et al.* Neuropathologic findings in patients with REM sleep behavior disorder and a neurodegenerative disorder. *Neurology.* 2001; **56**:A299.

12. Boeve B, Silber M, Ferman T *et al.* REM sleep behavior disorder in Parkinson's disease, dementia with Lewy bodies, and multiple system atrophy. In Bedard M, Agid Y, Chouinard S *et al.* (eds.) *Mental and Behavioral Dysfunction in Movement Disorders.* Totowa, NJ: Humana Press, 2003:383–397.

13. Aarsland D, Ballard C, Larsen J, McKeith I. A comparative study of psychiatric symptoms in dementia with Lewy bodies and Parkinson's disease with and without dementia. *Int J Geriatr Psychiatry.* 2001;**16**:528–536.

14. Marantz A, Verghese J. Capgras' syndrome in dementia with Lewy bodies. *J Geriatr Psychiatr Neurol.* 2002;**15**:239–241.

15. Boeve B, Silber M, Ferman T *et al.* Association of REM sleep behavior disorder and neurodegenerative disease. *Sleep.* 1999;**22**(Suppl 1):S72.

16. Boeve B, Silber M, Ferman T *et al.* Association of REM sleep behavior disorder and neurodegenerative disease may reflect an underlying synucleinopathy. *Mov Disord.* 2001;**16**:622–630.

17. Boeve B, Silber M, Ferman T. Current management of sleep disturbances in dementia. *Cur Neurol Neurosci Rep.* 2001;**2**:169–177.

18. Ballard C, Shaw F, McKeith I, Kenny R. High prevalence of neurovascular instability in neurodegenerative dementias. *Neurology.* 1998;**51**:1760–1762.

19. Hishikawa N, Hashizume Y, Yoshida M, Sobue G. Clinical and neuropathological correlates of Lewy body disease. *Acta Neuropathol (Berl).* 2003;**105**:341–350.

20. Thaisetthawatkul P, Boeve B, Benarroch E *et al.* Autonomic dysfunction in dementia with Lewy bodies. *Neurology.* 2004;**62**:1804–1809.

21. Pakiam AS, Bergeron C, Lang AE. Diffuse Lewy body disease presenting as multiple system atrophy. *Can J Neurol Sci.* 1999;**26**:127–131.

209

22. Hawkes C, Del Tredici K, Braak H. Parkinson's disease: a dual-hit hypothesis. *Neuropathol Appl Neurobiol.* 2007;**33**:599–614.

23. Walker Z, Stevens T. Dementia with Lewy bodies: clinical characteristics and diagnostic criteria. *J Geriatr Psychiatry Neurol.* 2002;**15**:188–194.

24. Walker M, Ayre G, Cummings J *et al.* The Clinician Assessment of Fluctuation and the One Day Fluctuation Assessment Scale. Two methods to assess fluctuating confusion in dementia. *Br J Psychiatry.* 2000; **177**:252–256.

25. Walker M, Ayre G, Cummings J *et al.* Quantifying fluctuation in dementia with Lewy bodies, Alzheimer's disease, and vascular dementia. *Neurology.* 2000; **54**:1616–1625.

26. Walker M, Ayre G, Perry E *et al.* Quantification and characterization of fluctuating cognition in dementia with Lewy bodies and Alzheimer's disease. *Dem Geriatr Cog Disord.* 2000;**11**:327–335.

27. Ferman T, Smith G, Boeve B *et al.* DLB fluctuations: specific features that reliably differentiate DLB from AD and normal aging. *Neurology.* 2004;**62**:181–187.

28. Emre M, Aarsland D, Brown R *et al.* Clinical diagnostic criteria for dementia associated with Parkinson's disease. *Mov Disord.* 2007;**22**:1689–1707.

29. Gjerstad M, Boeve B, Wentzel-Larsen T *et al.* Occurrence and clinical correlates of REM sleep behavior disorder in patients with Parkinson's disease over time. *J Neurol Neurosurg Psychiatry.* 2008; **79**(4); 387–391.

30. Fronczek R, Overeem S, Lee S *et al.* Hypocretin (orexin) loss in Parkinson's disease. *Brain.* 2007;**130**:1577–1585.

31. Thannickal T, Lai Y, Siegel J. Hypocretin (orexin) cell loss in Parkinson's disease. *Brain.* 2007;**130**:1586–1595.

32. Boeve B, Silber M, Ferman T. REM sleep behavior disorder in Parkinson's disease and dementia with Lewy bodies. *J Ger Psychiatr Neurol.* 2004;**17**:146–157.

33. Boeve B, Silber M. Sleep Disturbances in Parkinson's disease. In Martine R, Duda J (eds.) *Parkinson Disease: Mind, Mood, and Memory.* Miami, FL: National Parkinson Foundation, 2005:54–71.

34. Boeve B, Ferman T, Smith G *et al.* Mild cognitive impairment preceding dementia with Lewy bodies. *Neurology.* 2004;**62**:A86–A87.

35. Caviness J, Driver-Dunckley E, Connor D *et al.* Defining mild cognitive impairment in Parkinson's disease. *Mov Disord.* 2007;**22**:1272–1277.

36. Petersen R. Mild cognitive impairment as a diagnostic entity. *J Intern Med.* 2004;**256**:183–194.

37. Postuma R, Lang A, Massicotte-Marquez J, Montplaisir J. Potential early markers of Parkinson disease in idiopathic REM sleep behavior disorder. *Neurology.* 2006;**66**:845–851.

38. Boeve B, Saper C. REM sleep behavior disorder: a possible early marker for synucleinopathies. *Neurology.* 2006;**66**:796–797.

39. Boeve B, Dickson D, Olson E *et al.* Insights into REM sleep behavior disorder pathophysiology in brainstem-predominant Lewy body disease. *Sleep Med* 2007; **8**:60–64.

40. Fantini ML, Gagnon JF, Petit D *et al.* Slowing of electroencephalogram in rapid eye movement sleep behavior disorder. *Ann Neurol.* 2003;**53**:774–780.

41. Massicotte-Marquez J, Carrier J, Decary A *et al.* Slow-wave sleep and delta power in rapid eye movement sleep behavior disorder. *Ann Neurol.* 2005;**57**:277–282.

42. Eisensehr I, Linke R, Noachtar S *et al.* Reduced striatal dopamine transporters in idiopathic rapid eye movement sleep behavior disorder: comparison with Parkinson's disease and controls. *Brain.* 2000; **123**:1155–1160.

43. Eisensehr I, Linke R, Tatsch K *et al.* Increased muscle activity during rapid eye movement sleep correlates with decrease of striatal presynaptic dopamine transporters. IPT and IBZM SPECT imaging in subclinical and clinically manifest idiopathic REM sleep behavior disorder, Parkinson's disease, and controls. *Sleep.* 2003;**26**:507–512.

44. Mazza S, Soucy J, Gravel P *et al.* Assessing whole brain perfusion changes in REM sleep behavior disorder. *Neurology.* 2006;**67**:1618–1622.

45. Caselli R, Chen K, Bandy D *et al.* A preliminary fluorodeoxyglucose positron emission tomography study in healthy adults reporting dream-enactment behavior. *Sleep.* 2006;**29**:927–933.

46. Ferini-Strambi L, Di Gioia M, Castronovo V *et al.* Neuropsychological assessment in idiopathic REM sleep behavior disorder (RBD): does the idiopathic form of RBD really exist? *Neurology.* 2004;**62**:41–45.

47. Stiasny-Kolster K, Doerr Y, Möller J *et al.* Combination of "idiopathic" REM sleep behavior disorder and olfactory dysfunction as possible indicator for α-synucleinopathy demonstrated by dopamine transporter FP-CIT-SPECT. *Brain.* 2005; **128**:126–137.

48. Ferini-Strambi L, Oldani A, Zucconi M, Smirne S. Cardiac autonomic activity during wakefulness and sleep in REM sleep behavior disorder. *Sleep.* 1996;**19**:367–369.

49. Abbott R, Ross G, White L *et al.* Excessive daytime sleepiness and subsequent development of Parkinson disease. *Neurology.* 2005;**65**:1442–1446.

50. Oka H, Yoshioka M, Morita M *et al.* Reduced cardiac ^{123}I-MIBG uptake reflects cardiac sympathetic dysfunction in Lewy body disease. *Neurology.* 2007;**69**:1460–1465.

51. Miyamoto T, Miyamoto M, Inoue Y *et al.* Reduced cardiac ^{123}I-MIBG scintigraphy in idiopathic REM sleep behavior disorder. *Neurology.* 2006;**67**: 2236–2238.

52. Braak H, Ghebremedhin E, Rub U *et al.* Stages in the development of Parkinson's disease-related pathology. *Cell Tissue Res.* 2004;**318**:121–134.

53. Maurage C, Ruchoux M, de Vos R *et al.* Retinal involvement in dementia with Lewy bodies: a clue to hallucinations? *Ann Neurol.* 2003;**54**:542–547.

54. Litvan I, Agid Y, Calne D *et al.* Clinical research criteria for the diagnosis of progressive supranuclear palsy (Steele–Richardson–Olszewski syndrome): report of the NINDS–SPSP International Workshop. *Neurology.* 1996;**47**:1–9.

55. Josephs K, Duffy J, Strand E *et al.* Clinicopathological and imaging correlates of progressive aphasia and apraxia of speech. *Brain.* 2006;**129**:1385–1398.

56. Josephs K, Boeve B, Duffy J *et al.* Atypical progressive supranuclear palsy underlying progressive apraxia of speech and nonfluent aphasia. *Neurocase.* 2005; **11**:283–296.

57. Dubois B, Pillon B, Legault F *et al.* Slowing of cognitive processing in progressive supranuclear palsy. A comparison with Parkinson's disease. *Arch Neurol.* 1988;**45**:1194–1199.

58. Pillon B, Deweer B, Michon A *et al.* Are explicit memory disorders of progressive supranuclear palsy related to damage to striatofrontal circuits? Comparison with Alzheimer's, Parkinson's, and Huntington's diseases. *Neurology.* 1994;**44**:1264–1270.

59. Pillon B, Blin J, Vidailhet M *et al.* The neuropsychological pattern of corticobasal degeneration: comparison with progressive supranuclear palsy and Alzheimer's disease. *Neurology.* 1995;**45**:1477–1483.

60. Bak T, Crawford L, Hearn V *et al.* Subcortical dementia revisited: similarities and differences in cognitive function between progressive supranuclear palsy (PSP), corticobasal degeneration (CBD) and multiple system atrophy (MSA). *Neurocase.* 2005;**11**:268–273.

61. Rippon G, Boeve B, Parisi J *et al.* Late-onset frontotemporal dementia associated with progressive supranuclear palsy/argyrophilic grain disease/ Alzheimer's disease pathology. *Neurocase.* 2005; **11**:204–211.

62. Arnulf I, Merino-Andreu M, Bloch F *et al.* REM sleep behavior disorder and REM sleep without atonia in patients with progressive supranuclear palsy. *Sleep.* 2005;**28**:349–354.

63. Karnik N, D'Apuzzo M, Greicius M. Non-fluent progressive aphasia, depression, and OCD in a woman with progressive supranuclear palsy: neuroanatomical and neuropathological correlations. *Neurocase.* 2006;**12**:332–338.

64. Boeve B. Corticobasal degeneration. In Adler C, Ahlskog J (eds.) *Parkinson's Disease and Movement Disorders: Diagnosis and Treatment Guidelines for the Practicing Physician.* Totawa, NJ: Human Press, 2000:253–261.

65. Boeve B, Lang A, Litvan I. Corticobasal degeneration and its relationship to progressive supranuclear palsy and frontotemporal dementia. *Ann Neurol.* 2003; **54**:S15–S19.

66. Boeve B. Corticobasal degeneration: the syndrome and the disease. In Litvan I (ed.) *Atypical Parkinsonian Disorders.* Totawa, NJ: Humana Press, 2005:309–334.

67. Schneider J, Watts R, Gearing M *et al.* Corticobasal degeneration: neuropathologic and clinical heterogeneity. *Neurology.* 1997;**48**:959–969.

68. Boeve BF, Maraganore DM, Parisi JE *et al.* Pathologic heterogeneity in clinically diagnosed corticobasal degeneration. *Neurology.* 1999;**53**:795–800.

69. Massman P, Kreiter K, Jankovic J, Doody R. Neuropsychological functioning in cortical-basal ganglionic degeneration: differentiation from Alzheimer's disease. *Neurology.* 1996;**46**:720–726.

70. Lehman M, Duffy J, Boeve B *et al.* Speech and language disorders associated with corticobasal degeneration. *J Med Speech-Lang Pathol.* 2003;**11**:131–146.

71. Cummings J, Litvan I. Neuropsychiatric aspects of corticobasal degeneration. In Litvan I, Goetz C, Lang A (eds.) *Corticobasal Degeneration and Related Disorders,* Vol. 82. London: Lippincott, Williams & Wilkins, 2000:147–152.

72. Geda Y, Boeve B, Negash S *et al.* Neuropsychiatric features in 36 pathologically confirmed cases of corticobasal degeneration. *J Neuropsychiatry Clin Neurosci.* 2007;**19**:77–80.

73. Hutton M, Lendon CL, Rizzu P *et al.* Association of missense and 5′-splice-site mutations in tau with the inherited dementia FTDP-17. *Nature.* 1998;**393**:702–705.

74. Baker M, Mackenzie I, Pickering-Brown S *et al.* Mutations in progranulin cause tau-negative frontotemporal dementia linked to chromosome 17. *Nature.* 2006;**442**:916–919.

75. Poorkaj P, Grossman M, Steinbart E *et al.* Frequency of tau gene mutations in familial and sporadic cases of non-Alzheimer dementia. *Arch Neurol.* 2001;**58**: 383–387.

76. Microtubule-associated protein tau; MAPT http://www. ncbi.nlm.nih.gov/entrez/dispomim.cgi?id=157140.

77. Benussi L, Binetti G, Sina E *et al.* A novel deletion in progranulin gene is associated with FTDP-17 and CBS. *Neurobiol Aging* 2008;**29**:427–435.

78. Boeve B, Baker M, Dickson D *et al.* Frontotemporal dementia and parkinsonism associated with the IVS1+1G→A mutation in progranulin: a clinicopathologic study. *Brain.* 2006;**129**:3103–3114.

211

79. Cruts M, Gijselinck I, van der Zee J et al. Null mutations in progranulin cause ubiquitin positive frontotemporal dementia linked to chromosome 17q21. Nature. 2006;442:920–924.

80. Gass J, Cannon A, Mackenzie I et al. Mutations in progranulin are a major cause of ubiquitin-positive frontotemporal lobar degeneration. Hum Mol Genet. 2006;15:2988–3001.

81. Huey ED, Grafman J, Wassermann EM et al. Characteristics of frontotemporal dementia patients with a progranulin mutation. Ann Neurol. 2006;60: 374–380.

82. Mackenzie I, Baker M, Pickering-Brown S et al. The neuropathology of frontotemporal lobar degeneration caused by mutations in the progranulin gene. Brain. 2006;129:3081–3090.

83. Masellis M, Momeni P, Meschino W et al. Novel splicing mutation in the progranulin gene causing familial corticobasal syndrome. Brain. 2006; 129:3115–3123.

84. Mukherjee O, Pastor P, Cairns NJ et al. HDDD2 is a familial frontotemporal lobar degeneration with ubiquitin-positive, tau-negative inclusions caused by a missense mutation in the signal peptide of progranulin. Ann Neurol. 2006;60:314–322.

85. Pickering-Brown S, Baker M, Gass J et al. Mutations in progranulin explain atypical phenotypes with variants in MAPT. Brain. 2006;129:3124–3126.

86. Snowden J, Pickering-Brown S, Mackenzie I et al. Progranulin gene mutations associated with frontotemporal dementia and progressive non-fluent aphasia. Brain. 2006;129:3091–3102.

87. Neumann M, Sampathu D, Kwong L et al. Ubiquitinated TDP-43 in frontotemporal lobar degeneration and amyotrophic lateral sclerosis. Science. 2006;314:130–133.

88. Geschwind DH, Robidoux J, Alarcon M et al. Dementia and neurodevelopmental predisposition: cognitive dysfunction in presymptomatic subjects precedes dementia by decades in frontotemporal dementia. Ann Neurol. 2001;50:741–746.

89. Ferman TJ, McRae CA, Arvanitakis Z et al. Early and pre-symptomatic neuropsychological dysfunction in the PPND family with the N279K tau mutation. Park Relat Disord. 2003;9:265–270.

90. Frank A, Wszolek Z, Jack CR J, Boeve B. Distinctive MRI findings in pallido-ponto-nigral degeneration (PPND). Neurology. 2007;68:620–621.

91. Miller BL, Boone K, Cummings JL et al. Functional correlates of musical and visual ability in frontotemporal dementia. Br J Psychiatry. 2000;176:458–463.

92. Miller BL, Seeley WW, Mychack P et al. Neuroanatomy of the self: evidence from patients with frontotemporal dementia. Neurology. 2001;57:817–821.

93. Miller BL, Diehl J, Freedman M et al. International approaches to frontotemporal dementia diagnosis: from social cognition to neuropsychology. Ann Neurol. 2003;54:S7–S10.

94. Rankin KP, Kramer JH, Mychack P, Miller BL. Double dissociation of social functioning in frontotemporal dementia. Neurology. 2003;60:266–271.

95. Hodges JR. Frontotemporal dementia (Pick's disease): clinical features and assessment. Neurology. 2001; 56:S6–S10.

96. Woolley J, Gorno-Tempini M, Seeley W et al. Binge eating is associated with right orbitofrontal-insular-striatal atrophy in frontotemporal dementia. Neurology. 2007;69:1424–1433.

97. Arvanitakis Z, Witte R, Dickson D et al. Clinical–pathologic study of biomarkers in FTDP-17 (PPND family with N279K tau mutation). Park Relat Disord. 2007;13:230–239.

98. Boeve B, Tremont-Lukats I, Waclawik A et al. Longitudinal characterization of two siblings with frontotemporal dementia and parkinsonism linked to chromosome 17 associated with the S305N tau mutation. Brain. 2005;128:752–772.

99. Boeve B, Lin S-C, Strongosky A et al. Absence of REM sleep behavior disorder in eleven members of the PPND kindred. Arch Neurol. 2006;63:268–272.

100. Cheshire WP, Tsuboi Y, Wszolek ZK. Physiologic assessment of autonomic dysfunction in pallidopontonigral degeneration with N279K mutation in the tau gene on chromosome 17. Autonom Neurosci Basic Clin. 2002;102:71–77.

101. Wszolek ZK, Lagerlund TD, Steg RE, McManis PG. Clinical neurophysiologic findings in patients with rapidly progressive familial parkinsonism and dementia with pallido-ponto-nigral degeneration. Electroenceph Clin Neurophysiol. 1998;107:213–222.

Chapter 16

Dementia treatment

Bradley F. Boeve and Adam L. Boxer

Introduction

There is reason for optimism about future treatment of the most common causes of dementia. Advances in understanding the molecular pathologies that underlie the most common causes of neurodegenerative dementia are rapidly being translated into new treatments. At the same time, basic investigations into the neurophysiology of synaptic transmission, neuronal growth, development and survival have identified new receptors, genes and intracellular second messenger cascades that may serve as targets for new treatments for dementia. Whereas most currently approved medications that are used to treat dementia are effective only in ameliorating the symptoms of disease, in the near future, medications that modify the course of the disease by protecting the brain from dementia-related pathology may be available. New diagnostic tests will also help to identify accurately who is likely to benefit from such treatment and monitor their treatment response. This chapter will review the currently available treatments for the most common forms of dementia, focusing on clinical syndromes that are readily identifiable by practicing clinicians, as well as new treatments that are currently under investigation or new avenues for treatment suggested by recent advances in understanding the molecular pathologies of these disorders.

Background

Alzheimer's disease (AD) is the most common cause of dementia. Multi-infarct dementia, classically thought to be the second-most common untreatable cause, is now considered within the spectrum of vascular dementia; this category also includes Binswanger's disease and cerebral autosomal dominant arteriopathy with subcortical infarcts and leukoencephalopathy

The Behavioral Neurology of Dementia, eds. Bruce L. Miller and Bradley F. Boeve. Published by Cambridge University Press. © Cambridge University Press 2009.

(CADASIL). The prevalence of vascular dementia has been debated, and recent studies have suggested that pure vascular dementia probably accounts for fewer than 20% of those with dementia. With the application of immunocytochemical techniques in neuropathological examinations since the early 1990s, new categories of illnesses have emerged. Dementia with Lewy bodies (DLB) is now considered the second-most common irreversible cause of dementia, accounting for approximately 15% to 25% of cases. Its relationship to Parkinson's disease (PD) – another disorder with Lewy bodies – is still evolving. Because α-synuclein is a constituent of Lewy bodies and Lewy neurites and mutations in the gene for α-synuclein (*SNCA*) are associated with Lewy body parkinsonism, DLB and PD are considered "synucleinopathies." However, recent neuropathological data,[1] as well as neuroimaging data using positron emission tomography (PET) with amyloid-sensitive agents,[2] suggests that many individuals with DLB also have considerable AD pathology. This raises the possibility that new AD treatments directed at amyloid accumulation may also be effective for treating DLB.

Frontotemporal dementia (FTD) is a clinical syndrome manifested by behavioral/dysexecutive changes or progressive aphasia (or both). The most common neuropathological substrates for FTD include Pick's disease, corticobasal degeneration (CBD), or frontotemporal lobar degeneration (FTLD) with ubiquitin-positive inclusions (FTLD-U), which most frequently occurs in individuals with overlapping motor neuron disease pathology. Less common substrates are AD and progressive supranuclear palsy (PSP) and dementia lacking distinctive histology (DLDH). This category of disorders accounts for approximately 10% to 15% of cases of untreatable dementia. Both CBD and PSP are classically considered Parkinson-plus syndromes, but these disorders can present clinically as behavioral/dysexecutive changes or progressive aphasia. Abnormal accumulations of hyperphosphorylated tau in neurons or glia is characteristic of Pick's disease,

CBD and PSP, and mutations in the gene for microtubule-associated protein tau (*MAPT*) are associated with dementia or parkinsonism. Historically, these disorders and AD have been considered "tauopathies;" however, the recognition that FTLD-U is at least as common as tau deposition in many cases of FTLD, and that the chief protein constituent of these deposits is not tau but another protein called TAR DNA-binding protein (TDP-43),[3] suggests that this may no longer be appropriate. Creutzfeldt–Jacob disease (CJD), Gerstmann–Strausser–Schenker disease (GSS) and fatal familial insomnia (FFI) are rare; however, because prion protein dysfunction is common to them all, they can be considered "prionopathies."

The nomenclature for the vascular and non-Alzheimer dementing illnesses is confusing. Most of the literature includes terms for clinical syndromes (e.g. FTD, primary progressive aphasia [PPA] and so forth) as well as ones for presumably distinct histopathological disorders (e.g. DLDH and Pick's disease). Importantly, each syndrome is associated with a spectrum of histopathologically defined disorders, and each disorder can be manifested clinically as various syndromes. Although histopathological examination is required to establish a specific diagnosis in the vascular and degenerative dementing illnesses, several sets of clinical diagnostic criteria have been proposed, although none is entirely accurate. Because no currently available therapy targets any of the pathophysiological processes of these disorders, up to this point errors in the diagnosis of specific diseases generally do not affect management.

However, determining the neurochemical alterations or topographic distribution of brain dysfunction can influence management and prognosis. Many signs and symptoms are associated with known or presumed neurochemical alterations (e.g. impaired memory is associated with acetylcholine deficiency; psychomotor slowing and bradykinesia are associated with dopamine deficiency; and hallucinations and delusions are associated with dopamine excess) or with dysfunction in certain neuroanatomical regions (e.g. amnesia is associated with mesial temporal, midline diencephalic or basal forebrain dysfunction; non-fluent aphasia is associated with dominant hemisphere frontal opercular or insular dysfunction; and visuospatial dysfunction is associated with non-dominant parietal, with or without occipital, dysfunction). Symptomatic therapy involving agents that target such signs and symptoms can improve daily functioning, and this continues to be the mainstay of treatment for management of vascular and degenerative disorders.

As new therapies are developed that target specific dementia pathophysiological processes, it will become increasingly important to establish the underlying disorder. In addition, emerging evidence suggests that different symptomatic therapies, as well as the side-effects of other types of medication, may have beneficial or deleterious effects, depending on the underlying disease pathology. Finally, an appreciation of ontogeny of different dementia may be helpful in deciding when to initiate or withdraw specific therapy.

Alzheimer's disease and variants
Alzheimer-type dementia
Background
It is important to distinguish between the syndrome of Alzheimer-type dementia and the disorder of AD. The typical evolution of AD evolves through the syndrome of amnestic mild cognitive impairment (aMCI) and subsequently develops into a cortical Alzheimer-type dementia with dysfunction in language, visuospatial, gnosis and executive functioning. While anterograde memory dysfunction tends to involve both verbal and non-verbal stimuli, some patients present with far greater verbal or visual memory deficits.

Diagnosis
Several biomarkers are being analyzed to determine their sensitivity and specificity for underlying AD in the Alzheimer-type dementia syndrome, with imaging using labeled ligands for amyloid (magnetic resonance imaging [MRI] and PET) showing the most promise.[4] These agents may be able to detect presymptomatic AD pathology, leading to the possibility of AD prevention.[5–7] Blood or cerebrospinal fluid (CSF) tests that incorporate new proteomic technology also show promise for early detection and differential diagnosis of AD from other dementias.[8–10]

Management
The pharmacological management of AD is focused on removing medications with potential to further impair cognitive function, and adding medications that ameliorate or stabilize cognitive dysfunction. Common medications that may further impair cognition in AD are those which directly interfere with cholinergic neurotransmission, such as first-generation urinary incontinence medications (oxybutynin, tolterodine),

benzodiazipines, first-generation antihistamines (e.g. diphenhydramine) and certain antipsychotic drugs. Acetylcholinesterase inhibitors (donepezil, galantamine and rivastigmine) as well as the N-methyl-D-aspartate (NMDA) receptor antagonist memantine, alone or combination, are of modest benefit in stabilizing cognitive and behavioral decline. In a minority of patients, psychiatric symptoms, such as depression, anxiety and delusions may be prominent at the time of diagnosis. More frequently, agitated behavior, delusions and hallucinations occur in later stages of disease. Management of specific problem behaviors is reviewed at the end of the chapter.

Although none of the current medications approved by the US Food and Drug Administration (FDA) have any effects on modifying the underlying pathology that causes AD, a number of late-stage clinical trials are in progress or have recently been completed using a variety of approaches to clear β-amyloid from the brain or prevent its build up. One method for clearing AD from the brain involves generating an active central nervous system (CNS) immune response with a β-amyloid vaccine or infusing monoclonal antibodies or intravenous immunoglobulin, which may directly clear β-amyloid or generate a peripheral amyloid "sink."[11] Although one such amyloid vaccine study was halted owing to a high incidence of encephalitis,[12] subsequent clinical and neuropathological analyses showed some evidence of efficacy in those individuals who were able to mount an effective immune response.[13–15] Other approaches to interfering with β-amyloid toxicity include aggregation inhibitors,[16] or inhibition/modulation of the gamma secretase enzymes that help to generate β-amyloid.[17,18] An exciting possibility is that a combination of preclinical detection of AD pathology in normal elderly or individuals with MCI, using amyloid imaging or other new techniques, plus initiating an anti-amyloid agent could sufficiently slow or prevent the onset of clinical AD as well as other dementias.

Amnestic mild cognitive impairment
Background
Patients with prominent forgetfulness but not frank dementia that has evolved insidiously and progressively worsened very likely have dysfunction in one or both mesial temporal lobes, and such patients often have features in keeping with the syndrome of aMCI. While most individuals with aMCI likely have

evolving AD, argyrophilic grains and neurofibrillary tangles restricted in the mesial temporal lobes have been identified in such patients who have later undergone autopsy.[19] Pick's disease, FTLD-U, DLDH and CBD can rarely present with severe anterograde amnesia.[20]

Management
Several therapeutic trials have demonstrated that cholinesterase inhibitors fail to delay or prevent progression to dementia over long-term follow-up.[21,22] However, in one study there was a significant effect of donepezil treatment on conversion to dementia in carriers of the ε4 allele of the gene *APOE*, encoding apolipoprotein E, at 12 months.[21]

Posterior cortical atrophy, progressive visuoperceptual syndrome, progressive posterior cortical syndrome, progressive simultanagnosia and Balint syndrome
Background
Visual agnosia is related to dysfunction in the ventral, or "What," pathway of complex visual processing. All or parts of Balint syndrome correspond to dysfunction in the dorsal, or "Where," pathway. Overt visuoperceptual deficits are associated with abnormalities in the primary visual cortex or visual association cortex. Patients with simultanagnosia (the inability to grasp the gestalt of a visual image) or Balint syndrome (simultanagnosia, optic ataxia and ocular apraxia) often present to ophthalmologists complaining of blurred vision, poor depth perception, inability to follow lines while reading and so forth.[23] Those with frank visuoperceptual problems can experience micropsia (images appear smaller than they actually are), macropsia (images appear larger than they actually are), metmorphopsia (images appear to change shape or texture), illusions (objects appear to be images different from the actual objects, e.g. perceiving a chair to be an animal) and hallucinations. Occasionally, delusional overtones develop and a person's own reflection in a mirror may be interpreted as an intruder in the house, or Capgras syndrome evolves (believing a person has been replaced by an identical-appearing impostor). Visual field defects or cortical blindness develops in some patients. Several terms have been used to describe these conditions, including posterior cortical atrophy (PCA), progressive visuoperceptual

syndrome, progressive posterior cortical syndrome, progressive posterior cortical dysfunction, progressive simultanagnosia/Balint syndrome and visual variant of AD.[24,25] In typical AD, the neuritic plaques and neurofibrillary tangles are rarely most dense in the posterior cerebrum, but in patients with PCA, AD has been the most frequently identified histopathologic process. There are also reports of AD with Lewy body disease (LBD), non-specific histopathology, progressive subcortical gliosis, CBD, FFI and CJD.[24–29]

Diagnosis

Patients tend to be female, symptom onset is typically early and the course is very slowly progressive. Despite the prominent parieto-occipital pathology in those with PCA, visual hallucinations are rare.[30,31]

Management

Except for atypical neuroleptic drugs to manage hallucinations and delusions and antidepressant agents to treat depression (which is common in this syndrome because insight is often preserved),[32,33] no therapy has been shown to improve any of the features. Some place colored marks on kitchen and other items to help them to orient where to place their thumb and fingers so that they can hold and use objects correctly (e.g. telephone). Clinical experience indicates that some patients benefit from symptomatic therapy using cholinesterase inhibitors or memantine. Motor vehicle accidents and injuries relating to simply walking in public (and being struck by cars that are not seen) can be avoided by identifying this syndrome early and avoiding driving and walking alone in public.

Dementia with Lewy bodies and Parkinson's disease with dementia

Background

Several terms have been used to describe the condition of patients with known or suspected Lewy body lesions, including Lewy body disease, Lewy body dementia, the Lewy body variant of AD, diffuse Lewy body disease, cortical Lewy body disease, and senile dementia of the Lewy type. The Consortium on Dementia With Lewy Bodies developed consensus criteria for the clinical and neuropathological diagnoses of what is now termed *dementia with Lewy bodies*.[34] On the basis primarily of cases in hospital- and referral-based samples, the frequency of DLB is approximately 15–25% of those with irreversible

dementia. There is growing evidence that the cognitive and neuropsychiatric manifestations of PD with dementia (PDD) are related to cortical Lewy bodies.[35,36] Yet there is considerable debate regarding whether DLB and PDD should be considered as separate entities or variants of the same disease, differing primarily in the timing of when dementia and parkinsonism manifest. Since some recent clinical trials have enrolled DLB and PDD patients separately, DLB and PDD will be discussed separately where appropriate, although readers should consider DLB and PDD similar for purposes of management.[37]

Diagnosis

The criteria for the clinical diagnosis of DLB according to the Consortium on Dementia With Lewy Bodies were published originally in 1996,[38] minimally refined in 1999[39] and significantly revised in 2005.[1] Increasingly, data indicate that the neuropsychological pattern of impairment – poor verbal fluency, attention–concentration and visuospatial functioning – is distinct and different from that of AD, in which impairment is usually maximal in learning and memory and confrontational naming early in the course of the disease.[40,41] Rapid eye movement (REM) sleep-behavior disorder RBD (a parasomnia in which patients seemingly act out their dreams) has been associated with DLB, and the features of RBD can precede the development of dementia or parkinsonism (or both) by years or even decades.[42–47] Depression appears to be relatively common in DLB. Many patients have more of a postural than a rest tremor, and the parkinsonism can be more symmetrical than that typical of early PD. There appears to be less hippocampal atrophy on MRI scans in DLB than in AD and vascular dementia.[48] Other good sources regarding diagnosis and management can be found in references Boeve[47] and Burton et al.[49]

Management

Although limbic and neocortical neuronal loss occurs in DLB, the severity appears to be less than that in AD, FTD and other dementias.[50,51] Also, depletion of the cholinergic basal forebrain – classically viewed as characteristic of AD – is often even more profound in DLB.[36,50] Dopamine and serotonin depletion are also common in DLB. Thus, the marked neurotransmitter deficiencies but better preservation of viable neurons suggests that medical therapy may be as or more effective in DLB than in most other dementing disorders.

One approach that has proven useful in the management of DLB is to consider five principal aspects of symptomatology: cognitive impairment, neuropsychiatric issues, motor dysfunction, sleep disorders and autonomic dysfunction.[47] Several case series, open label studies and a few randomized clinical trials have shown that many medications can improve symptoms in one or more of these areas (Table 16.1). Improvement has been reported in cognitive functioning and neuropsychiatric symptoms of patients with DLB treated with any of the cholinesterase inhibitors, including tacrine, donepezil, rivastigmine, and galantamine.[48,52–57,59–62,73] What these large clinical studies do not elaborate on is the striking improvement that some patients with DLB experience (as exemplified in case 4–2 in Boeve[47]). In fact, any patient who appears to have probable AD but dramatically improves with a cholinesterase inhibitor must be considered to possibly harbor coexisting LBD. Rivastigmine has demonstrated efficacy and safety in DLB in randomized clinical trials,[58,62] but it is not yet clear if any of the cholinesterase inhibitors are superior to the others. A recent, preliminary study suggests that cholinesterase inhibitors may influence β-amyloid deposition in DLB, raising the possibility of some componenet of neuroprotection afforded by these agents.[74] Some individuals with advanced disease benefit from high-dose cholinesterase inhibitors, and for those who do not, a slow withdrawal of cholinesterase inhibitor is well tolerated[75] Carbidopa/levodopa treatment has no adverse effects on cognition and may help to improve neuropsychiatric status in DLB.[76] Psychostimulants, and dopamine agonists, can theoretically improve cognition, apathy and psychomotor slowing, but no controlled studies have been published to date demonstrating efficacy of these agents. For reasons that are not clear, increased parkinsonism occurs infrequently with the cholinesterase inhibitors.[77] Acute worsening of neuropsychiatric symptoms has been reported after switching from donepezil to galantamine.[78]

Clinical experience has shown some patients with DLB do benefit from memantine, but visual hallucinations, gait impairment and worsened cognition can occur; these typically resolve upon discontinuation of the drug.[79,80] The underlying cause for fluctuations in DLB is poorly understood, but this feature can improve with cholinesterase inhibitor therapy or, in some cases, following treatment of sleep disorders. Based on available data, clinicians should consider prescribing one of cholinesterase inhibitors

to patients with DLB who do not have a contraindication to its use.

Neuroleptic sensitivity, in which striking and irreversible parkinsonism can evolve shortly after use of neuroleptic drugs, has led to the strong recommendation that conventional neuroleptic drugs should be avoided in patients with DLB.[81] Neuroleptic sensitivity has been reported even with newer atypical neuroleptic agents. There are conflicting data on olanzapine in DLB[67,68] and more consistent data on quetiapine[69,70,82] (Tables 16.1 and 16.2). Since many of the newer atypical neuroleptic drugs have shown efficacy in PD patients with psychosis (see below), agents such as clozapine, quetiapine and olanzapine may be most appropriate; there is insufficient evidence on the efficacy of ziprasidone and aripiprazole in DLB or PDD.

The selective serotonin-reuptake inhibitors (SSRIs) are usually effective and well tolerated in patients with DLB for managing depression with or without anxiety. Owing to the anticholinergic properties of the tricyclic antidepressants, these agents should generally be avoided in DLB. Paroxetine also has anticholinergic effects and should be used cautiously in DLB. Electroconvulsive therapy can be effective for depression in some patients without significantly worsening cognition.[141]

Carbidopa/levodopa can be used in the management of parkinsonism, but this can exacerbate psychotic symptoms or orthostatism. In recent open-label studies, levodopa was generally well tolerated and was shown to improve motor functioning in a proportion of patients.[71,72] Orthostatic hypotension, likely caused by degenerative changes in the intermediolateral cell column of the spinal cord and peripheral autonomic system, can occur in DLB.[142–144] As in PD, management includes liberalizing salt in the diet, salt tablets, thigh-high compression stockings, fludrocortisone and midodrine.

Violent dreams and dream enactment behavior as part of RBD, which often precedes or accompanies dementia or parkinsonism in Lewy body-associated disorders, typically improve with clonazepam or melatonin therapy.[43,44,145–147] There are anecdotal reports that modafinil or methylphenidate improves hypersomnia in patients with DLB.

In summary, patients with DLB who have pronounced parkinsonism, psychosis and orthostatism are quite challenging to manage, but some clearly benefit from optimizing dosing of a cholinesterase inhibitor, carbidopa/levodopa and an atypical neuroleptic drug,

Table 16.1. Summary of published case series, open-label trials and randomized clinical trials in patients with dementia with Lewy bodies

Study	No.	Study type	Study duration	Main findings
Cholinesterase inhibitors for management of cognitive impairment and neuropsychiatric features				
Tacrine				
Lebert et al. (1998)[52]	19	OL	14 wks	Improvement in COG
Querfurth et al. (2000)[53]	6	OL	24 wks	Improvement in COG; worse EPS in some
Donepezil				
Shea et al. (1998)[54]	9	CS	12–24 wks	Improvement in COG and NP; worse EPS in 3 (33%)
Lanctot and Herrmann (2000)[55]	7	CS	24 wks	Improvement in COG and NP
Samuel et al. (2000)[56]	4	OL	26 wks	Improvement in COG and NP
Minett et al. (2003)[57]	8	OL	20 wks; 6 wk withdrawal	Improvement in COG and NP and no worsening of EPS; marked clinical worsening upon withdrawals of drug in most
Rivastigmine				
McKeith et al. (2000)[58]	11	OL	12 wks	Improvement in COG and NP
McKeith et al. (2000)[58]	120[a]	RCT	20 wks	Improvement in COG and NP
Grace et al. (2000)[59]	6	OL	12 wks	Improvement in COG and NP
Grace et al. (2001)[60]	29	OL	96 wks	Improvement in COG and NP
Maclean et al. (2001)[61]	8	CS	24 wks	Improvement in COG and NP and sleep parameters
Wesnes et al. (2002)[62]	120[a]	RCT	20 wks	Improvement in COG on computerized cognitive measures
Thomas et al. (2005)[63]	30	OL	20 wks	Improvement in COG and NP; no worsening of EPS
Rowan et al. (2007)[64]	22	OL	20 wks	Improvement in attention and reaction time
Galantamine				
Edwards et al. (2004)[65]	25	OL	24 wks	Improvement in COG and NP in many; no significant worsening in EPS
Edwards et al. (2007)[66]	50	OL	24 wks	Improvement in COG and NP in many; no significant worsening in EPS
Atypical neuroleptics for management of neuropsychiatric features				
Olanzapine				
Walker et al. (1999)[67]	8	OL	2 wks	Improvement in NP in 2 (25%); AEs leading to withdrawals in 3 (38%)
Cummings et al. (2002)[68]	27[a]	RCT	6 wks	Improvement in NP without worsening in COG or EPS
Quetiapine				
Fernandez et al. (2002)[69]	11	RetCR	n/a	Improvement in NP in 10 (90%); worsened EPS in 3 (27%)
Takahashi et al. (2003)[70]	9	OL	8 wks	Improvement in NP in 5 (55%); AEs leading to withdrawals in 3 (33%)
Agents for management of parkinsonism				
Levodopa				
Bonelli et al. (2004)[71]	20	OL	LDT[b]	15 (75%) had ≥ 10% improvement in motor score in LDT
Molloy et al. (2005)[72]	14	OL	LDT[b]	5 (36%) had significant improvement in motor score in LDT
Agents for management of REM sleep-behavior disorder				
Melatonin				
Boeve et al. (2003)[46]	7	OL	9+ months	Improvement in REM sleep-behavior disorder in 5 (71%); 2 were also treated with clonazepam

Notes:
AEs, adverse events; COG, cognition; CS, case series; EPS, extrapyramidal signs; LDT, levodopa test; NP, neuropsychiatric features; OL, open label trial; RetCR, retrospective chart review; RCT, randomized clinical trial.
[a]Approximately half of subjects treated with active drug.
[b]Clinical ratings performed in the fasting state in the morning as part of the levodopa test (LDT); n/a, not available.

Table 16.2. Summary of published case series, open-label trials and randomized clinical trials in patients with Parkinson's disease plus cognitive impairment/dementia and/or psychosis

Study	No.	Study type	Study duration	Main findings
Cholinesterase inhibitors for management of cognitive impairment and neuropsychiatric features				
Tacrine				
Hutchinson and Fazzini (1996)[83]	7	OL	8 wks	Improvement in COG, NP and EPS
Werber and Rabey (2001)[84]	7	OL	26 wks	Improvement in COG; EPS stable
Donepezil				
Werber and Rabey (2001)[84]	4	OL	26 wks	Improvement in COG; EPS stable
Fabbrini et al. (2002)[85]	8	OL	2 mo	Improvement in NP; worsened EPS in 2
Bergman and Lerner (2002)[86]	6	OL	6 wks	Improvement in NP in 5; EPS stable
Aarsland et al. (2002)[87]	14[a]	RCT	10 wks	Improvement in COG and NP and no worsening of EPS; marked clinical worsening upon withdrawals of drug in most
Minett et al. (2003)[57]	11	OL	20 wks, 6 wk withdrawal	Improvement in COG; AE leading to withdrawals in 4/7 (57%) treated with donepezil
Leroi et al. (2004)[88]	16[a]	RCT	18 wks	Slight improvement in COG; well tolerated.
Ravina, et al. (2005)[89]	22	RCT	10 wks	
Rivastigmine				
Reading et al. (2001)[90]	12	OL	6 wks	Improvement in COG and NP; EPS stable
Bullock and Cameron (2002)[91]	5	OL	Variable	Improvement in COG and NP
Giladi et al. (2003)[92]	28	OL	26 wks	Improvement in COG without worsening in EPS
Emre et al. (2004)[93]	541[a]	RCT	24 wks	Improvement in COG and NP; AEs (nausea, vomiting, tremor) more frequent than placebo
Galantamine				
Aarsland et al. (2004)[94]	16	OL	8 wks	Improvement in COG and NP; AEs leading to withdrawals in 3 (19%)
Atypical neuroleptics for management of neuropsychiatric features ± motor features				
Clozapine				
Ostergaard and Dupont (1988)[95]	16	OL	Variable	Improvement in NP in 14 (88%); frequent AEs
Friedman and Lannon (1989)[96]	6	CS	Variable	Improvement in NP in all; few AEs
Pfeiffer et al. (1990)[97]	5	OL	Variable	Improvement in NP in 3 (60%); AEs leading to withdrawals in 2
Wolters et al. (1990)[98]	6	RCT	40 days	While titrating levodopa, improvement in NP in 3 (50%); AEs leading to withdrawals in 3
Kahn et al. (1991)[99]	11	OL	Variable	Improvement in NP in 8 (72%); frequent AEs

Table 16.2. *(cont.)*

Study	No.	Study type	Study duration	Main findings
Wolk and Douglas (1992)[100]	5	OL	Variable	Improvement in NP in 3 (60%); AEs leading to withdrawals in 2
Greene et al. (1993)[101]	13	CS	Variable	Improvement in NP in 10 (77%); frequent AEs
Factor et al. (1994)[102]	17	OL	Variable	Improvement in NP in all; frequent AEs
Chacko et al. (1995)[103]	10	OL	Variable	Improvement in NP in all; few AEs
Rabey et al. (1995)[104]	27	CS	Variable	Improvement in NP in 25; AEs leading to withdrawals in 2
Rich et al. (1995)[105]	5	CS	Variable	Improvement in COG/NP/EPS in 4/5 patients switched from respiridone to clozapine
Wagner et al. (1996)[106]	49	CS	Up to 18 mo	Improvement in NP without worsening of EPS in over 34 (70%)
Bonuccelli et al. (1997)[107]	17[a]	RCT	Variable	Improvement in tremor in 15 (88%)
Ruggieri et al. (1997)[108]	36	OL	12 mo	Improvement in NP without worsening of EPS in all subjects
Widman et al. (1997)[109]	27	CS	Variable	Improvement in NP in most; AEs leading to withdrawals in 5
Friedman et al. (1998)[110]	12	CS	Variable	9 (75%) patients switched back to quetiapine after attempting olanzapine for psychosis
Pierelli et al. (1998)[111]	10	OL	4 mo	Improvement in levodopa-induced dyskinesias
Trosch et al. (1998)[112]	172	CS	Variable	Improvement in NP and motor features in most; AEs leading to withdrawals in 40 (23%)
French Clozapine Parkinson Study Group (1999)[113]	50[a]	RCT	4 wks	Improvement in NP and also tremor without worsening of EPS; AEs leading to withdrawals in 6 (3 placebo, 3 active drug) with one patient on active drug dropping out owing to leukopenia
French Clozapine Parkinson Study Group (1999)[113]	60[a]	RCT	4 wks	Improvement in NP, mild worsening of EPS in 7/32 (22%) treated with clozapine; no patients with leukopenia
Dewey and O'Suilleabhain (2000)[114]	9	CS	Variable	Switched from quetiapine; improvement in NP in 8 (89%)
Goetz et al. (2000)[115]	15	RCT	2 mo	Clozapine group improved in NP whereas olanzapine did not, and olanzapine group experienced worsening of EPS whereas clozapine did not
Ellis et al. (2000)[116]	10	RCT	3 mo	Clozapine and risperidone groups improved in NP; trend for worsening EPS in risperidone group and improving EPS in clozapine group
Factor et al. (2001)[117]	53[a]	RCT	12 wks	Improvement in NP without worsening of EPS
Morgante et al. (2002)[118]	10	OL	12 wks	Improvement in NP and motor features
Morgante et al. (2004)[119]	20	OL	12 wks	Improvement in NP and dyskinesias
Quetiapine				
Fernandez et al. (1999)[120]	24	CS	Variable	Improvement in NP, no worsening of EPS; AEs leading to withdrawals in 3
Dewey and O'Suilleabhain (2000)[114]	61	CS	Variable	Improvement in NP in 40 (66%), no worsening of EPS

220

Study	N	Design	Duration	Outcome
Targum and Abbott (2000)[121]	11	CS	Variable	Improvement in NP in 6 (55%), AEs leading to withdrawals in 4
Fernandez et al. (2002)[69]	87	CS	Variable	Improvement in NP in 70 (80%), mild worsening of EPS in 28 (32%)
Morgante et al. (2002)[118]	10	OL	12 wks	Improvement in NP without worsening of EPS
Reddy et al. (2002)[122]	43	CS	Variable	Improvement in NP in 35 (81%), mild worsening of EPS in 5 (13%)
Baron and Dalton (2003)[123]	22	CS	Variable	Improvement in levodopa-induced dyskinesias in 15 (68%)
Fernandez et al. (2003)[124]	106	CS	Variable	Improvement in NP in 87 (82%); mild worsening of EPS in 34 (32%)
Gimenez-Roldan et al. (2003)[125]	7	OL	16 wks	Improvement in NP and caregiver stress
Katzenschlager et al. (2004)[126]	9	RCT (double-blind cross-over) then OL	5 wks then 1 mo	No difference in dyskinesias during RCT phase; slight improvement in dyskinesias during OL phase at 50 mg/day; AEs leading to withdrawals in 4
Juncos et al. (2004)[127]	29	OL	24 wks	Improvement in NP and COG without worsening of EPS
Mancini et al. (2004)[128]	35	OL	12 mo	Improvement in NP, no worsening of COG or EPS
Morgante et al. (2004)[119]	20	OL	12 wks	Improvement in NP and dyskinesias
Kurlan et al. (2007)[82]	23	RCT	10 wks	Well tolerated; no worsening of EPS; trend toward decline in ADLs
Rabey et al. (2007)[129]	38	RCT	3 mo	No benefit on drug-induced psychosis, but low power to detect an effect
Risperidone				
Rich et al. (1995)[105]	6	CS	Variable	Improvement in NP without worsening of COG and EPS in 1; others switched to quetiapine with subsequent improvement
Meco et al. (1997)[130]	10	OL	Variable	Improvement in NP in most
Workman et al. (1997)[131]	9	CS	Variable	Improvement in NP in all without worsening of COG or EPS
Ellis et al. (2000)[116]	10	RCT	3 mo	Clozapine and risperidone groups improved in NP; trend for worsening EPS in risperidone group and improving EPS in clozapine group
Leopold (2000)[132]	39	OL	3–6 mo	Improvement in NP in 23 (59%); no change or worsening in 12 (31%)
Mohr et al. (2000)[133]	17	OL	12 wk	Improvement in NP without worsening of EPS; AEs leading to withdrawals in 2
Olanzapine				
Friedman et al. (1998)[110]	12	CS	Variable	3 (25%) patients successfully switched from quetiapine to olanzapine for psychosis
Graham et al. (1998)[134]	5	OL	9 days	Improvement in NP, but worsening of EPS; AEs leading to withdrawals in 2
Aarsland et al. (1999)[135]	21	OL	8 wks	Improvement in NP in 12/15 (80%); no change in COG or EPS; AEs leading to withdrawals in 6
Molho and Factor (1999)[136]	12	CS	Variable	Improvement in NP in 9 (75%), and worsening of EPS in 9 (75%)

222

Table 16.2. (cont.)

Study	No.	Study type	Study duration	Main findings
Goetz et al. (2000)[115]	15	RCT	2 mo	Clozapine group improved in NP whereas olanzapine did not; olanzapine group experienced worsening of EPS whereas clozapine did not
Brier et al. (2002)[137] USA study	41[a]	RCT	4 wks	No improvement in NP and worsening of EPS
Brier et al. (2002)[137] European study	49[a]	RCT	4 wks	No improvement in NP and worsening of EPS
Marsh et al. (2001)[138]	5	OL	6 wks	No improvement in NP; AEs leading to withdrawals in 4
Ondo et al. (2002)[139]	30[a]	RCT	9 wks	No improvement in NP and worsening of EPS
Aripiprazole				
Fernandez et al. (2004)[140]	8	OL	> 2 wks	Improvement in NP in 2 (25%); AE leading to withdrawals in 2 (25%)
Agents for management of parkinsonism				
Levodopa				
Bonelli et al. (2004)[71]	20	OL	LDT[b]	17 (85%) had ≥ 10% improvement in motor score in LDT
Molloy et al. (2005)[72]	30	OL	LDT[b]	7 (23%) had significant improvement in motor score in LDT
Molloy et al. (2006)[76]	27	OL	LDT[b]	No significant effects on COG

Notes:
AEs, adverse events; COG, cognition; CS, case series; EPS, extrapyramidal signs; LDT, levodopa test; mo, months; NP, neuropsychiatric features; OL, open-label trial; RCT, randomized clinical trial; wks, weeks; ADL, activities of daily living.
[a]Approximately half to two-thirds of subjects treated with active drug.
[b]Clinical ratings performed in the fasting state in the morning as part of the levodopa test (LDT).

and with treatment of orthostatism.[39,47,148] Specific treatment suggestions for the varying features in DLB are shown in the section on management of target symptoms.

Parkinson disease with dementia and/or psychosis

Background
Some degree of cognitive impairment exists in most individuals with PD, but when mild and early in the illness, this is usually not functionally disabling. However, approximately 80% of patients with PD develop dementia within 8 years,[149] and these cognitive and neuropsychiatric features are disturbing to patients as well as their caregivers.[135] "Psychosis" in patients with PD is typically considered related to levodopa therapy, although some with PD, regardless of whether they have dementia or not, experience hallucinations and/or delusions. As noted above, the distribution of Lewy body and Lewy neurite pathology and neurochemical alterations in DLB are very similar to those in PDD, and it, therefore, stands to reason why management is similar regardless of the clinical diagnosis.[150]

Diagnosis
Despite the wide acceptance that dementia often evolves in PD, there are no established criteria for the diagnosis of PDD. Since the diagnosis of DLB has been considered applicable to patients who develop dementia no more than 1 year after the onset of parkinsonism, by default, one could view the diagnosis of PDD as appropriate for those who develop dementia at least 1 year after the onset of parkinsonism.[1]

Management
Table 16.2 summarizes pertinent data regarding those studies involving patients with PD and cognitive impairment/dementia and/or psychosis. Cholinesterase inhibitors have been shown to improve cognition and neuropsychiatric features in PD patients.[57,83–93,149,151,152] As in DLB, some patients with PDD will experience dramatic improvement in cognition and neuropsychiatric features, although this is not common. Individuals with visual hallucinations show the largest responses to cholinesterase inhibitors.[153] Beneficial effects of cholinesterase inhibitors may be present even after 48 months of treatment.[154] The largest randomized clinical trial involved rivastigmine, but as with DLB, it is not yet known if one cholinesterase inhibitor is superior to any of the others. Smaller studies have been carried out with donepezil.[89] Similar efficacy

was seen in a head-to-head comparison of donepezil and rivastigmine for DLB/PDD.[63] Typical side-effects include nausea, vomiting and diarrhea. Worsening of parkinsonism occurs in a small minority of patients treated. Studies with relatively few patients have shown improvement with memantine therapy for parkinsonism in those with PD. The neuropsychiatric features of PD (with or without dementia), particularly visual hallucinations and delusions, can also improve with treatment with clozapine, quetiapine, risperidone, olanzapine, or aripiprizole.[69,95–134,136–138,140,155–158]

The atypical neuroleptics in the management of problematic neuropsychiatric features, particularly hallucinations and delusions, deserve further comment. As shown in Table 16.2, there are considerable data demonstrating efficacy for clozapine and quetiapine, and exacerbation of parkinsonism is rare and only mild when associated with either of these agents. Efficacy with risperidone and olanzapine has also been shown, but worsening of parkinsonism occurs with some frequency and can be quite severe in some patients. There are too few data to know how effective and tolerable aripiprazole is yet. While leukopenia is rare with clozapine, the need for frequent laboratory monitoring makes it unappealing for many patients. Therefore, based on the available data, treatment of psychosis with quetiapine is a reasonable choice; if dementia is also present, treatment with a cholinesterase inhibitor with or without quetiapine may be best.

Parkinsonism usually responds well to levodopa therapy.[71,72] Hallucinations and delusions occur frequently with the dopamine agonists, particularly in the setting of coexisting dementia, thus limiting their use in patients with PD plus dementia and/or psychosis. Tremor and dyskinesias can be ameliorated by clozapine.[107,111,119] Management of depression, autonomic dysfunction and sleep disorders is similar to that in DLB.

Diagnosis and management of vascular dementia

Background
Vascular dementia is an enigmatic area in dementia care and research. Although it is clear that infarcts in important structures such as the thalamus and various cortical regions can cause cognitive impairment, and impairment in the various cognitive domains correlates with the topographic distribution of infarcts, there are several lingering uncertainties.

Does the presence of two or more infarcts constitute vascular dementia if the course of cognitive decline has been progressive rather than stepwise? If leukoariosis is so common in the cognitively normal elderly, how does one interpret white matter abnormalities on MRI in patients with cognitive impairment? How does one interpret severe leukoariosis in patients who have no history of any vascular risk factor such as hypertension or diabetes mellitus? How are clinicians expected to diagnose vascular dementia if there is so much debate about what does and what does not constitute vascular dementia pathologically? These and many other questions must be answered to improve our understanding of the contribution of cerebrovascular disease-associated dementia and ultimately to develop treatments more effectively.

Diagnosis

All clinical schemes have limited sensitivity, owing, in part, to the considerable variability of infarct types, sizes, locations and presumed pathophysiology. Although the Hachinski Ischemic Scale was developed (in 1975) long before the others, it was shown recently to have the highest sensitivity.[159] The new term "subcortical ischemic vascular dementia" appears less heterogeneous, with the cognitive and behavioral features largely stemming from frontosubcortical neural network dysfunction.[160] This more consistent phenotype may facilitate the elucidation of which agents provide any benefit in the setting of cognitive impairment/dementia associated with subcortical cerebrovascular disease.

Management

Management can be divided into strategies for decreasing the risk of subsequent cerebrovascular disease, improving or stabilizing cognition once vascular dementia is present, and managing target symptoms. Hypertension, hyperlipidemia and diabetes mellitus should be optimally treated to minimize the risk of cerebrovascular events, and there is growing evidence that lowering blood pressure reduces the risk of dementia.[161–164] Patients with atrial fibrillation, congestive heart disease, patent foramen ovale, thoracic aortic debris or other risk factors should be given appropriate stroke prophylaxis. Tobacco use should be discouraged. Several randomized, double-blind, placebo-controlled trials have been completed in vascular dementia, with variable efficacy but usually good tolerability (Table 16.3).[160,165–192] The cholinesterase inhibitors have consistently shown mild

improvement in cognition and/or functional activities and neuropsychiatric features with minimal adverse effects of treatment.[197] Memantine and ginkgo biloba have also shown modest efficacy with tolerable side-effects. Hydergine has also been efficacious, but the studies involving hydergine included subjects diagnosed with cerebral insufficiency and other disorders that would not be considered compatible with current criteria for vascular dementia.[179,193] As yet there is sufficient evidence to consider hydergine for vascular dementia, and randomized clinical trials using current criteria are warranted. Most of the other agents tested have not been efficacious, or are being tested in larger randomized clinical trials. The more variable issue is whether any of these in isolation or in combination produce *clinically significant* effects in individual patients. Clinicians can also consider therapy for management of target symptoms.

Frontotemporal lobar degeneration

Clinically, FTLD presents either with changes in personality, behavioral problems and/or executive impairment or as PPA. The behavioral–dysexecutive presentation of FTD is often referred to as "frontal variant" FTD (fvFTD). The PPA associated with FTD pathology may be further subdivided into a fluent aphasia and a non-fluent aphasia. The fluent PPA has been referred to as semantic dementia (SD), reflecting a primary loss of knowledge about the world as the etiology of the aphasia, or as "temporal variant" FTD, reflecting the prominent anterior temporal lobe atrophy associated with this clinical FTD subtype. The non-fluent aphasia has been termed progressive non-fluent aphasia (PNFA).[198]

Several disorders can present with features of FTLD, especially disorders with tau-positive inclusions (e.g. Pick's disease, CBD, PSP, agyrophilic grain disease and FTDP-17), ubiquitin-positive inclusions (e.g. FTLD-U), non-specific histopathological features (e.g. DLDH, hippocampal sclerosis) and other rare conditions (e.g. neurofilament inclusion body disease or neuronal intermediate filament inclusion disease). Tau-positive inclusions are found most commonly in FTD and PNFA, whereas ubiquitin-positive inclusions are more common in SD.[199,200] The primary protein constituent of FTLD-U inclusions was recently identified to be TDP-43.[201] A family history positive for dementia, parkinsonism or motor neuron disease can often be elicited, and parkinsonism or motor neuron disease can develop in patients with FTD.

Table 16.3. Summary of published open-label and randomized clinical trials in patients with cognitive impairment/dementia as a result of cerebrovascular disease

Reference	No.	Study type	Study duration	Main findings
Cholinesterase inhibitors for management of cognitive impairment +/- neuropsychiatric features				
Donepezil				
Black et al. (2003)[166]	603[a]	RCT	24 wks	Improvement in COG and ADLs; AEs infrequent and mild
Wilkinson et al. (2003)[167]	616[a]	RCT	24 wks	Improvement in COG and ADLs; AEs infrequent and mild
Rivastigmine				
Kumar et al. (2000)[170]	319[a,b]	RCT	26 wks	Improvement in COG and NP; AEs infrequent and mild
Moretti et al. (2001)[168]	16[a]	RCT	12 mo	Improvement in COG and NP; AEs infrequent and mild
Moretti et al. (2002)[169]	8	OL	22 mo	Improvement in COG and NP; AEs infrequent and mild
Moretti et al. (2003)[171]	208[a]	RCT	12 mo	Slight improvement in COG and NP; AEs infrequent and mild
Moretti et al. (2004)[172]	64	OL	16 mo	Rivastigmine group (32) showed improvement in COG, NP and ADLs compared with aspirin plus nimodipine group (32)
Galantamine				
Erkinjuntti et al. (2002)[173]	592[a,b]	RCT	6 mo	Improvement or maintenance of COG, NP and ADLs; AEs infrequent and mild
Erkinjuntti et al. (2003)[174]	459[b]	OL	12 mo	Improvement or maintenance of COG and NP; AEs infrequent and mild (this study is OL extension of Erkinjuntti et al. [2002][174])
Other agents				
Memantine				
Orgogozo et al. (2002)[175]	321[a]	RCT	28 wks	Improvement in COG; AEs infrequent and mild
Wilcock et al. (2002)[176]	579[a]	RCT	28 wks	Improvement in COG; AEs infrequent and mild
Aspirin (antiplatelet agent)				
Meyer et al. (1989)[177]	70[a]	RCT	15 mo	Improvement or stabilization of COG and quality of life
Devine and Rands (2003)[178]	78[a]	RetCR	n/a	Survival from dementia onset to institutionalization and death not different between active drug and placebo
Hydergine (ergoloid mesylate)				
Schneider and Olin (1994)[193]	436	MA	4–52 wks	Improvement in COG and global ratings
Pentoxifylline (xantine derivative)				
Ghose (1987)[180]	36[a]	RCT	3 mo	Trend toward improvement in primary outcome measures of COG; subgroup/secondary analysis showed statistically significant improvement in COG
Black et al. (1992)[181]	64[a]	RCT	9 mo	Trend toward improvement in primary outcome measures of COG

Table 16.3. (cont.)

Reference	No.	Study type	Study duration	Main findings
Blume et al. (1992)[182]	80[a]	RCT	6 mo	Trend toward improvement in primary outcome measures of COG; subgroup/secondary analyses showed statistically significant improvements in COG
EPMIDSG (1996)[183]	239[a]	RCT	9 mo	Trend toward improvement in primary outcome measures of COG; subgroup/secondary analysis showed statistically significant improvement in COG
Propentofylline (xantine derivative)				
Marcusson et al. (1997)[184]	90[a]	RCT	12 mo	Improvement in COG and functional activities; AEs infrequent and mild
Posatirelin (neurotrophic agent)				
Parnetti et al. (1996)[185]	110[a]	RCT	12 wks	Improvement in COG; AEs infrequent and mild
Nicergoline (ergot derivative)				
Herrmann et al. (1997)[186]	136[a]	RCT	6 mo	Improvement in COG; AEs infrequent and mild
Nimodipine (calcium antagonist)				
Pantoni et al. (1996)[187]	31	OL	Up to 12 mo	Most remained stable or improved; AEs infrequent and mild
Pantoni et al. (2000a)[194]	251[a]	RCT	26 wks	No difference between active drug and placebo
Pantoni et al. (2000b)[195]	251[a]	RCT	26 wks	Improvement in COG only in those meeting criteria for subcortical vascular dementia
Pantoni et al. (2005)[188]	230[a]	RCT	52 wks	Slight improvement in COG; fewer vascular AEs in active drug group suggesting protective effect
Cytidine diphosphate choline (citicoline, nootropic agent)				
Cohen et al. (2003)[196]	30[a]	RCT	12 mo	No differences in neuropsychological performance or radiologic measures
Gingko biloba				
Le Bars et al. (2000)[190]	244[a,b]	RCT	26 wks	Modest improvement in COG and ADLs; AEs infrequent and mild
Kanowski et al. (2003)[191]	216[a,b]	RCT	24 wks	Modest improvement in COG and ADLs; AEs infrequent and mild
Olanzapine (atypical antipsychotic)				
Moretti et al. (2004)[192]	94	OL	6 mo	Olanzapine group showed improvement in anxiety compared with bromazepam group

Notes:
ADLs, activities of daily living; AEs, adverse events; COG, cognition; MA, meta-analysis; mo, months; NP, neuropsychiatric features; OL, open-label trial; RetCR, retrospective chart review; RCT, randomized clinical trial; wks, weeks; n/a, not available.
[a] Approximately half to two-thirds of subjects treated with active drug.
[b] Included patients diagnosed with vascular dementia as well as Alzheimer's disease with cerebrovascular disease.

Since the discovery of several mutations in *MAPT* in kindreds with FTD and/or FTDP-17, over 30 mutations have been identified.[202] All autopsied cases have had tau-positive neuronal and/or glial pathology, but the topography and qualitative features of the tau inclusions have been highly variable. Mutations in *MAPT* have also been found in individuals without a family history of any neurodegenerative disorder (i.e. genetic mosaicism); therefore, a genetically mediated disorder should be considered in anyone with early-onset FTD regardless of family history. Several kindreds with familial FTD have been linked to chromosome 17, chromosome 9[203,204] and chromosome 3.[205] Numerous other kindreds with autosomal dominant FTD do not have tau mutations.

An important cause of FTD in kindreds linked to chromosome 17 without mutations affecting tau are loss-of-function mutations within the gene for progranulin (*PGRN*), leading to haplo-insufficiency.[40,206] These patients may clinically resemble either fvFTD,[207] FTD with parkinsonism[208] or PPA.[209–211] All of these individuals show ubiquitin-positive neuronal inclusions at autopsy that also stain positive for TDP-43.[212]

Frontotemporal dementia: behavioral-dysexecutive subtype

Background
Several terms have been applied to a progressive neuropsychiatric syndrome indicative of frontal network dysfunction. These include *frontal lobe dementia, dementia of the frontal lobe type, dysexecutive syndrome* and, the term used most often, *frontotemporal dementia*. Here the subtype with a behavioral-dysexecutive presentation is discussed, fvFTD. The following section discusses the other subtype, PPA.

Diagnosis
In 1994, investigators in Sweden and England proposed clinical criteria for diagnosis of FTD.[213] These criteria were revised in 1998 with input from other clinicians.[198] Patients with marked degeneration in the non-dominant (usually right) frontotemporal cortex tend to exhibit more behavioral problems and neuropsychiatric features.[214] For reasons unknown, some patients with FTD develop artistic talent beyond what they exhibited before the onset of cognitive or behavioral symptoms.[215]

Management
No therapy has been developed that halts or delays the progression of neurodegeneration in the disorders that present with FTD, although numerous agents are

being tested in transgenic tau mice. For symptomatic therapy (Table 16.4), the results have been mixed with SSRIs, particularly paroxetine.[216,218,220–222] Trazodone was efficacious in many and generally well tolerated.[218] While cognition declined during an open-label trial with rivastigmine, there was improvement in neuropsychiatric features and caregiver burden.[172] More recent open-label data with donepezil suggest that cholinesterase inhibitors have the potential to worsen disinhibition and compulsive symptoms in FTD.[219] These agents should be used with caution in FTD.

In general, pharmacologic management of FTD is tailored to address symptoms. Various symptoms and behaviors can evolve and many can be very difficult to manage. Support for caregivers is critical. The atypical neuroleptic drugs are increasingly being used to manage problem behaviors in FTD, but their efficacy in this patient population have yet to be demonstrated in any clinical trial. The effects of therapeutic agents acting on different neurotransmitter systems in FTD have recently been reviewed in detatil.[220] Placebo-controlled trials are underway to test the efficacy of cholinesterase inhibitors and memantine in FTD; however, at best, these interventions may lead to modest symptomatic improvements.

As FTLD is further classified into clinical syndromes with prominent TDP-43 pathology at autopsy (a large proportion of FTD, most FTD with amyotrophic lateral sclerosis [ALS] and SD) versus those with prominent tau pathology at autopsy (some FTD and most PNFA), new avenues for potentially disease-modifying therapies have arisen. Future clinical trials of disease-modifying agents will likely focus on one pathological subtype of FTLD or the other. A small number of those with FTD and tau mutations have been treated with lithium, an agent known to affect second messenger systems that modify tau,[222] and larger studies are planned to investigate the effects of this medication in PNFA. Other evidence suggests that induction of heat shock protein pathways may protect cells from tau-related neurodegeneration.[223,224] A particularly exciting possibility is that restoration of progranulin protein levels in patients with FTD and *PGRN* mutations could significantly modify the course of this disease.

Frontotemporal dementia: primary progressive aphasia subtype

Background
In 1982, Mesulam[225] first described a series of patients who had aphasia without dementia, and later, he

Table 16.4. Summary of published open label and randomized clinical trials in patients with frontotemporal dementia[a]

Reference	Subjects	Study type	Study duration	Main findings
Selective serotonin-reuptake inhibitors				
Fluoxetine, sertraline, or paroxetine				
Swartz *et al.* (1997)[216]	11	OL	3 mo	Improvement in NP in more than half of patients
Paroxetine				
Moretti *et al.* (2001)[168]	16[b]	RCT	14 mo	Improvement in NP and caregiver stress; few AEs
Deakin *et al.* (2004)[217]	10	RCT (DBXO)	6 wks	No improvement in NP, mild worsening in COG
Other agents				
Trazodone				
Lebert *et al.* (2004)[218]	26	RCT (DBXO)	12 wks	Improvement in NP in many, stable COG; few AEs
Rivastigmine				
Moretti *et al.* (2004)[172]	20	OL	12 mo	Improvement in NP and caregiver burden, while COG declined
Donepezil				
Mendez *et al.* (2007)[219]	24	OL	6 mo	No difference in COG between treated/untreated; NP worse, reversible after drug removal in 33% of treated subjects

Notes:
AEs, adverse events; COG, cognition; DBXO, double-blind cross-over; mo, months; NP, neuropsychiatric features; OL, open-label trial; RCT, randomized clinical trial; wks, weeks.
[a]Further details in Huey *et al.* (2006)[220] and Huey (2006).[221]
[b]Approximately half the subjects were treated with active drug.

introduced the term *primary progressive aphasia*. Data have since been published on numerous other patients.[26,27,226] Although several subgroups of PPA have been described,[26,27] the clinical presentations fall into two main categories that are separable by fluency. Patients with non-fluent aphasia often have apraxia of speech and non-verbal oral apraxia and, in our experience, have a striking tendency to say "yes" for "no" and vice versa. Structural or functional neuroimaging studies show abnormalities involving the frontal opercular area (area of Broca) or insula in the dominant hemisphere. A similar spectrum of disorders that presents with FTD can manifest as progressive non-fluent aphasia–apraxia of speech. Patients with fluent aphasia typically have marked dysnomia. Semantic dementia refers to the features of fluent aphasia plus loss of word meaning (and hence agnosia), and imaging studies show prominent atrophy in the dominant temporal lobe (often most evident in the anterior inferolateral temporal cortex), which can be involved anywhere from the anterior pole to the posterior perirolandic area. The phenomenology of the language disturbance in many patients with fluent aphasia includes the terms *semantic dementia* and *semantic aphasia*.

Some patients develop difficulties recognizing objects (visual agnosia) or faces (prosopagnosia), but auditory cues, for example, shaking a ring of keys or having a person speak, allow the patient to recognize the object or person. It is important for clinicians to differentiate anomia from agnosia from visuoperceptual impairment in patients with impaired naming of objects or beings. Patients who cannot state the name of an object or a being but can demonstrate how the object is used or state identifying features of a being are likely to have anomia. Those who are unable to recognize an object or being but can describe the various aspects of an object or being are likely to have agnosia. Visual or associative agnosia refers to stimuli that are stripped of their meaning.

Controversy still exists about the minimal brain lesion necessary to cause prosopagnosia. For years, bilateral dysfunction of the inferior temporo-occipital cortex was considered necessary for prosopagnosia.[227] A detailed case report of a patient with prosopagnosia associated with right anterior temporal dysfunction (indicated by functional neuroimaging) suggests that this type of visual agnosia can occur with unilateral temporal lobe dysfunction.[228]

Alzheimer's disease occurs more frequently in patients with fluent aphasia, and the tauopathies and non-specific histopathology typically occur in those without AD. Some patients can have a protracted course, with features restricted to aphasia or agnosia, while others develop features of FTD or CBD or appear clinically indistinguishable from patients with AD in later stages. Parkinsonism or motor neuron disease can evolve; the latter portends a more rapid course.[23]

Management
The only pharmacologic study in patients with PPA ($n = 6$) showed mild slowing of language deterioration with bromocriptine therapy, but no alteration in the overall course of the disease.[229] Other treatments such as piracetam, amphetamine, donepezil and transcranial magnetic stimulation, which have shown some promise in aphasia caused by stroke (reviewed in detail by Berthier[230]) have not been evaluated in any of the progressive aphasia syndromes. Speech therapy can help some patients. For those with moderate to severe non-fluent aphasia, therapy with communication devices may be tried, but the patient's receptive language capabilities and functioning in non-language domains determine their utility. No drug treatment has been shown to improve agnosia.

Corticobasal degeneration
Background
In 1967, Rebeiz et al.[231] identified three patients who had progressive asymmetrical akinetic-rigid syndrome and apraxia and distinctive histopathological features. In these patients, achromatic neurons and degeneration of the cerebral cortex, substantia nigra and cerebellar dentate nucleus were found (leading to the term corticodentatonigral degeneration). Subsequently, findings in other patients were characterized by more basal ganglia than cerebellar degeneration (leading to such terms as cortical-basal ganglionic degeneration, corticobasal ganglionic degeneration and corticobasal degeneration). Most cases appear to be sporadic, although familial cases exist.

Diagnosis
Three sets of clinical criteria have been published for making the diagnosis of CBD.[232-234] Common to all three sets is the combination of progressive asymmetrical rigidity and apraxia, known as the PARA syndrome. This chapter has included CBD because neuropsychiatric morbidity occurs with the disorder,[235,236] and numerous patients have presented with progressive aphasia or dementia.[44,237] The patients with dementia typically present with features of FTD, although some have appeared clinically indistinguishable from those with AD. Importantly,

although these sets of clinical criteria have been developed to predict the underlying disease of CBD, antemortem diagnosis is about 50–60%.[238] Hence, these criteria should be considered similar to those for corticobasal syndrome (CBS; see below).

Management
The only report to consider specifically the effect of various pharmacological interventions in CBD is that of Kompoliti et al.[239] who found that no agent produced a consistent and prolonged benefit for any symptom or sign. Some patients have had some degree of improvement in parkinsonism with carbidopa/levodopa, but this has not been sustained. Valproic acid and clonazepam can improve myoclonus. Physical, occupational and speech therapy can be worthwhile. Depression and sleep disorders are also treatable. Other symptoms can improve with therapy directed toward target symptoms.

Corticobasal syndrome (also known as corticobasal degeneration syndrome, progressive perceptual-motor syndrome, progressive asymmetrical rigidity and apraxia syndrome)
Background
Although the core syndrome of progressive asymmetrical rigidity and apraxia has been considered characteristic of underlying CBD, approximately half the patients with this syndrome in one series were found to have CBD, whereas the others had either AD, Pick's disease, PSP, FTLD-U, DLDH, or CJD.[238,240] Presentation as CBS can also occur in NIBD.[241] Therefore, it is presumptive and often incorrect to label these patients with the pathological diagnosis of CBD, and syndromic nomenclature would be more appropriate. The term CBS is increasingly being used;[242] other terms for this syndrome include the progressive perceptual-motor syndrome, the PARA syndrome and corticobasal degeneration syndrome.

Management
As described in the section on CBD, the only report to consider specifically the effect of various pharmacological interventions in patients with clinically suspected CBD is that of Kompoliti et al.[239] who found that no agent produced a consistent and prolonged benefit for any symptom or sign. Some patients have

Table 16.5. Summary of published open-label and randomized clinical trials in patients with progressive supranuclear palsy

Reference	Subjects	Study type	Study duration	Main findings
Cholinesterase inhibitors for management of cognitive impairment				
Donepezil				
Fabbrini et al. (2001)[249]	6	OL	3 mo	No improvement in COG, motor or functional status
Litvan et al. (2001)[250]	21	RCT (DBXO)	13 wks	Modest improvement in COG; deleterious effects on mobility and ADLs
Cholinesterase inhibitors for management of dysphagia				
Physostigmine				
Frattali et al. (1999)[251]	8	RCT (DBXO)	10 days	No improvement in dysphagia
Agents for management of parkinsonism				
Efaroxan				
Rascol et al. (1998)[252]	14	RCT (DBXO)	12 wks	No improvement in motor status
Pramipexole				
Weiner et al. (1999)[253]	6	OL	2 mo	No improvement in motor status

Notes:
ADL, activities of daily living; COG, cognition; DBXO, double-blind crossover; mo, months; OL, open-label trial; RCT, randomized clinical trial; wks, weeks.

had some degree of improvement in parkinsonism with carbidopa/levodopa, but this has not been sustained. Valproic acid and clonazepam can improve myoclonus. Physical, occupational and speech therapy can be worthwhile, and constraint-induced movement therapy (CIMT) has been beneficial for some patients, albeit over several months and not several years. Depression and sleep disorders are also treatable.[238] Other symptoms can improve with therapy.

Progressive supranuclear palsy

Background
In 1964, Steele et al.[243] described the clinical features of a syndrome (which still bears their names) with degeneration of the brainstem, basal ganglia and cerebellum. Recent immunocytochemical studies have demonstrated characteristic tau-positive abnormalities, and PSP is also considered a four-repeat tauopathy. Dementia occurs frequently in PSP. Most cases are sporadic.

Diagnosis
The classic presentation of PSP is the constellation of supranuclear gaze palsy, postural instability and falls, and parkinsonism.[244] Numerous patients have had atypical features, including ones mistaken for CBD; those with no gaze palsy, gait impairment, or parkinsonism; and those presenting with progressive aphasia, FTD, or having obsessive–compulsive features.[200,245,246]

Management
Management of the cognitive, motor and gait aspects of PSP is challenging.[235,247,248] The results from the few open-label studies and randomized clinical trials (all placebo-controlled cross-over studies) have been disappointing (Table 16.5).[249–253] Parkinsonism responds poorly to carbidopa/levodopa, and gait assistance devices or confinement to a wheelchair is often necessary for management of gait impairment. The topography of cortical dysfunction tends to involve the frontal or frontosubcortical neural networks; consequently, apathy and executive dysfunction are often present. Disinhibition, dysphoria and anxiety are also common,[245] but agitation and obsessive–compulsive features are less frequent. Treatment is directed toward target symptoms. Physical and occupational therapy and gait-assistance devices are also indicated in many.

Diagnosis and management of the human prion disorders
Creutzfeldt–Jakob disease
Background
The diagnosis of CJD has been applied to patients with rapidly progressive dementia who subsequently

Table 16.6. Summary of published open label and randomized clinical trials in patients with Creutzfeldt–Jakob disease

Reference	Subjects	Study type	Study duration	Main findings
Quinacrine				
Nakajima *et al.* (2004)[257]	4	OL	3 months	Mild and transient improvement in clinical status
Haik *et al.* (2004)[259]	32	OL	Up to 265 days	No clear improvement in symptoms nor prolongation of survival
Flupertine				
Otto *et al.* (2004)[258]	28[a]	RCT	Up to 86 days	Less decline in COG but no difference in survival in those treated with active drug compared to placebo

Notes:
COG, cognition; OL, open label trial; RCT, randomized clinical trial.
[a]Approximately half the subjects were treated with active drug.

are found to have spongiform changes (and positive prion protein immunostaining on neuropathological examination). The term *prion* was coined by Prusiner for *pro*teinaceous *in*fectious particles that appear to induce conformational changes in the prion protein that all humans have and ultimately cause neuronal death. There are sporadic, familial and iatrogenic forms, and the so-called "new variant CJD" (nvCJD) appears to be related to the ingestion of products from animals that previously had been fed contaminated food. Three other prion disorders that affect humans are GSS, FFI and kuru.

Diagnosis

The typical features of CJD include rapidly progressive dementia (time from onset of symptoms to death is often less than 1 year), myoclonus and quasiperiodic sharp wave complexes on electroencephalography.[254] Atypical presentations include clinical manifestations that reflect the topography of signal abnormalities on MRI or the distribution of spongiform changes on neuropathological examination, for example progressive aphasia syndrome, frontal lobe dementia syndrome, progressive apraxia and rigidity (CBS), progressive visuoperceptual and visuospatial impairment syndrome (Heidenhain variant) and various neuropsychiatric presentations. Increased levels of 14-3-3 protein and neuron-specific enolase in CSF have been associated with CJD and may aid in diagnosis.[255] Importantly, elevations of both 14-3-3 protein and neuron-specific enolase reflect acute or subacute neuronal injury and are *not* specific for CJD. Increased signal changes on fluid attenuation inversion recovery (FLAIR) or, particularly, diffusion-weighted images (DWI) in MRI may also be diagnostically relevant, particularly when the basal ganglia or cortical ribbon is involved.

Management

Recent cell culture and animal experiments have suggested that certain acridine and phenothiazine derivatives, particularly quinacrine and chlorpromazine, may affect prion protein pathophysiology.[256] Flupertine has also shown some promise. Small numbers of patients with CJD have been treated with either quinacrine or flupertine (Table 16.6).[257,258] There have been mixed results with quinacrine, and flupertine appeared to decrease the degree of cognitive impairment but did not affect survival. Much larger clinical trials are underway. Otherwise, management is directed toward target symptoms or behaviors. In many cases, involvement of a hospice is appropriate.

New variant Creutzfeldt–Jakob disease

Background

Two cases of sporadic CJD in teenagers living in the UK were reported in 1995. Several additional cases with atypical clinical features were identified, with most of the patients residing in the UK or France. The neuropathological findings of prion protein deposition in the cerebral and cerebellar cortices and the presence of so-called florid and multicentric plaques were atypical of sporadic CJD.[260] The clinical and histological features led to the use of the term "new variant" for these cases. Analyses have established that the causative agent of the prion protein strain is bovine spongiform encephalopathy, also known as *mad cow disease*.[261] Cattle had been fed processed animal products that were unknowingly infected, and the cattle were then consumed by humans. This process of using animal products as cattle feed was banned in 1989, but because of the lengthy period from ingestion to clinical symptoms, nvCJD likely will continue to develop in humans for years to come. Only two individuals living in North America have been identified, both of whom had resided in the UK years earlier and when ingestion presumably occurred.

Diagnosis

Patients with nvCJD have tended to be younger than those with sporadic CJD, and the symptoms typically have been more "psychiatric," with depression, behavioral changes, apathy, delusions and hallucinations.[262] Sensory symptoms have been common. Dementia usually evolves, as does myoclonus.[263] The duration of symptoms has generally been longer than for typical CJD, with some exceeding 3 years from onset to death.[264] Electroencephalographic findings are abnormal, but the quasiperiodic pattern of sharp wave complexes is rare. In several cases, signal changes in the posterior thalamus have been documented on MRI.[265] Examination of brain tissue or, more recently, tonsil tissue, establishes the diagnosis.[264]

Management

Quinacrine, flupertine and other agents have been or will likely be used in nvCJD cases, but there are too few data to determine if these have been effective in this disorder. Consequently, management is directed toward target symptoms or behaviors. Involvement of a hospice is again appropriate. The advances in molecular genetics and molecular biology have led to remarkable changes in our understanding of degenerative and prion-related dementing illnesses. A major shift is evolving in which the pathophysiological processes are becoming increasingly relevant for drug development rather than clinical characterization.

Management of target symptoms in dementia

Since no currently available therapy directly and importantly alters the pathophysiological processes causing dementia, management of dementia, regardless of the cause, typically is tailored toward target symptoms. Although most reports on the available agents have involved patients with clinically suspected AD, many of these agents may be helpful in the management of non-AD disorders. Readers are encouraged to review some key articles and texts on the management of problematic symptoms and behaviors in dementia.[266–270]

In the office, a helpful exercise is to ask patients and their caregivers to cite and to rank by priority the symptoms or features they want most to alter. Initial therapy can be directed at the issue of top priority, and if this is better managed with therapy, then therapy can be directed toward the next most important issue, and so forth. Therapies for important symptoms and behaviors – categorized as cognitive and non-cognitive features – are described below; specific drugs and dosing suggestions are shown in Table 16.7.

Cognitive features

Amnesia and forgetfulness

Cholinesterase inhibitors were developed to improve memory; however, because in AD and DLB the cholinergic neurons of the basal forebrain degenerate, progressively less and less acetylcholine is available to modulate therapeutically as the illness worsens. Because neuronal death is comparatively less in DLB than in AD, the response to cholinesterase inhibitor therapy can be impressive in some patients with DLB.[56–62,65,67,81,271] Some individuals with FTD and other non-AD disorders may also experience cognitive improvement with cholinesterase inhibitors. Presumably, agents with nicotinic or muscarinic (or both) receptor agonist activity would be most likely to improve memory; however, preliminary studies have suggested that the systemic effects are too intolerable for many patients. Cholinergic agonists that are selective for the CNS may offer the most benefit for amnesia and forgetfulness. Some patients and their families have noticed improvement in forgetfulness with levodopa, modafinil or methylphenidate therapy. Memantine is another option, although the effects tend to be modest.

Aphasia

Aphasia can result from dysfunction of the frontal, temporal or parietal lobes of the dominant hemisphere as well as from lesions in the thalamus, basal ganglia, insula and arcuate fasciculus. Aphasia is the core feature of the progressive aphasia syndromes, and aphasia can occur with AD, Pick's disease, CBD, PSP, DLDH, CJD and cerebrovascular insults. Speech therapy can improve communicability for some aphasic patients. When expressive language functions are severely compromised, specially designed devices can be helpful. As noted above for progressive aphasia, bromocriptine is the only agent that has been tested, and the effect was modest.[229]

Agnosia

Agnosia (the inability to recognize the meaning of stimuli) is characteristic of the associative agnosia

Table 16.7. Symptoms, behaviors and disorders in dementia: selected medications with suggested dosing schedules[a]

Symptom/behavior/disorder	Medication	Starting dose	Suggested titrating schedule	Typical therapeutic range
Apathy or psychomotor slowing or subcortical dementia	Methylphenidate	2.5 mg qam	Increase in 2.5–5 mg increments q3–5 days in bid dosing (a.m. and noon)	5 mg qam–30 mg bid
	Amphetamine/dextroamphetamine	5 mg qam	Increase in 5 mg increments q7 days in qd–bid dosing (a.m. and noon) dosing, maximum 25 mg bid	5 mg qam–20 mg bid
	Modafinil	100 mg qam	Increase in 100 mg increments every morning weekly, up to 400 mg po qam	100–400 mg qam
	Carbidopa/levodopa	25/100 ½ tab tid	Increase in ½ tab increments over all 3 daily doses each week (take 1 h before or after meals)	1–3 tabs tid
	Donepezil	5 mg qam	Increase to 10 mg qam 4 weeks later	5–10 mg qam
	Rivastigmine	1.5 mg bid	Increase in 1.5 mg increments for both doses every 2–4 weeks, maximum 6 mg bid	1.5 mg bid to 6.0 mg bid
	Galantamine	4 mg bid	Increase in 4 mg increments for both doses every 4 weeks; maximum 12 mg bid	4 mg bid to 12 mg bid
	Memantine	5 mg qd	Increase gradually over 4 weeks up to 10 mg bid	5 mg qd to 10 mg bid
Forgetfullness	Donepezil	5 mg qam	Increase to 10 mg qam 4 weeks later	5–10 mg qam
	Rivastigmine	1.5 mg bid	Increase in 1.5 mg increments for both doses every 2–4 weeks; maximum 6 mg bid	1.5 mg bid to 6.0 mg bid
	Galantamine	4 mg bid	Increase in 4 mg increments for both doses every 4 weeks; maximum 12 mg bid	4 mg bid to 12 mg bid
	Memantine	5 mg qd	Increase gradually over 4 weeks up to 10 mg bid	5 mg qd to 10 mg bid
Depression or emotional lability/ pseudobulbar affect	Fluoxetine	10 mg qd	Increase to 20 mg 2–4 weeks later	10–40 mg qd
	Sertraline	25 mg qd	Increase to 50 mg 2 weeks later; titrate gradually up to maximum of 200 mg qd	50–100 mg qd
	Paroxetine	10 mg qd	Increase to 20 mg 2 weeks later; titrate gradually up to maximum of 50 mg/day	10–40 mg qd
	Citalopram	10 mg qd	Increase to 20 mg 2 weeks later; titrate gradually up to maximum of 60 mg/day	10–60 mg qd
Orthostatic hypotension	Fludrocortisone	0.1 mg qd	Increase in 0.1 mg increments q5–7 days; maximum 1.0 mg/day	0.1–0.3 mg qd
	Midodrine	5 mg tid	Increase up to 10 mg tid if necessary	5–10 mg tid
Parkinsonism	Carbidopa/levodopa	25/100 ½ tab tid		1–3 tabs tid

Table 16.7. (cont.)

Symptom/behavior/disorder	Medication	Starting dose	Suggested titrating schedule	Typical therapeutic range
Anxiety or obsessions/compulsions	Escitalopram	10 mg qd	Increase in ½ tab increments over all 3 daily doses each week (take 1 h before or after meals) Increase to 20 mg 2–4 weeks later; titrate gradually up to maximum of 40 mg qd	10–40 mg qd
	Sertraline	25 mg qd	Increase to 50 mg 2 weeks later; titrate gradually up to maximum of 200 mg qd	50–100 mg qd
	Paroxetine	10 mg qd	Increase to 20 mg 2 weeks later; titrate gradually up to maximum of 50 mg/day	10–40 mg qd
	Buspirone	5 mg bid	Increase in 5 mg increments in bid–tid dosing q3–5 days; maximum of 60 mg/day	5–10 mg tid
Insomnia	Trazodone	25 mg qhs	Increase in 25 mg increments q3–5 days	50–200 mg/night
	Chloral hydrate	500 mg qhs	Increase in 500 mg increments q5–7 days	500–1500 mg/night
	Melatonin	3 mg	Increase in 3 mg increments as necessary, up to 12 mg/night	3–12 mg/night
	Quetiapine	12.5 mg qhs	Increase in 12.5 to 25 mg increments as necessary, up to 100–200 mg qhs	12.5–200 mg qhs
	Zolpidem	2.5 mg qhs	Increase in 2.5 mg increments as necessary, up to 10 mg qhs	2.5–10 mg qhs
Restless legs syndrome/periodic limb movement disorder	Carbidopa/levodopa	25/100 or controlled release 25/100	1 tab qhs; increase to 2 tabs 1 week later if necessary	1–2 tabs qhs
	Pramipexole	0.125 mg qhs	Increase in 0.125 mg increments q2–3 days	0.25–0.75 mg/night
	Ropinirole	0.25 mg qhs	Increase in 0.25 mg increments q2–3 days	0.5–2 mg/night
	Gabapentin	100 mg qhs	Increase in 100 mg increments q2–3 days	300–1200 mg/night
Excessive day-time somnolence	Methylphenidate	2.5 mg qam	Increase in 2.5–5 mg increments q3–5 days in bid dosing (a.m. and noon)	5 mg qam to 30 mg bid
	Amphetamine/ dextroamphetamine	5 mg qam	Increase in 5 mg increments q7 days in qd–bid (a.m. and noon) dosing; maximum 25 mg bid	5 mg qam to 20 mg bid
	Modafinil	100 mg qam	Increase in 100 mg increments every morning weekly, up to 400 mg po qam	100–400 mg qam
REM sleep-behavior disorder	Clonazepam	0.25 mg qhs	Increase in 0.25 mg increments q7 days	0.25–1.0 mg/night
	Melatonin	3 mg	Increase in 3 mg increments q3–5 days up to 12 mg if necessary	3–12 mg/night
	Quetiapine	12.5 mg qhs	Increase in 12.5 to 25 mg increments as necessary, up to 100–200 mg qhs	12.5–200 mg qhs

Indication	Drug	Starting dose	Titration	Target dose
Hallucinations or delusions or behavioral dyscontrol or agitation/aggression or nocturnal wandering or disinhibition	Donepezil	5 mg qam	Increase to 10 mg qam 4 weeks later	5–10 mg qam
	Rivastigmine	1.5 mg bid	Increase in 1.5 mg increments for both doses every 4 weeks; maximum 6 mg bid	1.5 mg bid to 6.0 mg bid
	Galantamine	4 mg bid	Increase in 4 mg increments for both doses every 4 weeks; maximum 12 mg bid	4 mg bid to 12 mg bid
	Risperidone	0.5 mg qhs	Increase in 0.5 mg increments q7 days in bid dosing (a.m. and at bedtime)	0.5 mg qhs to 1.5 mg bid
	Olanzapine	5 mg qhs	Increase in 5 mg increments q7 days in bid dosing (a.m. and at bedtime)	5 mg qhs to 10 mg bid
	Clozapine	12.5 mg qhs	Increase in 12.5 mg increments q2–3 days	25 mg qhs–50 mg tid
	Quetiapine	25 mg qhs	Increase in 25 mg increments q3 days	25 mg qhs to 100 mg qam/400 mg qpm
	Valproic acid	125 mg qhs	Increase in 125 mg increments q3–7 days in bid to tid dosing	250 mg qhs to 500 mg tid
	Carbamazepine	100 mg qhs	Increase in 100 mg increments q3–7 days in bid to tid dosing	200 mg qhs to 200 mg tid
	Memantine	5 mg qd	Increase gradually over 4 weeks up to 10 mg bid	5 mg qd to 10 mg bid

Notes:
Bid, twice daily; po, oral; qX, every X period of time; qam, every morning; qd, every day; qhs, every hour of sleep; qpm, every night; tab, tablet; tid, three times a day.
[a]Disclaimer and important points. The choice of which agents to use and which dosing schedules to recommend must be individualized. It is the responsibility of the clinician to consider potential side-effects, drug interactions, allergic response, life-threatening reactions (e.g. leukopenia with clozapine), dosing changes required in renal or hepatic dysfunction, etc. before administering any drug to any patient, including those listed above. The authors, the Mayo Foundation and the publisher will not be responsible for any adverse reactions of any kind to any patient regarding the content of this information. The US Food and Drug Administration (FDA) has issued warnings about the increased frequency of hyperglycemia/diabetes, stroke and mortality associated with some or all of the atypical neuroleptics; increased mortality associated with galantamine in patients with mild cognitive impairment and other warnings (refer to the FDA website: www.fda.gov). Clinicians, patients and their families must carefully weigh the risks and benefits before commencing any of these agents. Periodic laboratory monitoring is necessary when using some agents; refer to guidelines provided by manufacturer.

syndrome, and it can occur in any of the cortical dementing disorders. No drug has been shown to improve agnosia.

Apraxia

Limb apraxia is a core feature of the CBS, and apraxia can occur in other syndromes and disorders with prominent parietofrontal neural networks dysfunction. Carbidopa/levodopa can improve apraxia slightly and for a period of months in select patients. Experience at our center has shown that CIMT, in which the "good" limb is restrained for hours every day and thus forcing the person to use the "bad" limb, has resulted in impressive improvement of limb functionality in some patients with CBS. The challenge is identifying therapists trained in CIMT, and strong motivation by the patient is critical for CIMT to be potentially helpful.

Visuospatial and visuoperceptual dysfunction

Dysfunction in complex visual processing is characteristic of PCA, and such dysfunction can occur in patients with DLB, CBD, AD, CJD or DLDH. Ophthalmological consultation is reasonable for all patients with visuospatial and visuoperceptual dysfunction so that any potential ocular cause of visual impairment can be evaluated and treated. Otherwise, patients with marked impairment should not be allowed to drive or to operate machinery, and measures should be taken to minimize the potential for injury around the house. For patients who experience illusions, changing the illumination in rooms or removing problematic items from the house may minimize the illusions. Misidentification errors, particularly if they involve the spouse and children, can be troubling to family members; counseling the family on the dysfunction in complex visual processing may reduce the anxiety related to these errors. For those patients who are troubled by their own reflections in mirrors, covering the mirrors can suffice. Rarely, patients have shown improvement functionally and on neuropsychometric testing with cholinesterase inhibitor and levodopa therapy. No drug has been shown in clinical studies to improve visuospatial and visuoperceptual dysfunction.

Executive dysfunction

Difficulties in judgement, insight, reasoning, complex decision making and performing sequential tasks all reflect dysfunction in frontosubcortical neural networks. While executive dysfunction is at the core of FTD, such dysfunction tends to occur in almost all other syndromes and disorders at some point in the course. While no studies have been performed and published about any pharmacologic therapies for executive dysfunction per se, many of the drugs that affect acetylcholine, dopamine, serotonin and norepinephrine could theoretically improve executive functioning. Recent analyses using neuropsychological testing and PET suggests that cholinesterase inhibitors activate frontosubcortical networks, at least in patients with mild cognitive impairment.[272]

Non-cognitive features

Agitation, aggression and behavioral dyscontrol

Agitation, verbally and physically aggressive behavior, as well as psychotic features, sleep disturbances, and wandering, are often collectively termed as "behavioral and psychological symptoms of dementia" and abbreviated BPSD.[273] These BPSD are a major cause of institutionalization, and even for 24 hour care facilities. The management of BPSD can be very challenging, and the costs associated with BPSD are staggering.[274] While intervention should always be focused specifically on target symptoms and behaviors (see the specific targets of hallucinations and delusions, and sleep disturbances, below), the concept of BPSD has been useful for designing treatment trials. Traditionally, treatment has been with conventional neuroleptics and benzodiazepines, but several randomized clinical trials and meta-analyses involving atypical neuroleptic drugs, cholinesterase inhibitors, memantine, antidepressants, carbamazepine and valproic acid have been completed (Table 16.8).[73,78,87,173,189,275–295] The focus with these studies has been on the constellation of problematic behaviors more so than the underlying disorder. As shown in Table 16.8, efficacy and tolerability have been shown in most studies involving atypical neuroleptic drugs, cholinesterase inhibitors and memantine; the results from the trials using antidepressants, carbamazepine and valproic acid have not shown efficacy in most open-label and randomized clinical trials. Yet lack of superiority of any drug over placebo in clinical trials does *not* translate into futility in individual patients. The suggestions and findings in Tables 16.7 and 16.8 are, therefore, presented to allow clinicians to consider options and evidence-based data before deciding what agents, if any, should be used for select patients.

Table 16.8. Summary of open-label trials, randomized clinical trials and meta-analyses for managing behaviors and problem symptoms in dementia (BPSD)[a]

Reference	Subjects	Study type	Study duration	Main findings
Conventional neuroleptics				
Haloperidol, thioridazine, perphenazine				
Stotsky et al. (1984)[275] *"Senile" dementia*	358	RCT	4 wks	Improvement in NP (particularly anxiety and agitation) in thioridazine group
Schneider et al. (1990)[276] *"Senile" dementia, VaD*	252	MA	3–8 wks	Less than 20% improved
Lonergan et al. (2002)[277] *AD, VaD*	573	MA	3–16 wks	Improvement in NP (particularly aggression) in haloperidol group; AEs frequent
Pollock et al. (2002)[278] *AD, VaD, mixed AD/VaD and DLB*	54	RCT	17 days	No improvement demonstrated with perphenazine; withdrawals frequent
Atypical neuroleptics				
Risperidone, Olanzepine and Quetiapine				
Schneider et al. (2006)[296] *AD*	421	RCT	36 wks.	AEs offset efficacy of all three drugs; discontinuations owing to AEs highest with olanzepine and risperdone
Risperidone				
De Deyn et al. (1999)[279] *AD, VaD and mixed AD/VaD*	344	RCT	12 wks	Improvement in NP secondary outcome measures but not primary; more frequent AEs
Katz et al. (1999)[280] *AD, VaD and mixed AD/VaD*	625	RCT	12 wks	Improvement in NP primary outcome measure; more frequent withdrawals and AEs higher (especially EPS)
Brodaty et al. (2003)[189] *AD, VaD and mixed AD/VaD*	345	RCT	12 wks	Improvement in NP (particularly aggression); more frequent AEs, including stroke
Olanzapine				
Satterlee et al. (1995) *AD*	238	RCT	12 wks	No significant improvement in NP (mean dose upon study completion only 2.7 mg/day)
Street et al. (2000)[281] *AD*	206	RCT	6 wks	Improvement in NP (particularly agitation/aggression, hallucinations, delusions); more frequent withdrawals and AEs
Meehan et al. (2002)[282] *AD, VaD and mixed AD/VaD*	204	RCT	1 day	Improvement in NP; few AEs
De Deyn et al. (2004)[283] *AD*	652	RCT	10 wks	No improvement demonstrated, more frequent AEs
Quetiapine				
Schneider et al. (1999) *AD + psychosis*	78	OL	52 wks	Improvement in NP
Tariot et al. (2000)[284] *Dementia + psychosis*	184	OL	52 wks	Improvement in NP; mild to moderate, tolerable AEs; no worsening of EPS
Tariot et al. (2006)[297] *AD + psychosis*	284	RCT	10 wks	Improvement in NP (particularly agitation, anergia) and functional abilities
Aripiprazole				
De Deyn et al. (2005)[298] *AD + psychosis*	208	RCT	10 wks	Improvement in NP on secondary but not primary outcome measure

Table 16.8. (cont.)

Reference	Subjects	Study type	Study duration	Main findings
Cholinesterase inhibitors				
Donepezil				
Feldman et al. (2001)[22] *AD*	290	RCT	24 wks	Improvement in most measures; withdrawals similar; AEs more frequent
Tariot et al. (2001)[299] *AD*	208	RCT	24 wks	No improvement demonstrated; withdrawals similar; AEs more frequent
Courtney et al. (2004)[73] *AD and mixed AD/VaD*	565	RCT	Up to 4 years	No improvement demonstrated; withdrawals and AEs more frequent
Holmes et al. (2004)[286] *AD*	96	RCT	12 wks	Improvement in most measures; withdrawals and AEs similar
Rivastigmine				
McKeith et al. (2000)[58] *DLB*	120	RCT	20 wks	Improvement in NP; AEs more frequent; no worsening of EPS
Emre et al. (2004)[93] *PDD*	541	RCT	24 wks	Improvement in NP; AEs more frequent, including tremor
Galantamine				
Erkinjunnti et al. (2002)[173] *VaD and mixed VaD/AD*	592	RCT	24 wks	Improvement or stabilization in most measures; withdrawals and AEs more frequent
Olin and Schneider (2002)[300] *AD*	1364	MA	12–20 wks	Improvement dose related (16 mg); withdrawals and AEs more frequent for doses ≥ 16 mg
N-Methyl-D-aspartate (NMDA) antagonists				
Memantine				
Reisberg et al. (2003)[301] *AD*	252	RCT	28 wks	No improvement demonstrated; withdrawals and AEs more frequent in *placebo* group
Tariot et al. (2004)[269] *AD (plus donepezil)*	404	RCT	24 wks	Improvement in NP; withdrawals more frequent in *placebo* group
Gauthier et al. (2005)[287] *AD*	656	MA	24–28 wks	Improvement in NP; particularly agitation/aggression
Antidepressants				
Citalopram				
Pollock et al. (2002)[278] *AD, VaD, mixed AD/VaD and DLB*	52	RCT	17 days	Improvement in NP, particularly agitation and lability; frequent AEs in both groups; many withdrawals in both groups from either AEs or poor efficacy
Fluoxetine				
Auchus and Bissey-Black (1997)[288] *AD*	15	RCT	6 wks	No improvement demonstrated; AEs more frequent
Sertraline				
Lyketsos et al. (2003)[289] *AD*	44	RCT	12 wks	No improvement in BPSD demonstrated, but improvement *was* shown for depression; AEs similar
Finkel et al. (2004)[290] *AD*	245	RCT	12 wks	No improvement demonstrated; AEs moderate

	N			
Trazodone				
Teri et al. (2000)[291] *AD*	73	RCT	16 wks	No improvement demonstrated; AEs and withdrawals similar
Mood stabilizers				
Carbamazepine				
Tariot et al. (1998)[292] *AD and mixed AD/VaD*	51	RCT	6 wks	Improvement in agitation; AEs and withdrawals more frequent in active drug group
Olin et al. (2001)[293] *AD*	21	RCT	6 wks	No improvement demonstrated; AEs similar
Divalproex sodium				
Porsteinsson et al. (2001)[294] *AD and mixed AD/VaD*	56	RCT	6 wks	No improvement demonstrated; AEs more frequent in active drug group
Tariot et al. (2001)[299] *AD, VaD and mixed AD/VaD*	172	RCT	6 wks	No improvement demonstrated; AEs more frequent in active drug group
Sival et al. (2002)[295] *AD, VaD, mixed AD/VaD and dementia associated with PD*	42	RCT	3 wks	No improvement demonstrated; AEs infrequent and similar

Notes:

AD, Alzheimer's disease; AEs, adverse events; DLB, dementia with Lewy bodies; EPS, extrapyramidal signs; MA, meta–analysis; mo, months; NP, neuropsychiatric features; OL, open-label study; PD, Parkinson's disease; PDD, Parkinson's disease with dementia; RCT, randomized clinical trial; VaD, vascular dementia; wks, weeks.

[a]RCTs typically had one-third to half the subjects using placebo; efficacy, withdrawals and AEs in active treatment group are compared with placebo.

While the data substantiating efficacy of the atypical neuroleptic drugs in the management of BPSD is firmly growing, the US FDA has issued warnings of concern regarding the increased risk of cerebrovascular events[301] and hyperglycemia/diabetes,[302] and in April of 2005 of slightly increased mortality associated with atypical neuroleptic use in patients with dementia.[303] The warning on increased mortality was based on data with an atypical neuroleptic from 17 placebo-controlled trials.[304] The implications of this warning are worrisome; atypical neuroleptic drugs should be used with great caution, and other agents such as conventional neuroleptic agents and benzodiazepines may be safer and hence better options for managing problem behaviors in dementia. Most experts still regard atypical neuroleptic drugs as preferable to conventional neuroleptics and benzodiazepines, provided that families are aware of these risks. Results from the Clinical Antipsychotic Trials of Intervention Effectiveness (CATIE) suggest that adverse effects offset advantages in the efficacy of atypical antipsychotic drugs for the treatment of psychosis, aggression or agitation in patients with Alzheimer's disease;[296] however, problems with study design and drug dosing limit the applicability of these results to general practice.

Before instituting any drug in patients with dementia, it is important to ensure that sources of pain, another medical illness (e.g. urinary tract infection), effects of other medications, and so on have been evaluated and addressed. Patients, caregivers and the clinicians involved in their care should weigh the advantages and disadvantages of specific drugs and make a joint decision on which drug is most appropriate for specific target symptoms. A drug should be commenced at a low dose and titrated up slowly, with the aim of decreasing the target behaviors to a tolerable level. If one drug is not efficacious or leads to intolerable side-effects, it should be discontinued and another agent should be discussed and instituted. Inherent in this trial and error approach is the risk–benefit ratio, with improvement in problem behaviors and quality of life often considered by caregivers as much or more important than prolonging life in their loved ones who are suffering from diseases that are universally and ultimately fatal.

One important caveat regarding clinical trials in BPSD must be emphasized. Evidence-based medicine necessitates unbiased, randomized, double-blind, placebo-controlled clinical trials be performed to demonstrate any drug is superior to placebo for any clinical disorder. Patients with moderate to severe BPSD are probably rarely enrolled in clinical trials, as the clinicians and particularly the caregivers may be wary of participating in trials when life is so challenging and there is a 33% or 50% chance of their relative getting placebo. Therefore, essentially by default, patients with mild BPSD are enrolled, and the data from randomized clinical trials cannot be extrapolated to all patients with dementia and problem behaviors. If agitated depression is suspected, referral to a psychiatrist for consideration of electroconvulsive therapy is warranted.

Apathy

Apathy is common in FTD, but it also occurs with most dementing disorders. For example, a patient may look through a window or watch a monotonous TV channel for hours, or rarely initiate conversation or spontaneously perform activities around the house. Experience has shown that apathy can improve with treatment with psychostimulants, amantadine, levodopa, the dopamine agonists, buproprion, selegiline or cholinesterase inhibitors, as well as antidepressants when the apathy is part of depression.[305,306]

Disinhibition and socially inappropriate behavior

Inappropriate comments or gestures are the dread of many caregivers, particularly ones that have a sexual theme or are directed at children. Disinhibition is characteristic of FTD but can occur in other syndromes and diseases in which the frontal networks are dysfunctional. Atypical neuroleptic drugs, antidepressants (particularly SSRIs), cholinesterase inhibitors and anxiolytics can be effective.[307–310] If ineffective, avoidance of social settings may be the only way to minimize embarrassment owing to inappropriate behavior.

Hallucinations and delusions

Hallucinations and delusions are common in DLB and FTD, but they can occur in many other disorders and syndromes. Visual hallucinations are rarely present in CBD, and when they are associated with cognitive impairment and parkinsonism, their presence may suggest DLB rather than CBD.[310] If hallucinations or delusions are mild and visual and hearing impairment has been excluded as a cause, simple reassurance of the patient may be all that is necessary. When hallucinations or delusions are a problem, treatment with atypical neuroleptic agents and cholinesterase inhibitors can be beneficial. Melatonin taken before bedtime has improved or eliminated visual hallucinations in some patients. Levodopa, dopamine agonists, psychostimulants, amantadine and selegiline should be used with caution, because each can aggravate psychotic features.

Anxiety

Anxiety can occur in all the syndromes and disorders, and management can be challenging. Anxiolytics, antidepressants, cholinesterase inhibitors, and atypical neuroleptics, or some combination of these, may be beneficial.

Depression

Depression is common to all dementing disorders, and numerous effective antidepressant agents are available, although few have shown efficacy in randomized, double-blind, placebo-controlled trials in dementia.[311] All these agents can have adverse cognitive or behavioral effects. Agents with anticholinergic properties should be avoided, particularly tricyclic antidepressants, and paroxetine also must be used with caution owing to its anticholinergic effects. The presence of dementia should not preclude the use of electroconvulsive therapy if other therapies have not been effective.

Emotional lability and pseudobulbar affect

Frontosubcortical network dysfunction regardless of the underlying histopathological process can lead to emotional lability, with tearfulness induced by minimally emotional stimuli (pseudobulbar affect) being more common than excessive jocularity. If emotional lability is socially embarrassing, treatment with SSRIs can be effective; lithium therapy has also been suggested.[312–315] Although tricyclic antidepressants also minimize a pseudobulbar affect, the benefit must be weighed against the anticholinergic effects. While a combination of dextromethorphan and quinidine was not effective for slowing progression in ALS, the impressive improvement in pseudobulbar affect has led to continued clinical trials with this combination therapy.[316] Treatment trials for pseudobulbar affect have recently been reviewed.[317]

Hyperphagia

Hyperphagia is particularly problematic in FTD, especially involving sweets and ice cream, and gains of 100 pounds or more can occur in some patients if no intervention is successful. Restricting access to food by locking cupboards and the refrigerator may be effective in some, but agitation can result. There

are no clinical trials showing efficacy for hyperphagia related to dementia, but clinical experience has shown that topiramate can be effective in some, presumably owing to its poorly understood weight loss tendancies.

Urinary incontinence

The supratentorial control of continence has strong input from the frontal lobes; as a result, incontinence often occurs in patients with frontal lobe dysfunction. Nearly all patients with dementia develop incontinence terminally. If urinary studies exclude an infection and urological evaluation does not reveal a treatable cause in the genitourinary structures, agents with anticholinergic properties can improve incontinence, but the improvement must be considered in the context of possible diminished cholinergic activity in the cerebral cortex.[318–321] Scheduled voiding attempts, whereby the patient is encouraged to attempt to urinate even if no urge is apparent every 4 hours while awake, can greatly minimize incontinence during the day. If cognitive impairment is mild to moderate but urinary incontinence seriously affects quality of life, placement of a suprapubic catheter may be warranted.

Insomnia

In patients, insomnia can result from primary insomnia (includes psychophysiological insomnia and inadequate sleep hygiene), restless legs syndrome or central sleep apnea syndrome. In a caregiver, insomnia can be caused by the same spectrum of disorders in addition to disruptive snoring, obstructive sleep apnea/hypopnea syndrome, periodic limb movement disorder or nocturnal wandering in their cognitively impaired bedpartner. Diagnosis requires a detailed sleep disorders interview, physical examination and, in some cases, polysomnography. Primary insomnia can improve with treatment with trazodone, chloral hydrate or melatonin.[268,322–326] Carbidopa/levodopa, dopamine agonists such as pergolide or pramipexole, gabapentin or opiates are generally effective for restless legs syndrome and periodic limb movement disorder. Nasal continuous positive airway pressure (CPAP), if calibrated to the correct pressure and used nightly, eliminates disruptive snoring and obstructive sleep apnea. Central sleep apnea syndrome can be difficult to treat, often requiring various combinations of CPAP, bilevel positive airway pressure, supplemental oxygen and benzodiazepines. Referral to a sleep medicine specialist can be helpful.

Hypersomnia

Hypersomnia can result from restless legs syndrome, periodic limb movement disorder, central sleep apnea syndrome, obstructive sleep apnea, insufficient sleep, narcolepsy or idiopathic hypersomnia. Consultation with a sleep disorders specialist and polysomnography with or without a multiple sleep latency test can be fruitful. Psychostimulants can be safe and effective in elderly patients.[327]

Parasomnia

Parasomnias refer to unpleasant nocturnal experiences or behaviors. Probably the most common parasomnia among the elderly is RBD, which also occurs in PD, DLB and multiple system atrophy.[42–45,330] Patients seemingly "act out their dreams," and the dream content often involves a chasing or attacking theme. Polysomnography is often necessary to investigate nocturnal seizures or obstructive sleep apnea (a history identical to that of RBD can occur in severe obstructive sleep apnea). Treatment with a low dose of clonazepam or melatonin is often effective for reducing the chance of injury to patients and their bedpartners.[68,314] Quetiapine can improve RBD in some patients.[44,45] Patients and bedpartners can also be counseled, for example to move potentially injurious objects away from the bed and to place a mattress on the floor next to the bed.[329]

"Sundowning"

Delirium, confusion, disorganized thinking, impaired attention, wandering, agitation, insomnia, hypersomnia, hallucinations, illusions, delusions, anxiety, restlessness, hyperactivity and anger have all been considered features of the *sundowning syndrome*.[330,331] The term implies that problem symptoms or behaviors develop during the evening or night, although few data support that this occurs.[328] The term is nebulous, and more descriptive terms such as "agitation" or "wandering" are more appropriate. Several therapies have been suggested to improve various elements of the sundowning syndrome.[332] We suggest that clinicians identify specifically which symptoms are a problem and treat them accordingly. Our clinical experience has shown that diagnosis and management of the primary sleep disorders with or without a scheduled nap after the noon meal can markedly improve symptoms or behaviors that are most bothersome in the afternoon or evening.

Acknowledgements

Bradley Boeve is supported by grants P50 AG16574, U01 AG06786, RO1 AG 23195, P01 NS 40256, and the Robert H. and Clarice Smith and Abigail Van Buren Alzheimer's Disease Research Program of the Mayo Foundation (B.F.B). Adam Boxer is supported by grant K23NS48855 and the John Douglas French Foundation.

References

1. McKeith IG, Dickson DW, Lowe J et al. Diagnosis and management of dementia with Lewy bodies: third report of the DLB Consortium. *Neurology.* 2005;**65**:1863–1872.

2. Rowe CC, Ng S, Ackermann U et al. Imaging beta-amyloid burden in aging and dementia. *Neurology.* 2007;**68**:1718–1725.

3. Neumann M, Mackenzie IR, Cairns NJ et al. TDP-43 in the ubiquitin pathology of frontotemporal dementia with VCP gene mutations. *J Neuropathol Exp Neurol.* 2007;**66**:152–157.

4. Johnson KA. Amyloid imaging of Alzheimer's disease using Pittsburgh Compound B. *Curr Neurol Neurosci Rep.* 2006;**6**:496–503.

5. Small GW, Kepe V, Ercoli LM et al. PET of brain amyloid and tau in mild cognitive impairment. *N Engl J Med.* 2006;**355**:2652–2663.

6. Mintun MA, Larossa GN, Sheline YI et al. [^{11}C]PIB in a nondemented population: potential antecedent marker of Alzheimer disease. *Neurology.* 2006;**67**:446–452.

7. Kemppainen NM, Aalto S, Wilson IA et al. PET amyloid ligand [^{11}C]PIB uptake is increased in mild cognitive impairment. *Neurology.* 2007;**68**:1603–1606.

8. Hye A, Lynham S, Thambisetty M et al. Proteome-based plasma biomarkers for Alzheimer's disease. *Brain.* 2006;**129**:3042–3050.

9. Simonsen AH, McGuire J, Hansson O et al. Novel panel of cerebrospinal fluid biomarkers for the prediction of progression to Alzheimer dementia in patients with mild cognitive impairment. *Arch Neurol.* 2007;**64**:366–370.

10. Finehout EJ, Franck Z, Choe LH et al. Cerebrospinal fluid proteomic biomarkers for Alzheimer's disease. *Ann Neurol.* 2007;**61**:120–129.

11. Weiner HL, Frenkel D. Immunology and immunotherapy of Alzheimer's disease. *Nat Rev Immunol.* 2006;**6**:404–416.

12. Bayer AJ, Bullock R, Jones RW et al. Evaluation of the safety and immunogenicity of synthetic Abeta42 (AN1792) in patients with AD. *Neurology.* 2005;**64**:94–101.

13. Lee M, Bard F, Johnson-Wood K et al. Abeta42 immunization in Alzheimer's disease generates Abeta N-terminal antibodies. *Ann Neurol.* 2005;**58**:430–435.

14. Fox NC, Black RS, Gilman S *et al.* Effects of Abeta immunization (AN1792) on MRI measures of cerebral volume in Alzheimer disease. *Neurology.* 2005; **64**:1563–1572.

15. Gilman S, Koller M, Black RS *et al.* Clinical effects of Abeta immunization (AN1792) in patients with AD in an interrupted trial. *Neurology.* 2005;**64**:1553–1562.

16. Aisen PS, Saumier D, Briand R *et al.* A Phase II study targeting amyloid-beta with 3APS in mild to moderate Alzheimer disease. *Neurology.* 2006;**67**:1757–1763.

17. Siemers ER, Quinn JF, Kaye J *et al.* Effects of a gamma-secretase inhibitor in a randomized study of patients with Alzheimer disease. *Neurology.* 2006;**66**:602–604.

18. Eriksen JL, Sagi SA, Smith TE *et al.* NSAIDs and enantiomers of flurbiprofen target gamma-secretase and lower Abeta 42 in vivo. *J Clin Invest.* 2003; **112**:440–449.

19. Petersen RC, Parisi JE, Dickson DW *et al.* Neuropathologic features of amnestic mild cognitive impairment. *Arch Neurol.* 2006;**63**:665–672.

20. Graham A, Davies R, Xuereb J *et al.* Pathologically proven frontotemporal dementia presenting with severe amnesia. *Brain.* 2005;**128**:597–605.

21. Petersen RC, Thomas RG, Grundman M *et al.* Vitamin E and donepezil for the treatment of mild cognitive impairment. *N Engl J Med.* 2005;**352**:2379–2388.

22. Feldman HH, Ferris S, Winblad B *et al.* Effect of rivastigmine on delay to diagnosis of Alzheimer's disease from mild cognitive impairment: the InDDEx study. *Lancet Neurol.* 2007;**6**:501–512.

23. Caselli RJ, Windebank AJ, Petersen RC *et al.* Rapidly progressive aphasic dementia and motor neuron disease. *Ann Neurol.* 1993;**33**:200–207.

24. Tang-Wai DF, Graff-Radford NR, Boeve BF *et al.* Clinical, genetic, and neuropathologic characteristics of posterior cortical atrophy. *Neurology.* 2004; **63**:1168–1174.

25. Renner JA, Burns JM, Hou CE *et al.* Progressive posterior cortical dysfunction: a clinicopathologic series. *Neurology.* 2004;**63**:1175–1180.

26. Caselli R. Focal and asymmetric cortical degeneration syndromes. *Neurologist.* 1995;**1**:1–19.

27. Caselli RJ. Asymmetric cortical degeneration syndromes. *Curr Opin Neurol.* 1996;**9**:276–280.

28. Benson DF, Davis RJ, Snyder BD. Posterior cortical atrophy. *Arch Neurol.* 1988;**45**:789–793.

29. Tang-Wai DF, Josephs KA, Boeve BF *et al.* Pathologically confirmed corticobasal degeneration presenting with visuospatial dysfunction. *Neurology.* 2003;**61**:1134–1135.

30. Furuya H, Ikezoe K, Ohyagi Y *et al.* A case of progressive posterior cortical atrophy (PCA) with vivid hallucination: are some ghost tales vivid hallucinations in normal people? *J Neurol Neurosurg Psychiatry.* 2006;**77**:424–425.

31. Josephs KA, Whitwell JL, Boeve BF *et al.* Visual hallucinations in posterior cortical atrophy. *Arch Neurol.* 2006;**63**:1427–1432.

32. Wolf RC, Schonfeldt-Lecuona C. Depressive symptoms as first manifestation of posterior cortical atrophy. *Am J Psychiatry.* 2006;**163**:939–940.

33. Mendez MF, Ghajarania M, Perryman KM. Posterior cortical atrophy: clinical characteristics and differences compared to Alzheimer's disease. *Dement Geriatr Cogn Disord.* 2002;**14**:33–40.

34. McKeith IG, Galasko D, Kosaka K *et al.* Consensus guidelines for the clinical and pathologic diagnosis of dementia with Lewy bodies (DLB): report of the consortium on DLB International Workshop. *Neurology.* 1996;**47**:1113–1124.

35. Grace J, McKeith IG. Decline in cognitive function in Parkinson's disease may be due to dementia with Lewy bodies. *BMJ.* 1998;**316**:1022.

36. Apaydin H, Ahlskog JE, Parisi JE *et al.* Parkinson disease neuropathology: later-developing dementia and loss of the levodopa response. *Arch Neurol.* 2002; **59**:102–112.

37. Galvin JE, Pollack J, Morris JC. Clinical phenotype of Parkinson disease dementia. *Neurology.* 2006;**67**: 1605–1611.

38. McKeith IG. Consensus guidelines for the clinical and pathologic diagnosis of dementia with Lewy bodies (DLB): report of the Consortium on DLB International Workshop. *J Alzheimers Dis.* 2006;**9**:417–423.

39. McKeith IG, Perry EK, Perry RH. Report of the Second Dementia with Lewy Body International Workshop: diagnosis and treatment. Consortium on Dementia with Lewy Bodies. *Neurology.* 1999;**53**:902–905.

40. Baker M, Mackenzie IR, Pickering-Brown SM *et al.* Mutations in progranulin cause tau-negative frontotemporal dementia linked to chromosome 17. *Nature.* 2006;**442**:916–919.

41. Ferman TJ, Smith GE, Boeve BF *et al.* Neuropsychological differentiation of dementia with Lewy bodies from normal aging and Alzheimer's disease. *Clin Neuropsychol.* 2006;**20**:623–636.

42. Boeve BF, Silber MH, Saper CB *et al.* Pathophysiology of REM sleep behaviour disorder and relevance to neurodegenerative disease. *Brain.* 2007;**130**:2770–2778.

43. Boeve BF, Silber MH, Ferman TJ *et al.* REM sleep behavior disorder and degenerative dementia: an association likely reflecting Lewy body disease. *Neurology.* 1998;**51**:363–370.

44. Olson EJ, Boeve BF, Silber MH. Rapid eye movement sleep behaviour disorder: demographic, clinical and laboratory findings in 93 cases. *Brain.* 2000;**123** (Pt 2):331–339.

45. Boeve BF, Silber MH, Ferman TJ *et al.* Association of REM sleep behavior disorder and neurodegenerative disease may reflect an underlying synucleinopathy. *Mov Disord.* 2001;**16**:622–630.

46. Boeve BF, Silber MH, Parisi JE *et al.* Synucleinopathy pathology and REM sleep behavior disorder plus dementia or parkinsonism. *Neurology.* 2003;**61**:40–45.

47. Boeve B. Dementia with Lewy bodies. In Peterson R (ed.) *Continuum*, Vol. 10. Minneapolis: American Academy of Neurology, 2004: 81–112.

48. Barber R, Ballard C, McKeith IG *et al.* MRI volumetric study of dementia with Lewy bodies: a comparison with AD and vascular dementia. *Neurology.* 2000; **54**:1304–1309.

49. Burton EJ, McKeith IG, Burn DJ *et al.* Cerebral atrophy in Parkinson's disease with and without dementia: a comparison with Alzheimer's disease, dementia with Lewy bodies and controls. *Brain.* 2004;**127**:791–800.

50. Dickson DW, Crystal H, Mattiace LA *et al.* Diffuse Lewy body disease: light and electron microscopic immunocytochemistry of senile plaques. *Acta Neuropathol (Berl).* 1989;**78**:572–584.

51. Dickson DW. Dementia with Lewy bodies: neuropathology. *J Geriatr Psychiatry Neurol.* 2002;**15**:210–216.

52. Lebert F, Pasquier F, Souliez L, Petit H. Tacrine efficacy in Lewy body dementia. *Int J Geriatr Psychiatry.* 1998;**13**:516–519.

53. Querfurth HW, Allam GJ, Geffroy MA *et al.* Acetylcholinesterase inhibition in dementia with Lewy bodies: results of a prospective pilot trial. *Dement Geriatr Cogn Disord.* 2000;**11**:314–321.

54. Shea C, MacKnight C, Rockwood K. Donepezil for treatment of dementia with Lewy bodies: a case series of nine patients. *Int Psychogeriatr.* 1998;**10**:229–238.

55. Lanctot KL, Herrmann N. Donepezil for behavioural disorders associated with Lewy bodies: a case series. *Int J Geriatr Psychiatry.* 2000;**15**:338–345.

56. Samuel W, Caligiuri M, Galasko D *et al.* Better cognitive and psychopathologic response to donepezil in patients prospectively diagnosed as dementia with Lewy bodies: a preliminary study. *Int J Geriatr Psychiatry.* 2000; **15**:794–802.

57. Minett TS, Thomas A, Wilkinson LM *et al.* What happens when donepezil is suddenly withdrawn? An open label trial in dementia with Lewy bodies and Parkinson's disease with dementia. *Int J Geriatr Psychiatry.* 2003;**18**:988–993.

58. McKeith I, Del Ser T, Spano P *et al.* Efficacy of rivastigmine in dementia with Lewy bodies: a randomised, double-blind, placebo-controlled international study. *Lancet.* 2000;**356**:2031–2036.

59. Grace JB, Walker MP, McKeith IG. A comparison of sleep profiles in patients with dementia with Lewy

bodies and Alzheimer's disease. *Int J Geriatr Psychiatry.* 2000;**15**:1028–1033.

60. Grace J, Daniel S, Stevens T *et al.* Long-Term use of rivastigmine in patients with dementia with Lewy bodies: an open-label trial. *Int Psychogeriatr.* 2001;**13**:199–205.

61. Maclean LE, Collins CC, Byrne EJ. Dementia with Lewy bodies treated with rivastigmine: effects on cognition, neuropsychiatric symptoms, and sleep. *Int Psychogeriatr.* 2001;**13**:277–288.

62. Wesnes KA, McKeith IG, Ferrara R *et al.* Effects of rivastigmine on cognitive function in dementia with Lewy bodies: a randomised placebo-controlled international study using the cognitive drug research computerised assessment system. *Dement Geriatr Cogn Disord.* 2002;**13**:183–192.

63. Thomas AJ, Burn DJ, Rowan EN *et al.* A comparison of the efficacy of donepezil in Parkinson's disease with dementia and dementia with Lewy bodies. *Int J Geriatr Psychiatry.* 2005;**20**:938–944.

64. Rowan E, McKeith IG, Saxby BK *et al.* Effects of donepezil on central processing speed and attentional measures in Parkinson's disease with dementia and dementia with Lewy bodies. *Dement Geriatr Cogn Disord.* 2007;**23**:161–167.

65. Edwards KR, Hershey L, Wray L *et al.* Efficacy and safety of galantamine in patients with dementia with Lewy bodies: a 12-week interim analysis. *Dement Geriatr Cogn Disord.* 2004;**17**(Suppl 1):40–48.

66. Edwards KR, Royall D, Hershey L *et al.* Efficacy and safety of galantamine in patients with dementia with Lewy bodies: a 24-week open-label study. *Dement Geriatr Cogn Disord.* 2007;**23**:401–405.

67. Walker Z, Grace J, Overshot R *et al.* Olanzapine in dementia with Lewy bodies: a clinical study. *Int J Geriatr Psychiatry.* 1999;**14**:459–466.

68. Cummings JL, Street J, Masterman D, Clark WS. Efficacy of olanzapine in the treatment of psychosis in dementia with Lewy bodies. *Dement Geriatr Cogn Disord.* 2002;**13**:67–73.

69. Fernandez HH, Trieschmann ME, Burke MA, Friedman JH. Quetiapine for psychosis in Parkinson's disease versus dementia with Lewy bodies. *J Clin Psychiatry.* 2002;**63**:513–515.

70. Takahashi H, Yoshida K, Sugita T *et al.* Quetiapine treatment of psychotic symptoms and aggressive behavior in patients with dementia with Lewy bodies: a case series. *Prog Neuropsychopharmacol Biol Psychiatry.* 2003;**27**:549–553.

71. Bonelli SB, Ransmayr G, Steffelbauer M *et al.* L-dopa responsiveness in dementia with Lewy bodies, Parkinson disease with and without dementia. *Neurology.* 2004;**63**:376–378.

72. Molloy S, McKeith IG, O'Brien JT, Burn DJ. The role of levodopa in the management of dementia with

Lewy bodies. *J Neurol Neurosurg Psychiatry*. 2005; **76**:1200–1203.

73. Courtney C, Farrell D, Gray R *et al.* Long-term donepezil treatment in 565 patients with Alzheimer's disease (AD2000): randomised double-blind trial. *Lancet*. 2004;**363**:2105–2115.

74. Ballard CG, Chalmers KA, Todd C *et al.* Cholinesterase inhibitors reduce cortical Abeta in dementia with Lewy bodies. *Neurology*. 2007;**68**:1726–1729.

75. Pakrasi S, Thomas A, Mosimann UP *et al.* Cholinesterase inhibitors in advanced dementia with Lewy bodies: increase or stop? *Int J Geriatr Psychiatry*. 2006;**21**:719–721.

76. Molloy SA, Rowan EN, O'Brien JT *et al.* Effect of levodopa on cognitive function in Parkinson's disease with and without dementia and dementia with Lewy bodies. *J Neurol Neurosurg Psychiatry*. 2006;**77**: 1323–1328.

77. Miyasaki JM, Shannon K, Voon V *et al.* Practice parameter: evaluation and treatment of depression, psychosis, and dementia in Parkinson disease (an evidence-based review): report of the Quality Standards Subcommittee of the American Academy of Neurology. *Neurology*. 2006;**66**:996–1002.

78. Bhanji NH, Gauthier S. Emergent complications following donepezil switchover to galantamine in three cases of dementia with Lewy bodies. *J Neuropsychiatry Clin Neurosci*. 2005;**17**:552–555.

79. Ridha BH, Josephs KA, Rossor MN. Delusions and hallucinations in dementia with Lewy bodies: worsening with memantine. *Neurology*. 2005;**65**:481–482.

80. Sabbagh MN, Hake AM, Ahmed S, Farlow MR. The use of memantine in dementia with Lewy bodies. *J Alzheimers Dis*. 2005;**7**:285–289.

81. McKeith I, Fairbairn A, Perry R *et al.* Neuroleptic sensitivity in patients with senile dementia of Lewy body type. *BMJ*. 1992;**305**:673–678.

82. Kurlan R, Cummings J, Raman R, Thal L. Quetiapine for agitation or psychosis in patients with dementia and parkinsonism. *Neurology*. 2007;**68**:1356–1363.

83. Hutchinson M, Fazzini E. Cholinesterase inhibition in Parkinson's disease. *J Neurol Neurosurg Psychiatry*. 1996;**61**:324–325.

84. Werber EA, Rabey JM. The beneficial effect of cholinesterase inhibitors on patients suffering from Parkinson's disease and dementia. *J Neural Transm*. 2001;**108**:1319–1325.

85. Fabbrini G, Barbanti P, Aurilia C *et al.* Donepezil in the treatment of hallucinations and delusions in Parkinson's disease. *Neurol Sci*. 2002;**23**:41–43.

86. Bergman J, Lerner V. Successful use of donepezil for the treatment of psychotic symptoms in patients with Parkinson's disease. *Clin Neuropharmacol*. 2002; **25**:107–110.

87. Aarsland D, Laake K, Larsen JP, Janvin C. Donepezil for cognitive impairment in Parkinson's disease: a randomised controlled study. *J Neurol Neurosurg Psychiatry*. 2002;**72**:708–712.

88. Leroi I, Brandt J, Reich SG *et al.* Randomized placebo-controlled trial of donepezil in cognitive impairment in Parkinson's disease. *Int J Geriatr Psychiatry*. 2004;**19**:1–8.

89. Ravina B, Putt M, Siderowf A *et al.* Donepezil for dementia in Parkinson's disease: a randomised, double blind, placebo controlled, crossover study. *J Neurol Neurosurg Psychiatry*. 2005;**76**:934–939.

90. Reading PJ, Luce AK, McKeith IG. Rivastigmine in the treatment of parkinsonian psychosis and cognitive impairment: preliminary findings from an open trial. *Mov Disord*. 2001;**16**:1171–1174.

91. Bullock R, Cameron A. Rivastigmine for the treatment of dementia and visual hallucinations associated with Parkinson's disease: a case series. *Curr Med Res Opin*. 2002;**18**:258–264.

92. Giladi N, Shabtai H, Gurevich T *et al.* Rivastigmine (Exelon) for dementia in patients with Parkinson's disease. *Acta Neurol Scand*. 2003;**108**:368–373.

93. Emre M, Aarsland D, Albanese A *et al.* Rivastigmine for dementia associated with Parkinson's disease. *N Engl J Med*. 2004;**351**:2509–2518.

94. Aarsland D, Hutchinson M, Larsen JP. Cognitive, psychiatric and motor response to galantamine in Parkinson's disease with dementia. *Int J Geriatr Psychiatry*. 2003;**18**:937–941.

95. Ostergaard K, Dupont E. Clozapine treatment of drug-induced psychotic symptoms in late stages of Parkinson's disease. *Acta Neurol Scand*. 1988; **78**:349–350.

96. Friedman JH, Lannon MC. Clozapine in the treatment of psychosis in Parkinson's disease. *Neurology*. 1989; **39**:1219–1221.

97. Pfeiffer RF, Kang J, Graber B *et al.* Clozapine for psychosis in Parkinson's disease. *Mov Disord*. 1990;**5**:239–242.

98. Wolters EC, Hurwitz TA, Mak E *et al.* Clozapine in the treatment of parkinsonian patients with dopaminomimetic psychosis. *Neurology*. 1990; **40**:832–834.

99. Kahn N, Freeman A, Juncos JL *et al.* Clozapine is beneficial for psychosis in Parkinson's disease. *Neurology*. 1991;**41**:1699–1700.

100. Wolk SI, Douglas CJ. Clozapine treatment of psychosis in Parkinson's disease: a report of five consecutive cases. *J Clin Psychiatry*. 1992;**53**:373–376.

101. Greene P, Cote L, Fahn S. Treatment of drug-induced psychosis in Parkinson's disease with clozapine. *Adv Neurol*. 1993;**60**:703–706.

102. Factor SA, Brown D, Molho ES, Podskalny GD. Clozapine: a 2-year open trial in Parkinson's

disease patients with psychosis. *Neurology.* 1994;
44:544–546.

103. Chacko RC, Hurley RA, Harper RG et al. Clozapine for acute and maintenance treatment of psychosis in Parkinson's disease. *J Neuropsychiatry Clin Neurosci.* 1995;**7**:471–475.

104. Rabey JM, Treves TA, Neufeld MY et al. Low-dose clozapine in the treatment of levodopa-induced mental disturbances in Parkinson's disease. *Neurology.* 1995;**45**:432–434.

105. Rich SS, Friedman JH, Ott BR. Risperidone versus clozapine in the treatment of psychosis in six patients with Parkinson's disease and other akinetic-rigid syndromes. *J Clin Psychiatry.* 1995;**56**:556–559.

106. Wagner ML, Defilippi JL, Menza MA, Sage JI. Clozapine for the treatment of psychosis in Parkinson's disease: chart review of 49 patients. *J Neuropsychiatry Clin Neurosci.* 1996;**8**:276–280.

107. Bonuccelli U, Ceravolo R, Salvetti S et al. Clozapine in Parkinson's disease tremor. Effects of acute and chronic administration. *Neurology.* 1997;**49**: 1587–1590.

108. Ruggieri S, De Pandis MF, Bonamartini A et al. Low dose of clozapine in the treatment of dopaminergic psychosis in Parkinson's disease. *Clin Neuropharmacol.* 1997;**20**:204–209.

109. Widman LP, Burke WJ, Pfeiffer RF, McArthur-Campbell D. Use of clozapine to treat levodopa-induced psychosis in Parkinson's disease: retrospective review. *J Geriatr Psychiatry Neurol.* 1997;**10**:63–66.

110. Friedman JH, Goldstein S, Jacques C. Substituting clozapine for olanzapine in psychiatrically stable Parkinson's disease patients: results of an open label pilot study. *Clin Neuropharmacol.* 1998;**21**:285–288.

111. Pierelli F, Adipietro A, Soldati G et al. Low dosage clozapine effects on L-dopa induced dyskinesias in parkinsonian patients. *Acta Neurol Scand.* 1998;**97**:295–299.

112. Trosch RM, Friedman JH, Lannon MC et al. Clozapine use in Parkinson's disease: a retrospective analysis of a large multicentered clinical experience. *Mov Disord.* 1998;**13**:377–382.

113. The French Clozapine Parkinson Study Group. Clozapine in drug-induced psychosis in Parkinson's disease. *Lancet.* 1999;**353**:2041–2042.

114. Dewey RB, Jr., O'Suilleabhain PE. Treatment of drug-induced psychosis with quetiapine and clozapine in Parkinson's disease. *Neurology.* 2000;**55**:1753–1754.

115. Goetz CG, Blasucci LM, Leurgans S, Pappert EJ. Olanzapine and clozapine: comparative effects on motor function in hallucinating PD patients. *Neurology.* 2000;**55**:789–794.

116. Ellis T, Cudkowicz ME, Sexton PM, Growdon JH. Clozapine and risperidone treatment of psychosis in

Parkinson's disease. *J Neuropsychiatry Clin Neurosci.* 2000;**12**:364–369.

117. Factor SA, Friedman JH, Lannon MC et al. Clozapine for the treatment of drug-induced psychosis in Parkinson's disease: results of the 12 week open label extension in the PSYCLOPS trial. *Mov Disord.* 2001;**16**:135–139.

118. Morgante L, Epifanio A, Spina E et al. Quetiapine versus clozapine: a preliminary report of comparative effects on dopaminergic psychosis in patients with Parkinson's disease. *Neurol Sci.* 2002;**23**(Suppl 2): S89–S90.

119. Morgante L, Epifanio A, Spina E et al. Quetiapine and clozapine in parkinsonian patients with dopaminergic psychosis. *Clin Neuropharmacol.* 2004;**27**:153–156.

120. Fernandez HH, Friedman JH, Jacques C, Rosenfeld M. Quetiapine for the treatment of drug-induced psychosis in Parkinson's disease. *Mov Disord.* 1999;**14**:484–487.

121. Targum SD, Abbott JL. Efficacy of quetiapine in Parkinson's patients with psychosis. *J Clin Psychopharmacol.* 2000;**20**:54–60.

122. Reddy S, Factor SA, Molho ES, Feustel PJ. The effect of quetiapine on psychosis and motor function in parkinsonian patients with and without dementia. *Mov Disord.* 2002;**17**:676–681.

123. Baron MS, Dalton WB. Quetiapine as treatment for dopaminergic-induced dyskinesias in Parkinson's disease. *Mov Disord.* 2003;**18**:1208–1209.

124. Fernandez HH, Trieschmann ME, Burke MA et al. Long-term outcome of quetiapine use for psychosis among Parkinsonian patients. *Mov Disord.* 2003;**18**:510–514.

125. Gimenez-Roldan S, Navarro E, Mateo D. [Effects of quetiapine at low doses on psychosis motor disability and stress of the caregiver in patients with Parkinson's disease.] *Rev Neurol.* 2003;**36**:401–404.

126. Katzenschlager R, Manson AJ, Evans A et al. Low dose quetiapine for drug induced dyskinesias in Parkinson's disease: a double blind cross over study. *J Neurol Neurosurg Psychiatry.* 2004;**75**:295–297.

127. Juncos JL, Roberts VJ, Evatt ML et al. Quetiapine improves psychotic symptoms and cognition in Parkinson's disease. *Mov Disord.* 2004;**19**:29–35.

128. Mancini F, Tassorelli C, Martignoni E et al. Long-term evaluation of the effect of quetiapine on hallucinations, delusions and motor function in advanced Parkinson disease. *Clin Neuropharmacol.* 2004;**27**:33–37.

129. Rabey JM, Prokhorov T, Miniovitz A, Dobronevsky E et al. Effect of quetiapine in psychotic Parkinson's disease patients: a double-blind labeled study of 3 months' duration. *Mov Disord.* 2007;**22**:313–318.

130. Meco G, Alessandri A, Giustini P, Bonifati V. Risperidone in levodopa-induced psychosis in advanced Parkinson's disease: an open-label, long-term study. *Mov Disord.* 1997;**12**:610–612.

131. Workman RH, Jr., Orengo CA, Bakey AA et al. The use of risperidone for psychosis and agitation in demented patients with Parkinson's disease. *J Neuropsychiatry Clin Neurosci.* 1997;**9**:594–597.

132. Leopold NA. Risperidone treatment of drug-related psychosis in patients with parkinsonism. *Mov Disord.* 2000;**15**:301–304.

133. Mohr E, Mendis T, Hildebrand K, De Deyn PP. Risperidone in the treatment of dopamine-induced psychosis in Parkinson's disease: an open pilot trial. *Mov Disord.* 2000;**15**:1230–1237.

134. Graham JM, Sussman JD, Ford KS, Sagar HJ. Olanzapine in the treatment of hallucinosis in idiopathic Parkinson's disease: a cautionary note. *J Neurol Neurosurg Psychiatry.* 1998;**65**:774–777.

135. Aarsland D, Larsen JP, Lim NG, Tandberg E. Olanzapine for psychosis in patients with Parkinson's disease with and without dementia. *J Neuropsychiatry Clin Neurosci.* 1999;**11**:392–394.

136. Molho ES, Factor SA. Worsening of motor features of parkinsonism with olanzapine. *Mov Disord.* 1999;**14**:1014–1016.

137. Brier A, Sutton VK, Feldman PD et al. Olanzapine in the treatment of dopamimetic-induced psychosis in patients with Parkinson's disease. *Biol Psychiatry.* 2002;**52**:438–445.

138. Marsh L, Lyketsos C, Reich SG. Olanzapine for the treatment of psychosis in patients with Parkinson's disease and dementia. *Psychosomatics.* 2001;**42**:477–481.

139. Ondo WG, Levy JK, Vuong KD et al. Olanzapine treatment for dopaminergic-induced hallucinations. *Mov Disord.* 2002;**17**:1031–1035.

140. Fernandez HH, Trieschmann ME, Friedman JH. Aripiprazole for drug-induced psychosis in Parkinson disease: preliminary experience. *Clin Neuropharmacol.* 2004;**27**:4–5.

141. Rasmussen KG, Jr., Russell JC, Kung S et al. Electroconvulsive therapy for patients with major depression and probable Lewy body dementia. *J ECT.* 2003;**19**:103–109.

142. Thaisetthawatkul P, Boeve BF, Benarroch EE et al. Autonomic dysfunction in dementia with Lewy bodies. *Neurology.* 2004;**62**:1804–1809.

143. Benarroch EE, Schmeichel AM, Low PA et al. Involvement of medullary regions controlling sympathetic output in Lewy body disease. *Brain.* 2005;**128**:338–344.

144. Allan LM, Ballard CG, Allen J et al. Autonomic dysfunction in dementia. *J Neurol Neurosurg Psychiatry.* 2007;**78**:671–677.

145. Boeve BF, Silber MH, Ferman TJ. Melatonin for treatment of REM sleep behavior disorder in neurologic disorders: results in 14 patients. *Sleep Med.* 2003;**4**:281–284.

146. Boeve BF, Silber MH, Ferman TJ. REM sleep behavior disorder in Parkinson's disease and dementia with Lewy bodies. *J Geriatr Psychiatry Neurol.* 2004; **17**:146–157.

147. Massironi G, Galluzzi S, Frisoni GB. Drug treatment of REM sleep behavior disorders in dementia with Lewy bodies. *Int Psychogeriatr.* 2003;**15**:377–383.

148. McKeith I, Mintzer J, Aarsland D et al. Dementia with Lewy bodies. *Lancet Neurol.* 2004;**3**:19–28.

149. Aarsland D, Andersen K, Larsen JP et al. Prevalence and characteristics of dementia in Parkinson disease: an 8-year prospective study. *Arch Neurol.* 2003;**60**: 387–392.

150. Lippa CF, Duda JE, Grossman M et al. DLB and PDD boundary issues: diagnosis, treatment, molecular pathology, and biomarkers. *Neurology.* 2007; **68**:812–819.

151. Wesnes KA, McKeith I, Edgar C et al. Benefits of rivastigmine on attention in dementia associated with Parkinson disease. *Neurology.* 2005;**65**:1654–1656.

152. Muller T, Welnic J, Fuchs G et al. The DONPAD-study: treatment of dementia in patients with Parkinson's disease with donepezil. *J Neural Transm Suppl.* 2006:27–30.

153. Burn D, Emre M, McKeith I et al. Effects of rivastigmine in patients with and without visual hallucinations in dementia associated with Parkinson's disease. *Mov Disord.* 2006;**21**:1899–1907.

154. Poewe W, Wolters E, Emre M et al. Long-term benefits of rivastigmine in dementia associated with Parkinson's disease: an active treatment extension study. *Mov Disord.* 2006;**21**:456–461.

155. The Parkinson Study Group. Low-dose clozapine for the treatment of drug-induced psychosis in Parkinson's disease. *N Engl J Med.* 1999;**340**:757–763.

156. Fernandez HH, Lannon MC, Friedman JH, Abbott BP. Clozapine replacement by quetiapine for the treatment of drug-induced psychosis in Parkinson's disease. *Mov Disord.* 2000;**15**:579–581.

157. Aarsland D, Larsen JP, Karlsen K et al. Mental symptoms in Parkinson's disease are important contributors to caregiver distress. *Int J Geriatr Psychiatry.* 1999;**14**:866–874.

158. Ananth H, Popescu I, Critchley HD et al. Cortical and subcortical gray matter abnormalities in schizophrenia determined through structural magnetic resonance imaging with optimized volumetric voxel-based morphometry. *Am J Psychiatry.* 2002;**159**:1497–1505.

159. Chui HC, Mack W, Jackson JE et al. Clinical criteria for the diagnosis of vascular dementia: a multicenter study of comparability and interrater reliability. *Arch Neurol.* 2000;**57**:191–196.

160. Erkinjuntti T, Inzitari D, Pantoni L *et al.* Research criteria for subcortical vascular dementia in clinical trials. *J Neural Transm Suppl.* 2000;**59**:23–30.

161. Forette F, Seux ML, Staessen JA *et al.* Prevention of dementia in randomised double-blind placebo-controlled Systolic Hypertension in Europe (Syst-Eur) trial. *Lancet.* 1998;**352**:1347–1351.

162. Forette F, Seux ML, Staessen JA *et al.* The prevention of dementia with antihypertensive treatment: new evidence from the Systolic Hypertension in Europe (Syst-Eur) study. *Arch Intern Med.* 2002;**162**: 2046–2052.

163. Tzourio C, Anderson C, Chapman N *et al.* Effects of blood pressure lowering with perindopril and indapamide therapy on dementia and cognitive decline in patients with cerebrovascular disease. *Arch Intern Med.* 2003;**163**:1069–1075.

164. Feigin V, Ratnasabapathy Y, Anderson C. Does blood pressure lowering treatment prevent dementia or cognitive decline in patients with cardiovascular and cerebrovascular disease? *J Neurol Sci.* 2005; **229–230**:151–155.

165. Meyer JS, Chowdhury MH, Xu G *et al.* Donepezil treatment of vascular dementia. *Ann N Y Acad Sci.* 2002;**977**:482–486.

166. Black S, Roman GC, Geldmacher DS *et al.* Efficacy and tolerability of donepezil in vascular dementia: positive results of a 24-week, multicenter, international, randomized, placebo-controlled clinical trial. *Stroke.* 2003;**34**:2323–2330.

167. Wilkinson D, Doody R, Helme R *et al.* Donepezil in vascular dementia: a randomized, placebo-controlled study. *Neurology.* 2003;**61**:479–486.

168. Moretti R, Torre P, Antonello RM, Cazzato G. Rivastigmine in subcortical vascular dementia: a comparison trial on efficacy and tolerability for 12 months follow-up. *Eur J Neurol.* 2001;**8**:361–362.

169. Moretti R, Torre P, Antonello RM *et al.* Rivastigmine in subcortical vascular dementia: an open 22-month study. *J Neurol Sci.* 2002;**203–204**:141–146.

170. Kumar V, Anand R, Messina J *et al.* An efficacy and safety analysis of Exelon in Alzheimer's disease patients with concurrent vascular risk factors. *Eur J Neurol.* 2000;**7**:159–169.

171. Moretti R, Torre P, Antonello RM *et al.* Rivastigmine in subcortical vascular dementia: a randomized, controlled, open 12-month study in 208 patients. *Am J Alzheimers Dis Other Demen.* 2003; **18**:265–272.

172. Moretti R, Torre P, Antonello RM *et al.* Rivastigmine in frontotemporal dementia: an open-label study. *Drugs Aging.* 2004;**21**:931–937.

173. Erkinjuntti T, Kurz A, Gauthier S *et al.* Efficacy of galantamine in probable vascular dementia and

Alzheimer's disease combined with cerebrovascular disease: a randomised trial. *Lancet.* 2002;**359**: 1283–1290.

174. Erkinjuntti T, Kurz A, Small GW *et al.* An open-label extension trial of galantamine in patients with probable vascular dementia and mixed dementia. *Clin Ther.* 2003;**25**:1765–1782.

175. Orgogozo JM, Rigaud AS, Stoffler A *et al.* Efficacy and safety of memantine in patients with mild to moderate vascular dementia: a randomized, placebo-controlled trial (MMM 300). *Stroke.* 2002;**33**:1834–1839.

176. Wilcock G, Mobius HJ, Stoffler A. A double-blind, placebo-controlled multicentre study of memantine in mild to moderate vascular dementia (MMM500). *Int Clin Psychopharmacol.* 2002;**17**:297–305.

177. Meyer JS, Rogers RL, McClintic K *et al.* Randomized clinical trial of daily aspirin therapy in multi-infarct dementia. A pilot study. *J Am Geriatr Soc.* 1989; **37**:549–555.

178. Devine ME, Rands G. Does aspirin affect outcome in vascular dementia? A retrospective case-notes analysis. *Int J Geriatr Psychiatry.* 2003;**18**:425–431.

179. Olin J, Schneider L, Novit A, Luczak S. Hydergine for dementia. *Cochrane Database Syst Rev.* 2000; **1**: CD000359.

180. Ghose K. Oxpentifylline in dementia: a controlled study. *Arch Gerontol Geriatr.* 1987;**6**:19–26.

181. Black RS, Barclay LL, Nolan KA *et al.* Pentoxifylline in cerebrovascular dementia. *J Am Geriatr Soc.* 1992;**40**:237–244.

182. Blume J, Ruhlmann KU, de la Haye R, Rettig K. Treatment of chronic cerebrovascular disease in elderly patients with pentoxifylline. *J Med.* 1992; **23**:417–432.

183. European Pentoxifylline Multi-Infarct Dementia Study. *Eur Neurol.* 1996;**36**:315–321.

184. Marcusson J, Rother M, Kittner B *et al.* A 12-month, randomized, placebo-controlled trial of propentofylline (HWA 285) in patients with dementia according to DSM III-R. The European Propentofylline Study Group. *Dement Geriatr Cogn Disord.* 1997;**8**:320–328.

185. Parnetti L, Ambrosoli L, Agliati G *et al.* Posatirelin in the treatment of vascular dementia: a double-blind multicentre study vs placebo. *Acta Neurol Scand.* 1996;**93**:456–463.

186. Herrmann WM, Stephan K, Gaede K, Apeceche M. A multicenter randomized double-blind study on the efficacy and safety of nicergoline in patients with multi-infarct dementia. *Dement Geriatr Cogn Disord.* 1997;**8**:9–17.

187. Pantoni L, Carosi M, Amigoni S *et al.* A preliminary open trial with nimodipine in patients with cognitive impairment and leukoaraiosis. *Clin Neuropharmacol.* 1996;**19**:497–506.

188. Pantoni L, del Ser T, Soglian AG *et al.* Efficacy and safety of nimodipine in subcortical vascular dementia: a randomized placebo-controlled trial. *Stroke.* 2005;**36**:619–624.

189. Brodaty H, Ames D, Snowdon J *et al.* A randomized placebo-controlled trial of risperidone for the treatment of aggression, agitation, and psychosis of dementia. *J Clin Psychiatry.* 2003;**64**:134–143.

190. Le Bars PL, Kieser M, Itil KZ. A 26-week analysis of a double-blind, placebo-controlled trial of the ginkgo biloba extract EGb 761 in dementia. *Dement Geriatr Cogn Disord.* 2000;**11**:230–237.

191. Kanowski S, Hoerr R. Ginkgo biloba extract EGb 761 in dementia: intent-to-treat analyses of a 24-week, multi-center, double-blind, placebo-controlled, randomized trial. *Pharmacopsychiatry.* 2003;**36**:297–303.

192. Moretti R, Torre P, Antonello RM *et al.* Rivastigmine superior to aspirin plus nimodipine in subcortical vascular dementia: an open, 16-month, comparative study. *Int J Clin Pract.* 2004;**58**:346–353.

193. Schneider LS, Olin JT. Overview of clinical trials of hydergine in dementia. *Arch Neurol.* 1994;**51**:787–798.

194. Pantoni L, Bianchi C, Beneke M *et al.* The Scandinavian Multi-Infarct Dementia Trial: a double-blind, placebo-controlled trial on nimodipine in multi-infarct dementia. *J Neurol Sci.* 2000;**175**: 116–123.

195. Pantoni L, Rossi R, Inzitari D *et al.* Efficacy and safety of nimodipine in subcortical vascular dementia: a subgroup analysis of the Scandinavian Multi-Infarct Dementia Trial. *J Neurol Sci.* 2000;**175**:124–134.

196. Cohen RA, Browndyke JN, Moser DJ *et al.* Long-term citicoline (cytidine diphosphate choline) use in patients with vascular dementia: neuroimaging and neuropsychological outcomes. *Cerebrovasc Dis.* 2003;**16**:199–204.

197. Demaerschalk BM, Wingerchuk DM. Treatment of vascular dementia and vascular cognitive impairment. *Neurologist.* 2007;**13**:37–41.

198. Neary D, Snowden JS, Gustafson L *et al.* Frontotemporal lobar degeneration: a consensus on clinical diagnostic criteria. *Neurology.* 1998;**51**:1546–1554.

199. Forman MS, Farmer J, Johnson JK *et al.* Frontotemporal dementia: clinicopathological correlations. *Ann Neurol.* 2006;**59**:952–962.

200. Josephs KA, Petersen RC, Knopman DS *et al.* Clinicopathologic analysis of frontotemporal and corticobasal degenerations and PSP. *Neurology.* 2006;**66**:41–48.

201. Neumann M, Sampathu DM, Kwong LK *et al.* Ubiquitinated TDP-43 in frontotemporal lobar degeneration and amyotrophic lateral sclerosis. *Science.* 2006;**314**:130–133.

202. Wszolek ZK, Tsuboi Y, Farrer M *et al.* Hereditary tauo-pathies and parkinsonism. *Adv Neurol.* 2003;**91**:153–163.

203. Vance C, Al-Chalabi A, Ruddy D *et al.* Familial amyotrophic lateral sclerosis with frontotemporal dementia is linked to a locus on chromosome 9p13.2–21.3. *Brain.* 2006;**129**:868–876.

204. Morita M, Al-Chalabi A, Andersen PM *et al.* A locus on chromosome 9p confers susceptibility to ALS and frontotemporal dementia. *Neurology.* 2006;**66**:839–844.

205. Cannon A, Baker M, Boeve B *et al.* CHMP2B mutations are not a common cause of frontotemporal lobar degeneration. *Neurosci Lett.* 2006;**398**:83–84.

206. Cruts M, Gijselinck I, van der Zee J *et al.* Null mutations in progranulin cause ubiquitin-positive frontotemporal dementia linked to chromosome 17q21. *Nature.* 2006;**442**:920–924.

207. Spina S, Murrell JR, Huey ED *et al.* Clinicopathologic features of frontotemporal dementia with progranulin sequence variation. *Neurology.* 2007;**68**:820–827.

208. Boeve BF, Baker M, Dickson DW *et al.* Frontotemporal dementia and parkinsonism associated with the IVS1+1G→A mutation in progranulin: a clinicopathologic study. *Brain.* 2006;**129**:3103–3114.

209. Mesulam M, Johnson N, Krefft TA *et al.* Progranulin mutations in primary progressive aphasia: the PPA1 and PPA3 families. *Arch Neurol.* 2007;**64**:43–47.

210. Mukherjee O, Pastor P, Cairns NJ *et al.* HDDD2 is a familial frontotemporal lobar degeneration with ubiquitin-positive, tau-negative inclusions caused by a missense mutation in the signal peptide of progranulin. *Ann Neurol.* 2006;**60**:314–322.

211. Behrens MI, Mukherjee O, Tu PH *et al.* Neuropathologic heterogeneity in HDDD1: a familial frontotemporal lobar degeneration with ubiquitin-positive inclusions and progranulin mutation. *Alzheimer Dis Assoc Disord.* 2007;**21**:1–7.

212. Cairns NJ, Neumann M, Bigio EH *et al.* TDP-43 in familial and sporadic frontotemporal lobar degeneration with ubiquitin inclusions. *Am J Pathol.* 2007;**171**(1): 227–240.

213. The Lund and Manchester Groups. Clinical and neuropathological criteria for frontotemporal dementia. *J Neurol Neurosurg Psychiatry.* 1994;**57**: 416–418.

214. Miller BL, Chang L, Mena I *et al.* Progressive right frontotemporal degeneration: clinical, neuropsychological and SPECT characteristics. *Dementia.* 1993;**4**:204–213.

215. Miller BL, Cummings J, Mishkin F *et al.* Emergence of artistic talent in frontotemporal dementia. *Neurology.* 1998;**51**:978–982.

216. Swartz JR, Miller BL, Lesser IM, Darby AL. Frontotemporal dementia: treatment response to

249

serotonin selective reuptake inhibitors. *J Clin Psychiatry*. 1997;**58**:212–216.

217. Deakin JB, Rahman S, Nestor PJ *et al.* Paroxetine does not improve symptoms and impairs cognition in frontotemporal dementia: a double-blind randomized controlled trial. *Psychopharmacology (Berl)*. 2004;**172**:400–408.

218. Lebert F, Stekke W, Hasenbroekx C, Pasquier F. Frontotemporal dementia: a randomised, controlled trial with trazodone. *Dement Geriatr Cogn Disord*. 2004;**17**:355–359.

219. Mendez MF, Shapira JS, McMurtray A, Licht E. Preliminary findings: behavioral worsening on donepezil in patients with frontotemporal dementia. *Am J Geriatr Psychiatry*. 2007;**15**:84–87.

220. Huey ED, Putnam KT, Grafman J. A systematic review of neurotransmitter deficits and treatments in frontotemporal dementia. *Neurology*. 2006;**66**:17–22.

221. Moretti R, Torre P, Antonello RM *et al.* Frontotemporal dementia: paroxetine as a possible treatment of behavior symptoms. A randomized, controlled, open 14-month study. *Eur Neurol*. 2003;**49**:13–19.

222. Noble W, Planel E, Zehr C *et al.* Inhibition of glycogen synthase kinase-3 by lithium correlates with reduced tauopathy and degeneration in vivo. *Proc Natl Acad Sci USA*. 2005;**102**:6990–6995.

223. Dickey CA, Yue M, Lin WL *et al.* Deletion of the ubiquitin ligase CHIP leads to the accumulation, but not the aggregation, of both endogenous phospho- and caspase-3-cleaved tau species. *J Neurosci*. 2006;**26**:6985–6996.

224. Dickey CA, Kamal A, Lundgren K *et al.* The high-affinity HSP90-CHIP complex recognizes and selectively degrades phosphorylated tau client proteins. *J Clin Invest*. 2007;**117**:648–658.

225. Mesulam M. Primary progressive aphasia without generalized dementia. *Ann Neurol*. 1982;**11**:592–598.

226. Duffy JR PR. Primary progressive aphasia. *Aphasiology*. 1992;**6**:1–15.

227. Damasio A. Disorders of complex visual processing: agnosias, achromatopsia, Balint's syndrome, and related difficulties of orientation and construction. In Mesulam M-M (ed.) *Principles of Behavioral Neurology*. Philadelphia, PA: F.A. Davis, 1985: 259–288.

228. Evans JJ, Heggs AJ, Antoun N, Hodges JR. Progressive prosopagnosia associated with selective right temporal lobe atrophy. A new syndrome? *Brain*. 1995;**118**:1–13.

229. Reed DA, Johnson NA, Thompson C *et al.* A clinical trial of bromocriptine for treatment of primary progressive aphasia. *Ann Neurol*. 2004;**56**:750.

230. Berthier ML. Poststroke aphasia: epidemiology, pathophysiology and treatment. *Drugs Aging*. 2005;**22**:163–182.

231. Rebeiz JJ, Kolodny EH, Richardson EP, Jr. Corticodentatonigral degeneration with neuronal achromasia: a progressive disorder of late adult life. *Trans Am Neurol Assoc*. 1967;**92**:23–26.

232. Maraganore DM, Ahlskog JE, Petersen RC. Progressive asymmetric rigidity with apraxia: a distinctive clinical entity (abstract). *Mov Disord*. 1992;**7**(Suppl 1):80.

233. Lang AERD, Bergeron C. Cortical-basal ganglionic degeneration. In Calne DB (ed.) *Neurodegenerative Diseases*. Philadelphia, PA: WB Saunders, 1994:877–894.

234. Kumar RBC, Pollanen MS, Lang AE. Cortical-basal ganglionic degeneration. In Jankovic JTE (ed.) *Parkinson's Disease and Movement Disorders*. 3rd edn. Baltimore, MD: Williams & Wilkins, 1998: 297–316.

235. Kompoliti K, Goetz CG, Litvan I *et al.* Pharmacological therapy in progressive supranuclear palsy. *Arch Neurol*. 1998;**55**:1099–1102.

236. Geda Y, Boeve B, Parisi J *et al.* Neuropsychiatric features in 20 cases of pathologically-confirmed corticobasal degeneration. *Mov Disord*. 2000; **15**(Suppl 3):229.

237. Grimes DA, Lang AE, Bergeron CB. Dementia as the most common presentation of cortical-basal ganglionic degeneration. *Neurology*. 1999;**53**:1969–1974.

238. Boeve B. Corticobasal degeneration: the syndrome and the disease. In Litvan I (ed.) *Atypical Parkinsonian Disorders*. Totowa, NJ: Humana Press, 2005:309–334.

239. Kompoliti K, Goetz CG, Boeve BF *et al.* Clinical presentation and pharmacological therapy in corticobasal degeneration. *Arch Neurol*. 1998;**55**:957–961.

240. Boeve BF, Maraganore DM, Parisi JE *et al.* Pathologic heterogeneity in clinically diagnosed corticobasal degeneration. *Neurology*. 1999;**53**:795–800.

241. Josephs KA, Holton JL, Rossor MN *et al.* Neurofilament inclusion body disease: a new proteinopathy? *Brain*. 2003;**126**:2291–2303.

242. Boeve BF, Lang AE, Litvan I. Corticobasal degeneration and its relationship to progressive supranuclear palsy and frontotemporal dementia. *Ann Neurol*. 2003;**54**(Suppl 5):S15–S19.

243. Steele JC, Richardson JC, Olszewski J. Progressive supranuclear palsy. A heterogeneous degeneration involving the brain stem, basal ganglia and cerebellum with vertical gaze and pseudobulbar palsy, nuchal dystonia and dementia. *Arch Neurol*. 1964;**10**:333–359.

244. Litvan I, Agid Y, Calne D *et al.* Clinical research criteria for the diagnosis of progressive supranuclear palsy (Steele–Richardson–Olszewski syndrome): report of the NINDS–SPSP International Workshop. *Neurology*. 1996;**47**:1–9.

245. Litvan I, Mega MS, Cummings JL, Fairbanks L. Neuropsychiatric aspects of progressive supranuclear palsy. *Neurology.* 1996;**47**:1184–1189.

246. Rippon G, Boeve B, Parisi J, Dickson D *et al.* Atypical progressive supranuclear palsy presenting as frontotemporal dementia. *Neurocase.* 2005;**11**:1–8.

247. Nieforth KA, Golbe LI. Retrospective study of drug response in 87 patients with progressive supranuclear palsy. *Clin Neuropharmacol.* 1993;**16**:338–346.

248. Cole DG, Growdon JH. Therapy for progressive supranuclear palsy: past and future. *J Neural Transm Suppl.* 1994;**42**:283–290.

249. Fabbrini G, Barbanti P, Bonifati V *et al.* Donepezil in the treatment of progressive supranuclear palsy. *Acta Neurol Scand.* 2001;**103**:123–125.

250. Litvan I. Diagnosis and management of progressive supranuclear palsy. *Semin Neurol.* 2001;**21**:41–48.

251. Frattali CM, Sonies BC, Chi-Fishman G, Litvan I. Effects of physostigmine on swallowing and oral motor functions in patients with progressive supranuclear palsy: a pilot study. *Dysphagia.* 1999;**14**:165–168.

252. Rascol O, Sieradzan K, Peyro-Saint-Paul H *et al.* Efaroxan, an alpha-2 antagonist, in the treatment of progressive supranuclear palsy. *Mov Disord.* 1998;**13**:673–676.

253. Weiner WJ, Minagar A, Shulman LM. Pramipexole in progressive supranuclear palsy. *Neurology.* 1999; **52**:873–874.

254. Human transmissible spongiform encephalopathies. *Wkly Epidemiol Rec.* 1998;**73**:361–365.

255. Collinge J. New diagnostic tests for prion diseases. *N Engl J Med.* 1996;**335**:963–965.

256. Korth C, May BC, Cohen FE, Prusiner SB. Acridine and phenothiazine derivatives as pharmacotherapeutics for prion disease. *Proc Natl Acad Sci USA.* 2001;**98**:9836–9841.

257. Nakajima M, Yamada T, Kusuhara T *et al.* Results of quinacrine administration to patients with Creutzfeldt–Jakob disease. *Dement Geriatr Cogn Disord.* 2004;**17**:158–163.

258. Otto M, Cepek L, Ratzka P *et al.* Efficacy of flupirtine on cognitive function in patients with CJD: a double-blind study. *Neurology.* 2004;**62**:714–718.

259. Haïk S, Brandel JP, Salomon D *et al.* Compassionate use of quinacrine in Creutzfeldt-Jakob disease fails to show significant effects. *Neurology.* 2004;**63**: 2413–2415.

260. Ironside JW. Neuropathological findings in new variant CJD and experimental transmission of BSE. *FEMS Immunol Med Microbiol.* 1998;**21**:91–95.

261. Scott MR, Will R, Ironside J *et al.* Compelling transgenetic evidence for transmission of bovine spongiform encephalopathy prions to humans. *Proc Natl Acad Sci USA.* 1999;**96**:15137–15142.

262. Zeidler M, Johnstone EC, Bamber RW *et al.* New variant Creutzfeldt–Jakob disease: psychiatric features. *Lancet.* 1997;**350**:908–910.

263. Zeidler M, Stewart GE, Barraclough CR *et al.* New variant Creutzfeldt–Jakob disease: neurological features and diagnostic tests. *Lancet.* 1997;**350**:903–907.

264. Will RG, Zeidler M, Stewart GE *et al.* Diagnosis of new variant Creutzfeldt–Jakob disease. *Ann Neurol.* 2000;**47**:575–582.

265. Coulthard A, Hall K, English PT *et al.* Quantitative analysis of MRI signal intensity in new variant Creutzfeldt–Jakob disease. *Br J Radiol.* 1999;**72**:742–748.

266. Carlson DL, Fleming KC, Smith GE, Evans JM. Management of dementia-related behavioral disturbances: a nonpharmacologic approach. *Mayo Clin Proc.* 1995;**70**:1108–1115.

267. Knopman DS, Sawyer-DeMaris S. Practical approach to managing behavioral problems in dementia patients. *Geriatrics.* 1990;**45**:27–30, 35.

268. Boeve BF, Silber MH, Ferman TJ. Current management of sleep disturbances in dementia. *Curr Neurol Neurosci Rep.* 2002;**2**:169–177.

269. Tariot PN, Profenno LA, Ismail MS. Efficacy of atypical antipsychotics in elderly patients with dementia. *J Clin Psychiatry.* 2004;**65**(Suppl 11):11–15.

270. Sink KM, Holden KF, Yaffe K. Pharmacological treatment of neuropsychiatric symptoms of dementia: a review of the evidence. *JAMA.* 2005;**293**:596–608.

271. McKeith IG, Grace JB, Walker Z *et al.* Rivastigmine in the treatment of dementia with Lewy bodies: preliminary findings from an open trial. *Int J Geriatr Psychiatry.* 2000;**15**:387–392.

272. Saykin AJ, Wishart HA, Rabin LA *et al.* Cholinergic enhancement of frontal lobe activity in mild cognitive impairment. *Brain.* 2004;**127**:1574–1583.

273. Finkel SI. Behavioral and psychological symptoms of dementia: a current focus for clinicians, researchers, and caregivers. *J Clin Psychiatry.* 2001;**62**(Suppl 21):3–6.

274. Beeri MS, Werner P, Davidson M, Noy S. The cost of behavioral and psychological symptoms of dementia (BPSD) in community dwelling Alzheimer's disease patients. *Int J Geriatr Psychiatry.* 2002;**17**:403–408.

275. Stotsky B. Multicenter study comparing thioridazine with diazepam and placebo in elderly, nonpsychotic patients with emotional and behavioral disorders. *Clin Ther.* 1984;**6**:546–559.

276. Schneider LS, Pollock VE, Lyness SA. A metaanalysis of controlled trials of neuroleptic treatment in dementia. *J Am Geriatr Soc.* 1990;**38**:553–563.

277. Lonergan E, Luxenberg J, Colford J. Haloperidol for agitation in dementia. *Cochrane Database Syst Rev.* 2002;**4**:CD002852.

251

278. Pollock BG, Mulsant BH, Rosen J et al. Comparison of citalopram, perphenazine, and placebo for the acute treatment of psychosis and behavioral disturbances in hospitalized, demented patients. *Am J Psychiatry.* 2002;**159**:460–465.

279. De Deyn PP, Rabheru K, Rasmussen A et al. A randomized trial of risperidone, placebo, and haloperidol for behavioral symptoms of dementia. *Neurology.* 1999;**53**:946–955.

280. Katz IR, Jeste DV, Mintzer JE et al. Comparison of risperidone and placebo for psychosis and behavioral disturbances associated with dementia: a randomized, double-blind trial. Risperidone Study Group. *J Clin Psychiatry.* 1999;**60**:107–115.

281. Street JS, Clark WS, Gannon KS et al. Olanzapine treatment of psychotic and behavioral symptoms in patients with Alzheimer disease in nursing care facilities: a double-blind, randomized, placebo-controlled trial. The HGEU Study Group. *Arch Gen Psychiatry.* 2000;**57**:968–976.

282. Meehan KM, Wang H, David SR et al. Comparison of rapidly acting intramuscular olanzapine, lorazepam, and placebo: a double-blind, randomized study in acutely agitated patients with dementia. *Neuropsychopharmacology.* 2002;**26**:494–504.

283. De Deyn PP, Carrasco MM, Deberdt W et al. Olanzapine versus placebo in the treatment of psychosis with or without associated behavioral disturbances in patients with Alzheimer's disease. *Int J Geriatr Psychiatry.* 2004;**19**:115–126.

284. Tariot PN, Salzman C, Yeung PP et al. Long-term use of quetiapine in elderly patients with psychotic disorders. *Clin Ther.* 2000;**22**:1068–1084.

285. Feldman H, Gauthier S, Hecker J et al. A 24-week, randomized, double-blind study of donepezil in moderate to severe Alzheimer's disease. *Neurology.* 2001;**57**:613–620.

286. Holmes C, Wilkinson D, Dean C et al. The efficacy of donepezil in the treatment of neuropsychiatric symptoms in Alzheimer disease. *Neurology.* 2004; **63**:214–219.

287. Gauthier S, Wirth Y, Mobius HJ. Effects of memantine on behavioural symptoms in Alzheimer's disease patients: an analysis of the Neuropsychiatric Inventory (NPI) data of two randomised, controlled studies. *Int J Geriatr Psychiatry.* 2005;**20**:459–464.

288. Auchus AP, Bissey-Black C. Pilot study of haloperidol, fluoxetine, and placebo for agitation in Alzheimer's disease. *J Neuropsychiatry Clin Neurosci.* 1997;**9**:591–593.

289. Lyketsos CG, DelCampo L, Steinberg M et al. Treating depression in Alzheimer disease: efficacy and safety of sertraline therapy, and the benefits of depression reduction: the DIADS. *Arch Gen Psychiatry.* 2003;**60**:737–746.

290. Finkel SI, Mintzer JE, Dysken M et al. A randomized, placebo-controlled study of the efficacy and safety of sertraline in the treatment of the behavioral manifestations of Alzheimer's disease in outpatients treated with donepezil. *Int J Geriatr Psychiatry.* 2004;**19**:9–18.

291. Teri L, Logsdon RG, Peskind E et al. Treatment of agitation in AD: a randomized, placebo-controlled clinical trial. *Neurology.* 2000;**55**:1271–1278.

292. Tariot PN, Erb R, Podgorski CA et al. Efficacy and tolerability of carbamazepine for agitation and aggression in dementia. *Am J Psychiatry.* 1998;**155**:54–61.

293. Olin JT, Fox LS, Pawluczyk S et al. A pilot randomized trial of carbamazepine for behavioral symptoms in treatment-resistant outpatients with Alzheimer disease. *Am J Geriatr Psychiatry.* 2001;**9**:400–405.

294. Porsteinsson AP, Tariot PN, Erb R et al. Placebo-controlled study of divalproex sodium for agitation in dementia. *Am J Geriatr Psychiatry.* 2001;**9**:58–66.

295. Sival RC, Haffmans PM, Jansen PA et al. Sodium valproate in the treatment of aggressive behavior in patients with dementia–a randomized placebo controlled clinical trial. *Int J Geriatr Psychiatry.* 2002;**17**:579–585.

296. Schneider LS, Tariot PN, Dagerman KS et al. Effectiveness of atypical antipsychotic drugs in patients with Alzheimer's disease. *N Engl J Med.* 2006;**355**:1525–1538.

297. Tariot PN, Schneider L, Katz IR et al. Quetiapine treatment of psychosis associated with dementia: a double-blind, randomized, placebo-controlled clinical trial. *Am J Geriatr Psychiatry.* 2006;**14**:767–776.

298. De Deyn P, Jeste DV, Swanink R et al. Aripiprazole for the treatment of psychosis in patients with Alzheimer's disease: a randomized, placebo-controlled study. *J Clin Psychopharmacol.* 2005;**25**:463–467.

299. Tariot PN, Cummings JL, Katz IR et al. A randomized, double-blind, placebo-controlled study of the efficacy and safety of donepezil in patients with Alzheimer's disease in the nursing home setting. *J Am Geriatr Soc.* 2001;**49**:1590–1599.

300. Olin J, Schneider L. Galantamine for Alzheimer's disease. *Cochrane Database Syst Rev.* 2002;(3):CD001747.

301. Reisberg B, Doody R, Stöffler A et al. Memantine Study Group. Memantine in moderate-to-severe Alzheimer's disease. *N Engl J Med.* 2003;**348**:1333–1341.

302. MedWatch F. *Safety Alerts for Drugs, Biologics, Medical Devices, and Dietary Supplements.* Rockville, MD: US Food and Drug Administration, 2003, 2005.

303. MedWatch F. *Safety Alerts for Drugs, Biologics, Medical Devices, and Dietary Supplements.* Rockville, MD: US Food and Drug Administration, 2004.

304. Research FCfDEa. *FDA Public Health Advisory: Deaths with Antipsychotics in Elderly Patients with Behavioral Disturbances.* Rockville, MD: US Food and Drug Administration, 2005.

305. Schneider LS, Dagerman KS, Insel P. Risk of death with atypical antipsychotic drug treatment for dementia: meta-analysis of randomized placebo-controlled trials. *JAMA.* 2005;**294**:1934–1943.

306. Marin RS, Fogel BS, Hawkins J *et al.* Apathy: a treatable syndrome. *J Neuropsychiatry Clin Neurosci.* 1995;**7**:23–30.

307. van Reekum R, Stuss DT, Ostrander L. Apathy: why care? *J Neuropsychiatry Clin Neurosci.* 2005;**17**:7–19.

308. MacKnight C, Rojas-Fernandez C. Quetiapine for sexually inappropriate behavior in dementia. *J Am Geriatr Soc.* 2000;**48**:707.

309. Stewart JT, Shin KJ. Paroxetine treatment of sexual disinhibition in dementia. *Am J Psychiatry.* 1997;**154**:1474.

310. Leo RJ, Kim KY. Clomipramine treatment of paraphilias in elderly demented patients. *J Geriatr Psychiatry Neurol.* 1995;**8**:123–124.

311. Tiller JW, Dakis JA, Shaw JM. Short-term buspirone treatment in disinhibition with dementia. *Lancet.* 1988;**2**:510.

312. Lopez OL, Jagust WJ, Dulberg C *et al.* Risk factors for mild cognitive impairment in the Cardiovascular Health Study Cognition Study: part 2. *Arch Neurol.* 2003;**60**:1394–1399.

313. Lauterbach EC, Schweri MM. Amelioration of pseudobulbar affect by fluoxetine: possible alteration of dopamine-related pathophysiology by a selective serotonin reuptake inhibitor. *J Clin Psychopharmacol.* 1991;**11**:392–393.

314. Messiha FS. Fluoxetine: a spectrum of clinical applications and postulates of underlying mechanisms. *Neurosci Biobehav Rev.* 1993;**17**:385–396.

315. Shader RI. Does lithium both cause and treat pseudobulbar affect? *J Clin Psychopharmacol.* 1992;**12**:360.

316. Seliger GM, Hornstein A. Serotonin, fluoxetine, and pseudobulbar affect. *Neurology.* 1989;**39**:1400.

317. Brooks BR, Thisted RA, Appel SH *et al.* Treatment of pseudobulbar affect in ALS with dextromethorphan/ quinidine: a randomized trial. *Neurology.* 2004;**63**:1364–1370.

318. Rosen HJ, Cummings J. A real reason for patients with pseudobulbar affect to smile. *Ann Neurol.* 2007; **61**:92–96.

319. Skelly J, Flint AJ. Urinary incontinence associated with dementia. *J Am Geriatr Soc.* 1995;**43**:286–294.

320. Kay GG, Abou-Donia MB, Messer WS Jr *et al.* Antimuscarinic drugs for overactive bladder and their potential effects on cognitive function in older patients. *J Am Geriatr Soc.* 2005;**53**:2195–2201.

321. Ouslander JG, Zarit SH, Orr NK, Muira SA. Incontinence among elderly community-dwelling dementia patients. Characteristics, management, and impact on caregivers. *J Am Geriatr Soc.* 1990;**38**:440–445.

322. Ouslander JG, Uman GC, Urman HN, Rubenstein LZ. Incontinence among nursing home patients: clinical and functional correlates. *J Am Geriatr Soc.* 1987; **35**:324–330.

323. Mishima K, Okawa M, Hozumi S, Hishikawa Y. Supplementary administration of artificial bright light and melatonin as potent treatment for disorganized circadian rest-activity and dysfunctional autonomic and neuroendocrine systems in institutionalized demented elderly persons. *Chronobiol Int.* 2000; **17**:419–432.

324. Asplund R. Sleep disorders in the elderly. *Drugs Aging.* 1999;**14**:91–103.

325. Brusco LI, Fainstein I, Marquez M, Cardinali DP. Effect of melatonin in selected populations of sleep-disturbed patients. *Biol Signals Recept.* 1999;**8**:126–131.

326. Campbell SS, Terman M, Lewy AJ *et al.* Light treatment for sleep disorders: consensus report. V. Age-related disturbances. *J Biol Rhythms.* 1995;**10**:151–154.

327. Gerner RH. Geriatric depression and treatment with trazodone. *Psychopathology.* 1987;**20** Suppl 1:82–91.

328. Gurian B, Rosowsky E. Low-dose methylphenidate in the very old. *J Geriatr Psychiatry Neurol.* 1990;**3**:152–154.

329. Schenck CH, Mahowald MW. REM sleep behavior disorder: clinical, developmental, and neuroscience perspectives 16 years after its formal identification in SLEEP. *Sleep.* 2002;**25**:120–138.

330. Vitiello MV, Bliwise DL, Prinz PN. Sleep in Alzheimer's disease and the sundown syndrome. *Neurology.* 1992;**42**:83–93; discussion 93–84.

331. Bliwise DL, Carroll JS, Lee KA *et al.* Sleep and "sundowning" in nursing home patients with dementia. *Psychiatry Res.* 1993;**48**:277–292.

332. McGaffigan S, Bliwise DL. The treatment of sundowning. A selective review of pharmacological and nonpharmacological studies. *Drugs Aging.* 1997; **10**:10–17.

Dementia and cognition in the oldest-old

Kristin Kahle-Wrobleski, María M. Corrada and Claudia H. Kawas

Introduction

Fueled by medical and technological advances, average life expectancy in the USA has increased by more than 25 years over the past century. A consequence of increased longevity and the aging of the "baby boomers" is that the oldest-old (age 90 or older) have become the fastest growing segment of the US population. Currently, there are fewer than 2 million Americans aged 90 and older, but this number will increase to approximately 10 million by 2050.[1] In terms of percentage of the population, those aged 90 and older presently represent 0.5% of the population in the USA, while by the middle of the twenty-first century, they will form about 2.5% of the population[2] as depicted in Fig. 17.1. Moreover, the increases in the oldest-old population are occurring worldwide. Countries including Japan, France, Italy and Germany are expected to have between 3 and 5% of their population aged 90 and over by 2050.[3]

Cognition in the oldest-old: key questions

- What is the prevalence of dementia in the oldest-old?
- What are the causes of dementia in the oldest-old?
- How can we screen for dementia in this population and what challenges must we overcome in the cognitive assessment of this age group?
- What are the clinical–pathological correlates of dementia in the oldest-old?

The rapidly growing population over the age of 90 signals a need to understand aging and age-related conditions in the oldest-old. Many issues require investigation in these pioneers of aging. Estimates of dementia prevalence vary as described in more detail below. More precise estimates and a better understanding of the causes of dementia are crucial for understanding the public health impact of this rapidly growing group. The present chapter presents a brief overview of our knowledge regarding dementia and cognition in the oldest-old and describes preliminary findings from the 90+ Study, a population-based study of individuals aged 90–108 years of age.

The 90+ Study

To address the dearth of information regarding dementia and cognition in the oldest-old, The 90+ Study was established in 2003. The study is composed of survivors from the Leisure World Cohort Study, which was established in the early 1980s when 13 978 residents (8877 women and 5101 men) of a California retirement community (Leisure World, Laguna Woods) completed a postal health survey.[4,5] The cohort is mostly white and well educated. Basic demographic information is summarized in Table 17.1 and a summary of participants' medical histories is shown in Fig. 17.2.

The 90+ Study invited all 1151 members of the Leisure World Cohort Study who were aged 90 years and older on January 1, 2003 to participate in this longitudinal study of aging and dementia. Cohort members were asked to undergo a comprehensive evaluation either at our clinic or their residence, including a neuropsychological evaluation, neurological examination and self-administered as well as informant questionnaires. A list of neuropsychological tests is provided in Table 17.2. Participants are evaluated in-person every 6 months and informant information is updated annually. As of December 1, 2006, information had been ascertained on 948 (82%) of the 90+ Study cohort.

Dementia prevalence

Although estimates of dementia prevalence are reasonably well established for individuals under the age of 85 years, they have not been well defined for those

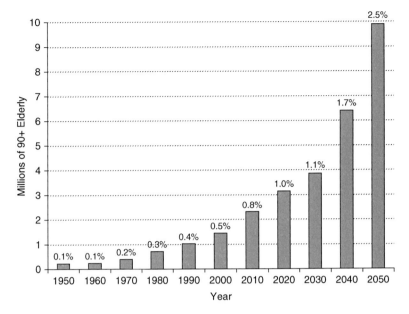

Fig. 17.1. Oldest-old population in the USA from 1950 to 2050. Figures over bars are percentage of US population. (Sources: US Census Bureau 1950–2000[1] and US Census Bureau Population Projections Middle Series, 2002[2].)

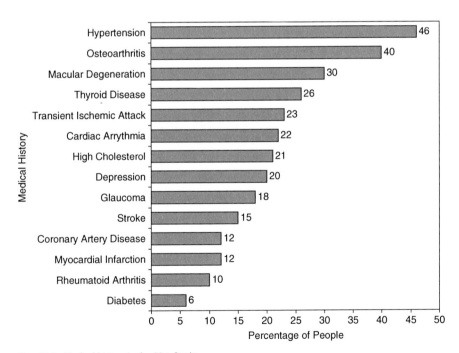

Fig. 17.2. Medical history in the 90+ Study.

in their tenth and eleventh decades of life. It is not clear if the prevalence of dementia, which doubles every 5 years of life between ages 65 and 85, continues this exponential increase in the tenth decade. Figure 17.3 shows available studies of dementia prevalence in people over age 90. Some studies have found that prevalence continues to increase with age after 90,[19,20,22] whereas others suggest that prevalence plateaus in the tenth decade.[23,30] Estimates of prevalence for people over age 90 vary from approximately 30%

Table 17.1. Baseline demographic characteristics of participants in the 90+ Study (n = 948)

Characteristic	Percentage
Sex	
Women	77
Men	23
Marital status	
Widowed	76
Married	14
Never married	6
Separated or divorced	4
Education	
High school or less	31
Some college or vocational school	29
College graduate or more	40
Type of residence	
At home alone	28
At home with spouse	11
At home with relatives or friends	7
At home with paid caregiver	10
Nursing or group home	44
Cognitive diagnosis from neurological examination	
Normal	32
Cognitively impaired not demented	34
Demented	34
Use of assistive devices	
None	29
Cane	31
Walker	51
Wheelchair	37
Average age (years [range])	94.9 (90–106)

Table 17.2. Neuropsychological assessment battery of the 90+ Study

Domain	Test	Reference
Global cognition	Modified Mini-Mental State Examination (3MS)	6
	Mini-Mental State Examination (MMSE)	7
Language	Boston Naming Test (BNT) 15-item	8,9
	Animal Fluency	10,11
Visuoconstruction	CERAD constructions	11
	Clock Drawing	12,13
Verbal memory	California Verbal Memory Test (CVLT) 9-item	14
Attention/ Executive Function	Digit Span (Forward and Backward) from Wechsler Adult Intelligence Scale, 3rd edn	15
	Trail Making Test A	16,17
	Trail Making Test B	16,17
	Clock Drawing	12,13
	Letter F Fluencies	10,11
Motor speed	Trail Making Test C	18

to approximately 60%, essentially a two-fold difference between estimates. When specifically considering prevalence rates of centenarians, the percentages also vary widely, with estimates ranging from 42% to 88%.[19,31–35] Moreover, the confidence intervals of all estimates in the oldest-old are wide, reflecting the lack of precision of these estimates.

Owing to small numbers, most studies of the oldest-old estimate prevalence for all subjects aged 90 and older as a combined group. Only a handful of publications have reported age- and gender-specific estimates for ages 90 and above.[19,20,22,25] In these studies, estimates for ages 90–94 range from approximately 32%

to 48% and increase modestly from approximately 40% to 60% for ages 95+. Although prevalence estimates for women are fairly consistent in terms of magnitude and direction (all appear to increase with age after age 90), the estimates for men are discrepant. When comparing prevalence between ages 90–94 and 95+ in men, one study shows a dramatic increase,[19] another shows a striking decrease[20] and the remaining two studies have similar estimates for the age groups.[19,22] Consequently, precise estimates of the prevalence of dementia have been elusive in the oldest-old, with insufficient numbers of subjects in most studies.

The 90+ Study is to our knowledge the largest prevalence investigation in a population-based sample of those 90+ years of age and, therefore, allows more precise estimates than previously published. Preliminary results obtained from 911 participants show an overall prevalence of all-cause dementia of 41%. Estimates of prevalence were higher in women than in men (45% versus 28%) and continued to increase with age in women but appeared to level off in men (Fig. 17.4). The 90+ Study suggests that dementia prevalence rates, particularly in women, continue to

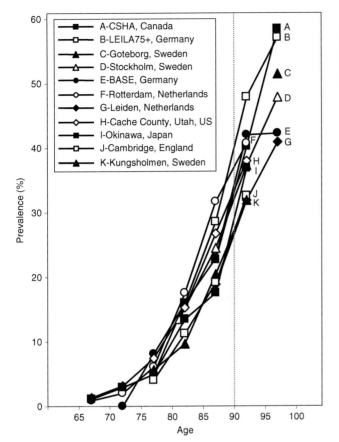

Fig. 17.3. Age-specific prevalence of dementia in studies with subjects aged 90+ years. Studies A-CSHA, Canada;[19] B-LEILA75+, Germany;[20] C-Goteborg, Sweden;[21] D-Stockholm, Sweden;[22] E-BASE, Germany;[23] F-Rotterdam, the Netherlands;[24] G-Leiden, the Netherlands;[25] H-Cache County, Utah;[26] I-Okinawa, Japan;[27] J-Cambridge, England;[28] K-Kungsholmen, Sweden.[29]

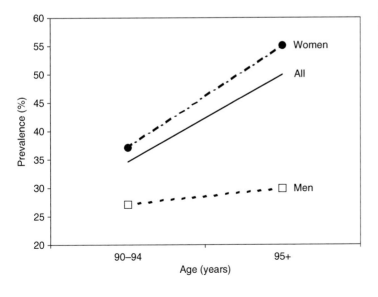

Fig. 17.4. Age- and sex-specific prevalence of all-cause dementia in the 90+ Study.

Table 17.3. Mini-Mental State Examination (MMSE): cutoff scores for dementia by education group in the 90+ Study

Age (years)	High school or less		College or more	
	MMSE cutoff score	Sensitivity/specificity	MMSE cutoff score	Sensitivity/specificity
90–93	≤ 23	0.87/0.94	≤ 25	0.82/0.80
94–96	≤ 23	0.90/0.93	≤ 24	0.85/0.80
97+	≤ 22	0.80/0.76	≤ 22	0.89/0.90

From Kahle-Wrobleski et al. (2007)[40] with permission.

rise across the tenth decade. Because women make up more than three-quarters of all individuals over age 90, we can expect increasing numbers of persons with dementia in the growing population of oldest-old.

Screening for dementia

With high rates of prevalent dementia in the oldest-old, determining the utility of dementia screening instruments for this age group is essential. Perhaps the most widely used dementia screening instrument, the Mini-Mental State Examination (MMSE),[7] does not have published cutoffs for persons over age 90. Scores on the MMSE generally decline with age,[36,37] and failure to adjust cutoffs for older age groups may reduce the specificity of this instrument,[38,39] resulting in more oldest-old patients or participants inaccurately being labeled as having dementia.

Table 17.3 shows results from the 90+ Study, suggesting the MMSE is an accurate screening tool for identifying dementia in those aged 90+ years when used with age- and education-adjusted cutoff points.[40] Even across the tenth decade, cutoff values need to be adjusted downward with increasing age to preserve the balance between sensitivity and specificity, a crucial first step in characterizing dementia in nonagenarians and centenarians.

Normative neuropsychological data

Limited age-appropriate normative data are available when assessing persons over age 90 for impairments in specific domains of cognition. Common normative datasets, such as those published for the Halstead–Reitan Neuropsychological Battery[41] or the Wechsler Adult Intelligence Scale, 3rd edition[15] do not include adults over the age of 90 in their samples. The Mayo Older Adults Normative Study does include those aged 90+ years but has relatively few individuals (less than 30).[42] One recently published study provided norms

on the neuropsychological battery of the Consortium to Establish a Registry for Alzheimer's Disease (CERAD) drawn from 196 individuals aged 85 years and older.[43] The authors found a strong effect of education and age on most tests, concluding that norms drawn from younger populations are not appropriate for the oldest-old and might lead to misclassification of participants as demented.[43]

To establish a set of normative data for the oldest-old using the largest number of subjects to date, data were compiled from 339 non-demented participants in the 90+ Study. These norms are available in the public domain[44] and include age-specific means, standard deviations, and percentiles for several standardized and widely used tests, listed in Table 17.2. When comparing mean scores of our oldest-old participants with previous studies of younger individuals, age effects are easily noted (Figure 17.5). The oldest-old performed less well, on average, than their younger counterparts on both timed and untimed tasks. Further analyses within our group aged 90+ years showed that cognitive test performance was inversely related to age.[44] Tests with an age effect included the Modified Mini-Mental Status Examination (3MS), Boston Naming Test – 15 item, Animal Fluency, California Verbal Learning Test, Trail Making Tests A and B, Clock Drawing Test, and Digit Span Backward. As seen in Figure 17.5, cognitive performance across age groups for those aged 90+ decreased at nearly twice the magnitude as differences across the younger age groups. For example, mean time to complete the Trail Making Test A was nearly 30 seconds slower for the 95+ age group than in the group aged 90–91 years. In contrast, the mean time to complete the test in the group aged 76–85 years was only 10 seconds slower than completion time for the group aged 71–75 years. Results from the 90+ Study suggest that the performance of non-demented nonagenarians and centenarians continues to decline and

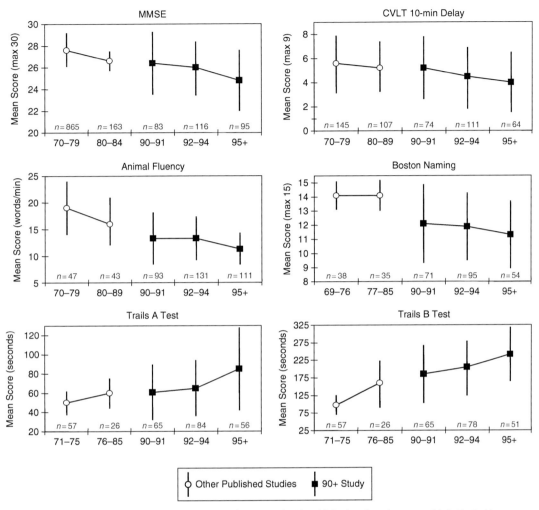

Fig. 17.5. Mean cognitive test scores from the 90+ Study compared with published studies of younger elderly. Vertical bars represent ±1 standard deviation. MMSE, Mini-Mental State Examination; CVLT, California Verbal Learning Test; BNT, Boston Naming Test. Source for other published studies: MMSE,[37] CVLT,[14] Animal Fluency,[45] BNT,[46] Trail Making Tests A and B.[47]

possibly even accelerates past the age of 90. Whether these findings reflect latent disease processes or other age-associated processes requires further investigation.

Challenges in the cognitive assessment of the oldest-old

Factors affecting validity and reliability of clinical assessments are magnified when working with the oldest-old. In particular, sensory deficits, fatigue and motor limitations influence how cognitive tests must be administered and interpreted in studies such as the 90+ Study. A majority (72%) of the participants in the 90+ Study had significant hearing loss, vision loss,

or both. Some sensory limitations are overcome with personal devices, such as hearing aids and eyeglasses. However, degenerative conditions such as macular degeneration and glaucoma lead to untreatable visual loss and affect the choice and presentation of neuropsychological tests, as well as interpretation of results.

In addition, our experience shows that fatigue is a pressing concern when working with individuals over the age of 90. Frequent breaks are required and subjects often are slow to complete procedures. Although the cognitive assessment battery of the 90+ Study does not usually take more than 45 minutes to complete, approximately 20% of participants omit at least one test because of fatigue.

Fatigue in those aged 90+ may be attributable to a wide variety of factors. For some participants, sensory deficits may demand additional effort to perceive the stimulus. For instance, participants with macular degeneration often report during the examination that their eyes are tired from the strain, and visually based tests such as the Boston Naming Test or Trail Making Tests cannot be completed. Other likely sources of fatigue include comorbid medical conditions, medications and frailty.

Diagnostic considerations

The effects of sensory deficits, fatigue and medical comorbidities present a challenge for determining if dementia or cognitive impairment should be diagnosed in a person aged 90 or older. For individuals who cannot complete cognitive testing, it is often challenging to determine the nature and extent of cognitive difficulties. Against a background of medical illnesses and sensory losses, it is frequently difficult to determine if functional losses have occurred as a result of cognitive loss. Moreover, informant reports are constrained by different individual and cultural notions of what impairment or decline looks like in the oldest-old. In addition, current diagnostic criteria for dementia were developed with populations under the age of 90, somewhat limiting their applicability to the oldest-old.

Assigning a diagnosis of dementia or mild cognitive impairment is difficult in the oldest-old, and identifying an etiology is a further challenge. The effect of medical comorbidities on cognitive test performance or on the brain itself is not well understood in this advanced age group. Careful consideration must be made of the medical history and medication usage, with an understanding that nonagenarians and centenarians may have less reserve energy and an increased sensitivity to medication interactions and side-effects compared with younger adults.

Neuropathology of dementia in the oldest-old

The association between clinical dementia and neuropathological features is inconsistent In the oldest-old, unlike younger age groups where the association between cognitive functioning and β-amyloid plaque and neurofibrillary tangle neuropathology has been well established.[48] Approximately half of nonagenarians have clinically diagnosed dementia without any measured neuropathology generally associated with

dementia.[49,50] The inverse has also been found in the oldest-old: individuals with no significant cognitive impairment have sufficient neuropathology meeting criteria for Alzheimer's disease.[50–52]

Consistent with previous reports, approximately half of the participants in the 90+ Study diagnosed with dementia on clinical evaluation subsequently did not meet pathological criteria for Alzheimer's disease or other known conditions associated with dementia.[53] Yet the study has also identified several individuals with no cognitive impairments but very high levels of plaque and tangle pathology.[54] If amyloid deposition is not related to cognitive loss and dementia in extreme aging, anti-amyloid therapies currently under development may have little utility in our oldest citizens. The development of therapies and neuropathological diagnostic criteria in this age group requires considerable research before we can understand the substrates of cognitive loss in the oldest-old.

Successfully assessing cognition in the oldest-old

The inherent difficulties of working with a population with high rates of sensory impairment and fatigue, and limited mobility, do not preclude working successfully with the oldest-old. On the contrary, the 90+ Study provides us with a framework for improving our understanding of how best to capture the cognitive status of persons over the age of 90.

Based on our experiences with the oldest-old, we recommend the development of printed instructions to supplement oral instructions. We also suggest using abbreviated versions of tests when available to minimize fatigue and maximize the number of cognitive domains assessed. In considering the diagnostic difficulties of working with the oldest-old, we recommend that assessments include information from informants, medical records and other sources to optimize understanding of cognitive and functional abilities of those aged 90+ years.

Research considerations

With the challenges described above, missing data are frequently unavoidable; such missing data are unlikely to be missed at random. The reasons for non-completion are informative, and research studies should consider coding schemes that can capture reasons for non-completion, such as sensory impairments and fatigue. Order of administration also

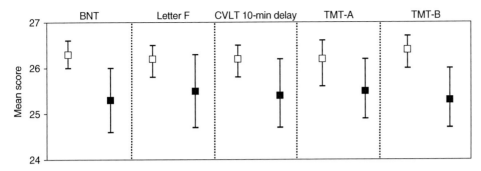

Fig. 17.6. Mean score on the Mini-Mental State Examination for participants who completed (□) or did not complete (■) neuropsychological tests. BNT, Boston Naming Test; Letter F, Letter F fluency; CVLT, California Verbal Learning Test 9-item 10 min delay; TMT, Trail Making Test. Vertical bars indicate 95% confidence interval.

impacts rates of missing data, as does declining cognition. Figure 17.6 demonstrates that those participants who complete a test had a higher global cognition score than non-completers on the same test. As individuals experience cognitive decline, they may be more likely to refuse, may experience fatigue more rapidly in the testing environment and may be less likely to complete some components of the neuropsychological battery.

Conclusions

The oldest-old are the fastest growing segment of the population in most of the world. Age is the primary risk factor for dementia, and the rising number of nonagenarians and centenarians portends an impending crisis for public health. The cost of caring for the rising number of those aged 90+ years who develop dementia in the coming decades will more than double from the approximately US$1 billion currently spent.[55]

Compounding this challenge, the etiology and diagnosis of dementia in this age group is poorly understood. Screening and diagnostic instruments require modifications and present challenges for interpretation. Pathologically, levels of amyloid deposition do not correlate with cognition after age 90, and about half of demented individuals in this age group do not have obvious pathologies, such as amyloid plaques, neurofibrillary tangles or strokes, to explain their cognitive loss. Population studies in the oldest-old, particularly those enriched with clinical pathological investigations, will be essential as we seek to understand the neurobiology of extreme aging.

Investigations such as the 90+ Study are helping to expand our knowledge of dementia and cognitive functioning in our oldest citizens. Determining causes of dementia and identifying risk and protective factors associated with dementia in the oldest-old will be key to the development of successful intervention strategies for this rapidly growing segment of our population.

Acknowledgement

This research was funded by grants from the National Institutes of Health (R01CA32197 and R01AG21055) and the Al and Trish Nichols Chair in Clinical Neuroscience.

References

1. US Census Bureau. *Census 2000 Summary File 2.* Washington, DC: US Census Bureau, 2001.

2. US Census Bureau. *Population Projections (Middle Series).* Washington, DC: US Census Bureau, 2002.

3. United Nations Population Division. *World Population Prospects: The 2004 Revision Population Database.* New York: United Nations, 2005 http://esa.un.org/unpp.

4. Paganini-Hill A, Ross RK, Henderson BE. Prevalence of chronic disease and health practices in a retirement community. *J Chronic Dis.* 1986;**39**:699–707.

5. Paganini-Hill A, Chao A, Ross RK, Henderson BE. Exercise and other factors in the prevention of hip fracture: the Leisure World study. *Epidemiology.* 1991; **2**:16–25.

6. Teng EL, Chui HC. The Modified Mini-Mental State (3MS) Examination. *J Clin Psychiatry.* 1987;**48**:314–318.

7. Folstein MF, Folstein SE, McHugh PR. "Mini-mental state." A practical method for grading the cognitive state of patients for the clinician. *J Psychiatr Res.* 1975; **12**:189–198.

8. Kaplan EF, Goodglas H, Weintraub S. *The Boston Naming Test.* Boston, MA: Kaplan and Goodglass, 1978.

9. Mack WJ, Freed DM, Williams BW, Henderson VW. Boston Naming Test: shortened version for use in Alzheimer's disease. *J Gerontol.* 1992;**47**:164–168.

10. Benton AL, Hamsher K, Sivan AB. *Multilingual Aphasia Examination*, 3rd edn. Iowa City, IA: AJA Associates, 1983.

11. Morris JC, Mohs R, Rogers H, Fillenbaum G, Heyman A. Consortium to establish a registry for Alzheimer's disease (CERAD): clinical and neuropsychological assessment of Alzheimer's Disease. *Psychopharmacol Bull*. 1988;**24**:641–652.

12. Rouleau I, Salmon DP, Butters N, Kennedy C, McGuire K. Quantitative and qualitative analyses of clock face drawings in Alzheimer's and Huntington's diseases. *Brain Cogn*. 1992;**18**:70–87.

13. Freedman M, Kaplan E, Delis D, Morris R. *Clock Drawing: A Neuropsychological Analysis*. New York: Oxford University Press, 1994.

14. Delis DC, Kramer JH, Kaplan E, Ober BA. *California Verbal Learning Test*, 2nd edn. San Antonio, TX: Psychological Corporation, 2000.

15. Wechsler D. *WAIS-III Administration and Scoring Manual*. San Antonio, TX: The Psychological Corporation and Harcourt Brace, 1997.

16. US War Department. *Army Individual Test Battery: Manual of Directions and Scoring*. Washington, DC: War Department, Adjutant General's Office, 1944.

17. Reitan RM, Wolfson D. *The Halstead–Reitan Neuropsychological Battery*. Tucson, AZ: Neuropsychological Press, 1985.

18. Delis D, Kaplan E, Kramer JH. *The Delis–Kaplan Executive Function System (DK-EFS)*. San Antonio, TX: Psychological Corporation, 2001.

19. Ebly EM, Parhad IM, Hogan DB, Fung TS. Prevalence and types of dementia in the very old: results from the Canadian Study of Health and Aging. *Neurology*. 1994;**44**:1593–1600.

20. Riedel-Heller SG, Busse A, Aurich C, Matschinger H, Angermeyer MC. Prevalence of dementia according to DSM-III-R and ICD-10: results of the Leipzig Longitudinal Study of the Aged (LEILA75+) Part 1. *Br J Psychiatry*. 2001;**179**:250–254.

21. Borjesson-Hanson A, Edin E, Gislason T, Skoog I. The prevalence of dementia in 95 year olds. *Neurology*. 2004;**63**:2436–2438.

22. von Strauss E, Viitanen M, de Ronchi D, Winblad B, Fratiglioni L. Aging and the occurrence of dementia: findings from a population-based cohort with a large sample of nonagenarians. *Arch Neurol*. 1999; **56**:587–592.

23. Wernicke TF, Reischies FM. Prevalence of dementia in old age: Clinical diagnoses in subjects aged 95 years and older. *Neurology*. 1994;**44**:250–253.

24. Ott A, Breteler MM, van Harskamp F, *et al*. Prevalence of Alzheimer's disease and vascular dementia: association with education. The Rotterdam study. *BMJ*. 1995;**310**:970–973.

25. Heeren TJ, Lagaay AM, Hijmans W, Rooymans HG. Prevalence of dementia in the "oldest old" of a Dutch community. *J Am Geriatr Soc*. 1991;**39**:755–759.

26. Breitner JC, Wyse BW, Anthony JC, *et al*. APOE-epsilon4 count predicts age when prevalence of AD increases, then declines: the Cache County Study. *Neurology*. 1999;**53**:321–331.

27. Ogura C, Nakamoto H, Uema T *et al*. Prevalence of senile dementia in Okinawa, Japan. COSEPO Group. Study Group of Epidemiology for Psychiatry in Okinawa. *Int J Epidemiol*. 1995;**24**:373–380.

28. O'Connor DW, Pollitt PA, Hyde JB, *et al*. The prevalence of dementia as measured by the Cambridge Mental Disorders of the Elderly Examination. *Acta Psychiatr Scand*. 1989;**79**:190–198.

29. Fratiglioni L, Grut M, Forsell Y, *et al*. Prevalence of Alzheimer's disease and other dementias in an elderly urban population: relationship with age, sex, and education. *Neurology*. 1991;**41**:1886–1892.

30. Ritchie K, Kildea D. Is senile dementia "age-related" or "ageing-related"? Evidence from meta-analysis of dementia prevalence in the oldest old. *Lancet*. 1995;**346**:931–934.

31. Jensen GD, Polloi AH. The very old of Palau: health and mental state. *Age Ageing*. 1988;**17**:220–226.

32. Asada T, Yamagata Z, Kinoshita T *et al*. Prevalence of dementia and distribution of *ApoE* alleles in Japanese centenarians: an almost-complete survey in Yamanashi Prefecture, Japan. *J Am Geriatr Soc*. 1996;**44**:151–155.

33. Ravaglia G, Forti P, de Ronchi D *et al*. Prevalence and severity of dementia among northern Italian centenarians. *Neurology*. 1999;**53**:416–418.

34. Blansjaar BA, Thomassen R, van Schaick HW. Prevalence of dementia in centenarians. *Int J Geriatr Psychiatry*. 2000;**15**:219–225.

35. Dewey ME, Copeland JR. Dementia in centenarians. *Int J Geriatr Psychiatry*. 2001;**16**:538–539.

36. O'Connor DW, Pollitt PA, Treasure FP, Brook CPB, Reiss BB. The influence of education, social class, and sex on Mini-Mental State scores. *Psychol Med*. 1989;**19**:771–776.

37. Crum RM, Anthony JC, Bassett SS, Folstein MF. Population-based norms for the Mini-Mental State Examination by age and educational level. *JAMA*. 1993;**269**:2386–2391.

38. Tombaugh TN, McDowell I, Kristjansson B, Hubley AM. Mini-Mental State Examination (MMSE) and the Modified MMSE (3MS): a psychometric comparison and normative data. *Psychol Assess*. 1996;**8**:48–59.

39. Iverson G. Interpretation of Mini-Mental State Examination scores in community-dwelling elderly and geriatric neuropsychiatry patients. *Int J Geriat Psychiatry*. 1998;**13**:661–666.

40. Kahle-Wrobleski K, Corrada MM, Li B, Kawas CH. Sensitivity and specificity of the mini-mental state examination for identifying dementia in the oldest-old: the 90+ Study. *J Am Geriatr Soc*. 2007;**55**:284–289.

41. Heaton RK, Grant I, Matthews C. *Comprehensive Norms for an Expanded Halstead-Reitan Neuropsychological Battery: Demographic Corrections, Research Findings, and Clinical Applications*. Odessa, FL: Psychological Assessment Resources, 1991.

42. Ivnik RJ, Malec JF, Smith GE, Tangalos EG, Petersen RC. Neuropsychological tests' norms above age 55: COWAT, BNT, MAE Token, WRAT-R Reading, AMNART, STROOP, TMT, and JLO. *Clin Neuropsychol*. 1996;**10**:262–278.

43. Beeri MS, Schmeidler J, Sano M, *et al*. Age, gender, and education norms on the CERAD neuropsychological battery in the oldest old. *Neurology*. 2006;**67**:1006–1010.

44. Whittle C, Corrada MM, Dick M, *et al*. Neuropsychological data in nondemented oldest-old: the 90+ Study. *J Clin Exp Neuropsychol*. 2007;**29**:290–299.

45. Kozora E, Cullum CM. Generative naming in normal aging: total output of qualitative changes using phonemic and semantic constraints. *Clin Neuropsychol*. 1995; **9**:313–320.

46. Fastenau PS, Denburg NL, Mauer BA. Parallel short forms for the Boston Naming Test: psychometric properties and norms for older adults. *J Clin Exp Neuropsychol*. 1998;**20**:828–834.

47. van Gorp WG, Satz P, Mitrashina M. Neuropsychological processes associated with normal aging. *Dev Neuropsychol*. 1990;**6**:279–290.

48. Blennow K, de Leon MJ, Zetterberg H. Alzheimer's disease. *Lancet*. 2006;**368**:387–403.

49. Crystal HA, Dickson D, Davies P *et al*. The relative frequency of "dementia of unknown etiology" increases with age and is nearly 50% in nonagenarians. *Arch Neurol*. 2000;**57**:713–719.

50. Polvikoski T, Sulkava R, Myllykangas L *et al*. Prevalence of Alzheimer's disease in very elderly people: a prospective neuropathological study. *Neurology*. 2001;**56**:1690–1696.

51. Katzman R, Terry RD, DeTeresa R *et al*. Clinical, pathological, and neurochemical changes in dementia: a subgroup with preserved mental status and numerous neocortical plaques. *Ann Neurol*. 1988; **23**:138–144.

52. Crystal H, Dickson D, Fuld P *et al*. Clinico-pathologic studies in dementia: nondemented subjects with pathologically confirmed Alzheimer's disease. *Neurology*. 1988;**38**:1682–1687.

53. Corrada MM, Head E, Kim R, Kawas C. Braak and Braak staging and dementia in the oldest-old: preliminary results from the 90+ Study. In *Proceedings of the 57th Annual American Academy of Neurology Meeting*, April 9–16, 2005, Miami, FL.

54. Berlau DJ, Kahle-Wrobleski K, Head EMG, Kim R, Kawas C. A case of dissociation between neuropathology and cognition in the oldest-old: a protective role of APOE-ε2. *Arch Neurol*. 2007;**64**:1193–1196.

55. Alzheimer's Association. *Alzheimer's Disease Facts and Figures*. Chicago, IL: Alzheimer's Association, 2007.

Slowly progressive dementias
Semantic dementia

John R. Hodges, R. Rhys Davies and Karalyn Patterson

Introduction

Semantic dementia (SD; also known as progressive fluent aphasia) is regarded as a part of the spectrum of non-Alzheimer dementias that produce selective atrophy of the anterior temporal and/or orbitomedial frontal lobes; these conditions are referred to collectively as either the frontotemporal dementias (FTD) or frontotemporal lobar degeneration (FTLD) (Neary, 1994; Neary et al., 1998). Although previously thought to be rare, FTD in fact has about the same prevalence as Alzheimer's disease (AD) below the age of 65 (Ratnavalli et al., 2002). Three clinical presentations of FTD are commonly described: a behavioral variant (bv-FTD), and two language variants, SD and progressive non-fluent aphasia (PNFA) (Hodges and Miller, 2001a,b). Since the mid 1990s, research on SD has produced a great deal of information about the clinical and neuropsychological features, progression, anatomy and neuropathology of the condition, which we attempt to review and synthesize here.

Early history

Although the term "semantic dementia" is recent (Snowden et al., 1989), the syndrome has been recognized under different labels for over a century. Between 1892 and 1904, Arnold Pick (1892, 1904) reported a series of remarkable cases characterized by progressive amnesic aphasia and changes in behavior; at autopsy these patients had marked atrophy of the left temporal lobe. Pick was perhaps the first neuroscientist to draw attention to the fact that progressive brain atrophy may lead to focal symptoms. He also made specific and, as we will see below, highly perceptive predictions regarding the role of the mid-temporal region of the left hemisphere in the representation of word meaning. Many other similar cases were

reported in the early twentieth century (Rosenfeld, 1909; Mingazzini, 1913; Stertz, 1926; Schneider, 1927); however, following the early flurry of reports, interest gradually faded, and Pick's disease was for a long period regarded as a medical rarity, and furthermore was specifically (and erroneously) associated with frontal lobe dysfunction.

A renaissance of interest began in the 1970s. The neuropsychological world became re-acquainted with the syndrome through the landmark study of Elizabeth Warrington (1975) who proposed a unifying explanation for the cognitive deficits exhibited by such patients. Warrington recognized that the associative agnosia, anomia and impaired word comprehension in her three patients reflected a fundamental and selective loss of semantic memory (or knowledge). Semantic memory is the term applied to the component of long-term memory that represents our knowledge about things in the world and their inter-relationships, facts and concepts as well as words and their meanings (Rogers et al., 2004a).

In the neurological literature, interest in focal dementia syndromes causing predominant language impairment was re-awakened by Marsel Mesulam's 1982 report of five patients with progressive loss of ability to communicate for which he coined the term primary progressive aphasia (PPA). Many case reports quickly followed and it became apparent that PPA actually forms a relatively bimodal distribution (Mehler et al., 1986; Basso et al., 1988; Poeck and Luzzatti, 1988; Grossman and Ash, 2004): patients with effortful speech and progressive breakdown in the syntactic and phonological aspects of language (PNFA), and those with effortless and phonologically accurate but empty speech. Like most bimodal distibutions in the real world, this one also contains at least a smattering of mixed cases.

In 1989, Julie Snowden and colleagues proposed the term "semantic dementia" for patients with progressive fluent aphasia and a loss of comprehension. Our 1992 report of five cases further clarified the

The Behavioral Neurology of Dementia, eds. Bruce L. Miller and Bradley F. Boeve. Published by Cambridge University Press.
© Cambridge University Press 2009.

Table 18.1. Key clinical, neuropsychological and radiological findings in semantic dementia

Area	Features
Clinical	Loss of memory for words
	Anomia
	Impaired word comprehension
	Impaired person recognition (particularly right cases)
	Personality changes, notably rigidity, apathy and social withdrawal
	Obsessions and stereotyped behaviors
	Changes in eating patterns
	Good day-to-day memory and spatial abilities
Neuropsychological	Impaired category fluency, naming (semantic errors) and word comprehension
	Loss of specific fine-grained knowledge with preservation of broad superordinate knowledge
	Preservation of non-verbal problem solving, perceptual and spatial ability and working memory
	Good episodic memory for non-verbal materials and recent autobiographical memory
Neuroradiological	Asymmetric anterior temporal lobe atrophy (typically left > right) involving temporal pole, parahippocampal and fusiform gyri plus amygdala and anterior hippocampus

clinical and neuropsychological features (Hodges *et al.*, 1992). Since 1992, we have studied almost 100 such patients and have confirmed the association with focal atrophy of the temporal lobe involving the temporal pole and inferolateral neocortex. In many cases, the atrophy is strikingly asymmetric and usually more severe on the left, but it is always bilateral (Garrard and Hodges, 2000; Thompson *et al.*, 2003). Other major developments since the mid 1990s have been refinement of the cognitive profile of SD, particularly the impact on reading/writing, object recognition/use, episodic memory and perceptual abilities; clearer specification of the distribution of changes on magnetic resonance imaging (MRI); and the pathological basis of the condition. In addition there is increasing realization that most, if not all, patients exhibit behavioral changes, which may be subtle at presentation but have major consequences for caregivers as the disease progresses. Another important advance has been the description of the right-dominant temporal variant of SD, which has some unique cognitive and behavioral features.

Clinical features

Patients with SD almost invariably complain of difficulty finding words, often expressed as a "loss of memory for words." Insight into these problems is variable, with a curious distinction between production and comprehension – patients frequently think that the latter is preserved. Carers may report subtle

behavioral changes at or soon after onset, especially in patients with right-predominant atrophy. Table 18.1 summarizes the key clinical, neuropsychological and imaging findings in SD.

Anomia

Anomia is perhaps the defining feature of SD, and it is made especially salient by the fact that the unavailable content words (specific nouns, verbs, adjectives) are replaced and surrounded by speech that is correctly pronounced and has normal grammatical structure (though syntax is somewhat simplified relative to that of normal speakers: (Patterson and MacDonald, 2006). In SD speech, specific and lower-frequency words such as "kettle" or "zebra" are replaced by more general and higher-frequency terms like "thing" and "animal." Anomia always raises the possibility that the patient knows about *kettles* and *zebras* but cannot find the specific names for them and so must settle for more general terms; but in the case of SD, this interpretation would be incorrect. Although patients with SD (like normal speakers) may occasionally fail to find a word whose meaning they know, word-retrieval failure in SD is mainly caused by impoverished semantic knowledge about the object or concept to be named. There are several bases for this claim. (1) A normal speaker in a temporary state of anomia is very likely to think of the word or name a few minutes later, and to produce it without hesitation the next time it is wanted; SD patients, by contrast, are highly consistent in their failures to retrieve specific names/words (Lambon Ralph and Howard, 2000). (2) Normal speakers can often be cued, with the initial sound or two, to retrieve a recalcitrant word; patients with SD receive strikingly little benefit, even from cueing with large chunks of the target word's sound (Graham *et al.*, 1995). (3) Normal speakers, and even patients with other types of aphasia with a less semantic source of anomia, can provide lots of correct conceptual information about the elusive target word (Lambon Ralph *et al.*, 2000); such information is rarely if ever forthcoming from a patient with SD. (4) Sometimes the comments of a patient with SD reveal how little they know about the things they fail to name. Patient PS, for example, when asked to name a picture of a zebra, said "It's a horse, isn't it?" And then, pointing to the zebra's stripes, she added "But what are these funny things for?"

As the above explanation of anomia (in terms of impoverished knowledge) might predict, the patient's profound anomia is mirrored by problems in comprehending content words. This deficit is often not obvious in conversation, as at first it affects only less-common words. Furthermore, normal conversation has a lot of redundancy and in any case does not rely on every single word being understood. Complex sentences made up of simple words are usually understood well by those with SD; but less-common words invariably cause problems, and eventually the patients even lose all sense of familiarity with many words (this has been called *word alienation* [Poeck and Luzzatti, 1988]). A useful clinical test is to ask the patient first to repeat a long, unusual word such as "hippopotamus" or "chrysanthemum," and then to define it. Repetition is almost always normal and rapid, but the definition will be generalized, lacking in detail and, sometimes, frankly uninformative.

A typical conversation between clinician and patient illustrates some of these features:

Clinician: "Antelope" – can you say that?
Patient: Antelope, sorry no idea what that is
Clinician: No idea on that one?
Patient: Antelope, it might be an animal
Clinician: Can you describe it?
Patient: No, sorry I can't remember anything about it.

Although many patients with SD complain of *memory* loss, this does not reflect a true amnesia. Their ability to encode and remember day-to-day events in basic content and temporal/spatial context is, in fact, fairly well preserved, as will be discussed in more detail below. To the extent that knowledge – of words and concepts and facts – is a kind of memory, however, the patients and their carers are not wrong to complain of a memory problem.

As a disorder of concepts, SD also affects *object use*, although this is often subtle in the beginning. Carers typically report that the patients function normally with everyday objects at home; and although formal tests of object knowledge can often reveal impairment, even at an early stage, the carers' reports are once again not incorrect. There are two reasons for this apparent discrepancy. First, the objects that the patients use appropriately at home are mostly very common ones, like forks and combs and socks; when presented with such common objects in formal tests, the patients are also likely to demonstrate their uses correctly. It is less-familiar objects, such as a corkscrew or a stethoscope, on which they fail in formal assessments. Second, it is now well established that patients with SD are significantly better at recognizing and using their own familiar exemplars of everyday objects than the equally good but unfamiliar exemplars with which they are confronted in testing (see below for fuller discussion).

Behavior and personality change

Behavioral and personality changes are common in SD. Degraded social functioning results from a combination of emotional withdrawal, depression, disinhibition, apathy and/or irritability, as well as the obvious difficulty in dealing with certain aspects of social events that might depend on understanding the things people say and do. Changes in eating behavior are common, and often seem to reveal themselves in the development or exacerbation of a sweet tooth. Usually there is a restriction of food preferences, or bizarre food choices, rather than the overeating seen typically in bv-FTD. Loss of physiological drives is common and includes poor appetite, weight loss and decreased libido. A new sense of religiosity and/or eccentricity of dress have also been reported (Edwards Lee *et al.*, 1997). The right temporal variant of SD, which appears to have only one-third the prevalence of left-dominant SD, seems to be more convincingly associated with behavioral disturbance than the left (Edwards Lee *et al.*, 1997; Perry *et al.*, 2001; Thompson *et al.*, 2003; Seeley *et al.*, 2005).

Stereotyped interests

Stereotyped interests often verging on obsessions are a prominent, but delayed feature, and may reflect the predominant temporal lobe involved. A recent study suggested that in patients with left-predominant SD, visual objects such as coins or buttons are likely to become the target stimulus while in the right-sided variant, the focus is on letters, words and symbols (e.g. word puzzles, and writing notes to doctors) (Seeley *et al.*, 2005), although we have observed the latter in patients with the common left atrophy form. Clockwatching and an intense interest in jigsaws is very common (Thompson *et al.*, 2002). *Lack of empathy* and *mental inflexibility* are also commonly reported by caregivers.

Person recognition

Deficits in person recognition frequently occur at some stage in the disease (Thompson *et al.*, 2003). Difficulty with proper names is a ubiquitous feature, independent of the side of predominant atrophy, but patients with the rarer right-predominant pattern may *present* with a profound difficulty in recognizing people as well as naming them. Over time, again largely independent of the balance of left/right hemisphere atrophy, there is cross-modal loss of person knowledge involving face, name and voice recognition (Evans *et al.*, 1995; Kitchener and Hodges, 1999; Gainotti *et al.*, 2003; Thompson *et al.*, 2003).

Maintained skills

All of our description so far has, quite naturally, emphasized the impairments in SD; however, an understanding of the nature of any disorder also requires specification of what is right as well as what is wrong. Patients with SD have good orientation and recall of recent life events, together with preserved visuospatial and topographical abilities. They are typically able to engage in complex hobbies such as playing golf or card games and show good practical skills.

Neuropsychological findings

Patients with SD are (by definition) impaired on tests of semantic memory. This is most apparent on tasks that require verbal output such as object/picture naming, category fluency (in which subjects are asked to produce as many examples as possible in 1 minute from a specified conceptual category, such as animals or musical instruments), and the generation of verbal definitions to words and pictures. The pattern of errors on these tasks reflects a loss of fine-grained or attribute knowledge, with relative preservation of broad superordinate information. Where anomia in

SD has been studied longitudinally (e.g. Hodges *et al.*, 1995; Patterson *et al.*, 2008), it seems to evolve in the following sequence, which fits the description of gradually deteriorating differentiation amongst related concepts. First the target object may be named as a semantically similar category coordinate (e.g. zebra → "giraffe"); then as a much higher-familiarity member of the category (e.g. zebra → "horse"); then as the superordinate category name (e.g. zebra → "animal"); and then as a rather vague circumlocution, often with a personal context (e.g. zebra → "it's one of those things, I saw them on the television last night"); the late stage is characterized by an inability to say anything at all (zebra → "I don't know"). Although tests that require speech output are most sensitive at early and middle stages of SD, it is other tests – involving forced-choice responding in a comprehension task such as word–picture, word–word or picture–picture matching on a semantic basis – that can track the continued decline of conceptual knowledge once the patients can no longer name almost any objects.

The semantic memory battery developed in Cambridge involves a single set of items (64 in the current version) that are used to assess the status of conceptual knowledge via different modalities of input and output. The tasks in the battery include category fluency, picture naming, naming in response to verbal descriptions, word–picture matching, picture and word sorting and a probed semantic attribute questionnaire. The battery has proven useful in the evaluation of patients with all forms of FTD as well as AD (Hodges and Patterson, 1995, 1996; Hodges *et al.*, 1996, 1999a; Rogers *et al.*, 2006).

Non-verbal semantic knowledge is always less easy to assess. In the Pyramids and Palm Trees Test (Howard and Patterson, 1992), the subject is asked to select one of two response pictures on the basis of its associative relationship to a third, target picture (e.g. on one trial, the correct choice to go with the tree is the apple rather than the onion – both roundish things to eat – because apples but not onions grow on trees). This test certainly reveals deficits for patients with SD who are moderately or severely impaired but is not especially sensitive to mild impairment. In order to demonstrate that the semantic impairment even early in SD indeed represents deterioration of central, cross-modal knowledge, and is not simply a language disorder, we have developed a range of other non-verbal tasks, including (1) a more difficult version of Pyramids and Palmtrees (the Camel and Cactus test); (2) matching of object pictures to their

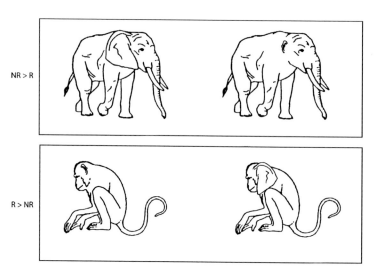

NR > R

R > NR

Fig. 18.1. Examples of stimulus pictures used to assess object decision in patients with semantic dementia. The NR > R pairs, like the two elephants, are cases where the non-real picture is more typical of the concept's domain than the real version. In R > NR pairs, like the two monkeys, typicality favors the real rather than the non-real picture. (From Rogers *et al.* [2004b] with permission from Informa http://www.informaworld.com.)

characteristic sounds; (3) matching of manufactured artefacts (like a vegetable peeler or a hammer) to their typical recipients or to other objects that could be used for the same purpose; (4) coloring in of line drawings of objects with characteristic colors; (5) selecting the correctly colored animal/object; (6) selecting the correct version of a pictured object or animal from two alternatives when one has been altered in some way (e.g. an elephant with a monkey's ears); (7) delayed copying of line drawings; and so on. Patients with even very early SD, who have minimally or even unimpaired performance on easy semantic tasks such as picture-to-word matching, invariably show deficits on many of these non-verbal tasks (Hodges *et al.*, 2000; Bozeat *et al.*, 2002a,b, 2003; Rogers *et al.*, 2003, 2004b; Ikeda *et al.*, 2006; Patterson *et al.*, 2006).

Tests of these kinds for patients with SD, whether verbal or non-verbal, should wherever possible be designed in a fashion that takes account/advantage of the patients' well-established sensitivity to the typicality structure of any domain of knowledge (Patterson *et al.*, 2006). For example, two trials of our object decision task (task (6) above) are illustrated in Fig. 18.1. In each pair of animals, one is pictured with an elephant's ears and one with a monkey's ears, and it should be apparent to the reader which item in each pair is the correct choice! What may be less apparent is the following. Small (monkey) ears are typical of mammals, whereas large, floppy (elephant) ears are very unusual. Of course each animal becomes incorrect when it dons the other one's ears; but this ear-swap makes

the monkey *less* typical of its animal brethren but makes the elephant *more* typical. As we predicted, and as shown in Fig. 18.2a, this manipulation has a major impact on the success of patients with SD when they are asked to decide which picture is the real thing. If their inclination to accept typical things coincides with the correct answer, they perform well; but if correct and typical are pitted against one another, the patients – especially the ones with more severe dysfunction, and especially when they are asked to recognize lower-familiarity objects – are often lured away from the correct to the typical.

These three factors – (1) the frequency or familiarity of the whole item, (2) the extent to which the components of the item have a structure typical of the domain, and (3) the severity of the patient's semantic deficit – turn out to be powerful and pervasive predictors of cognitive performance by patients with SD in virtually every cognitive ability that we have been able to assess (Rogers *et al.*, 2004a; Patterson *et al.*, 2006). For example, as shown in Fig. 18.2 along with object decision performance, the same pattern holds true for the task known as lexical decision. In our version of this task, the patient looks at two variations of a printed word, one real and one made-up, with the same manipulation as the one described for the pictures of elephants and monkeys, but here in the orthographic domain. That is, in one condition (e.g. SHOOT and SHUIT) the real word has a more typical spelling pattern than the non-word alternative; in the contrasting condition (e.g. FRUIT and FROOT) the real word is less typical of English spelling.

(A)

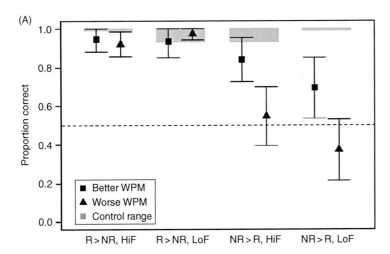

(B)

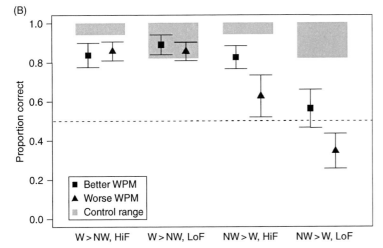

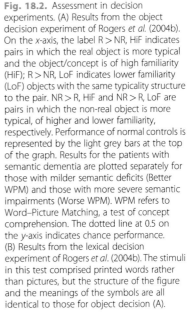

Fig. 18.2. Assessment in decision experiments. (A) Results from the object decision experiment of Rogers *et al.* (2004b). On the *x*-axis, the label R > NR, HiF indicates pairs in which the real object is more typical and the object/concept is of high familiarity (HiF); R > NR, LoF indicates lower familiarity (LoF) objects with the same typicality structure to the pair. NR > R, HiF and NR > R, LoF are pairs in which the non-real object is more typical, of higher and lower familiarity, respectively. Performance of normal controls is represented by the light grey bars at the top of the graph. Results for the patients with semantic dementia are plotted separately for those with milder semantic deficits (Better WPM) and those with more severe semantic impairments (Worse WPM). WPM refers to Word–Picture Matching, a test of concept comprehension. The dotted line at 0.5 on the *y*-axis indicates chance performance. (B) Results from the lexical decision experiment of Rogers *et al.* (2004b). The stimuli in this test comprised printed words rather than pictures, but the structure of the figure and the meanings of the symbols are all identical to those for object decision (A).

As Fig. 18.2 demonstrates, this manipulation has a marked impact on performance by patients with SD. The more severely affected patients are so strongly drawn to typicality that, for lower-frequency words, the FRUIT/FROOT condition actually results in *below*-chance performance. The relevance of word-specific semantic knowledge to this phenomenon is attested not only by the strong correlation with severity of semantic decline, but also by the occasional comment of patients with SD when they are asked to perform this lexical decision task, for example "I don't know what that word means, so how can I say if it is real?" As demonstrated in Patterson *et al.* (2006), the same three factors determine levels of success in other simple tasks like reading words aloud, writing them to dictation and turning stem (present-tense)

forms of verbs into their past-tense forms. Here the patient is lured not by a more typical alternative presented by the experimenter but by his/her own knowledge of the typicality structure of the relevant domain. Thus, again, especially for lower frequency words and more semantically impaired patients, atypical or irregular words are very often "regularized": for example, the written word PINT is read aloud as if it rhymed with "mint;" the spoken word "fruit" is written FROOT or FRUTE; and when patients with SD are asked to put the sentence "Today I grind the coffee" into the past tense, they are very likely to say "Yesterday I grinded the coffee."

We have been discussing SD deficits on verbal and non-verbal tasks as if they were all part of the same general phenomenon, which is indeed our

269

interpretation. In other words, we argue that, within the widespread semantic network in the brain, the anterior temporal lobe represents the component that coordinates and links information from all modalities of input and to all modalities of output, and whose deterioration will, therefore, have similar consequences for both objects and words. By contrast, other cognitive theorists maintain that object and word knowledge are represented in separate brain systems/regions, and they would, therefore, conclude that patients with SD revealing impairments of both have two separate deficits (Mesulam, 2001). In one study designed to yield evidence germane to these contrasting views, we evaluated definitions of concrete concepts provided by patients with SD in response to either the name or the picture of the same item from our semantic battery. The view that there are separate verbal and visual semantic systems predicts no striking item-specific similarities across the two conditions. In keeping with our expectation, however, there was a highly significant concordance between definition success to words and pictures referring to/depicting the same item. The number of definitions containing *no* appropriate semantic information was significantly greater for words than for the corresponding pictures, which theorists preferring the multiple-systems view might interpret as indicating relative preservation of visual semantics; however, we argue that it is open to the following alternative account (Lambon Ralph *et al.*, 1999, 2001; Rogers *et al.*, 2004a). The mapping between an object (or picture of it) and its conceptual representation is inherently different from the mapping between word and concept. Although not everything about objects can be inferred from their physical characteristics, there is a systematic relationship between many of the sensory features of an object or picture and its meaning. Such systematicity is totally lacking for words: phonological forms bear a purely arbitrary relationship to meaning. When conceptual knowledge is degraded, it, therefore, seems understandable that there should be a number of instances where a patient would be able to provide some, even though impoverished, information in response to the picture but draw a complete blank in response to the object's name.

Recent investigations of object usage in SD shed further light on this debate. Some theorists have claimed that there is a separate "action semantic" system, which can be spared when there is insufficient knowledge to drive other forms of response: not only naming but even non-verbal kinds of responding like sorting, word–picture matching or associative matching of pictures or words (e.g. Rothi *et al.*, 1991; Buxbaum *et al.*, 1997; Lauro-Grotto *et al.*, 1997). This view is promoted by anecdotal reports that patients with SD who fail a whole range of laboratory-based tasks of the latter kind still function fairly normally in everyday life (e.g. Snowden *et al.*, 1995). Systematic examination of object usage reveals a more complex and interesting pattern. Patients with SD were asked to demonstrate the use of everyday objects such as a bottle opener, a potato peeler, a box of matches. The patients also performed a series of other semantic tasks involving these same objects, including naming, matching a picture of the object to a picture of the location in which it is typically found (a potato peeler with a picture of a kitchen rather than a garden) or to the normal recipient of the object's action (a potato peeler with a potato rather than an egg). Additionally, the patients performed the novel tool test designed by Goldenberg and Hagmann (1998), in which successful performance must rely on problem solving and general visual affordances of the tools and their recipients, since none of these corresponds to real, familiar objects. We found both a striking degree of impairment in the use of these objects and a strong concordance between the patients' ability to use a specific object and their conceptual knowledge of it as indexed by performance on the other semantic tasks (Hodges *et al.*, 1999b, 2000; Bozeat *et al.*, 2002b). Apart from the predictability offered by the patients' residual semantic knowledge of the objects, degree of success/ failure in using objects appears to be explicable in terms of two other factors. First, the parts and structure of some (but not all) objects give good clues to their function, and patients with SD usually have good problem-solving skills. Even in the face of degraded object-specific knowledge, therefore, the patients can often work out how to use those objects that have a systematic relationship between structure and function. Second, as mentioned in the clinical features above, success with objects is significantly modulated by factors of exemplar-specific familiarity and context. As demonstrated by the ingenious experiments of Snowden *et al.* (1994), a patient who knows how to use her own familiar kettle in the kitchen may fail to recognize and use the experimenter's (equally kettle-like but unfamiliar) kettle in the kitchen, or even the patient's own kettle when it is encountered out of familiar context, for example in the bedroom. This effect of object familiarity was replicated by

Bozeat *et al.* (2002a), who were also able to retrain a patient to use a set of everyday items in her own home that she had "forgotten" how to use. Disappointingly, however, such re-acquired knowledge in SD appears not to generalize well and to last for a few weeks only unless constantly practiced (Graham *et al.*, 1999a; Bozeat *et al.*, 2002b).

As mentioned in the clinical features above, patients with SD are characteristically well orientated and have reasonably good recall of recent personal events (Graham *et al.*, 1999b). This distinctive preservation is, however, not so easy to document empirically. Performance on tests of verbal anterograde memory, such as logical memory (story recall) and word-list learning, is uniformly poor and is, in part, secondary to the patients' poor semantic knowledge of the words to be encoded; however, semantic impairment is perhaps not the whole explanation for the impaired verbal memory in SD. Graham *et al.* (2002) compared the ability of patients with SD to learn and remember two lists of words selected individually for each of seven patients. For each patient, one list consisted of "known" words for which he or she could still provide quite a lot of appropriate information; another list of "degraded" words, matched for frequency with the "known" words, consisted of items for which the patients had at best only partial understanding. Although there was the expected advantage in both recall and recognition for "known" over "degraded" words, the patients' verbal memory even for "known" words was considerably impaired relative to controls. This result is in keeping with the anatomical finding of left hippocampal atrophy and hypometabolism in SD (Galton *et al.*, 2001; Nestor *et al.*, 2002; Davies *et al.*, 2004).

By contrast, patients with SD often score within the normal range on non-verbal memory tests such as recall of the Rey Complex Figure (Hodges *et al.*, 1999a). They also show excellent recognition memory when realistic pictures of objects are used as the stimuli, although it has been recently demonstrated that the patients' success in this task relies heavily upon perceptual information. Graham *et al.* (2000) assessed recognition memory, again for "known" and "degraded" items, this time with pictures and with an additional experimental manipulation. For some of the target items, the two pictures of the item presented at study and at test were perceptually identical (e.g. the same telephone); for others, two different exemplars (i.e. telephones of different colors/shapes) were viewed at study and test. Patients with SD

showed near perfect recognition memory for both known and degraded items in the perceptually identical condition, but were significantly impaired in recognizing perceptually different pictures of objects for which they had degraded conceptual knowledge. Similar results were obtained using photographs of "known" and "degraded" famous faces (Simons *et al.*, 2001). Both of these studies concluded that patients with SD are unusually reliant upon perceptual inputs to medial temporal episodic memory structures, whereas normal subjects can use both semantic and perceptual features to encode new information. This account also helps to explain the poor recognition memory for words in SD, even those still relatively "known" to the patients: words have very little distinctive perceptual content/quality.

On tests of autobiographical memory, patients with SD show a unique pattern. Whereas patients with the amnesic syndrome resulting from hippocampal damage (following anoxic brain damage or in the early stages of AD) typically have significantly impaired memory for their recent life events but relatively preserved autobiographical memory for earlier phases of their lives (Greene *et al.*, 1995), patients with SD show a reversal of this typical temporal gradient: that is, in SD, memory for remote events is most vulnerable (Graham and Hodges, 1997, 1999; Hodges and Graham, 1998; Nestor *et al.*, 2002). This finding has been somewhat controversial, with some authors claiming that the reverse gradient is artefactual and is more a reflection of the patients' language capacity than their memory, while other groups have confirmed the original finding (Piolino *et al.*, 2003; Westmacott *et al.*, 2004).

One simple interpretation of this outcome is that old episodic and semantic memories are essentially the same type of memory. A number of theorists have argued that repeatedly rehearsed episodes have the status of semantic knowledge and that general semantic information is merely the residue of numerous episodes (McClelland *et al.*, 1995). This proposal awaits further analysis and experimental evaluation, although researchers' efforts to devise comparable tests of semantic versus episodic memory are always hampered by fundamental differences in the nature of the information about general concepts/facts versus personal events. In any case, the relatively preserved recent autobiographical memory observed in SD suggests that the mechanisms for encoding new episodic memories may not be disrupted in SD. If true, this would run counter to Tulving's (1995) influential

271

theory of long-term memory organization, which asserts that episodic memory is essentially a subsystem of semantic memory, and that new episodic learning is dependent upon semantic knowledge of the items/concepts involved in the episode (Hodges and Graham, 2001; Simons *et al.*, 2002).

Structural and functional imaging studies

The most striking and consistent neuroanatomical finding in SD is focal, often severe, often asymmetric (typically left more than right) atrophy of the anterior portion of the temporal lobe. Early studies, based upon visual inspection, suggested involvement of the polar and inferolateral regions with relative sparing of the superior temporal gyrus and of the hippocampal formation (Hodges *et al.*, 1992). More recent studies using methods of quantification (both voxel-based morphometry and manual volumetry of defined anatomical structures) have clarified a number of issues. First, although defects may *appear* to be strikingly unilateral, volumetric assessment establishes that, even if asymmetric, atrophy is bilateral in all cases, even early in the course of the disease (Chan *et al.*, 2001; Galton *et al.*, 2001; Davies *et al.*, 2004). Second, the regions most profoundly affected are the temporopolar and perirhinal cortices (Galton *et al.*, 2001; Rosen *et al.*, 2002; Davies *et al.*, 2004; Gorno-Tempini *et al.*, 2004). Third, the degree of anterior temporal atrophy correlates with the extent of semantic impairment (Galton

et al., 2001; Davies *et al.*, 2004; Williams *et al.*, 2005). Typical MRI images are shown in Fig. 18.3.

The status of the hippocampus and functionally related parahippocampal structures (notably the entorhinal cortex) has been a topic of debate, particularly given relatively good episodic memory in SD. Despite previous reports of relative sparing of the hippocampus (Mummery *et al.*, 1999), volumetric analyses have shown asymmetric atrophy of the hippocampus, which, on the left, is typically as severe if not more so in SD than in AD when patients are matched for disease duration (Galton *et al.*, 2001; Davies *et al.*, 2004). The appearance of "relative" preservation of medial temporal structures results from the profound atrophy of surrounding structures: in SD, the volume loss of the temporopolar and perirhinal cortex averages 50%, compared with 20% for the hippocampal region. In AD, by contrast, the 20% loss of hippocampi stands out against the relatively normal polar and inferolateral structures (Galton *et al.*, 2001). There is also a rostral–caudal (front–back) difference between SD and AD. In AD, the loss of volume tends to be symmetrical in terms of both left–right and rostral–caudal distribution. In SD, by contrast, there is both lateralized asymmetry (usually, though not always, left more than right) and front–back asymmetry (virtually always rostral greater than caudal) (Chan *et al.*, 2001; Davies *et al.*, 2004). The entorhinal cortex, which constitutes a major component of the parahippocampal gyrus, is also severely affected in SD, particularly in the rostral portion (Davies *et al.*, 2004). The perirhinal cortex has a complex anatomy in

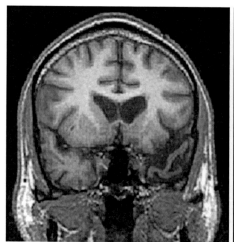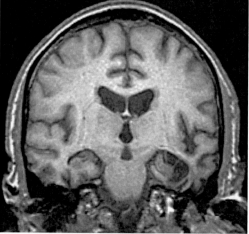

Fig. 18.3. Representative magnetic resonance imaging (MRI). (A) Coronal MRI brain slice showing temporopolar atrophy, more severe on the left. (B) More posterior slice showing atrophy of inferior temporal regions including the perirhinal cortex

humans, occupying the banks of the collateral sulcus and medial aspect of the temporal lobe (Insausti *et al.*, 1998). It is cytoarchitectonically continuous with the temporopolar cortex, which should be considered as part of the same cortical region in terms of connectivity (Insausti *et al.*, 1998). We have shown that the temporopolar–perirhinal cortex is severely affected in SD but spared in early AD (Davies *et al.*, 2004). The amygdala is also consistently involved in SD (Rosen *et al.*, 2002).

Neuropathology

The neuropathology of FTD has become an increasingly complex issue, with the recent identification of four basic patterns (McKhann *et al.*, 2001; Cairns *et al.*, 2004; Hodges *et al.*, 2004; Knopman *et al.*, 2005; Mott *et al.*, 2005). The first is a tau-positive subgroup, which is also made up of further subdivisions: classic Pick's disease with tau- and ubiquitin-positive spherical cortical inclusions best seen in the hippocampal dentate gyrus and frontotemporal cortex; familial FTD with characteristic tau-positive inclusions in neurons and glial cells; and corticobasal degeneration with tau-positive inclusions, swollen acromatic neurons and astrocytic plaques. A second subgroup is characterized by ubiquitin-positive inclusions, initially reported in the context of motor neuron disease (MND) but subsequently found in many cases of FTD without MND in vivo; these ubiquitin inclusions are typically found in cortical layer II and hippocampal dentate granule cells. The third subgroup is neuronal intermediate filament inclusion disease and, finally, there is microvacular degeneration and gliosis lacking distinctive inclusions.

Until recently, data on the neuropathological basis of SD was extremely sparse, consisting largely of single case reports (Garrard and Hodges, 2000; Hodges *et al.*, 2004; Davies *et al.*, 2005). It was generally assumed to represent a form of FTD, but positive evidence for this was largely lacking. We have recently reported the findings in 18 patients from Cambridge and Sydney, all of whom were studied longitudinally. The majority, 13/18, had ubiquitin-positive pathology. Interestingly, one of these patients developed clinical MND late in the course of his illness, and another had a family history of MND. Of the five not characterized by ubiquitin pathology, three had classic Pick body-positive FTD and two had Alzheimer pathology. With the benefit of hindsight, one of the two whose autopsy revealed AD pathology should probably not have

been included in an SD sample since his MRI was atypical, showing extensive white matter pathology in the temporal lobe as well as an unusual degree of posterior extension of the atrophy. He had severe AD pathology with congophilic angiopathy. He was included in the series because the consensus criteria are, at present, entirely clinical and do not mandate any particular radiological changes. We have suggested that inclusion criteria for SD should perhaps now include the typical pattern of anterior temporal lobe atrophy (Davies *et al.*, 2005). Since the completion of this study, the two further patients with SD who have died in Cambridge both had ubiquitin-positive pathology. Therefore, based on our personal experience, the association of SD with ubiquitin-positive FTD is strong, with about an 80% probability. Representative illustrations of the pathology in SD are shown in Fig. 18.4.

Prognosis

The prognosis of FTD in general is highly variable from patient to patient. In a series of 61 mixed FTD cases coming to autopsy from Sydney and Cambridge, the mean age of diagnosis was 61.5 years (±7.7), with an average of 3 years of symptoms prior to diagnosis (Hodges *et al.*, 2003). Survival averaged 4 years from diagnosis, resulting in an average of 7 years from symptom onset to death. This large FTD series contained only nine with SD, but their survival statistics were identical to that of the overall group. In a subsequent extension of this series to 18 autopsy-confirmed SD cases, the survival from symptom onset varied from 2 to 19 years, with a mean of 9.3 years, suggesting a slightly less rapid course than was apparent from the earlier study (Davies *et al.*, 2005).

Management

There is, at present, no effective disease-modifying treatment for patients with this devastating and progressive disorder. Associated affective and behavioral symptoms may require drug treatment with either a selective serotonin-reuptake inhibitor or low-dose neuroleptic medication. In all cases, a multidisciplinary approach is required with support for the patient, spouse and other family members. With progression of the dementia, input from professions allied to medicine (speech and language and occupational therapy) is vital. The issue of whether patients benefit from a cognitive rehabilitation approach is open

273

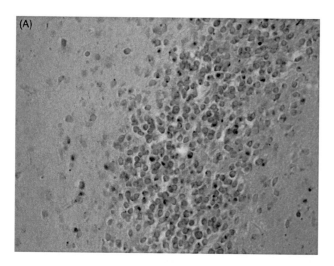

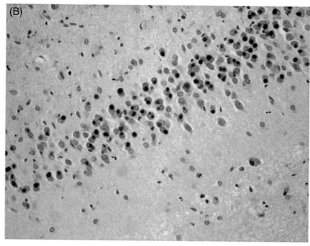

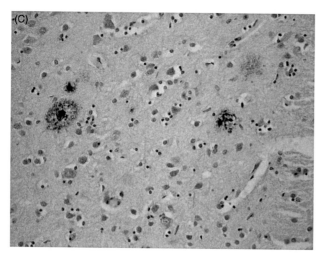

Fig. 18.4. Microscopic photographs (× 200) showing the pathological features of semantic dementia. (A) Frontotemporal dementia with ubiquitin inclusions: ubiquitin immunohistochemistry preparation of hippocampal dentate gyrus showing intraneuronal deposits (motor neuron disease inclusions). (B) Pick's disease: tau immunohistochemistry preparation of hippocampal dentate gyrus showing Pick bodies. (C) Alzheimer's disease: β-amyloid 4 immunohistochemistry preparation of neocortex showing amyloid plaques.

to debate since little empirical research has been conducted. Single case studies have shown that patients can relearn "lost" vocabulary and regain some knowledge of object usage, but the benefit is short lived and appears not to generalize beyond the specific training situation (Graham *et al.*, 1999a; Bozeat *et al.*, 2004). Clearly much more work is required on ways to help these patients.

References

Basso A, Capitani E, Laiacona M (1988). Progressive language impairment without dementia: a case with isolated category specific semantic defect. *Journal of Neurology, Neurosurgery and Psychiatry* **52**: 1201–1207.

Bozeat S, Lambon Ralph MA, Patterson K, Hodges JR (2002a). The influence of personal familiarity and context on object use in semantic dementia. *Neurocase* **8**:127–134.

Bozeat S, Lambon Ralph MA, Patterson K, Hodges JR (2002b). When objects lose their meaning: what happens to their use? *Cognitive, Affective and Behavioural Neuroscience* **2**:236–251.

Bozeat S, Lambon Ralph MA, Graham KS *et al.* (2003). A duck with four legs: investigating the structure of conceptual knowledge using picture drawing in semantic dementia. *Cognitive Neuropsychology* **20**:27–47.

Bozeat S, Patterson K, Hodges JR (2004). Re-learning object use in semantic dementia. *Neuropsychological Rehabilitation* **14**:351–363.

Buxbaum LJ, Schwartz MF, Carew TG (1997). The role of semantic memory in object use. *Cognitive Neuropsychology* **14**:219–254.

Cairns NJ, Grossman M, Arnold SE *et al.* (2004). Clinical and neuropathologic variation in neuronal intermediate filament inclusion disease. *Neurology* **63**:1376–1384.

Chan D, Fox NC, Scahill RI *et al.* (2001). Patterns of temporal lobe atrophy in semantic dementia and Alzheimer's disease. *Annals of Neurology* **49**:433–442.

Davies R, Graham KS, Xuereb JH, Williams GB, Hodges JR (2004). The human perirhinal cortex and semantic memory. *European Journal of Neuroscience* **20**: 2441–2446.

Davies R, Hodges JR, Kril J *et al.* (2005). The pathological basis of semantic dementia. *Brain* **128**:1985–1995.

Edwards Lee T, Miller B, Benson F *et al.* (1997). The temporal variant of frontotemporal dementia. *Brain* **120**:1027–1040.

Evans JJ, Heggs AJ, Antoun N, Hodges JR (1995). Progressive prosopagnosia associated with selective right temporal lobe atrophy: a new syndrome? *Brain* **118**:1–13.

Gainotti G, Barbier A, Marra C (2003). Slowly progressive defect in recognition of familiar people in a patient with right anterior temporal atrophy. *Brain* **126**: 792–803.

Galton CJ, Patterson K, Graham KS *et al.* (2001). Differing patterns of temporal atrophy in Alzheimer's disease and semantic dementia. *Neurology* **57**:216–225.

Garrard P, Hodges JR (2000). Semantic dementia: clinical, radiological and pathological perspectives. *Journal of Neurology* **247**:409–422.

Goldenberg G, Hagmann S (1998). Tool use and mechanical problem solving in patients with apraxia. *Neuropsychologia* **36**:581–589.

Gorno-Tempini ML, Dronkers NF, Rankin KP (2004). Cognition and anatomy in three variants of primary progressive aphasia. *Annals of Neurology* **55**:335–346.

Graham KS, Hodges JR (1997). Differentiating the roles of the hippocampal complex and the neocortex in long-term memory storage: evidence from the study of semantic dementia and Alzheimer's disease. *Neuropsychology* **11**:77–89.

Graham KS, Hodges JR (1999). Episodic memory in semantic dementia: implications for the roles played by the perirhinal and hippocampal memory systems in new learning. *Behavioural and Brain Sciences* **22**: 452–453.

Graham KS, Patterson K, Hodges JR (1995). Progressive pure anomia: insufficient activation of phonology by meaning. *Neurocase* **1**:25–38.

Graham KS, Patterson K, Pratt KH, Hodges JR (1999a). Relearning and subsequent forgetting of semantic category exemplars in a case of semantic dementia. *Neuropsychology* **13**:359–380.

Graham KS, Patterson K, Hodges JR (1999b). Episodic memory: new insights from the study of semantic dementia. *Current Opinion in Neurobiology* **9**: 245–250.

Graham KS, Simons JS, Pratt KH, Patterson K, Hodges JR (2000). Insights from semantic dementia on the relationship between episodic and semantic memory. *Neuropsychologia* **38**:313–324.

Graham KS, Patterson K, Powis J, Drake J, Hodges JR (2002). Multiple inputs to episodic memory in semantic dementia: words tell another story. *Neuropsychology* **16**:380–389.

Greene JDW, Hodges JR, Baddeley AD (1995). Autobiographical memory and executive function in early dementia of Alzheimer type. *Neuropsychologia* **33**:1647–1670.

Grossman M, Ash S (2004). Primary progressive aphasia: a review. *Neurocase* **10**:3–18.

Hodges JR, Graham KS (1998). A reversal of the temporal gradient for famous person knowledge in semantic dementia: implications for the neural organisation of long-term memory. *Neuropsychologia* **36**:803–825.

Hodges JR, Graham KS (2001). Episodic memory: insights from semantic dementia. *Philosophical Transactions of the Royal Society of London Series B: Biological Sciences* **356**:1423–1434.

Hodges JR, Miller BL (2001a). The neuropsychology of frontal variant FTD and semantic dementia. Introduction to the special topic papers: Part II. *Neurocase* 7:113–121.

Hodges JR, Miller BL (2001b). The classification, genetics and neuropathology of frontotemporal dementia (FTD). Introduction to the special topic papers: Part I. *Neurocase* 7:31–35.

Hodges JR, Patterson K (1995). Is semantic memory consistently impaired early in the course of Alzheimer's disease? Neuroanatomical and diagnostic implications. *Neuropsychologia* **33**:441–459.

Hodges JR, Patterson K (1996). Non-fluent progressive aphasia and semantic dementia: a comparative neuropsychological study. *Journal of the International Neuropsychological Society* 2:511–524.

Hodges JR, Patterson K, Oxbury S, Funnell E (1992). Semantic dementia: progressive fluent aphasia with temporal lobe atrophy. *Brain* **115**:1783–1806.

Hodges JR, Patterson K, Graham N, Dawson K (1996). Naming and knowing in dementia of Alzheimer's type. *Brain and Language* **54**:302–325.

Hodges JR, Patterson K, Ward R *et al.* (1999a). The differentiation of semantic dementia and frontal lobe dementia (temporal and frontal variants of frontotemporal dementia) from early Alzheimer's disease: a comparative neuropsychological study. *Neuropsychology* **13**:31–40.

Hodges JR, Spatt J, Patterson K (1999b). What and how: evidence for the dissociation of object knowledge and mechanical problem solving skills in the human brain. *Proceedings of the National Academy of Sciences USA* **96**:9444–9448.

Hodges JR, Bozeat S, Lambon Ralph MA, Patterson K, Spatt J (2000). The role of conceptual knowledge in object use: evidence from semantic dementia. *Brain* **123**: 1913–1925.

Hodges JR, Davies R, Xuereb J, Kril J, Halliday G (2003). Survival in frontotemporal dementia. *Neurology* **61**:349–354.

Hodges JR, Davies R, Xuereb J *et al.* (2004). Clinicopathological correlates in frontotemporal dementia. *Annals of Neurology* **56**:399–406.

Howard D, Patterson K (1992). *Pyramids and Palm Trees: A Test of Semantic Access From Pictures and Words.* Bury St Edmunds, UK: Thames Valley Test Company.

Ikeda M, Patterson K, Graham KS, Lambon Ralph MA, Hodges JR (2006). "A horse of a different colour": do patients with semantic dementia recognise different versions of the same object as the same? *Neuropsychologia* **44**:566–575.

Insausti R, Juottonen K, Soininen H *et al.* (1998). MR volumetric analysis of the human entorhinal, perirhinal, and temporopolar cortices. *American Journal of Neuroradiology* **19**:659–671.

Kitchener E, Hodges JR (1999). Impaired knowledge of famous people and events and intact autobiographical knowledge in a case of progressive right temporal lobe degeneration: implications for the organization of remote memory. *Cognitive Neuropsychology* **16**:589–607.

Knopman DS, Boeve BF, Parisi JE *et al.* (2005). Antemortem diagnosis of frontotemporal lobar degeneration. *Annals of Neurology* **57**:480–488.

Lambon Ralph MA, Howard D (2000). Gogi aphasia or semantic dementia? Simulating and assessing poor verbal comprehension in a case of progressive fluent aphasia. *Cognitive Neuropsychology* **17**:437–465.

Lambon Ralph M, Graham KS, Patterson K, Hodges JR (1999). Is a picture worth a thousand words? Evidence from concept definitions by patients with semantic dementia. *Brain and Language* **70**:309–335.

Lambon Ralph MA, Sage K, Roberts J (2000). Classical anomia: a neuropsychological perspective on speech production. *Neuropsychologia* **38**:186–202.

Lambon Ralph MA, McClelland JL, Patterson K, Galton CJ, Hodges JR (2001). No right to speak? The relationship between object naming and semantic impairment: neuropsychological evidence and a computational model. *Journal of Cognitive Neuroscience* **13**:341–356.

Lauro-Grotto R, Piccini C, Shallice T (1997). Modality-specific operations in semantic dementia. *Cortex* **33**:593–622.

McClelland JL, McNaughton BL, O'Reilly RC (1995). Why there are complementary learning systems in the hippocampus and neocortex: insights from the successes and failures of connectionist models of learning and memory. *Psychological Review* **102**:419–457.

McKhann GM, Albert MS, Grossman M *et al.* (2001). Clinical and pathological diagnosis of frontotemporal dementia: report of the Working Group on Frontotemporal Dementia and Pick's Disease. *Archives of Neurology* **58**:1803–1809.

Mehler MF, Dickson D, Davies P, Horoupian DS (1986). Primary dysphasic dementia: clinical, pathological, and biochemical studies. *Annals of Neurology* **20**:126.

Mesulam M-M (1982). Slowly progressive aphasia without generalised dementia. *Annals of Neurology* **11**:592–598.

Mesulam M-M (2001). Primary progressive aphasia. *Annals of Neurology* **49**:425–432.

Mingazzini G (1913). On aphasia due to atrophy of the cerebral convolutions. *Brain* **36**:493–524.

Mott RT, Dickson DW, Trojanowski JQ *et al.* (2005). Neuropathologic, biochemical, and molecular characterization of the frontotemporal dementias. *Journal of Neuropathology and Experimental Neurology* 64:420–428.

Mummery CJ, Patterson K, Wise RJS *et al.* (1999). Disrupted temporal lobe connections in semantic dementia. *Brain* 122:61–73.

Neary D (1994). Neuropsychological correlates of frontotemporal cerebral atrophy. *Japanese Journal of Neuropsychology* 10:11–17.

Neary D, Snowden JS, Gustafson L *et al.* (1998). Frontotemporal lobar degeneration: a consensus on clinical diagnostic criteria. *Neurology* 51:1546–1554.

Nestor PJ, Graham KS, Bozeat S, Simons JS, Hodges JR (2002). Memory consolidation and the hippocampus: further evidence from the study of autobiographical memory in semantic dementia and the frontal variant of frontotemporal dementia. *Neuropsychologia* 40:633–654.

Patterson J, MacDonald MC (2006). Sweet nothings: narrative speech in semantic dementia. In Andrews S (ed.) *From Inkmarks to Ideas: Challenges and Controversies about Word Recognition and Reading.* Hove, UK: Psychology Press, pp. 299–317.

Patterson K, Lambon Ralph MA, Jefferies E *et al.* (2006). "Pre-semantic" cognition in semantic dementia: six deficits in search of an explanation. *Journal of Cognitive Neuroscience* 18:169–183.

Patterson K, Graham NL, Lambon-Ralph MA, Hodges JR (2008). Varieties of silence: the impact of neurodegenerative diseases on language systems in the brain. In Pomerantz JR (ed.) *Topics in Integrated Neuroscience: From Cells to Cognition.* Cambridge, UK: Cambridge University Press, pp. 181–205.

Perry RJ, Rosen HR, Kramer JH *et al.* (2001). Hemispheric dominance for emotions, empathy and social behaviour: evidence from right and left-handers with frontotemporal dementia. *Neurocase* 7:145–160.

Pick A (1892). Uber die Beziehungen der senilen Hirnatrophie zur Aphasie. *Prager Medische Wochenschrift* 17:165–167.

Pick A (1904). Zur symptomatologie der linksseitigen Schlafenlappenatrophie. *Monatschrift für Psychiatrie und Neurologie* 16:378–388.

Piolino P, Desgranges B, Belliard S *et al.* (2003). Autobiographical memory and autonoetic consciousness: triple dissociation in neurodegenerative diseases. *Brain* 126:2203–2219.

Poeck K, Luzzatti C (1988). Slowly progressive aphasia in three patients: the problem of accompanying neuropsychological deficit. *Brain* 111:151–168.

Ratnavalli E, Brayne C, Dawson K, Hodges JR (2002). The prevalence of frontotemporal dementia. *Neurology* 58:1615–1621.

Rogers TT, Lambon Ralph MA, Hodges JR, Patterson K (2003). Object recognition under semantic impairment: the effects of conceptual regularities on perceptual decisons. *Language and Cognitive Processes* 18:625–662.

Rogers TT, Lambon Ralph MA, Garrard P *et al.* (2004a). The structure and deterioration of semantic memory: a neuropsychological and computational investigation. *Psychological Review* 111:205–235.

Rogers TT, Lambon Ralph MA, Hodges JR, Patterson K (2004b). Natural selection: the impact of semantic impairment on lexical and object decision. *Cognitive Neuropsychology* 21:331–352.

Rogers TT, Ivanoiu A, Patterson K, Hodges JR (2006). Semantic memory in Alzheimer's disease and the fronto-temporal dementias: a longitudinal study of 236 patients. *Neuropsychology* 20:319–335.

Rosen HJ, Gorno-Tempini ML, Goldman WP *et al.* (2002). Patterns of brain atrophy in frontotemporal dementia and semantic dementia. *Neurology* 58:198–208.

Rosenfeld M (1909). Die partielle Gorsshirnatrophie. *Journal für Psychologie und Neurologie* 14:115–130.

Rothi LJG, Ochipa C, Heilman KM (1991). A cognitive neuropsychological model of limb praxis. *Cognitive Neuropsychology* 8:443–458.

Schneider C (1927). Uber Picksche Krankheit. *Monatschrift für Psychologie und Neurologie* 65:230–275.

Seeley WW, Bauer AM, Miller BL *et al.* (2005). The natural history of temporal variant frontotemporal dementia. *Neurology* 64:1384–1390.

Simons JS, Graham KS, Galton CJ, Patterson K, Hodges JR (2001). Semantic knowledge and episodic memory for faces in semantic dementia. *Neuropsychology* 15:101–114.

Simons J, Graham K, Hodges JR (2002). Perceptual and semantic contributions to episodic memory: evidence from semantic dementia and Alzheimer's disease. *Journal of Memory and Language* 47:197–213.

Snowden JS, Goulding PJ, Neary D (1989). Semantic dementia: a form of circumscribed cerebral atrophy. *Behavioural Neurology* 2:167–182.

Snowden JS, Griffiths HL, Neary D (1994). Semantic dementia: autobiographical contribution to preservation of meaning. *Cognitive Neuropsychology* 11:265–288.

Snowden JS, Griffiths HL, Neary D (1995). Autobiographical experience and word meaning. *Memory* 3:225–246.

Stertz G (1926). Uber die Picksche atrophie. *Aeitschrift für die Gesamte Neurologie und Psychiatrie* 101: 729–747.

277

Thompson SA, Graham KS, Patterson K, Sahakian BJ, Hodges JR (2002). Is knowledge of famous people disproportionately impaired in patients with early Alzheimer's disease? *Neuropsychology* 16:344–358.

Thompson SA, Patterson K, Hodges JR (2003). Left/right asymmetry of atrophy in semantic dementia: behavioural cognitive implications. *Neurology* 61:1196–1203.

Tulving E (1995). Organization of memory: quo vadis. In Gazzaniga MS (ed.) *The Cognitive Neurosciences* Cambridge, MA: MIT Press, pp. 839–847.

Warrington EK (1975). Selective impairment of semantic memory. *Quarterly Journal of Experimental Psychology* 27:635–657.

Westmacott R, Black SE, Freedman M, Moscovitch M (2004). The contribution of autobiographical significance to semantic memory: evidence from Alzheimer's disease, semantic dementia, and amnesia. *Neuropsychologia* 42:25–48.

Williams GB, Nestor PJ, Hodges JR (2005). The neural correlates of semantic and behavioural deficits in frontotemporal dementia. *NeuroImage* 24:1042–1051.

Chapter 19

Progressive non-fluent aphasia

Jennifer Ogar and Maria Luisa Gorno-Tempini

Introduction

Aphasia has long been recognized as a common language disorder typically resulting from acute left hemisphere lesions, often caused by strokes. A progressive form of aphasia was first described over a century ago by Arnold Pick, the famed Prague neurologist, who detailed the language deficits in his initial group of patients (Pick 1892). The modern term, *progressive aphasia*, was introduced by Marsel Mesulam in 1982 in a landmark paper in which he described six patients who presented with language deficits in the absence of other behavioral abnormalities. This progressive disorder was clinically distinct from other dementing processes, such as Alzheimer's disease (AD), because language complaints, rather than memory problems, were the most salient symptoms. Speech or language deficits remained the only impairment for the first 2 years in these patients, but as the disease progressed more generalized states of dementia became apparent.

Since then, numerous cases of what is now termed primary progressive aphasia (PPA) have been described, in which patients present with both fluent and non-fluent variants of the disorder (Deleceuse *et al.*, 1990; Weintraub *et al.*, 1990; Snowden *et al.*, 1992, 1996; Mesulam 2001; Gorno-Tempini *et al.*, 2004a). The non-fluent variant, known as progressive non-fluent aphasia (PNFA), is important clinically because speech problems are often the first symptoms of neurodegenerative diseases, such as frontotemporal lobar dementia (FTLD) and corticobasal degeneration (CBD) (Tyrrell *et al.*, 1991; Broussolle *et al.*, 1996; Chapman *et al.*, 1997; Gorno-Tempini *et al.*, 2004b).

Currently, PNFA is a clinical diagnosis used to describe patients who initially show isolated speech or language problems that result in non-fluent language

output (Neary *et al.*, 1998). Speech is generally slow, halting and effortful and patients arrive at clinics typically complaining of articulation or word-finding problems (Grossman *et al.*, 1996; Hodges and Patterson 1996; Neary *et al.*, 1998). Memory, visuospatial skills and judgement, which can be impaired in other dementias such as AD, are spared in patients with PNFA, at least initially. Among the PPA variants, PNFA (or "PPA with agrammatism") is the most common (Mesulam and Weintraub 1992; Mesulam *et al.*, 2003).

In the years since Mesulam's initial paper (1982), there has been much confusion surrounding the classification of PPA, often because the name serves only as a clinical diagnosis and does not specify an underlying etiology. The causes of PPA vary. Some have argued that the disorder should be considered a variant of AD, CBD or FTLD, because patients with PPA have been found at autopsy to have all these neuropathologies. Recent reports have suggested that CBD is the most common clinical evolution and pathological diagnosis associated with PNFA (Gorno-Tempini *et al.*, 2004b; Kertesz 2005). However, other neuropathologies are not uncommon and include dementia lacking distinctive histopathology (DLDH) (Turner *et al.*, 1996) and Pick's disease, characterized by tau-positive neuronal inclusions (Mesulam and Weintraub 1992; Galton *et al.*, 2000). Patients with PNFA have also shown unusual distributions of the senile plaques and neurofibrillary tangles seen in AD (Galton *et al.*, 2000).

This chapter will provide a basic definition of PNFA and diagnostic criteria for the disorder, as well as classic clinical presentations. Basic demographic information, neuroimaging correlates and pathological diagnosis associated with PNFA will also be reviewed, along with current treatment options. Variants of PPA will be described, and finally, a case study will illustrate the manifestations of PNFA in a patient who evolved to have corticobasal degeneration syndrome (CBDS).

The Behavioral Neurology of Dementia, eds. Bruce L. Miller and Bradley F. Boeve. Published by Cambridge University Press.
© Cambridge University Press 2009.

Progressive non-fluent aphasia
Basic definition and diagnostic criteria

Progressive non-fluent aphasia is characterized by slow spontaneous speech, agrammatism in production and/or comprehension, anomia and phonemic paraphasias, in the presence of relatively spared word comprehension (Hodges and Patterson 1996; Grossman et al., 1996; Neary et al., 1998; Gorno-Tempini et al., 2004a). Patients may present with a Broca's-like aphasia, using simplified sentences of decreased phrase length. Speech is slow and apraxia of speech and/or stuttering are common complaints. Patients often describe word-finding deficits, although it is difficult to determine if this symptom is the result of a semantic/lexical impairment or an underlying speech production problem. Sentence comprehension may be impaired for the most difficult syntactic constructions, such as negative passives (e.g. "The girl was not hit by the boy"). As the disease progresses, patients can begin to show signs of a frontal executive disorder: poor thought organization, severe frustration, depression and mild disinhibition may accompany predominant speech and language symptoms (Neary et al., 1998).

Researchers have noted that PPA symptoms are often misattributed to stress, anxiety or depression (Mesulam 1982). In an effort to improve the recognition of variants of FTLD, of which PNFA is one presentation, widely-used diagnostic criteria for PNFA were agreed upon by Neary and colleagues in 1998 (Table 19.1). Other clinical forms of FTLD include: frontotemporal dementia (FTD), which is characterized by progressive behavioral changes, and semantic dementia (SD), which is associated with loss of word, face or object meaning, with preserved fluency and syntactic abilities (Table 19.1).

To clarify the meaning of the core diagnostic features associated with PNFA, Neary and colleagues (1998) included explicit descriptions of commonly used characteristics. "Non-fluent speech," as defined by the criteria, refers to hesitant, effortful production with reduced speaking rate. "Agrammatism" refers to the omission or inappropriate use of grammatical words such as articles, prepositions and auxiliary verbs. Patients with PNFA may retain some simplified syntax, so that the term "mild grammatism" may be more descriptive than the more complete agrammatism, which characterizes patients with Broca's aphasia caused by stroke. In one study, only 6.4% of 47 patients with PNFA presented with agrammatism (Clark et al.,

Table 19.1. Clinical diagnostic features of progressive non-fluent aphasia

Features	
Core diagnostic features	A. Insidious onset and gradual progression
	B. Non-fluent spontaneous speech with at least one of the following: agrammatism, phonemic paraphasias, anomia
Supportive diagnostic features	A. Speech and language
	1. Stuttering or oral apraxia
	2. Impaired repetition
	3. Alexia, agraphia
	4. Early preservation of word meaning
	5. Late mutism
	B. Behavior
	1. Early preservation of social skills
	2. Late behavioral changes similar to frontotemporal dementia
	C. Physical signs: late contralateral primitive reflexes, akinesia, rigidity and tremor
	D. Investigations
	1. Neuropsychology: non-fluent aphasia in the absence of severe amnesia or perceptuospatial disorder
	2. Electroencephalography: normal or minor asymmetric slowing
	3. Brain imaging (structural and/or functional): asymmetric abnormality predominantly affecting the dominant (usually left) hemisphere

2005). These authors raise the possibility that non-fluency in progressive aphasia may arise from articulation deficits, as opposed to the true linguistic agrammatism that characterizes non-fluent Broca's aphasia (Clark et al., 2005).

Agrammatism is often apparent in conversation or in structured tasks such as a picture description. For example, when asked to describe the picnic scene from the Western Aphasia Battery (WAB) (Kertesz 1980), one patient with PNFA, gave the following narrative:

Um ... a boy flying kite ... a dog is (unintelligible) by him. The sailboat is in the water. The jetski is um ... in the water ... The bucket and pail ... um ... sand, the sand. The flag is on the pole, um, the uh, the couples on the blanket ... The tree, beyond the tree, below the tree, the radio is going ...

Phonemic paraphasias, also typically heard in the speech of PNFA patients, are errors in which the incorrect sound is used within a word (e.g. "tittle" for "little," or "label" for "table"). Anomia refers to the naming deficit. Patients with anomia have difficulty finding the correct word, which results in long pauses during spontaneous speech or the selection of a wrong word (Neary *et al.*, 1998). The most typical clinical presentation of PPA often begins with anomia, which then progresses to a non-fluency (Kertesz *et al.* 2003). In fact, Mesulam's initial patients presented with anomic aphasia (Mesulam 1982). Often it can be difficult to discern whether speech errors are caused by motor speech problems, such as speech apraxia or dysarthria, or whether they result from anomic hesitations and pauses. The following WAB picnic scene description from another patient with PNFA illustrates anomic production, with phonemic paraphasias in a structured speech task:

> The b,boy fly, flying a kite. The t ... dog and maybe the kite might come back down here and maybe the dog to try and catch it and these people on the /se/, sailboat ... Then I don't know what there, there ... There's a /banket/ in /spe/ and a bucket ... a ... a ... shes p ... p ... pouring coke for a ... a ... um ... like the ...

Patients with PNFA may present with alexia (impaired reading) and/or agraphia (impaired writing) (Neary *et al.*, 1998). Neuropsychological testing can be difficult to interpret, particularly the Mini-Mental Status Examination (MMSE), since such tests have verbal instructions or require verbal responses (Mesulam *et al.*, 2003). Also, traditional aphasia batteries such as the WAB, or the Boston Diagnostic Aphasia Evaluation (BDAE), originally created for vascular aphasic patients, often fail to distinguish between variants of PPA.

Neuroimaging and the neurological evaluation

Neuroimaging, using magnetic resonance imaging (MRI), single-photon emission computed tomography (SPECT) or positron emission tomography (PET), is typically part of the diagnostic work-up for possible PNFA, with MRI being particularly sensitive to temporal neocortical atrophy and SPECT helping to reveal functional, blood flow changes prior to atrophy. At times, results from these studies are normal, or they may identify lateralized, bilateral or diffuse damage (Westbury and Bub 1997). Neuroimaging

helps to exclude other potential causes of neurologic change, such as tumor, stroke or arteriovenous malformations.

Typically, specific regions within the speech and language network are damaged in PNFA. Left frontal hypometabolism has been documented in PNFA by a number of investigators using PET (Tyrrell *et al.*, 1990, 1991; Grossman *et al.*, 1998; Nestor *et al.*, 2003). Studies using voxel-based morphometry (VBM) have found atrophy in the left inferior and middle frontal gyri, motor and premotor cortex and anterior insula regions (Nestor *et al.*, 2003; Gorno-Tempini *et al.*, 2004c). These regions are thought to underlie motor speech and syntactic processing. Apraxia of speech, a common symptom of PNFA, has been associated with damage to the left precentral gyrus of the insula in stroke patients (Dronkers 1996). Left insular neuronal loss was also reported in a patient with PNFA and AD pathology (Harasty *et al.*, 2001).

Though studies support left greater than right hemisphere damage in PNFA, it is important to note that bilateral damage is common (Westbury and Bub 1997). For example, in a review of the literature, Westbury and Bub (1997) found that functional imaging showed changes that were restricted to the left hemisphere in only 69% of patients with PPA, meaning that 31% had bilateral damage. Such a finding suggests that the diseases causing PNFA are not restricted to the left hemisphere.

The neurological evaluation often reveals mild motor symptoms in PNFA, usually localized to the right hand or the right side of the body (Kertesz *et al.*, 2003; Kertesz and Munoz 2004). Patients with PNFA may show diffuse motor slowing, reduced dexterity and mild rigidity. Limb apraxia is a relatively frequent finding and is one of the two non-language symptoms (along with acalculia) that can be present early in the disease (Neary *et al.*, 1998). Impaired gestural imitation (apraxia) is consistent with disruption to a left parietofrontal network (Joshi *et al.*, 2003). A number of studies have described a progression that involves extrapyramidal symptoms with dystonia and alien limb phenomenon, providing further evidence that PNFA and CBDS can present in the same patient at different stages of the same disease (Gorno-Tempini *et al.*, 2004c; Kertesz *et al.*, 2003; Kertesz 2005; Knibb *et al.*, 2006). Buccofacial apraxia and dysarthria can also co-occur in patients with PNFA (Tyrrell *et al.*, 1990; Caselli and Jack 1992; Grossman *et al.*, 1996).

281

Table 19.2. Demographic information for PNFA progressive non-fluent aphasia

Feature	Data	Source
Age of onset (years)	63	Johnson et al. (2005)
	62	Westbury and Bub (1997)
	65	Duffy and Peterson (1992)
Gender ratio (M:F)	1:2	Westbury and Bub (1997); Duffy and Peterson (1992)
	4:9	Clark et al. (2005)
Duration of isolated speech and/or language symptoms (years)	4.3	Rogers and Alarcon (1999)
Percentage evolving to have cognitive deficits	37	Rogers and Alarcon (1999)
Average time from symptom onset to death (years)	6.8	Rogers and Alarcon (1999)

Pathology

Autopsy studies have found numerous neuropathological changes associated with PNFA, with tauopathies being the most common (Kertesz et al., 2003; Kertesz 2005; Josephs et al., 2006; Knibb et al., 2006). Diseases associated with tauopathies include: CBD, classic Pick's disease, progressive supranuclear palsy (PSP), familial tauopathies linked to chromosome 17 and argyrophilic grain disease. In CBD, patients initially presented with anomia or speech problems that progressed to mutism and an extrapyramidal syndrome, characterized by alien limb phenomenon and dystonia (Kertesz and Munoz 2003; Gorno-Tempini et al., 2004b; Knibb et al., 2006). In PSP, symptoms are initially consistent with PNFA, but as the disease progresses, postural instability, behavioral abnormalities and dysphagia also emerge (Caselli et al., 1993; Bak et al., 2001; Mochizuki et al., 2003).

Alzheimer's disease is another common pathology associated with PNFA (Green et al., 1990; Kempler et al., 1990; Karbe et al., 1993; Galton et al., 2000; Li et al., 2000; Godbolt et al., 2004; Kertesz et al., 2005; Josephs et al., 2006; Knibb et al., 2006). There is some controversy surrounding the relationship between AD and PNFA, with some researchers emphasizing the distinct clinical profile typically seen in each (e.g. speech impairments in PNFA versus memory deficits in AD [Mesulam 2001]). Despite a distinct clinical presentation, a growing number of reports suggest that as much as 30% of PNFA is caused by AD pathology (Knibb et al., 2006). The distribution of neuritic plaques and neurofibrillary tangles is atypical in many of these patients, with the frontal and temporal lobes being most affected (as opposed to the parietal lobes in more typical AD) (Galton et al., 2000; Mesulam et al., 2003; Knibb et al., 2006). Mesulam et al. (2003) noted that the true role of AD in progressive aphasia

may be overestimated because patients may come to autopsy decades after the onset of their disease, when plaques and tangles are more typical in an elderly age group.

Progressive non-fluent aphasia has also been linked to non-specific cellular changes, DLDH (Snowden et al. 1992; Turner et al., 1996), where no tau- synuclein- or ubiquitin-containing inclusions are seen. Some estimates have suggested that roughly 60% of PPA is caused by DLDH, which is distinguished by neuronal loss, gliosis and mild spongiform changes in the superficial cortical layers (Mesulam et al., 2003). Autopsy studies have also confirmed Creutzfeldt–Jakob disease (Mandell et al., 1989; Neary et al., 1998), Lewy body disease (Caselli et al., 2002) and FTD with motor neuron disease (FTD-MND) (Caselli et al., 1993) as other neuropathologies associated with PNFA.

Demographics

Demographic information suggests that those with PNFA are more likely to be female and that, on average, they may present with isolated speech or language symptoms for over 4 years before other non-linguistic cognitive domains become affected (Table 19.2). In some cases, language symptoms may remain isolated for up to 14 years (Mesulam et al., 2003). In this way, PNFA progresses more slowly than other variants of PPA (Rogers and Alarcon 1999). The disproportionate amount of PNFA among women has been reported in a number of studies (Hodges et al., 2003; Clark et al., 2005; Johnson et al., 2005). Some have speculated that the predominace of PNFA in women and FTD in men may reflect different cortical vulnerabilities between the sexes; in particular, the left frontal lobes may be more vulnerable in women, while the right frontal lobe may be more prone to neurodegeneration in men (Johnson et al., 2005).

Patients with PNFA may have a later age of onset than patients with other FTLD diagnoses (Johnson et al., 2005; Kertesz et al., 2005). In one study that detailed the demographic characteristics of over 350 patients with FTLD, the authors found that those with PNFA had a later age of onset than those with SD and FTD, with PNFA having a mean age of onset of 63 years, compared with 57.5 years in FTD and 59.3 years in SD. Other studies have found an equal sex distribution among the variants of FTD (Chow et al., 1999; Hodges et al., 2003; Rosso et al., 2003; Kertesz et al., 2005).

Kertesz and collegues (2005) found no significant differences in gender distribution, disease duration or education between patients with different FTLD variants. Some reports have suggested that FTLD may progress rapidly compared with other degenerative diseases, such as Parkinson's disease. For example, one study found that 19% of patients with FTLD died in less than 5 years after the onset of their initial symptoms, suggesting a relatively rapid course for the disease (Johnson et al., 2005) (Table 19.2).

Other variants of primary progressive aphasia

At least two other clinical variants of progressive aphasia have been described in addition to PNFA: SD and logopenic progressive aphasia (LPA). All three variants are associated with distinct behavioral, anatomical and genetic differences (Gorno-Tempini et al., 2004a).

Semantic dementia

Patients with SD often present with the most distinct cognitive profile (Gorno-Tempini et al., 2004a). Whereas articulation is most notably affected in PNFA, spontaneous speech is fluent in SD, with no signs of motor speech impairments (Hodges et al., 1992; Snowden et al., 1992). Anomia is particularly severe in SD owing to a prominent semantic memory impairment, and patients slowly lose the meaning of common words and objects (Hodges et al., 1992). For example, one patient with SD who remained an avid golfer heard the word "golf," looked puzzled and said, " 'golf,'? I know I should know that word, but I don't.' " Interestingly, though comprehension is impaired for single words, patients with SD typically do well on tests of complex syntax comprehension, at least initially (Gorno-Tempini et al., 2004a).

Semantic paraphasias (i.e. substituting a related word for the target word, such as "table" for "chair") are common in SD, and as the disease progresses speech output becomes empty, devoid of nouns and with an over-reliance on fillers such as "thing" and "that" (Gorno-Tempini et al., 2004a). For example, one patient with moderately severe SD produced the following when asked to describe the WAB picnic scene.

> Well I remember seeing this … because there are people right here and there are people going here. To me, I thought this was pretty interesting … You see these students coming here … and these guys were going down here and he's going high up on that one …

As the disease progresses, patients with SD are also prone to behavioral changes such as depression, overeating, loss of insight and emotional blunting (Rosen et al., 2002; Thompson et al., 2003). Anatomically, SD is associated with left anterior temporal lobe damage (Gorno-Tempini et al., 2004a), an area thought to underlie semantic memory (Rosen et al., 2002). In SD, unlike the other variants, MND is the most common pathology (Knibb et al., 2006). When motor deficits are present, the term FTD-MND is used, while frontotemporal lobar degeneration with ubiquitin inclusions (FTLD-U) or MND inclusion dementia (MNDID) are appropriate when motor symptoms are absent (Rossor et al., 2000; Hodges et al., 2004; Davies et al., 2005).

Logoponic progressive aphasia

The third variant of progressive aphasia, LPA, is characterized by slow speech, impaired comprehension of complex syntax and word-finding deficits (Gorno-Tempini et al., 2004a). The term logopenic refers to the halting, anomic quality of spontaneous speech, which is marked by hesitations and pauses and with sentences with simplified but accurate syntactic structure (Gorno-Tempini et al., 2004a). Comprehension (for all but the most simple morphosyntactic sentences) and repetition is impaired for patients with LPA (Gorno-Tempini et al., 2004a). A pronounced auditory-verbal short-term memory (AVSTM) is thought to underlie these comprehension and repetition deficits (Gorno-Tempini et al., 2004a). As the disease progresses, this core deficit can make conversation difficult to follow for the patient with LPA, as AVSTM is needed to derive meaning from speech. A recent study also noted marked acalculia as another LPA symptom. Anatomically, LPA is characterized by atrophy in the left posterior temporal

283

cortex and inferior parietal lobe, an area associated with AVSTM (Gorno-Tempini *et al.*, 2004a).

Distinguishing variants of primary progressive aphasia

Genetically, PPA variants show differences as well, as measured by the frequency of the ε4 allele of *APOE*, encoding apolipoprotein E. In a recent study comparing the variants, the frequency of this haplotype was 67% in LPA, 0% in SD and 20% in PNFA (Gorno-Tempini *et al.*, 2004a). The high frequency of ε4 haplotype in LPA suggests that many of these patients may have an atypical form of AD (Gorno-Tempini *et al.*, 2004a).

Though variants are differentiated in the literature, the question of how best to conceptualize PPA has yet to be answered. Mesulam and colleagues (2003) have proposed that PPA should reflect a unitary disease process, particularly because so many of its underlying neuropathologies (CBD, PSP, etc.) are related to mutations affecting tau. Others support the classification of PPA into two distinct clinical variants: PNFA and SD (Knibb *et al.*, 2006), while some groups recognize three subgroups: PNFA, SD and LPA (Snowden *et al.*, 1992; Kertesz *et al.*, 2003; Gorno-Tempini *et al.*, 2004a). One of the central issues in PPA classification revolves around the term "fluency." For some practitioners, non-fluency implies agrammatism, while for others it refers to abnormally slow speech. So, for example, in some studies both slow-speaking and agrammatic patients are classified as PNFA (Knibb *et al.*, 2006), while in others, PNFA designates agrammatic patients and LPA is applied to those presenting with slow, anomic speech.

Pure motor speech disorder

Recently, there has been some support for the recognition of a separate disorder, affecting speech more than language. A syndrome called progressive aphemia, progressive isolated motor speech disorder, slowly progressive anarthria or primary progressive apraxia was described in the 1990s, in which patients presented primarily with apraxia of speech and dysarthria (Cohen *et al.*, 1993; Broussolle *et al.*, 1996; Fukui *et al.*, 1996; Chapman *et al.*, 1997; Kertesz *et al.*, 2003). The course of the disease is similar in these cases, with speech disturbance being the most prominent early sign. It remains unclear whether this "pure motor speech" presentation is a separate entity or an early PNFA (Josephs *et al.*, 2006).

Treatment options

Patients with PNFA often report that they benefit from working with a speech-language pathologist to improve communication deficits that arise. Traditional speech therapy, aimed at maintaining skills as the disease progresses, as well as the use of augmentative/alternative communication (AAC) devices (e.g. "talking computers") are two types of treatment that are typically used with PNFA. To date, few treatment studies have examined the efficacy of therapy with patients with progressive aphasia.

In the first study designed to assess the efficacy of a treatment with a patient with PPA and spastic dysarthria, aphasia and oral apraxia, McNeil and colleagues (1995) found improved word-finding skills when that was the focus of the treatment. The most effective treatment, according to the study, combined behavioral therapy with the administration of dextroamphetamine. Other language modalities that were not treated continued to decline. In another study, Schneider and colleagues (1996) used a combination of speech and gesturing to improve oral sentence production.

A series of treatments for a single patient with PNFA with stuttering, dysarthria and word-finding complaints was described in an uncontrolled case study by Murray (1998). The treatments evolved over 2.5 years to meet the patient's changing needs. Initially, therapy focused on traditional drills designed to facilitate auditory and reading comprehension. The second phase of intervention involved teaching the patient a drawing technique to improve communication, while the third focused on the training and use of an AAC device (Murray 1998).

Selective serotonin-reuptake inhibitors (SSRIs) have been prescribed to address behavioral and mood changes that occur in PPA, but to date, no study has assessed the effects of these drugs specifically on speech or language. In a recent double-blind, placebo-controlled study, six patients with PPA showed mild slowing of progression in language symptoms when the dopamine agonist bromocriptine was used over the course of 7 weeks (Reed *et al.*, 2004). Box 19.1 describes the progression of a patient with PNFA.

Summary

The early recognition of PNFA is important in clinical settings, as patients may benefit from behavioral treatments appropriate for this distinct disorder. Also, the speech and language symptoms indicative of

---

Box 19.1 Case report of a patient with progressive non-fluent aphasia

AS, a 53-year-old business executive, presented with halting, slow speech in the presence of intact language comprehension and naming skills. Initially, no cognitive or behavioral changes were noted, and her neurological evaluation was normal. She was pleasant and cooperative upon examination. AS complained that she had trouble "expressing her thoughts," and spoke in simple sentences. Her husband commented that she was "not as conversant" as she had once been, although she was still functioning adequately in her job. These symptoms initially led to a diagnosis of a functional disorder, arising from depression. Unhappy with this assessment, AS sought a second opinion at a neurology clinic, where she was followed over the course of 4 years.

Speech-language neuropsychological tests were performed annually and MRI scans were also obtained yearly over the 4 years. At the time of her first visit, testing was normal, except for mild impairment noted on the verbal agility subtest of the BDAE and slow performance on executive tasks, such as the Trailmaking and Stroop tests. AS had no significant past medical or family history. Over the course of her annual visits, testing revealed apraxia of speech, progressing from mild to severe within 1 year. Dysarthia was also apparent by the fourth year. AS's speech became progressively more non-fluent, and she began to have some difficulty with comprehension of complex syntax. These symptoms led to a diagnosis of PNFA.

Seven years after first noticing speech problems, AS's symptoms had worsened to the point that she was no longer able to work and she retired. Compulsive behaviors eventually surfaced, after 6 years of isolated speech complaints. Neurological examination revealed mild slowing of fine finger movements on the right hand, progressing to right-sided limb apraxia severe enough to impair cooking and dressing. AS began to show poor judgement, as evidenced by aggressive driving and inappropriate behavior at restaurants (sweeping up other patrons' dishes). Other cognitive skills, though initially intact, declined gradually as well. Initially she scored 29/30 on the MMSE, but by her fourth annual evaluation she scored 16/30. Scores on executive tasks also progressively fell, as did scores on verbal memory subtests from the California Verbal Memory Test-Mental Status (CVLT-MS).

Annual MRI scans were analyzed using VBM. On her first scan, though no area showed decreased gray matter volume compared with controls at a corrected level of significance, the left inferior frontal gyrus, insula, frontal and temporal poles and medial frontal lobes showed significant volume loss. Over the next 3 years, more extensive atrophy in these areas was seen, with additional volume loss noted in left inferior premotor regions, the thalamus, the posterior inferior temporal gyrus and the superior parietal lobule. AS's last scan showed extension into left prefrontal areas and medial frontal regions, including the supplementary motor area.

Comment

AS's case is particularly interesting from a longitudinal perspective, as her symptoms evolved from those consistent with a PNFA diagnosis to one of a classic CBDS. For the first 3 years of her evaluations at a neurology clinic, AS presented with an isolated, progressive speech and language disorder consistent with a diagnosis of PNFA. At her fourth evaluation, 10 years after her first symptoms, AS showed a severe, right-sided extrapyramidal syndrome (limb apraxia, dystonia, alien limb phenomenon), which led to a diagnosis of CBDS. For a more detailed description of this case please see Gorno-Tempini *et al.* (2004c).

PNFA may be early signs of left hemisphere neurodegenerative diseases, particularly CBDS. Thorough speech and language testing, as well as neuroimaging, can help to diagnose PNFA and to distinguish the disorder from other PPA variants, namely SD and LPA.

References

Bak T H, Antoun N, Balan K, Hodges J R (2001). Memory lost, memory regained: neuropsychological findings and neuroimaging in two cases of paraneoplastic limbic encephalitis with radically different outcomes. *J Neurol Neurosurg Psychiatry* 71:40–7.

Broussolle E, Bakchine S, Tommasi M *et al.* (1996). Slowly progressive anarthria with late anterior opercular syndrome: a variant form of frontal cortical atrophy syndromes. *J Neurol Sci* 144(1–2):44–58.

Caselli R J, Jack C R, Jr (1992). Asymmetric cortical degeneration syndromes. A proposed clinical classification. *Arch Neurol* 49(7):770–80.

Caselli R J, Windebank A J, Petersen R C *et al.* (1993). Rapidly progressive aphasic dementia and motor neuron disease. *Ann Neurol* 33(2):200–7.

Caselli R J, Beach T G, Sue L I, Conner D J, Sabbagh M N (2002). Progressive aphasia with Lewy bodies. *Dement Geriatr Cogn Disord* 14(2):55–8.

Chapman S B, Rosenberg R N, Weiner M F, Shobe A (1997). Autosomal dominant progressive syndrome of motor-speech loss without dementia. *Neurology* 49(5):1298–306.

285

Chow T W, Miller B L, Hayashi V N, Geschwind D H (1999). Inheritance of frontotemporal dementia. *Arch Neurol* **56**(7):817–22.

Clark D G, Charuvastra A, Miller B L, Shapira J S, Mendez M F (2005). Fluent versus nonfluent primary progressive aphasia: a comparison of clinical and functional neuroimaging features. *Brain Lang* **94**(1):54–60.

Cohen L, Benoit N, Van Eeckhout P, Ducarne B, Brunet P (1993). Pure progressive aphemia. *J Neurol Neurosurg Psychiatry* **56**(8):923–4.

Davies R R, Hodges J R, Kril J J et al. (2005). The pathological basis of semantic dementia. *Brain* **128**(Pt 9):1984–95.

Deleceuse F, Andersen A R, Waldemar G et al. (1990). Cerebral blood flow in progressive aphasia without dementia. *Brain* **113**:1395–404.

Dronkers N F (1996). A new brain region for coordinating speech articulation. *Nature* **384**(6605):159–61.

Duffy J R, Peterson R C (1992). Primary progressive aphasia. *Aphasiology* **6**, 1–15

Fukui T, Sugita K, Kawamura M, Shiota J, Nakano I (1996). Primary progressive apraxia in Pick's disease: a clinicopathologic study. *Neurology* **47**(2):467–73.

Galton C J, Patterson K, Xuereb J H, Hodges J R (2000). Atypical and typical presentations of Alzheimer's disease: a clinical, neuropsychological, neuroimaging and pathological study of 13 cases. *Brain* **123**(Pt 3):484–98.

Godbolt A K, Beck J A, Collinge J et al. (2004). A presenilin 1 R278I mutation presenting with language impairment. *Neurology* **63**(9):1702–4.

Gorno-Tempini M L, Dronkers N F, Rankin K P et al. (2004a). Cognition and anatomy in three variants of primary progressive aphasia. *Ann Neurol* **55**(3):335–46.

Gorno-Tempini M L, Murray R C, Rankin K P, Weiner M W, Miller B L (2004b). Clinical, cognitive and anatomical evolution from nonfluent progressive aphasia to corticobasal syndrome: a case report. *Neurocase* **10**(6):426–36.

Gorno-Tempini M L, Murray R C, Rankin K P, Weiner M W and Miller B L (2004c). Clinical, cognitive and anatomical evolution from non-fluent progressive aphasia to corticobasal syndrome: a case report. *Neurocase* **10**(6):426–36.

Green J, Morris J C, Sandson J, McKeel D W, Jr., Miller J W (1990). Progressive aphasia: a precursor of global dementia? *Neurology* **40**(Pt 1):423–9.

Grossman M, Mickanin J, Onishi K et al. (1996). Progressive non-fluent aphasia: language, cognitive and PET measures contrasted with probable Alzheimer's disease. *J Cogn Neurosci* **8**:135–54.

Grossman M, Payer F, Onishi K et al. (1998). Language comprehension and regional cerebral defects in frontotemporal degeneration and Alzheimer's disease. *Neurology* **50**(1):157–63.

Harasty J A, Halliday G M, Xuereb J et al. (2001). Cortical degeneration associated with phonologic and semantic language impairments in AD. *Neurology* **56**(7):944–50.

Hodges J R, Patterson K (1996). Nonfluent progressive aphasia and semantic dementia: a comparative neuropsychological study. *J Int Neuropsychol Soc* **2**(6):511–24.

Hodges J R, Patterson K, Oxbury S, Funnell E (1992). Semantic dementia. Progressive fluent aphasia with temporal lobe atrophy. *Brain* **115**(Pt 6):1783–806.

Hodges J R, Davies R, Xuereb J, Kril J, Halliday G (2003). Survival in frontotemporal dementia. *Neurology* **61**(3):349–54.

Hodges J R, Davies R R, Xuereb J H et al. (2004). Clinicopathological correlates in frontotemporal dementia. *Ann Neurol* **56**(3):399–406.

Johnson J K, Diehl J, Mendez M F et al. (2005). Frontotemporal lobar degeneration: demographic characteristics of 353 patients. *Arch Neurol* **62**(6):925–30.

Josephs K A, Duffy J R, Strand E A et al. (2006). Clinicopathological and imaging correlates of progressive aphasia and apraxia of speech. *Brain* **129**:1385–98.

Joshi A, Roy E A, Black S E, Barbour K (2003). Patterns of limb apraxia in primary progressive aphasia. *Brain Cogn* **53**(2):403–7.

Karbe H, Kertesz A, Polk M (1993). Profiles of language impairment in primary progressive aphasia. *Arch Neurol* **50**(2):193–201.

Kempler D, Metter E J, Riege W H et al. (1990). Slowly progressive aphasia: three cases with language, memory, CT and PET data. *J Neurol Neurosurg Psychiatry* **53**(11):987–93.

Kertesz A (1980). *Western Aphasia Battery*. London, Ontario: University of Western Ontario Press.

Kertesz A (2005). Frontotemporal dementia: one disease, or many? probably one, possibly two. *Alzheimer Dis Assoc Disord* **19**(Suppl 1):S19–24.

Kertesz A, Munoz D G (2003). Primary progressive aphasia and Pick complex. *J Neurol Sci* **206**(1):97–107.

Kertesz A, Munoz D (2004). Relationship between frontotemporal dementia and corticobasal degeneration/progressive supranuclear palsy. *Dement Geriatr Cogn Disord* **17**(4):282–6.

Kertesz A, Davidson W, McCabe P, Takagi K, Munoz D (2003). Primary progressive aphasia: diagnosis, varieties, evolution. *J Int Neuropsychol Soc* **9**(5):710–19.

Kertesz A, McMonagle P, Blair M, Davidson W, Munoz D G (2005). The evolution and pathology of frontotemporal dementia. *Brain* **128**(Pt 9):1996–2005.

Knibb J A, Xuereb J H, Patterson K, Hodges J R (2006). Clinical and pathological characterization of progressive aphasia. *Ann Neurol* **59**(1):156–65.

286

Li F, Iseki E, Kato M, Adachi Y, Akagi M, Kosaka K (2000). An autopsy case of Alzheimer's disease presenting with primary progressive aphasia: a clinicopathological and immunohistochemical study. *Neuropathology* **20**(3): 239–45.

McNeil M R, Small S L, Masterson R J, Fossett T RD (1995). Behavioral and pharmacological treatment of lexical–semantic deficits in a single patient with primary progressive aphasia. *Am J Speech Lang Pathol* **4**:76–87.

Mandell A M, Alexander M P, Carpenter S (1989). Creutzfeldt–Jakob disease presenting as isolated aphasia. *Neurology* **39**(1):55–8.

Mesulam M M (1982). Slowly progressive aphasia without generalized dementia. *Ann Neurol* **11**(6):592–8.

Mesulam M M (2001). Primary progressive aphasia. *Ann Neurol* **49**(4):425–32.

Mesulam M M, Weintraub S (1992). Spectrum of primary progressive aphasia. *Baillières Clin Neurol* **1**(3):583–609.

Mesulam M M, Grossman M, Hillis A, Kertesz A, Weintraub S (2003). The core and halo of primary progressive aphasia and semantic dementia. *Ann Neurol* **54**(Suppl 5):S11–14.

Mochizuki A, Ueda Y, Komatsuzaki Y *et al.* (2003). Progressive supranuclear palsy presenting with primary progressive aphasia: clinicopathological report of an autopsy case. *Acta Neuropathol* **105**(6):610–14.

Murray L L (1998). Longitudinal treatment of primary progressive aphasia: a case study. *Aphasiology* **12**:651–72.

Neary D, Snowden J S, Gustafson L, *et al.* (1998). Frontotemporal lobar degeneration: a consensus on clinical diagnostic criteria. *Neurology* **51**(6):1546–54.

Nestor P J, Graham N L, Fryer T D *et al.* (2003). Progressive non-fluent aphasia is associated with hypometabolism centred on the left anterior insula. *Brain* **126**(Pt 11):2406–18.

Pick A (1892). Uber die Beziehungen der senilen Hirnatrophie zur Aphasie. *Prager Med Wochenschr* **17**:165–7.

Reed D A, Johnson N A, Thompson C, Weintraub S, Mesulam M M (2004). A clinical trial of bromocriptine for treatment of primary progressive aphasia. *Ann Neurol* **56**(5):750.

Rogers M A, Alarcon N B (1999). Characteristics and management of primary progressive aphasia. *Neurophysiol Neurogen Speech Lang Disord (ASHA Special Interest Division)* **9**(4):12–26.

Rosen H J, Kramer J H, Gorno-Tempini M L *et al.* (2002). Patterns of cerebral atrophy in primary progressive aphasia. *Am J Geriatr Psychiatry* **10**(1):89–97.

Rosso S M, Landweer E J, Houterman M *et al.* (2003). Medical and environmental risk factors for sporadic frontotemporal dementia: a retrospective case–control study. *J Neurol Neurosurg Psychiatry* **74**(11):1574–6.

Rossor M N, Revesz T, Lantos P L, Warrington E K (2000). Semantic dementia with ubiquitin-positive tau-negative inclusion bodies. *Brain* **123**(Pt 2):267–6.

Schneider S L, Thompson C K, Luring B (1996). Effects of verbal plus gestural training on sentence production in a patient with primary progressive aphasia. *Aphasiology* **10**(3):297–317.

Snowden J S, Neary D, Mann D M, Goulding P J, Testa H J (1992). Progressive language disorder due to lobar atrophy. *Ann Neurol* **31**(2):174–83.

Snowden J S, Neary D, Mann D MA (1996). Fronto-temporal dementia. In *Fronto-temporal Lobar Degeneration: Fronto-temporal Dementia, Progressive Aphasia, Semantic Dementia*. New York: Churchill Livingstone, pp. 9–41.

Thompson S A, Patterson K, Hodges J R (2003). Left/right asymmetry of atrophy in semantic dementia: behavioral–cognitive implications. *Neurology* **61**(9):1196–203.

Turner R S, Kenyon L C, Trojanowski J Q, Gonatas N, Grossman M (1996). Clinical, neuroimaging, and pathologic features of progressive nonfluent aphasia. *Ann Neurol* **39**(2):166–73.

Tyrrell P J, Warrington E K, Frackowiak R S J, Rossor M N (1990). Heterogeneity in progressive aphasia due to focal cortical atrophy. A clinical and PET study. *Brain* **113**:1321–36.

Tyrrell P J, Kartsounis L D, Frackowiak R S, Findley L J, Rossor M N (1991). Progressive loss of speech output and orofacial dyspraxia associated with frontal lobe hypometabolism. *J Neurol Neurosurg Psychiatry* **54**(4):351–7.

Weintraub S, Rubin N P, Mesulam M-M (1990). Primary progressive aphasia: longitudinal course, neuropsychological profile, and language features. *Arch Neurol* **47**:1329–35.

Westbury C, Bub D (1997). Primary progressive aphasia: a review of 112 cases. *Brain Lang* **60**(3):381–406.

Chapter 20

Cognition in corticobasal degeneration and progressive supranuclear palsy

Paul McMonagle and Andrew Kertesz

Introduction

Progressive supranuclear palsy (PSP) and corticodentatonigral degeneration, later renamed as corticobasal degeneration (CBD), were originally described as unitary clinicopathologic entities and defined primarily as motor disorders with atypical parkinsonism lacking levodopa response, though the pathologic resemblance to Pick's disease was acknowledged for CBD. We now know that the relationship between these clinical entities and the pathology is not uniform, and nomenclature has changed as a result. The corticobasal degeneration syndrome (CBDS) is so named to distinguish it from the pathologic entity and has core features of asymmetric apraxia (cortical) and rigidity (basal ganglionic) with additional findings from each region such as cortical sensory loss, alien limb behavior, myoclonus or bradykinesia, dystonia, tremor. Pathology in CBD is characterized by lobar atrophy, which is mainly superior parietal and frontal with relative sparing of the occipital and temporal lobes (Munoz 1998). Microscopically, the cortex contains swollen achromatic neurons, tau-positive glial plaques (the most characteristic feature of CBD) and rounded/fibrillary neuronal inclusions, also positive for tau. Another distinctive feature of CBD is the strong silver staining of the rounded inclusions with the Gallyas method, separating this pathology from the otherwise very similar findings in Pick's disease. Subcortical structures (mainly basal ganglia but also thalamus) demonstrate significant neuronal depletion, and rounded/fibrillary neuronal inclusions are seen here also. By comparison, PSP is typified by its symmetry, with limb and axial rigidity, a supranuclear gaze palsy and early falling. Pathologically, PSP is characterized by the abnormal accumulation of tau protein in neurons and, less

commonly but distinctively, in glial cells as thorny astrocytes (Ikeda et al. 1995) accompanied by neuronal loss and gliosis. Tau-containing globose neurofibrillary tangles are frequent in subcortical structures, particularly basal ganglia and oculomotor nuclei where the density contributes to pathologic diagnosis (Hauw et al. 1994; Litvan et al. 1996a). Extension of tangles to the cortex is well documented and though identical to CBD subcortically, the tangles in cortex are morphologically distinct (Munoz 1998).

There is significant overlap between CBDS and PSP clinically in terms of the movement disorder, pathologically in view of the shared 4-repeat (4R) tau-positive pathology and genetically with the A0 polymorphism and H1 haplotype association for both (Sha et al. 2006). After the initial reports from movement disorder clinics, these patients began to appear in cognitive clinics with varied descriptions of cognitive deficits. In particular, reports of evolving aphasia and frontal features in patients with these akinetic rigid disorders define the prototypical cognitive profile in our experience (Kertesz et al. 2000), though other forms, in particular visuospatial variants in CBD (Tang Wai et al. 2003), are well recognized. The converse situation wherein patients with classical features of the behavioral variant of frontotemporal dementia (bv-FTD) or primary progressive aphasia (PPA) are shown to have tau-positive CBD or PSP pathology at autopsy shows that CBD(S) and PSP overlap not only with each other but also with the FTD spectrum or Pick complex (Kertesz et al. 2005). In this chapter, we describe the varied cognitive findings in these patients and in particular emphasize the overlap with FTD.

Corticobasal degeneration
The history of overlap with frontotemporal dementia

Precedence for the first description of CBDS may lie with Lhermitte (Ballan and Tison 1997), who in 1925

The Behavioral Neurology of Dementia, eds. Bruce L. Miller and Bradley F. Boeve. Published by Cambridge University Press. © Cambridge University Press 2009.

described a 67-year-old carpenter with a progressive right-sided, rigid-apractic disorder. Even here, we find the movement disorder combined with mild aphasic errors and word finding difficulty. Descriptions of extrapyramidal involvement in Pick's disease followed somewhat later (Löwenberg 1936) before the combination of aphasia and rigidity in Pick's disease was subsequently identified by Akelaitis (1944). Rebeiz and colleagues (1968) recognized the pathologic similarity of CBD to Pick's disease but felt it was distinct to the aphasic/behavioral clinical presentation of Pick's disease, observing that "mental faculties were relatively preserved" in their cases. Following this report, no new cases of CBD were added to the literature for almost 20 years (Scully et al. 1985; Watts et al. 1985) and though a careful reading of these early detailed cases does reveal evidence of dementia and dysphasia, the emphasis remained on the movement disorder with the belief that higher cognitive function was "relatively preserved" (Rinne et al. 1994). Reflecting this perspective, the first diagnostic criteria for CBD included "early dementia" as an exclusion (Lang et al. 1994). Soon afterwards, the same authors described cognitive presentations of CBD pathology (Bergeron et al. 1996) and later found that dementia was, in fact, the most common presentation in their pathologic series of CBD (Grimes et al. 1999).

Reports of patients attending cognitive clinics with overlapping aphasic and asymmetric extrapyramidal syndromes began appearing in the late 1980s. The Manchester group described a patient with progressive aphasia with a right-sided extrapyramidal syndrome combined with limb apraxia, upgaze palsy, primitive reflexes and prominent left temporoparietal atrophy on CT (Goulding et al. 1989). Pathology of CBD was confirmed as a substrate for PPA by Lippa and colleagues (1991), who described a 69-year-old man with a 3 year history of PPA defined as a transcortical motor aphasia who went on to develop rigidity and posturing of the right arm after the first year. Additional cases of PPA with CBD pathology followed, most (Lang 1992; Arima et al. 1994; Ikeda et al. 1996; Sakuri et al. 1996; Ferrer et al. 2003) but not all (Mimura et al. 2001) showing signs of extrapyramidal involvement at some stage before death. Kertesz and colleagues (1994) described similar patients with PPA, overlapping extrapyramidal signs and behavioral disturbance, who had Pick pathology and CBD at autopsy, leading to the suggestion that both CBD and PPA should be included with frontal lobe dementia under the rubric of Pick complex.

At a molecular level, insights from tau biology also highlight the overlap. Tau-positive inclusions in neurons and glia are frequent in FTD and characteristic of Pick's disease, while the astrocytic plaques, neuronal inclusions and intracellular coiled bodies of CBD also stain positively for tau in the 4R form. Mutations in the gene for tau on chromosome 17 cause genetic forms of CBD, with the apparent paradox of the same mutation causing bv-FTD in the father and CBDS in the son (Bugiani et al. 1999). The overlap is not confined to tau biology and also extends to the other major pathologic entity of FTD: the ubiquitinated inclusions. Here also CBDS phenotypes are recognized (Godbolt et al. 2005; Kertesz et al. 2005) and familial cases reported caused by mutations in the recently discovered gene PGRN, encoding progranulin (Maselis et al. 2006) with a similar phenotypic heterogeneity to tau in that the same mutation can result in CBDS or bv-FTD (Benussi et al. 2008).

In recent years, cognitive and language disturbances have become recognized as integral to CBD (Frattali et al. 2000; Kertesz et al. 2000; Graham et al. 2003a), causing increased awareness of the significant overlap with bvFTD and PPA (Kertesz and Martinez-Lage 1998; Kertesz et al. 2000; Mathuranath et al. 2000). To an extent, the wheel has come full circle in that aphasia and signs of focal or lateralized cognitive deficits are now considered among core inclusion criteria (Boeve et al. 2003) for CBDS. These patients are as likely to be seen by cognitive neurologists as movement disorders specialists, and CBD pathology is now regarded as a common substrate for PPA (Kertesz and Munoz 2003; Kertesz et al. 2005; Knopman et al. 2005).

In describing the cognitive and behavioral changes in CBDS, a distinction can be made between patients with first symptoms of a movement disorder (motor onset) followed by behavior change/aphasia or the reverse situation, where the motor disorder appears after a cognitive onset (Kertesz et al. 2000). The experience in our clinic with these two patterns of presentation, motor onset and cognitive onset, are summarized in Figs. 20.1 and 20.2, respectively, and illustrated in Boxes 20.1 and 20.2, respectively.

Frontal/behavioral change

Behavior change in CBDS overlaps to a large extent with that seen in bv-FTD in our experience (see Boxes 20.1 and 20.2). Using the Frontal Behavioral Inventory (FBI), a questionnaire specifically designed for the spectrum of apathy and disinhibition displayed

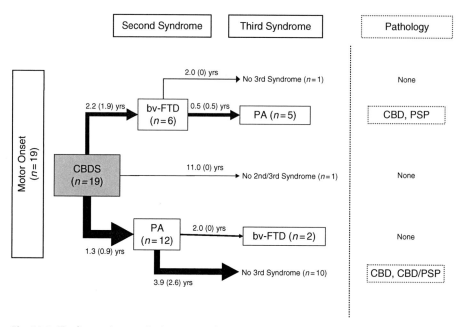

Fig. 20.1. The first syndrome and subsequent evolution through second and third syndromes in patients from our center with an initial motor presentation of corticobasal degeneration syndrome (CBDS). Final pathology is shown where available. Patients developed symptoms meeting criteria for the behavioral variant of frontotemporal dementia (bv-FTD) and progressive aphasia (PA). The size of the arrows is in proportion to the number of patients at each stage, and the average interval in years (SD) between the syndromes is indicated. CBD, corticobasal degeneration; PSP, progressive supranuclear palsy; CBD/PSP, transitional features of both.

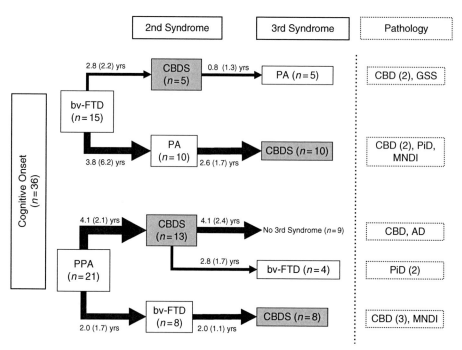

Fig. 20.2. The first syndrome and subsequent evolution through second and third syndromes in patients who developed corticobasal degeneration syndrome (CBDS) after an initial presentation with the behavioral presentation of frontotemporal dementia (bv-FTD) or primary progressive aphasia (PPA). Final pathology is shown where available. Aphasia developing secondarily is indicated as PA. The average interval in years (SD) between the syndromes is indicated. CBD, corticobasal degeneration; GSS, Gerstmann–Straussler–Scheinker disease; PiD, Pick's disease; AD, Alzheimer's disease; MNDI, FTD with motor neuron disease-type inclusions.

Box 20.1 Motor-onset corticobasal degeneration syndrome followed by cognitive change

A 63-year-old right-handed engineer developed stiffness in his right arm. His writing deteriorated and he was unable to control his lawn mower. Six months later he was holding his right arm at his side, like a patient after a stroke. Around that time, his speech diminished; he had word finding difficulty, and he lost interest in friends and daily activities. He became perseverative and had difficulty organizing complex activities. He began to lose his balance and fall forward. Parkinson's disease was diagnosed; levodopa plus carbidopa and selegiline hydrochloride were started but were ineffective.

One year after onset the patient was reassessed. Computed tomography (CT) and magnetic resonance imaging (MRI) showed asymmetrical atrophy, primarily in the left parietal lobe. At that time, it was noted that his right hand was interfering with his left hand as if it belonged to someone else. His right hand was also very apractic on testing. About 2.5 years after onset, the patient was noted to be abulic, apractic and aphasic. His right hand showed unusual posturing but he seemed to ignore it. The diagnosis of CBDS was made. Although he remained polite in public, he became preoccupied with sex, watching erotic videos, masturbating and demanding sex daily. His speech became perseverative. He could not put a sentence together, searched for words and used phrases unrelated to the discussion. He became angry and frustrated when not understood.

About 3 years after onset, he developed urinary incontinence. His right leg became stiff and the fingers of his right hand curled. Three and a half years after onset he was admitted to a chronic care hospital and had to be fed because he was unable to use his right arm. Four years after onset he became mute and dysphagic. He responded to teasing with a giggle and he still watched television and tapped his foot to music. He died 6 years after onset, following a urinary tract infection and sepsis at age 74 years. Just before his death, he had bilateral rigidity, severe immobility, vertical gaze palsy and total mutism. Pathology of CBD was confirmed at autopsy, with characteristic silver staining and tau-positive neuronal inclusions in cortex and basal ganglia. This is an example of CBDS diagnosed in life, with almost simultaneous onset of behavioral symptoms amounting to bvFTD and later progressive aphasia, having confirmed CBD pathology. This pattern or presentation is summarized in Fig. 20.1.

Box 20.2 Cognitive onset followed by corticobasal degeneration syndrome later

A 61-year-old female store clerk had gradual onset of behavioral symptoms initially. She began obsessively closing windows and barring doors. She had difficulty organizing her time, household chores and shopping. She would call her husband frequently at work just to make sure he was there. She also had difficulty concentrating, making change and remembering and knowing which cards to play in euchre or bridge. Later she would interrupt a conversation or make inappropriate comments. About 18 months after onset, she showed decreased interest in her environment and decreasing spontaneous speech; her responses became simpler and more slurred. Two years after symptoms began, she stopped speaking spontaneously; she began moaning and was only able to follow simple commands and repeat simple statements.

At the end of the second year of her illness, she developed some stiffness on the right side, mostly in her arm, with mild tremor. She had several admissions to the hospital, the first when she fell a year after the onset of her illness and the second a year later when she was diagnosed as having Alzheimer's disease. Neuropsychological testing showed a memory quotient of 103, which was average. Oral fluency was very poor. She failed to sort cards by category. She had difficulty with common sense judgements on the comprehension subtest of the Wechsler Adult Intelligence Scale and sequencing a series of cards from drawings (picture arrangement). In addition to the deficits of frontal lobe functioning, limitation of upward and lateral gaze was noted, suggesting a diagnosis of PSP. Her writing became very small. She walked with a shuffle and had increased tone on the right side. She was noted to be echolalic and at times her speech was unintelligible. On the two admissions CT scans showed frontal lobe atrophy.

By the third year of her illness, she was incontinent, unable to feed herself and needed help with dressing. On examination, she appeared in a fetal position, staring with repetitive moaning and had no spontaneous speech. She followed some simple commands with her limbs and was able to repeat very short sentences with slurred and nasal speech. She answered a few questions with an occasional word, such as her name. Upgaze impairment was noted again. She had a positive jaw jerk and palmomental, labial and glabellar tap reflexes. Electroencephalography showed bitemporal dysrhythmia that was prominent on the left side. Neuropathology in 1986 suggested subcortical degeneration possibly related to postencephalitic parkinsonism, revised to CBD subsequently with novel staining techniques. Our clinic experience for this scenario is summarized in Fig. 20.2.

by patients with FTD (Kertesz *et al.* 1997), we have previously described the behavior change in CBDS with motor and cognitive onsets (Kertesz *et al.* 2000). The significant personality changes consisted of apathy, disinhibition, perseveration, inattention or executive dysfunction, the core symptoms of FTD (Neary *et al.* 1998). Not all of these symptoms appeared in all patients, however. Using the Neuropsychiatric Inventory (NPI; Cummings 1994), Litvan *et al.* (1998) described high levels of depression in CBDS but also apathy, irritability, anxiety and disinhibition. Tests of executive function used in CBDS typically include phonemic and semantic fluency (Frattali *et al.* 2000; Mathuranath *et al.* 2000; Graham *et al.* 2003a), card sorting, Trails A and B, Stroop and abstraction, with consistent impairments described (Graham 2003a). Frontal lobe dysfunction with behavioral disturbances, or poor performance on frontal lobe tests, is described in at least 50% of the patients with CBD for whom case reports were available in the literature (Reibeiz *et al.* 1968; Clark *et al.* 1986; Gibb *et al.* 1989; Riley *et al.* 1990; Rinne *et al.* 1994; Frisoni *et al.* 1995; Wenning *et al.* 1998). Most of these reports contain descriptions of symptoms rather than quantitative neuropsychological results.

Language

Though not emphasized in early reports a focused reading of historical accounts of CBDS makes clear the aphasic deficits in CBDS. There may be several reasons for this. Mild anomia or aphasia may be overlooked in the face of motor presentations, and at times attributed to the dysarthria of the extrapyramidal disease or to generalized dementia. Cross-sectional studies without significant follow-up may not notice insidious language loss. There is also a reluctance to label progressive loss of language as "aphasia" because this term is generally used for sudden deficits. Nevertheless, the language loss, when examined formally, has the features of aphasia from other causes. Despite the now recognized overlap between CBDS and PPA, there has been little direct comparison of language performance in both. Except for a few studies (Mimura *et al.* 2001; Kertesz and Munoz 2003; Gorno-Tempini *et al.* 2004), reports of aphasia in CBDS tend to be cross-sectional rather than longitudinal, tend not to reflect the evolution from PPA and/or FTD to CBDS, or compare between motor and cognitive presentations of CBDS.

We recently reviewed our cohort with CBDS (McMonagle *et al.* 2006a) and identified 19 patients

with the movement disorder of CBDS as a first syndrome and another larger group of 36 patients who developed CBDS after an initial onset with a cognitive disorder aphasic or behavioral (Figs 20.1 and 20.2). All patients with cognitive-onset CBDS and all bar two with motor-onset CBDS developed aphasia during the course of their illness. Previously, we have shown that general cognitive and behavioral measures are similar for each presentation but language scores are lower in those with cognitive-onset disorder (Kertesz *et al.* 2000), reflecting the frequency of aphasic presentations. The change in language for patients with cognitive CBDS was identical to our other patients with PPA based on the Western Aphasia Battery (WAB; Kertesz 1982) save for a trend towards worse repetition in CBDS. Initially these patients are significantly anomic, but with time they develop problems with expressive language while receptive language and single-word comprehension are relatively preserved, corresponding to deficits in progressive non-fluent aphasia (PNFA) (Grossman *et al.* 1996). Over time, the picture changes, with normal and anomic patients becoming non-fluent, developing Broca's, conduction and global aphasias. Our longitudinal follow-up showed that both cognitive CBDS and PPA are distinct from motor CBDS at first, but by the fourth year of illness the motor-onset group had also begun to develop significant aphasia paralleling the cognitive CBDS group but lagging behind.

Although non-fluent aphasia was the predominant pattern, two of our patients had striking preservation of repetition consistent with transcortical sensory aphasia while another two had relatively fluent receptive aphasias classified as Wernicke's by the WAB, both uncommon findings in the CBDS literature (Ikeda *et al.* 1996; Graham *et al.* 2003b). One patient, in particular, with CBD pathology confirmed at autopsy, began with word-finding difficulty, progressing to prominent deficits in object recognition, comprehension and naming, with fluent but markedly circumlocutory speech containing frequent semantic paraphasias. He subsequently showed apraxia and behavioral change characterized by mental rigidity, irritability, aggression, gluttony, hoarding and utilization behavior. Extrapyramidal signs were late and atypical for CBDS because of bilateral rigidity and he died in a psychiatric hospital 10 years after onset. Imaging with CT and single-photon emission computed tomography (SPECT) revealed predominant left-sided frontotemporal atrophy and thinning of the left perisylvian, parietal and anterior temporal regions. This patient was seen in the mid 1980s before semantic dementia was delineated as a variant of FTD with associative agnosia (Snowden *et al.* 1989; Hodges *et al.* 1992) as distinct from fluent subtypes of PPA with sensory aphasia and preserved repetition. Tests for semantic memory impairment and visual agnosia were not performed; however, in retrospect, the clinical picture is consistent with criteria for semantic dementia (Neary *et al.* 1998). Our patient is of particular interest as this variant of FTD has so far been associated with the tau-negative pathology of FTD with MND type inclusions and on occasion the tau-positive pathology of Pick's disease but not CBD (Davies *et al.* 2005).

Emotional prosody, mediated by both the right hemisphere (Tucker *et al.* 1977; Ross 1981) and the basal ganglia (Cancelliere and Kertesz 1990), has not been systematically studied in CBDS though flat aprosodic speech is mentioned in some case reports of aphasic patients with CBD pathology before the emergence of rigidity (Arima *et al.* 1994; Kertesz and Munoz 2003). It is not known whether this distinguishes CBD pathology from other causes of PPA, but limited assessments to date suggest the preservation of expressive emotional prosody in otherwise typical PPA (Tsao *et al.* 2004). Apraxia of speech with or without PNFA is a feature of CBD and other tau-positive diseases such as PSP (Josephs *et al.* 2006a); see below.

Asymmetry and laterality

Despite the striking asymmetry inherent in CBDS there has been no study of whether the side of motor disorder influences the language disorder or indeed determines the pattern of patient presentation, though it is generally assumed that left hemisphere involvement and right-sided motor disturbance accompanies the aphasia (Mesulam 2001). We found no measurable difference in WAB scores for patients with right- versus left-sided motor onset or for left versus right hemisphere atrophy. Another study (Frattali *et al.* 2000) has used the WAB to examine language function in a cross-sectional study of patients with CBDS. Although the authors did not set out to analyze performance according to the motor side this can be calculated from their paper and also shows no difference in WAB scores. Nonetheless, that the vast majority (3:1) in our cohort had right-sided motor change and left hemisphere atrophy does suggest a predisposition to aphasia in such patients, though once present the severity of aphasia

is the same regardless of the laterality. Among patients with motor-onset CBDS, 32% had left-sided akinesia while the proportion in cognitive-onset CBDS was smaller, at 19%. In early reviews, the experience from movement disorders clinics suggested an over-representation of left-sided symptoms in CBDS (Lang *et al.* 1994) while our study suggests the opposite. It may be that patients with right-sided motor disturbances are more likely to present to cognitive disorders clinics because of predominant left hemisphere involvement, while those with left-sided akinesia present to movement disorders clinics since the "less eloquent" right hemisphere is involved.

Apraxia

Apraxia is the hallmark phenomenon of CBDS and a core component common to all diagnostic criteria (Boeve *et al.* 2003; Litvan *et al.* 2003), but determining the actual prevalence is difficult. Leiguarda and colleagues (1994) estimated the frequency at 70% in clinically defined CBDS, and though apraxia is present in all the early descriptions, there are cases of pathologically confirmed CBD without apraxia in retrospective case series, though the authors acknowledge that this sign is not routinely looked for by many neurologists (Wenning *et al.* 1998). In our own experience (Kertesz *et al.* 2000), ideomotor apraxia, which is apraxia on command and imitation, was the most common form and was equally frequent in motor and cognitive onsets. In fact, all our patients developed significant and severe apraxia, with the exception of one retrospectively added case where it was not documented. In many cases, ideational or object-use apraxia, where the conceptual system for action is disrupted, was also prominent. The definition of ideational apraxia is controversial but we used it here as object-use apraxia and as such found it occurred even without ideomotor apraxia on occasion, an unusual dissociation we have observed only in degenerative disease, particularly CBDS. Our findings of these apraxias in CBDS have also been described by others (Leiguarda *et al.* 1994; Spatt *et al.* 2002; Merians *et al.* 1999).

The nosology of limb kinetic apraxia, where fine distal movements are impaired for all movements, remains controversial (Zadikoff and Lang 2005), with some authors regarding it as a mild corticospinal or elemental motor deficit (Quencer *et al.* 2007). It was reported in CBDS initially as an uncommon finding (Leiguarda *et al.* 1998) but later recognized as frequent and in some cases the dominant form (Okuda

293

and Tochibana *et al.* 1994; Leiguarda *et al.* 2003; Soliveri *et al.* 2005). Similar variability applies to reports of buccofacial apraxia in CBDS. Leiguarda and colleagues found it absent in their series of ten patients (Leiguarda *et al.* 1994) while Ozsancak report it for all ten of theirs (Ozsancak *et al.* 2000). Others report orofacial apraxia and articulatory difficulty (verbal apraxia) as a presenting feature of CBD with pathology centered on Broca's area (Lang 1992; Zadikoff and Lang 2005).

Visuospatial impairment

Case series of CBDS emphasize pronounced deficits on visuospatial and visuoconstructive components of standardized tasks such as the Dementia Rating Scale or the Addenbrooke's Cognitive Examination (Kertesz *et al.* 2000; Bak *et al.* 2005a), which help to distinguish CBDS from other atypical parkinsonian disorders (Bak *et al.* 2005a). Certainly, impairment in handwriting and visuoconstructive tasks such as drawing and copying (constructional apraxia) are frequent in CBD/CBDS (Gibb *et al.* 1989; Lippa *et al.* 1991; Kertesz *et al.* 1994; Bergeron *et al.* 1996; Ikeda *et al.* 1996; Boeve *et al.* 1999) and typically felt to reflect the prominent parietal burden of pathology and limb apraxia. Visuoperceptual impairment as assessed with the Visual Object and Space Perception Battery is also prominent in patients with the clinically diagnosed disorder (Bak *et al.* 2006). A natural extension of this dorsal (where/action) stream involvement comes with the finding of overlapping cases of CBDS and Balint's syndrome (simultanagnosia, optic ataxia, oculomotor apraxia), as described by Mendez (2000), and the confirmation of CBD pathology in posterior cortical atrophy (Tang-Wai *et al.* 2003, 2004), which includes Balint's syndrome as a core feature (McMonagle *et al.* 2006b).

Other cognitive domains

Reports of episodic memory performance in CBDS vary, but forgetfulness does appear as a presenting symptom in those who subsequently have pathologically confirmed CBD (Boeve *et al.* 1999; Grimes *et al.* 1999), in some cases with the heaviest burden of pathology in the hippocampal structures (Bergeron *et al.* 1996). Formal assessment with story recall confirms objective deficits in episodic memory (Graham *et al.* 2003b), but in general logical memory performance is better for CBDS than for those with Alzheimer disease (AD) with similar scores on the Mini-Mental State Examination (MMSE) (Pillon *et al.* 1995;

Massman *et al.* 1996). The proposed mechanism for episodic memory deficits in CBDS lies with strategies for encoding and retrieval, reflecting frontosubcortical rather than hippocampal structures. Our own experience suggests similar performance for CBDS as with bv-FTD, PPA and semantic dementia, based on the memory component of the DRS (Kertesz *et al.* 2007).

Anomia in CBDS is very common owing to aphasia and may confound assessments of semantic memory. Tests using matching tasks of word to picture (Graham *et al.* 2003a) and name to famous face (Beatty *et al.* 1995), which minimize the effects of aphasia, typically show normal or borderline performance, suggesting relative preservation of semantic memory in these patients. Number knowledge can be regarded as a distinct domain of semantic memory, with features quite distinct from the attributes of objects. Halpern and colleagues (2004) have shown that patients with CBDS were consistently more impaired on tasks requiring number representations compared with object representations, and this was associated with atrophy in the right parietal cortex. Definitions of acalculia vary but difficulty manipulating numbers and performing arithmetic are pervasive in CBDS (Gibb *et al.* 1989; Lippa *et al.* 1991; Kertesz *et al.* 1994; Bergeron *et al.* 1996; Boeve *et al.* 1999).

Progressive supranuclear palsy
Historical aspects

Steele *et al.* (1964) recognized the cognitive features in the title of their paper describing the "vertical gaze and pseudobulbar palsy, nuchal dystonia and dementia" of PSP. As always it is instructive to read the original text, which clearly describes the cognitive impairment, behavior change and language difficulties present in all nine cases to variable degrees (summarized in Table 20.1). The first patient was summarized as "business executive (who) at age 50 developed mild intellectual impairment, indefinite visual difficulties and reactive depression." When he was examined at another center in the earliest stages, "the neurological examination was considered normal except for a mild organic dementia." In four patients, the cognitive impairment could be interpreted as remaining mild throughout, becoming moderate in one and prominent in four. Poor memory and recall, intellectual slowing, confusion, defects in abstract thought, calculation, attention, comprehension and apraxia (ideomotor defects) are all described. Personality and behavior change were evident and

Table 20.1. Summary of cognitive and behavioral findings from the original progressive supranuclear palsy cohort of Steele et al. (1964)

Case	Age (years)	First symptom(s)	Cognitive impairment	Behavior change	Language	Institution
I	50–56	Left hand motor control	"Slowed thinking" yr 2; still "reasonable and rational" yr 7	Depression (ECT), agitation, anxiety	Speech slowed	No
II[a]	56–59	"Unsteady, irritable, poor close vision"	"Moderate dementia" yr 2	Irritability, apathy, personal neglect	Slurred	In 2nd yr
III[b]	55–62	"Irritable, suspicious, dirty, confused" and falls	"Slight impairment" yr 2, but in same year was hospitalized for confusion, violence	Irritable, violent, suspicious, personal neglect, facile	Slurred	After 2 yrs
IV	62–67	Visual difficulty, dysarthria, dysphagia	"Mild intellectual impairment" in yr 3; no comment later	Jocular, facile, lability	Thick, explosive and abbreviated yr 4	Not stated
V[b]	69–72	"3 yr history of mental deterioration"	"Fairly severe dementia" by yr 3	"Personality change"	Speech slowed and monotonous	After 3 yrs
VI[a]	54–64	"Falls, irritable and unusually critical"	"Mild intellectual impairment" in yr 2; "dementia progressed" yr 5	Irritable, critical	Slurred	After 4 yrs
VII	57–64	"Tired easily and slower in various activities"	Interfering with work yr 4	Careless, irritable, violent outbursts	Monotonous, mute terminally	After 6 yrs
VIII[a,c]	54–64	"Mental deterioration and unsteadiness"	Still "pretty fair retention" after 10 yrs	None mentioned	Slow, slurred	After 8 yrs
IX[a,c]	58–62	"Mild personality change then unsteadiness"	Mild after 3 years	"Personality change"	Slurred	After 2 yrs

Notes:
ECT, electroconvulsive therapy; yr, year.
[a]Simultaneous cognitive/motor onset.
[b]Cognitive/behavioral onset.
[c]No pathology, still alive at time of report.

295

characterized by apathy, depression, poor personal hygiene, irritabililty, violent outbursts and facile, jocular affect. Behavioral or cognitive changes were the first symptoms in at least two patients but simultaneous with motor features in another five. For example patient 3 had been hospitalized with behavioral and cognitive change for a year before the gaze palsy and parkinsonism became apparent. Language and speech difficulties were typically described as dysarthric, with "slowed," "slurred" and "monotonous" speech. In patient 4 after 4 years of illness, "his speech had become thick, abbreviated and somewhat explosive," suggesting an emerging aphasia rather than dysarthria alone. Patient 7 became entirely mute terminally.

Albert and colleagues' (1974) used PSP as the prototype for "subcortical dementia," which became enshrined in the clinical phenotype. They defined a syndrome characterized by profound slowness of mentation, impaired memory retrieval and personality changes (mainly apathy with some outbursts of irritability), in the absence of "cortical" features of aphasia, agnosia and apraxia. The analysis used five cases of their own plus 42 from the literature with adequate data. Though the behavioral and cognitive features and the "striking clinical resemblance to dementia which occurs after bifrontal lobe disease" were emphasized, they likened it mainly to other subcortical processes such as thalamic tumors, olivopontocerebellar atrophy, progressive pallidal degeneration, Parkinson's disease and Wernicke–Korsakoff syndrome, feeling that the cognitive profile typified by PSP was distinct from cortical dementias. The distinction is less clear now and reports of cognitive phenomena initially considered unusual for PSP are now encountered with increasing regularity.

"Typical" cognitive impairment

A characteristic feature of cognitive impairment in PSP is the profound slowness of information-processing speed, similar to the bradyphrenia described by Naville (1922) after epidemic encephalitis. In the earliest descriptions, patients are described taking up to 5 minutes to respond (correctly) to a single question, creating an exaggerated impression of impairment, with performance improving by up to 50% if given adequate time to respond (Albert et al. 1974). The degree of cognitive slowing in PSP appears independent of motor slowing (Dubois et al. 1988; Pirtosek et al. 2001); and correlates with frontal lobe tests such

as the Wisconsin Card Sort and suggests striatofrontal dysfunction as a substrate (Dubois et al. 1988).

Frontal executive impairments are early and pervasive in PSP (Pillon et al. 1991; Bak and Hodges et al. 1998; Magherini and Litvan 2005). Though simple tests of attention and orientation are typically normal, more complex tasks of planning, attention set-shifting, abstraction and reasoning are significantly impaired (Robbins et al. 1994; Dubois et al. 2000). Set-shifting as measured with the Trail Making Test is impaired (Paviour et al. 2005) as is the Wisconsin Card Sort (Pillon et al. 1991; Monza et al. 1998; Soliveri et al. 2000; Paviour et al. 2005), with fewer categories sorted and more perseverative errors. Impairments are seen in non-verbal reasoning with Raven's progressive matrices (Dubois et al. 1988; Pillon et al. 1991; Robbins et al. 1994; Monza et al. 1998; Soliveri et al. 2000, 2005), similarities (Albert et al. 1974; Milberg and Albert 1989; Pillon et al. 1991; Dubois et al. 2000; Bak et al. 2005b; Paviour et al. 2005) and abstraction (Alberts et al. 1974; Dubois et al. 2000; Robinson et al. 2006). Particularly tasks of verbal fluency are greatly reduced in PSP (Dubois et al. 1988, 2000; Pillon et al. 1991; Esmonde et al. 1996; Monza et al. 1998; Bak et al. 2005b; Paviour et al. 2005; Soliveri et al. 2000, 2005), with poorer performance on letter than semantic fluency (Esmonde et al. 1996; Lange et al. 2003; Bak et al. 2005b; Paviour et al. 2005) exaggerating the pattern seen in normal controls and the reverse of that seen in AD (Bak et al. 2005b). Overall, patients with PSP score worse on these tasks of executive function than those with Parkinson's disease, multisystem atrophy and Huntington's disease (Dubois et al. 1988, 2000; Pillon et al. 1991; Monza et al. 1998; Soliveri et al. 2000; Bak et al. 2005b; Paviour et al. 2005) despite similar disease severity.

Memory complaints in PSP are usually mild and consist of impaired free recall with relatively preserved recognition memory (Pillon et al. 1995); this contrasts with the more profound deficit in AD, which also involves recognition (Milberg and Albert 1989). Inefficient storage and retrieval strategies lie behind the forgetfulness of PSP, which can be regarded as a dysexecutive phenomenon caused by disruption of striatofrontal circuits and is similar to that in Parkinson's and Huntington's diseases (Maher et al. 1985; Pillon et al. 1993, 1994). Patients with PSP demonstrate impaired working memory, disturbed learning and consistency of recall, and abnormal recognition, which were significantly improved by controlled encoding and cued recall (Pillon et al. 1994).

Personality and behavior change can be quite florid in PSP and may appear before the oculomotor and movement disorder. For example, in the original Steele *et al.* publication (1964) initial symptoms in Patient 3 were that "his wife noticed him becoming irritable, domineering, suspicious and rather dirty and untidy. He seemed confused at times and suffered some falls . . . His mood fluctuated and he tended to be argumentative, arrogant, and demanding . . . psychometric tests showed indices of slight intellectual impairment by way of defects of memory and abstract thought . . . because of increasing violence and confusion he was readmitted for permanent hospital care in 1955." Only after a further year of hospitalization did the gaze palsy and extrapyramidal disorder manifest itself. Litvan and colleagues (1996b) reported neuropsychiatric features in a cohort of PSP patients using the NPI and found apathy (91%) and disinhibition (36%) as the most common endorsements. Despite the prominence of apathy, depression scores were lower, a finding felt to distinguish PSP from CBDS where low mood was prominent. Psychotic symptoms, such as hallucinations and delusions, particularly Capgras syndrome and phantom boarder type, are uncommon in pathologically confirmed cases of PSP (Josephs and Dickson 2003), and indeed CBD and FTD, and should alert to the possibility of dementia with Lewy bodies or Parkinson's disease dementia (Ballard *et al.* 1999) as alternative diagnoses. Emotional blunting and disinhibition may also be seen in PSP, but these patients are less likely to demonstrate the other classical behaviors of frontotemporal degenerations such as stereotypies, rituals, gluttony, sweet tooth and altered pain response (Neary *et al.* 2005).

Cognitive impairment in PSP sufficient to be labeled "dementia" varies, with rates up to 70% reported. Daniel and colleagues (1995) used DSM-III-R criteria of the American Psychiatric Association (1987), which require memory impairment and hence are biased towards AD, and reported dementia in 10 of 17 with PSP subsequently confirmed pathologically. Pillon and colleagues (1991) found an identical rate if dementia was defined as global impairment 2 standard deviations below controls on a global composite including memory, rising to 71% if frontal tests were taken into account.

"Cortical" cognitive features

Initially a criterion of exclusion (Albert *et al.* 1974), limb apraxia in PSP is typically ideomotor, symmetrical and quite a common finding (40%) when studied systematically (Leiguarda *et al.* 1997; Pharr *et al.* 2001). Clinically defined series of PSP show transitive tasks performed more poorly than intransitive, with sequencing and complex gesture errors predominating while pantomime recognition is preserved (Leiguarda *et al.* 1997; Pharr *et al.* 2001; Soliveri *et al.* 2005). Apraxia scores correlate with levels of cognitive impairment, particularly frontal lobe tasks, suggesting frontal deafferentation as the cause (Leiguarda *et al.* 1997; Soliveri *et al.* 2005). Limb kinetic apraxia has not been systematically studied in PSP but is suggested in a subgroup of patients from earlier series (Zadikoff and Lang 2005).

Cases of PSP (and other) pathology mimicking the asymmetry of the corticobasal syndrome, and vice versa, abound (Hodges *et al.* 1992; Boeve *et al.* 1999; Kertesz *et al.* 2005; Knopman *et al.* 2005). It is difficult, therefore, to extrapolate these findings from clinically defined series into reliable discriminators between different pathologic entities. As a result, case series comparing parkinsonian syndromes without pathologic verification are somewhat circular, and this should be borne in mind for all discussions of cognitive findings in PSP and CBDS, but perhaps particularly for apraxia.

As in CBD, language and speech disorders are a feature of PSP, in particular PNFA caused by PSP pathology is well recognized (Josephs *et al.* 2006a,b; Kertesz *et al.* 2005; Knibb *et al.* 2006; Knopman *et al.* 2005). Logopenia or dynamic aphasia occurs with PSP (Esmonde *et al.* 1996) and refers to speech limited to short phrases or single words but otherwise grammatically correct and free of paraphasias. Adult-onset stammering was among the initial symptoms in Patient 1 from the case series of Albert and colleagues (1974) and may be a feature of parkinsonian disorders in general (Koller 1983). Apraxia of speech is a particular disorder of motor planning and programming of speech characterized by the inability to perform speech motor movements, typically with an intact ability to execute non-speech oral movements. Prosody is abnormal with distorted sound production and repeated articulatory trials. Apraxia of speech frequently accompanies PNFA, with or without dysarthria; however, it has also been reported as the initial manifestation of degenerative neurologic disease such as CBD (Lang 1992; Sakuri *et al.* 1996; Lehman *et al.* 2003) and PSP (Josephs *et al.* 2005) in the absence of aphasia. A recent study (Josephs *et al.* 2006b) examining clinicopathologic correlates in apraxia of speech

297

identified a strong relation between it and the presence of tau-positive pathology, such as CBD, PSP or Pick's disease, with important potential implications for predicting the underlying biochemistry.

Summary

There are many clinical and biological features in common in CBD and PSP, namely neurodegeneration with parkinsonism, oculomotor abnormalities, A0 polymorphism, H1H1 haplotype and tau-positive histology. Cases of one disorder mimicking the other abound in the literature, many of the case series quoted here do not have pathologic confirmation and so one must be cautious about using them to identify discriminating features. Nonetheless, some general statements can be made about the signature cognitive profiles of each disorder while acknowledging that many exceptions exist. Behavior change and non-fluent aphasia are common to both, but one can expect CBD to show more apraxia and visuospatial impairment while PSP is more classically dysexecutive, with "subcortical" slowing of cognition. Both overlap with bv-FTD and PPA clinically and pathologically, and while the orthodoxy for now is to maintain the distinction from the FTDs for PSP, the boundary for CBD becomes increasingly blurred.

References

Akelaitis AJ (1944). Atrophy of the basal ganglia in Pick's disease. *Arch Neurol Psychiatry* **51**:27–34.

Albert ML, Feldman RG, Willis AL (1974). The "subcortical dementia" of progressive supranuclear palsy. *J Neurol Neurosurg Psychiatry* **37**:121–30.

American Psychiatric Association (1987). *Diagnostic and Statistical Manual of Mental Disorders*, 3rd edn, revised. Washington, DC: American Psychiatric Association.

Arima K, Uesugi H, Fujita I *et al.* (1994). Corticonigral degeneration with neuronal achromasia presenting with primary progressive aphasia: ultrastructural and immunocytochemical studies. *J Neurol Sci* **127**:186–97.

Bak T, Hodges JR (1998). The neuropsychology of progressive supranuclear palsy: a review. *Neurocase* **4**:89–94.

Bak TH, Rogers TT, Crawford LM *et al.* (2005a). Cognitive bedside assessment in atypical parkinsonian syndromes. *J Neurol Neurosurg Psychiatry* **76**:420–2.

Bak TH, Crawford LM, Hearn VC *et al.* (2005b). Subcortical dementia revisited: similarities and differences in cognitive function between progressive supranuclear palsy (PSP), corticobasal degeneration (CBD) and multiple system atrophy (MSA). *Neurocase* **11**:268–73.

Bak TH, Caine D, Hearn VC, Hodges JR (2006). Visuospatial functions in atypical parkinsonian syndromes. *J Neurol Neurosurg Psychiatry* **77**:454–6.

Ballan G, Tison F (1997). A historical case of probable corticobasal degeneration? *Mov Disord* **12**:1073–4.

Ballard C, Holmes C, McKeith I *et al.* (1999). Psychiatric morbidity in dementia with Lewy bodies: a prospective clinical and neuropathological comparative study with Alzheimer's disease. *Am J Psychiatry* **156**:1039–45.

Beatty WW, Scott JG, Wilson DA, Prince JR, Williamson DJ (1995). Memory deficits in a demented patient with probable corticobasal degeneration. *J Geriatr Psychiatry Neurol* **8**:132–6.

Benussi L, Binetti G, Sina E *et al.* (2008). A novel deletion in progranulin gene is associated with FTDP-17 and CBS. *Neurobiol Aging* **29**:427–35.

Bergeron C, Pollanen MS, Weyer L *et al.* (1996). Unusual clinical presentations of cortical-basal ganglionic degeneration. *Ann Neurol* **40**:893–900.

Boeve BF, Maraganore DM, Parisi JE *et al.* (1999). Pathologic heterogeneity in clinically diagnosed corticobasal degeneration. *Neurology* **53**:795–800.

Boeve BF, Lang AE, Litvan I (2003). Corticobasal degeneration and its relationship to progressive supranuclear palsy and frontotemporal dementia. *Ann Neurol* **54**(Suppl 5):S15–19.

Bugiani O, Murrell JR, Giaccone G *et al.* (1999). Frontotemporal dementia and corticobasal degeneration in a family with a P301S mutation in tau. *J Neuropathol Exp Neurol* **58**:667–77.

Cancelliere AE, Kertesz A (1990). Lesion localization in acquired deficits of emotional expression and comprehension. *Brain Cogn* **13**:133–47.

Clark AW, Manz HJ, White III CL *et al.* (1986). Cortical degeneration with swollen chromatolytic neurons: its relationship to Pick's disease. *J Neuropathol Exp Neurol* **45**:268–84.

Cummings JL, Mega M, Gray K *et al.* (1994). The Neuropsychiatric Inventory: comprehensive assessment of psychopathology in dementia. *Neurology* **44**:2308–14.

Daniel SE, de Bruin VM, Lees AJ (1995). The clinical and pathological spectrum of Steele–Richardson–Olszewski syndrome (progressive supranuclear palsy): a reappraisal. *Brain* **118**:759–70.

Davies RR, Hodges JR, Kril JJ *et al.* (2005). The pathological basis of semantic dementia. *Brain* **128**:1984–95.

Dubois B, Pillon B, Legault F, Agid Y, Lhermitte F (1988). Slowing of cognitive processing in progressive supranuclear palsy. *Arch Neurol* **45**:1194–99.

Dubois B, Slachevsky A, Litvan I, Pillon B (2000). The FAB: a frontal assessment battery at bedside. *Neurology* **55**:1621–6.

Esmonde T, Giles E, Xuereb J, Hodges J (1996). Progressive supranuclear palsy presenting with dynamic aphasia. *J Neurol Neurosurg Psychiatry* **60**:403–10.

Ferrer I, Hernandez I, Boada M *et al.* (2003). Primary progressive aphasia as the initial manifestation of corticobasal degeneration and unusual tauopathies. *Acta Neuropathol* **106**:419–35.

Frattali CM, Grafman J, Patronas N *et al.* (2000). Language disturbances in corticobasal degeneration. *Neurology* **54**:990–2.

Frisoni GB, Pizzolato G, Zanetti O *et al.* (1995). Corticobasal degeneration: neuropsychological assessment and dopamine D_2 receptor SPECT analysis. *Eur Neurol* **35**:50–4.

Gibb WR, Luthert PJ, Marsden CD (1989). Corticobasal degeneration. *Brain* **112**:1171–92.

Godbolt AK, Josephs KA, Revesz T *et al.* (2005). Sporadic and familial dementia with ubiquitin-positive tau-negative inclusions: clinical features of one histopathological abnormality underlying frontotemporal lobar degeneration. *Arch Neurol* **62**: 1097–101.

Gorno-Tempini ML, Murray RC, Rankin KP, Weiner MW, Miller BL (2004). Clinical, cognitive and anatomical evolution from nonfluent progressive aphasia to corticobasal syndrome: a case report. *Neurocase* **10**:426–36.

Goulding PJ, Northen B, Snowden JS *et al.* (1989). Progressive aphasia with right-sided extrapyramidal signs: another manifestation of localized cerebral atrophy. *J Neurol Neurosurg Psychiatry* **52**:128–30.

Grafman J, Litvan I, Gomez C, Chase TN (1990). Frontal lobe function in progressive supranuclear palsy. *Arch Neurol* **47**:553–8.

Graham NL, Bak T, Patterson K, Hodges JR (2003a). Language function and dysfunction in corticobasal degeneration. *Neurology* **61**:493–9.

Graham NL, Bak TH, Hodges JR (2003b). Corticobasal degeneration as a cognitive disorder. *Mov Disord* **18**:1224–32.

Grimes DA, Lang AE, Bergeron CB (1999). Dementia as the most common presentation of cortical-basal degeneration. *Neurology* **53**:1969–74.

Grossman M, Mickanin J, Onishi K *et al.* (1996). Progressive non-fluent aphasia: language, cognitive and PET measures contrasted with probable Alzheimer's disease. *J Cogn Neurosci* **8**:135–54.

Halpern CH, Glosser G, Clark R *et al.* (2004). Dissociation of numbers and objects in corticobasal degeneration and semantic dementia. *Neurology* **62**:1163–9.

Hauw JJ, Daniel SE, Dickson D *et al.* (1994). Preliminary NINDS neuropathologic criteria for Steele–Richardson–Olszewski syndrome (progressive supranuclear palsy) *Neurology* **44**:2015–19.

Hodges JR, Patterson K, Oxbury S, Funnell E (1992). Semantic dementia. Progressive fluent aphasia with temporal lobe atrophy. *Brain* **115**:1783–806.

Ikeda K, Akiyama H, Kondo H *et al.* (1995). Thorn-shaped astrocytes: possibly secondarily induced tau-positive glial fibrillary tangles. *Acta Neuropathol* **90**:620–5.

Ikeda K, Akiyama H, Iritani S *et al.* (1996). Corticobasal degeneration with primary progressive aphasia and accentuated cortical lesion in superior temporal gyrus: case report and review. *Acta Neuropathol* **92**:534–9.

Josephs KA, Dickson DW (2003). Diagnostic accuracy of progressive supranuclear palsy in the Society for Progressive Supranuclear Palsy Brain Bank. *Mov Disord* **18**:1018–26.

Josephs KA, Boeve BF, Duffy JR *et al.* (2005). Atypical progressive supranuclear palsy underlying progressive apraxia of speech and nonfluent aphasia. *Neurocase* **11**:283–96.

Josephs KA, Petersen RC, Knopman DS *et al.* (2006a). Clinicopathologic analysis of frontotemporal and corticobasal degenerations and PSP. *Neurology* **66**:41–8.

Josephs KA, Duffy JR, Strand EA *et al.* (2006b). Clinicopathological and imaging correlates of progressive aphasia and apraxia of speech. *Brain* **129**:1385–98.

Kertesz A (1982). *The Western Aphasia Battery.* New York: Grune and Stratton.

Kertesz A, Munoz D (2003). Primary progressive aphasia and Pick complex. *J Neurol Sci* **206**(1):97–107.

Kertesz A, Hudson L, Mackenzie IRA, Munoz DG (1994). The pathology and nosology of primary progressive aphasia. *Neurology* **44**:2065–72.

Kertesz A, Davidson W, Fox H (1997). Frontal Behavioral Inventory. Diagnostic criteria for frontal lobe dementia. *Can J Neurol Sci* **24**:29–36.

Kertesz A, Martinez-Lage P (1998). Cognitive changes in corticobasal degeneration. In *Pick's Disease and Pick Complex*, eds. Kertesz A and Munoz DG. New York: Wiley, pp. 121–29.

Kertesz A, Martinez-Lage P, Davidson W, Munoz DG (2000). The corticobasal degeneration syndrome overlaps progressive aphasia and frontotemporal dementia. *Neurology* **55**:1368–75.

Kertesz A, McMonagle P, Blair M, Davidson W, Munoz DG (2005). The evolution and pathology of frontotemporal dementia. *Brain* **128**:1996–2005.

Kertesz A, Blair M, McMonagle P, Munoz DG (2007). The diagnosis and course of frontotemporal dementia. *Alzheimer Dis Assoc Disord* **21**:155–63.

Knibb JA, Xuereb JH, Patterson K, Hodges JR (2006). Clinical and pathological characterization of progressive aphasia. *Ann Neurol* **59**:156–65.

Knopman D, Boeve BF, Parisi JE *et al.* (2005). Antemortem diagnosis of frontotemporal lobar degeneration. *Ann Neurol* **57**:480–8.

299

Koller WC (1983). Dysfluency (stuttering) in extrapyramidal disease. *Arch Neurol* **40**:175–7.

Lang AE (1992). Cortico-basal ganglionic degeneration presenting with "progressive loss of speech output and orofacial dyspraxia." *J Neurol Neurosurg Psychiatry* **55**:1101.

Lang AE, Riley DE, Bergeron C (1994). Cortical-basal ganglionic degeneration. In *Neurodegenerative Diseases*, ed. Clane DB, Philadelphia, PA: WB Saunders, pp. 877–94.

Lange KW, Tucha O, Alders GL *et al.* (2003). Differentiation of parkinsonian syndromes according to differences in executive functions. *J Neural Transm* **110**:983–95.

Lehman M, Dufy J, Boeve B, Ahlskog J, Maraganore D (2003). Speech and language disorders associated with corticobasal degeneration. *J Med Speech Lang Pathol* **11**:131–46.

Leiguarda R, Lees AJ, Merello M, Starkstein S, Marsden CD (1994). The nature of apraxia in corticobasal degeneration. *J Neurol Neurosurg Psychiatry* **57**:455–9.

Leiguarda RC, Pramstaller PP, Merello M *et al.* (1997). Apraxia in Parkinson's disease, progressive supranuclear palsy, multiple system atrophy and neuroleptic-induced parkinsonism. *Brain* **120**:75–90.

Leiguarda R and Starkstein SE (1998). In *Pick's Disease and Pick Complex*, eds. Kertesz A and Munoz D. New York: Wiley-Liss, pp. 129–45.

Leiguarda RC, Merello M, Nouzeilles MI *et al.* (2003). Limb-kinetic apraxia in corticobasal degeneration: clinical and kinematic features. *Mov Disord* **18**:49–59.

Lippa CF, Cohen R, Smith TW, Drachman DA (1991). Primary progressive aphasia with focal neuronal achromasia. *Neurology* **41**:882–6.

Litvan I, Hauw JJ, Bartko JJ *et al.* (1996a). Validity and reliability of the preliminary NINDS neuropathologic criteria for progressive supranuclear palsy and related disorders. *J Neuropathol Exp Neurol* **55**:97–105.

Litvan I, Mega MS, Cummings JL, Fairbanks L (1996b). Neuropsychiatric aspects of progressive supranuclear palsy. *Neurology* **47**:1184–9.

Litvan I, Cummings JL, Mega M (1998). Neuropsychiatric features of corticobasal degeneration. *J Neurol Neurosurg Psychiatry* **65**:717–21.

Litvan I, Bhatia KP, Burn DJ for the Movement Disorders Society Scientific Issues Committee (2003). Movement Disorders Society Scientific Issues Committee Report: SIC Task Force appraisal of clinical diagnostic criteria for Parkinsonian disorders. *Mov Disord* **18**:467–86.

Löwenberg K (1936). Pick's disease: a clinicopathologic contribution. *Arch Neurol Psychiatr* **36**:768–89.

Magherini A, Litvan I (2005). Cognitive and behavioral aspects of PSP since Steele, Richardson and Olszewski's description of PSP 40 years ago and Albert's delineation of the subcortical dementia 30 years ago. *Neurocase* **11**:250–62.

Maher ER, Smith EM, Lees AJ (1985). Cognitive deficits in the Steele–Richardson–Olszewski syndrome (progressive supranuclear palsy). *J Neurol Neurosurg Psychiatry* **48**:1234–9.

Masellis M, Momeni P, Meschino W *et al.* (2006). Novel splicing mutation in the progranulin gene causing familial corticobasal syndrome. *Brain* **129**: 3115–23.

Massman PJ, Kreiter KT, Jankovic J, Doody RS (1996). Neuropsychological functioning in cortical-basal ganglionic degeneration: differentiation from Alzheimer's disease. *Neurology* **46**:720–6.

Mathuranath PS, Xuereb JH, Bak T, Hodges JR (2000). Corticobasal ganglionic degeneration and/or frontotemporal dementia? A report of two overlap cases and a review of literature. *J Neurol Neurosurg Psychiatry* **68**:304–12.

McMonagle P, Blair M, Kertesz A (2006a). Corticobasal degeneration and progressive aphasia. *Neurology* **67**:1444–51.

McMonagle P, Deering F, Berliner Y, Kertesz A (2006b). The cognitive profile of posterior cortical atrophy. *Neurology* **66**:331–8.

Mendez MF (2000). Corticobasal ganglionic degeneration with Balint's syndrome. *J Neuropsychiatry Clin Neurosci* **12**:273–5.

Merians AS, Clark M, Poizner H *et al.* (1999). Apraxia differs in corticobasal degeneration and left-parietal stroke: a case study. *Brain Cogn* **40**:314–35.

Mesulam MM (2001). Primary progressive aphasia. *Ann Neurol* **49**:425–32.

Milberg W, Albert M (1989). Cognitive differences between patients with progressive supranuclear palsy and Alzheimer's disease. *J Clin Exp Neuropsychol* **11**:605–14.

Mimura M, Oda T, Tsuchiya K *et al.* (2001). Corticobasal degeneration presenting with nonfluent primary progressive aphasia: a clinicopathological study. *J Neurol Sci* **183**:19–26.

Monza D, Soliveri P, Radice D *et al.* (1998). Cognitive dysfunction and impaired organization of complex motility in degenerative parkinsonian syndromes. *Arch Neurol* **55**:372–8.

Munoz D (1998). The pathology of Pick complex. In *Pick's Disease and Pick Complex*, eds. Kertesz A and Munoz D. New York: Wiley-Liss, pp. 211–43.

Naville F (1922). Les complications et les sequelles mentales de l'encephalite epidemique; la bradyphrenie. *Encephale* **17**:369–75.

Neary D, Snowden JS, Gustafson L *et al.* (1998). Frontotemporal lobar degeneration. A consensus on clinical diagnostic criteria. *Neurology* **51**:1546–54.

Neary D, Snowden J, Mann D (2005). Frontotemporal dementia. *Lancet Neurol* **4**:771–80.

Okuda B, Tachibana H (1994). The nature of apraxia in corticobasal degeneration. *J Neurol Neurosurg Psychiatry* **57**:1548–9.

Ozsancak C, Auzou P, Hannequin D (2000). Dysarthria and orofacial apraxia in corticobasal degeneration. *Mov Disord* **15**:905–10.

Paviour DC, Winterburn D, Simmonds S *et al.* (2005). Can the frontal assessment battery (FAB) differentiate bradykinetic rigid syndromes? Relation of the FAB to formal neuropsychological testing. *Neurocase* **11**:274–82.

Pharr V, Uttl B, Stark M *et al.* (2001). Comparison of apraxia in corticobasal degeneration and progressive supranuclear palsy. *Neurology* **56**:957–63.

Pillon B, Dubois B, Ploska A, Agid Y (1991). Severity and specificity of cognitive impairment in Alzheimer's, Huntington's, and Parkinson's diseases and progressive supranuclear palsy. *Neurology* **41**:634–43.

Pillon B, Deweer B, Agid Y, Dubois B (1993). Explicit memory in Alzheimer's, Huntington's, and Parkinson's diseases. *Arch Neurol* **50**:374–9.

Pillon B, Deweer B, Michon A *et al.* (1994). Are explicit memory disorders of progressive supranuclear palsy related to damage to striatofrontal circuits? Comparison with Alzheimer's, Parkinson's, and Huntington's diseases. *Neurology* **44**:1264–70.

Pillon B, Blin J, Vidailhet M *et al.* (1995). The neuropsychological pattern of corticobasal degeneration: comparison with progressive supranuclear palsy and Alzheimer's disease. *Neurology* **45**:1477–83.

Pirtosek Z, Jahanshahi M, Barrett G, Lees AJ (2001). Attention and cognition in bradykinetic-rigid syndromes: an event-related potential study. *Ann Neurol* **50**:567–73.

Quencer K, Okun MS, Crucian G *et al.* (2007). Limb-kinetic apraxia in Parkinson disease. *Neurology* **68**:150–1.

Rebeiz JJ, Kolodny EH, Richardson EP Jr. (1968). Corticodentatonigral degeneration with neuronal achromasia. *Arch Neurol* **18**:20–33.

Riley DE, Lang AE, Lewis MB *et al.* (1990). Cortical-basal ganglionic degeneration. *Neurology* **40**:1203–12.

Rinne JO, Lee MS, Thompson PD, Marsden CD (1994). Corticobasal degeneration: a clinical study of 36 cases. *Brain* **117**:1183–96.

Robbins TW, James M, Owen AM *et al.* (1994). Cognitive deficits in progressive supranuclear palsy, Parkinson's disease, and multiple system atrophy in tests sensitive to frontal lobe dysfunction. *J Neurol Neurosurg Psychiatry* **57**:79–88.

Robinson G, Shallice T, Cipolotti L (2006). Dynamic aphasia in progressive supranuclear palsy: a deficit in generating a fluent sequence of novel thought. *Neuropsychologia* **44**:1344–60.

Ross ED (1981). The aprosodias: functional–anatomic organization of the affective components of language in the right hemisphere. *Arch Neurol* **38**:561–9.

Sakuri Y, Hashida H, Uesugi H *et al.* (1996). A clinical profile of corticobasal degeneration presenting as primary progressive aphasia. *Eur Neurol* **36**:134–7.

Scully RE, Mark EJ, McNeely BU (1985). Case records of the Massachusetts General Hospital (case 38 – 1985). *N Engl J Med* **313**:739–48.

Sha S, Hou C, Viskontas IV, Miller BL (2006). Are frontotemporal lobar degeneration, progressive supranuclear palsy and corticobasal degeneration distinct diseases? *Nat Clin Pract Neurol* **2**:658–65.

Snowden JS, Goulding PJ, Neary D (1989). Semantic dementia: a form of circumscribed cerebral atrophy. *Behav Neurol* **2**:167–82.

Soliveri P, Monza D, Paridi D *et al.* (2000). Neuropsychological follow up in patients with Parkinson's disease, striatonigral degeneration-type multisystem atrophy, and progressive supranuclear palsy. *J Neurol Neurosurg Psychiatry* **69**:313–18.

Soliveri P, Piacentini S, Girotti F (2005). Limb apraxia in corticobasal degeneration and progressive supranuclear palsy. *Neurology* **64**:448–53.

Spatt J, Bak T, Bozeat S, Patterson K, Hodges JR (2002). Apraxia, mechanical problem solving and semantic knowledge: contributions to object usage in corticobasal degeneration. *J Neurol* **249**:601–8.

Steele JC, Richardson JC, Olszewski J (1964). Progressive supranuclear palsy. A heterogeneous degeneration involving the brain stem, basal ganglia and cerebellum with vertical gaze and pseudobulbar palsy, nuchal dystonia and dementia. *Arch Neurol* **10**:333–59.

Tang-Wai DF, Josephs KA, Boeve BF *et al.* (2003). Pathologically confirmed corticobasal degeneration presenting with visuospatial dysfunction. *Neurology* **61**:1134–5.

Tang-Wai DF, Graff-Radford NR, Boeve BF *et al.* (2004). Clinical, genetic, and neuropathologic characteristics of posterior cortical atrophy. *Neurology* **63**:1168–74.

Tsao JW, Dickey DH, Heilman KM (2004). Emotional prosody in primary progressive aphasia. *Neurology* **63**:192–3.

Tucker DM, Watson RT, Heilman KM (1977). Discrimination and intonation of affectively intoned speech in patients with right parietal disease. *Neurology* **27**:947–50.

Watts RL, Williams RS, Growden JD *et al.* (1985). Corticobasal ganglionic degeneration. *Neurology* **35**(S1):178.

Wenning GK, Litvan I, Jankovic J *et al.* (1998). Natural history and survival of 14 patients with corticobasal degeneration confirmed at postmortem examination. *J Neurol Neurosurg Psychiatry* **64**:184–9.

Zadikoff C, Lang AE (2005). Apraxia in movement disorders. *Brain* **128**:1480–97.

Chapter 21

Cognitive and behavioral abnormalities of vascular dementia

Jee H. Jeong, Eun-Joo Kim, Sang Won Seo and Duk L. Na

Introduction

Vascular dementia (VaD) is a cognitive syndrome caused by cerebrovascular disease with clinically apparent ischemic or hemorrhagic lesions. It is not synonymous with post-stroke dementia, which refers to any type of dementia developed after a clinical stroke, irrespective of the presumed cause for the dementia (Pasquier *et al.*, 1997). Unlike Alzheimer's disease (AD), which is accepted as the most common cause of dementia, reports on VaD show remarkably variable prevalence. Compared with western countries, the prevalence of VaD seems somewhat higher in eastern Asian countries such as China, South Korea and Japan, ranking second (Lee *et al.*, 2002; Zhang *et al.*, 2005; Dong *et al.*, 2007) or even approaching the prevalence of AD (Yanagihara 2002). As the occurrence of stroke rises exponentially with age, the contribution of vascular disease to the incidence, pathogenesis and clinical course of dementia is becoming more important in the elderly. Also, the incidence of AD doubles in stroke patients, confounding understanding of the relative contribution of the two conditions to clinical status and treatment (Kokmen *et al.*, 1996). Importantly, cognitive decline after stroke is common. In patients with a first stroke, fully one-fourth develop a newly diagnosed dementia within 1 year after the event (Andersen *et al.*, 1996). Similarly, the relative risk of new onset of dementia is 5.5 within 4 years after first ever stroke (Tatemichi *et al.*, 1994).

The clinical patterns of VaD differ, depending on the vessels involved (large versus small vessel), location of vascular lesions and the stages of disease. It is increasingly accepted that prevention of stroke protects cognitive reserve, diminishing the likelihood that dementia will occur. In this chapter, to aid in accurate diagnosis of vascular dementia, we aim to describe the behavioral and cognitive aspects of different subtypes of vascular dementia.

Diagnostic criteria for vascular dementia

The diagnostic key for identifying VaD is to determine the relevant neurological and neuropsychological findings and recognize the corresponding lesions on brain imaging. Clinical skills for detailed informant interview and neurological examination of the patients are essential.

There are several diagnostic working criteria in use. These include the *Diagnostic and Statistical Manual of Mental Disorders*, 4th edition (DSM-IV) (American Psychiatric Association 1994), the *International Classification of Diseases*, 10th revision (ICD-10) (World Health Organization 1993), criteria of the State of California Alzheimer's Disease Diagnostic and Treatment Centers (ADDTC) (Chui *et al.*, 1992) and the criteria of the National Institute of Neurological Disorders and Stroke and the Association Internationale pour la Recherche at L'Enseignement en Neurosciences (NINDS-AIREN) (Roman *et al.*, 1993a–c). The Hachinski Ischemic Score (HIS) incorporates the cardinal features of VaD to clinically differentiate it from AD (Hachinski *et al.*, 1975). The components of HIS including stepwise deterioration (odds ratio [OR], 6.0), fluctuating course (OR, 7.6), history of hypertension (OR, 4.3) and history of stroke (OR, 4.3) help to differentiate VaD from AD in pathologically confirmed cases (Moroney *et al.*, 1997). These criteria are not interchangeable; variation in definition and vascular cause leads to the identification of different subject groups and different types, confounding and complicating the interpretation of clinical trials results. Some of these criteria can be found in the Appendix at the end of this chapter.

Subtypes of vascular dementia

The differing etiologies for cerebrovascular disease have predilections for vessels of different sizes, giving rise to relatively distinctive clinical subtypes and syndromes, all placed under the category of VaD. Division can be into large vessel disease or small vessel disease based on the vessels involved. Vascular dementia associated with large vessel disease can be caused by single or multiple territory infarctions in cortical or subcortical locations. Small vessel disease usually involves subcortical structures such as deep gray matter (basal ganglia and thalamus) or cerebral white matter (periventricular and deep white matter), leading to subcortical vascular dementia (SVaD). If the lesions are predominantly located in deep gray matter, this type of SVaD is called lacunar state; if the lesions are predominantly located in white matter, it is called Binswanger's disease (Erkinjuntti et al., 2000).

In the earlier stages of VaD, the cognitive impairment can be mild enough so as not to interfere with daily functions. Researchers call this state vascular cognitive impairment with no dementia (VCIND) (Rockwood et al., 1999) or vascular mild cognitive impairment (MCI) (Petersen 2000; Rasquin et al., 2004). This topic is discussed in Ch. 12. If VCIND or vascular MCI is not successfully managed, it will eventually evolve into VaD associated with multiple recurrent cortical or subcortical territorial infarction, SVaD, or a combination of both.

Dementia associated with cortical territorial infarction

Single or multiple cortical infarct dementia

The concept of multi-infarct dementia (MID), as outlined in the NINDS-AIREN International Workgroup criteria, defines an illness in which multiple cognitive deficits occur with multiple large-vessel strokes involving cerebral cortical areas, resulting in a clinical dementia syndrome (Roman et al., 1993a–c). Dementia follows an obvious clinical history of stroke, and a temporal relationship between the stroke and dementia onset is required. Focal neurological deficits such as hemiparesis, lower facial weakness, Babinski sign, sensory deficit, hemianopsia and dysarthria typically accompany this type of VaD. Stepwise progression of cognitive deficits and the close association between clinical features and lesion locations usually make MID easy to

recognize (Hachinski et al., 1975). Box 21.1 describes a typical patient with MID and Fig. 21.1 shows the magnetic resonance images (MRI) for this patient.

The total lesion volume size, the number of lesions and the location of individual lesions are critical factors in the pathogenesis of MID (e.g. in general, the larger the infarct size, the more severe the dementia) (De Reuck et al., 1981; Erkinjuntti 1987). In contrast, quantitative correlations between the degree of cognitive deficits and lesion volumes or lesion locations has not been clearly elucidated (Erkinjuntti et al., 1999). The NINDS-AIREN criteria provide only a limited suggestion that bilateral anterior cerebral artery (ACA) distribution, posterior cerebral artery (PCA) distribution, parietotemporal and temporo-occipital association areas and superior frontal and parietal watershed territories are considered the major candidate areas for VaD (Roman et al., 1993a–c). Multiple infarctions of any combination of these restricted cortical regions can result in MID.

In contrast to MID, even a single cortical infarction can lead to dementia. Damage to critical regions such as the angular gyrus or anterior cingulate gyrus also may cause cognitive deficits that lead to VaD (Benson and Cummings 1982; Tatemichi et al., 1990). Therefore, the behavioral neurology of MID or single cortical infarct dementia requires understanding the cognitive and behavioral deficits following cerebral cortical infarction in distribution of ACA, PCA or middle cerebral artery (MCA), which we briefly review in this section.

Anterior cerebral artery territory infarction

The hemispheric branches of the ACAs supply the medial frontal surface (supplementary motor area; paracentral lobule, cingulate gyrus), the inferior frontal surface and part of the medial parietal lobes (anterior portion of precuneus). The pericallosal branches of the ACAs supply the anterior four-fifths of the corpus callosum (Brust et al., 2001). Therefore, ACA infarction mainly causes medial and inferior frontal dysfunction.

The functions of frontal lobe are too broad and complex to detail here but include elementary motor function, praxis, speech/language output, attention, working memory, executive function, social judgement and comportment (Absher and Cummings 1995). Consequently, frontal lobe damage may result in a variety of behavioral and cognitive disorders, which can be classified under three major categories: first, executive dysfunction followed by dorsolateral

Box 21.1 Multi-infarct dementia

A 65-year-old man with a history of hypertension and heart disease had a history of three strokes. After the first stroke (Fig. 21.1A), he experienced a sudden onset of comprehension deficits, which partially improved soon after; otherwise, his daily functioning and judgement were preserved. One year after this episode, he had the second stroke. According to his wife, his general cognitive dysfunction worsened at that time. He showed markedly decreased speech output and profound lethargy. He slept all day and expressed no interest in doing anything. He was not able to concentrate on watching TV programs and could not understand them. Three months later, his symptoms improved slightly but 6 months thereafter, new symptoms developed (third stroke). When having a meal, he was noted to eat food only from the right side of his plate. Walking down the hall, he travelled along the right side and upon reaching an intersection he always chose a path to the right. He had difficulty in wearing clothes, recalling the location of personal items and remembering his activities just the day before. He got lost on the way home. Neurological examinations revealed left facial weakness, left hemiparesis (grade IV), increased deep tendon reflex on the left upper and lower extremities, positive Babinski sign on the left, decreased arm swing on the left and left hemispatial neglect. His Korean version MMSE score was 17 out of 30. An MRI scan showed the infarct involving the left temporal area, the right frontal area as well as the right parietal area (Fig. 21.1C).

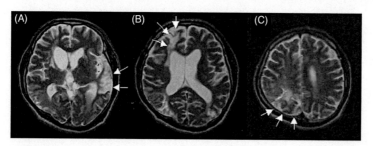

Fig. 21.1. Magnetic resonance T$_2$-weighted images of the patient described in Box 21.1, showing an infarct in left temporal area (A: first stroke), the other infarct in right frontal (B: second stroke) and the third in right parietal area (C).

Comment

This patient meets NINDS-AIREN criteria for probable VaD since there were impairments of memory and of two or more cognitive domains, evidence of cerebrovascular disease by focal signs on neurologic examinations and brain imaging, and a temporal relationship between the dementia and the strokes. At the first attack, he had mild language impairment that improved to the extent that he was able to manage his daily activities. After the second stroke, however, abnormal behavior and impaired judgement led him to withdraw from complex activities although this improved slightly over time. After the third stroke, he declined significantly and was no longer able to do basic activities such as dressing or eating. As we can see, there were clinical features of a stepwise deterioration over 2 years, with a fluctuating course associated with acute deficits followed by partial recovery. This was caused by three territorial infarctions without subcortical ischemic changes or lacunes and led to the diagnosis of MID.

frontal lobe damage; second, akinetic mutism or the apathy-abulia spectrum in medial frontal damage; and, third, disinhibition or aquired sociopathy in orbito-frontal damage (Cummings 1993, Fig. 21.2). Dorsolateral frontal lobe dysfunction will be discussed in the section on MCA infarctions.

Akinetic mutism, the sign of bilateral damage to the medial frontal lobe, is the most extreme form of a loss of spontaneity or initiative. Patients with akinetic mutism make no effort to communicate verbally or by gesture. Abulia, the minor form of akinetic mutism, can also follow medial frontal damage. The patient seems to be indifferent and less interested in the environment and people around him or her, has little spontaneous verbal output and responds to questions very briefly, often with prolonged response latencies. Left to his or her own devices, the patient stays indoors, seated and immobile.

Orbitofrontal lobe damage can produce disinhibition and impulsive behaviors. Impulse control failures result in excessive sexual drives, voracious appetites and addiction to alcohol, tobacco or drugs. Some patients exhibit compulsive behavior (e.g. cleaning, checking, arranging, ordering, hoarding or counting). One example would be a case reported by Hahm and his colleagues (2001). A 46-year-old patient showed a pathologic collecting behavior after a left orbitofrontal and caudate injury from an aneurysmal rupture of anterior communicating artery (Fig. 21.3A). Interestingly, his hoarding, an impulse control disorder or an

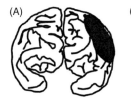 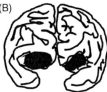 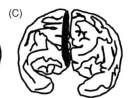

(A) (B) (C)

Fig. 21.2. Frontal lobe dysfunctions. (A) Dorsolateral frontal: executive dysfunction; (B) orbitofrontal: disinhibition or aquired sociopathy; (C) medial frontal: reduced motivation and spontaneity (akinetic mutism or abulia).

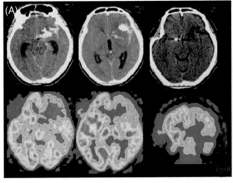 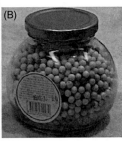

(A) (B)

Fig. 21.3. (A) Computed tomographic (CT) scans on admission (upper left two slices) shows subarachnoid hemorrhage with a hematoma involving the left orbitofrontal region, which became a low-density lesion on a CT scan performed 2 years after onset (upper right slice). Fluorodeoxyglucose [^{18}F]- positron emission tomography performed 2 years after onset (lower row) shows glucose hypometabolism in the left caudate and frontal lobe, mildly in the anterior temporal area and most prominent in the orbitofrontal region. (B) A sample bottle containing the toy bullets collected by the patient.

ego-syntonic compulsion, was restricted to one specific item (toy bullets) (Fig. 21.3B).

Other behavioral disorders associated with orbitofrontal damage may include utilization and imitation behaviors. Utilization behavior has been described as "a disturbance in responses to external stimuli, so that a patient with utilization behavior simply takes and uses the object presented to them" (Lhermitte *et al.,* 1986). Imitation behavior is characterized by "patients' imitating the gestures and behavior of the examiner without having been asked to do so, and continuing to imitate after being asked to stop" (Lhermitte *et al.,* 1986). These two "environmental dependency" syndromes are classified as a unilateral orbitofrontal symptom, without clear relation to the hemispheric dominance, and are interpreted as a release of the parietal approach behavior to visual and tactile stimulation from the outside world (Lhermitte 1983; Lhermitte *et al.,* 1986).

Acquired sociopathy is another frequent consequence of orbitofrontal damage (Tranel 1994). Orbitofrontal lobe, gyrus rectus and anterior cingulate gyrus serve to integrate sensory association cortex information (occipital lobe, temporal lobe and parietal lobe) with limbic cortical control of emotional responses. Normally, people can be affected by external stimuli that drive positive or negative emotions in order to make a proper decision, but the patient with orbitofrontal or anterior cingulate gyrus lesions may not be able to appropriately understand or respond to the external stimuli, such that he or she

cannot achieve normal social or emotional decision making (Gazzaniga *et al.,* 2002).

Heilman and Watson (1991) suggested that effective interaction with the environment required the presence of two critical motor systems, which they called the "how" system (praxis system) and the "when" system (intentional system). Disorders of the "how" or praxis program are called apraxias, while damage to the "when" or intentional programs are referred to as motor intentional disorder or action-intentional disorder. The pathophysiology for ideomotor apraxia is controversial. Damage to the anterior corpus callosum can result in left hand apraxia because it disconnects the left hemisphere language areas from the right movement control area for the left hand (language–motor disconnection; Wernicke 1874). Geschwind (1965a,b) postulated that auditory stimuli from primary auditory cortex (Heschl's gyrus) are conveyed to the auditory association cortex (Wernickes's area) in the left hemisphere, which is connected to premotor cortex by the arcuate fasciculus; the premotor cortex on the left is connected to the left primary motor cortex. The information in the left premotor cortex can also be conveyed to the right premotor cortex through the anterior corpus callosum. According to Geschwind's schema (Fig. 21.4), any lesions of this pathway (premotor cortex, anterior corpus callosum, arcuate fasciculus) can cause ideomotor apraxia.

Motor intentional disorder is divided into four different types: (1) akinesia, a failure of initiation of

305

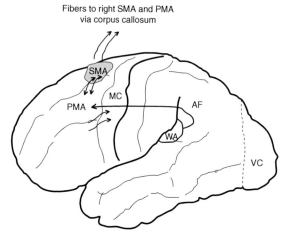

Fibers to right SMA and PMA
via corpus callosum

Fig. 21.4. Geschwind's (1965a,b) schema. AF, arcuate fasciculus; VC, visual cortex; PMA, premotor area; SMA, supplementary motor area; WA, Wernicke's area; MC, motor cortex.

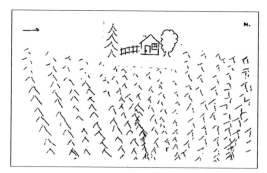

Fig. 21.5. Perseveration on the Ogden copying task by a 65-year-old man with acute left frontotemporal infarction.

movement in the absence of a corticospinal or motor neuron lesion; (2) hypokinesia, a delay in initiating a response; (3) motor impersistence, the inability to sustain a movement or posture; and (4) motor perseveration, the inability to stop a movement or an action program (Fig. 21.5). While ideomotor apraxias are usually associated with left hemisphere dysfunction (Heilman and Rothi, 1982), right hemisphere damage may be dominant for intentional control of the motor systems (Heilman and van den Abell 1979). Networks that mediate the intentional systems are widely distributed and have not been fully elucidated, but the fact that the frontal lobes play a critical role is supported by many human lesion studies and experimental animal studies: limb akinesia for medial frontal lesion (Meador *et al.*, 1986), directional limb hypokinesia for frontoparietal lesions (Heilman *et al.*, 1985), motor impersistence for dorsolateral frontal lesions (Kertesz *et al.*, 1985) and motor perseveration for frontal subcortical lesions (Sandson and Albert 1987).

Patients with infarctions of the anterior corpus callosum can display a callosal disconnection syndrome, including left hand ideomotor apraxia, left hand agraphia, left hand tactile anomia, right hand acopia and intermanual conflict (Kolb and Whishaw 2003). Recently, Seo *et al.* (2007) reported that after an infarction involving the right medial frontal lobe and corpus callosum, a 66-year-old right-handed man demonstrated right limb motor impersistence on bedside evaluation, which was substantiated experimentally. This suggested that following a callosal lesion, motor impersistence occurs more frequently in the

dominant than the non-dominant limb. Secondary mania featuring euphoria, pressured speech and hyperactivity is frequently associated with lesions of orbitofrontal cortex, almost always in the right hemisphere (Starkstein and Robinson 1991).

The elementary neurologic symptoms and signs of ACA stroke are contralateral to motor and sensory deficits (leg predominant weakness). Bilateral ACA occlusions can produce paraparesis with or without sensory loss. Pathologic reflexes such as grasp, groping, snout and sucking reflexes may appear unilaterally or bilaterally in hands, feet or around the mouth (Damasio and Anderson 2003). Urinary incontinence and disturbance of sphincter control have been described in superior frontal and cingulate gyrus damage (Andrew and Nathan 1964).

Middle cerebral artery territory infarction

Cortical areas supplied by the MCA include, superiorly, the frontal, parietal and occipital convexities and, inferiorly, the temporal convexity. Not surprisingly, cognitive and behavioral deficits resulting from MCA infarction are as variable as the location of the lesion.

As noted above, dorsolateral prefrontal cortex is a critical area for executive function (Fig. 21.2). Executive functions include planning, goal monitoring, and fluency and flexibility of thought in the generation of solutions. Patients with dorsolateral prefrontal damages may not be able to formulate a plan of action, consider possible different plans (impairment of mental fluency) or switch from one plan to another, which is required for success of ongoing actions (impairment of cognitive set-shifting). Motor intentional disorders such as directional hypokinesia, motor impersistence and motor perseveration have also been reported in dorsolateral prefrontal lesions, mostly when the right hemisphere is affected.

The typical clinical picture of superficial MCA territory infarctions include sudden onset of contralateral sensorimotor deficits, with aphasia in left hemispheric (dominant hemisphere) lesions and visuospatial impairment and neglect syndrome in right hemispheric (non-dominant hemisphere) lesions. The relative severity of motor deficits from mild hemiparesis to complete hemiplegia depends on the location and size of the infarction. Hemisensory loss affecting all sensory modalities can be produced, as can cortical sensory loss with agraphesthesia, astereognosis and failure of two-point discrimination. Approximately 90–95% of right-handed individuals have language dominance in the left hemisphere (Ropper *et al.*, 2005), so left MCA infarctions frequently cause aphasia syndromes. Rarely, right hemisphere lesions can produce aphasia in right handers (Zangwill 1979). Broca's aphasia consists of non-fluent, effortful speech with relatively preserved comprehension and follows damage to the left inferior frontal gyrus (Broca's area: pars opercularis and pars triangularis) and its adjacent areas. The hallmark of Wernicke's aphasia is fluent speech with disturbance of auditory comprehension, derived from the damage of the posterior one-third of the superior temporal gyrus and its adjacent areas. Global aphasia is caused by a large stroke encompassing Broca's and Wernicke's areas (Fig. 21.6). Patients with global aphasia have decreased spontaneous speech and comprehension and impaired repetition, reading and writing (Broca 1977; Damasio 1981; Benson 1988). Damage to the arcuate fasciculus, the fibers connecting the Broca's and Wernicke's areas, and the inferior parietal lobule (supramarginal gyrus) cause conduction aphasia characterized by impaired repetition and preserved comprehension (Damasio and Damasio 1983). Transcortical aphasias show preserved repetition. They result from the lesions affecting structures surrounding perisylvian language centers (Broca's and Wernicke's areas) with spared perisylvian cortex and arcuate fasciculus (Devinsky 1992). Destruction of the dominant supplementary motor area is a common pathogenic mechanism for transcortical motor aphasia (Freedman *et al.*, 1984) and lesions in the temporoparieto-occipital area for transcortical sensory aphasia (Alexander *et al.*, 1989).

Ideomotor apraxia is defined by the inability to perform previously learned or skilled movement in

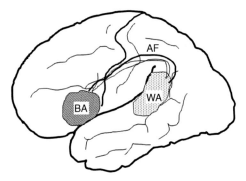

Fig. 21.6. Perisylvian language centers and their connections. BA, Broca's area; WA, Wernicke's area; AF, Arcuate fasciculus.

response to commands that cannot be explained by weakness, sensory loss, abnormal movement, poor comprehension or inattention. A lesion at any point along Geschwind's schema (1965a, b, see Fig. 21.4) can cause an ideomotor apraxia. Alternatively, Heilman and colleagues (1982) suggested that knowledge of motor skills, or the time–space motor representation (praxicon), is stored in the dominant parietal cortex (angular gyrus, supramarginal gyrus). Therefore, left parietal lesions can also produce ideomotor apraxia.

The posterior part of inferior parietal lobule (angular gyrus) is a heteromodal association cortex that responds to stimulation in more than one sensory modality (Mesulam *et al.*, 1977). Damage to this higher-order, supramodal cortex gives rise to impairments of multimodal interaction related to praxis (see above) and language, such as anomia, alexia and Gerstmann's syndrome (acalculia, agraphia, finger agnosia and right–left disorientation [Gerstmann 1940]), which together compose the angular gyrus syndrome.

Given that the right posterior parietal lobe is dominant for visuospatial integration and spatial attention (Benton *et al.*, 1978; Heilman and van den Abell 1980), lesions of the right parietal multimodal association cortex can yield visuospatial dysfunction and a neglect syndrome. Visuospatial function is categorized into visuoperceptual function, geographical orientation and visuoconstructive ability (Benton and Tranel 1993). Visuoperceptual function is considered as an ability to discriminate angles, shapes and colors of the presented object, or decide whether two faces are the same or different. Geographical orientation refers to the selective way-finding ability within a three-dimensional environment or two-dimensional map. The ability to copy, draw, or construct two- or three-dimensional figures or shapes can be defined

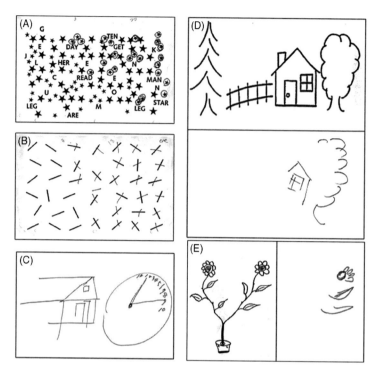

Fig. 21.7. Examples of left hemispatial neglect. A, star cancellation task (Halligan *et al.*, 1991); B, modified version of Albert's line cancellation task (Albert 1973); C, spontaneous drawing (house, clock); D, copying modified Ogden scene (Ogden 1985); E, copying two daisy figure (Marshall *et al.*, 1993).

as visuoconstructive function. Though visuospatial dysfunction predominantly follows right-sided posterior lesions, visuoperceptual and visuoconstructional impairments can follow bilateral posterior injury (Farah 2003).

Unilateral spatial neglect is a clinical syndrome in which patients are unaware of or fail to explore stimuli located in the contralesional half of extrapersonal space, even in the absence of primary sensory or motor deficit (Heilman and Rothi 2003a,b, Fig. 21.7). It can result from a variety of lesions, both cortical and subcortical, but the temporoparietal cortex is known to be one of the most critical anatomical substrates for hemispatial neglect (Mort *et al.*, 2003; Vallar *et al.*, 2003; Karnath *et al.*, 2004, 2005; Hillis *et al.*, 2005). Patients with neglect syndrome often exhibit reluctant or reduced movement toward the contralesional space, even though they have no sensory attentional problems. This type of neglect is called motor-intentional neglect, as opposed to sensory-attentional neglect (Heilman and Rothi 2003b). As mentioned above, since right frontal cortex is essential for motor intention, lesions causing intentional neglect usually include the right frontal area (Na *et al.*, 1998). Patients with neglect syndrome sometimes deny or fail to recognize their hemiplegia (anosognosia for hemiplegia; Babinski 1914) or

that their contralesional extremities are their own (personal neglect or asomatognosia; Beschin and Robertson 1997).

In addition to visuospatial function and spatial attention, the right parietal lobe is dominant for affective prosody. Consequently, patients with right hemisphere injury have greater difficulty regulating and understanding emotional components of language than patients with left hemispheric lesions (Tucker *et al.*, 1977; Ross 1981).

In terms of psychiatric symptoms, delirium or acute confusional state is most commonly associated with right MCA infarction involving right middle temporal gyrus or inferior parietal lobule (Mesulam *et al.*, 1976; Mori and Yamadori 1987). In contrast, post-stroke depression can be the prominent manifestation of left MCA infarction affecting the left fronto-opercular region (Starkstein *et al.*, 1987; Kim and Choi 2000).

Posterior cerebral artery territory infarction

The PCA arises from the terminal bifurcation of the basilar artery and has four main cortical branches: the anterior temporal, posterior temporal, parietooccipital and calcarine arteries, which supply the occipital lobes and the inferomedial portions of the temporal lobes. The most common neurological deficit in the

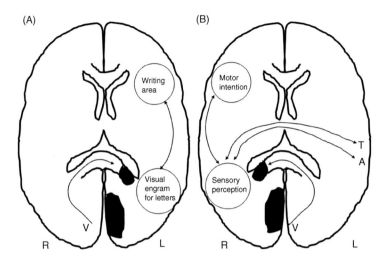

Fig. 21.8. (A) Alexia without agraphia. The visual information from right visual cortex cannot reach the left inferior parietal language area because of splenial lesion. (B) Left spatial neglect limited to visual modality and caused by right occipital plus splenium lesion. T, thalamus; V, ventricle; A, angular gyrus.

PCA infarction is a contralateral visual-field defect caused by the lesion of the primary visual cortex, the optic radiation or the lateral geniculate body (Fisher 1986). Complex visual abnormalities, such as simple or formed visual hallucinations localized to the affected visual field or visual perseveration (palinopsia and illusory visual spread) are often present in the PCA infarction (Critchley 1951; Lance 1976; Brust and Behrens 1977). Alexia without agraphia is a classic symptom that results from a lesion in the left calcarine cortex and adjacent splenium of the corpus callosum (De Renzi et al., 1987). It is usually accompanied by color anomia (Geschwind and Fusillo 1966). The symptomatology is interpreted as a disconnection of the visual input to the intact right visual cortex from the left language area (Fig. 21.8A). If the lesion extends to the left angular gyrus, alexia with agraphia, Gerstmann's syndrome (acalculia, agraphia, right-left confusion, finger agnosia) and ideomotor apraxia are often present. Patients with left PCA infarction may have transcortical sensory aphasia, although aphasia is not common in left PCA infarction (Kertesz et al., 1982).

Luders et al. (1991) observed that global aphasia was produced by electric stimulation of the dominant basal temporal region known as the basal temporal language area (BTLA). Interestingly, in the countries such as Korea or Japan where people use language that can be written in both ideogram (a graphic record of a meaning) and phonogram (a graphic record of a sound), dissociation between ideogram and phonogram impairment after brain injury has been reported.

Kwon et al. (2002) reported that a 64-year-old right-handed man, who used to be a Hanja (Korean ideogram) calligrapher, showed alexia with agraphia in Hanja (Korean ideogram) but preserved Hangul (Korean phonogram) reading and writing after a left posterior inferior temporal infarction (Fig. 21.9), a similar area to the BTLA. This was consistent with previous reports about dissociation between Kanji (Japanese ideogram) and Kana (Japanese phonogram) processing (Kawamura et al., 1987; Soma et al., 1989).

The posterior temporal branch of the PCA supplies medial temporal structures (including the hippocampus), and unilateral occlusion of this artery (especially left) causes infarction of the hippocampus and medial temporal lobe, which leads to temporary amnesia. However, bilateral occlusion can produce permanent amnesia (Benson et al., 1974). Prosopagnosia, the inability to recognize familiar faces, is rarely developed by damage to the right fusiform gyrus (fusiform face area) (Kanwisher et al., 1997). If PCA infarction extends to the right parietal or temporal lobe, visuoconstructional disability and geographical disorientation can occur (Piercy et al., 1960; Fisher 1982). Visuospatial neglect also can be elicited by a lesion combining the right occipital lobe and splenium, an analog lesion of the left occipital lobe and splenium injury associated with alexia without agraphia (Park et al., 2005) (Fig. 21.8B). This visual neglect might be related to a disconnection between the visual information processed by the left occipital lobe and the right posterior temporoinferior parietal areas that mediate attention in the left

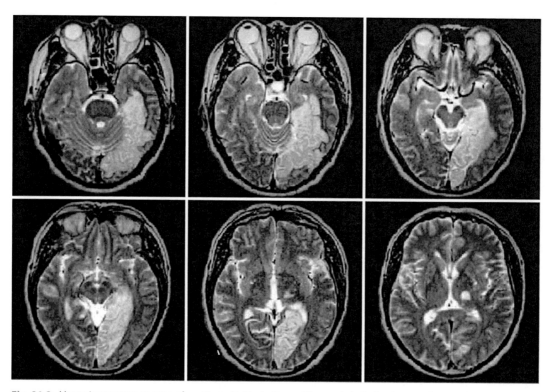

Fig. 21.9. Magnetic resonance imaging of a patient with Hanja (Korean ideogram) alexia showing an infarct involving the left lingual, fusiform and parahippocampal gyri and a lacune in the left thalamus.

hemispace. Additionally, in a large number of studies regarding hemispatial neglect in PCA infarction, it was reconfirmed that only the right occipital plus splenial lesion significantly influenced the frequency and severity of neglect (Park *et al.*, 2006). Bilateral destruction of primary visual cortex causes cortical blindness. Patients with cortical blindness are occasionally unaware of their visual loss. This is a phenomenon known as Anton's syndrome, or visual anosognosia. The mechanism and precise anatomy of visual anosognosia remains uncertain. On the contrary, patients with cortical blindness might have some residual visual function (blindsight) but are unaware of it and deny its existence (Poppel *et al.*, 1973; Aldrich *et al.*, 1987).

Ungerleider and Mishkin (1982) proposed that there are two parallel visual-processing pathways: a dorsal or occipitoparietal "where" pathway for spatial perception and visuomotor performance and a ventral or occipitotemporal "what" pathway for object discrimination and recognition. Patients with bilateral occipitoparietal lesion have Balint's syndrome, defined by a triad of simultanagnosia, the inability to recognize a picture or scene as a whole; optic ataxia, impaired

hand movement under visual guidance; and gaze apraxia, an inability to direct gaze voluntarily toward the peripheral field (Hecaen and de Ajuriaguerra 1954). Patients with bilateral occipitotemporal lesion have prosopagnosia, visual object agnosia (inability to identifying a visually presented object even with normal perception) and achromatopsia (acquired color blindness) (Albert *et al.*, 1979; Damasio *et al.*, 1980, 1982).

Ischemic-hypoperfusive vascular dementia
Behavioral and neuropsychological findings in borderzone infarction

There are two types of borderzone infarction: the anterior borderzone infarct is located between the superficial territories of the ACA and MCA while the posterior type is the infarction located between the superficial territories of the MCA and PCA (Fig. 21.10).

The anterior type located in the frontal parasagittal borderzone area manifests as somnolence and transcortical motor aphasia (Ringelstein *et al.*, 1983a,b; Bogousslavsky and Regli 1986, 1992). When the anterior borderzone infarct is located in the non-dominant

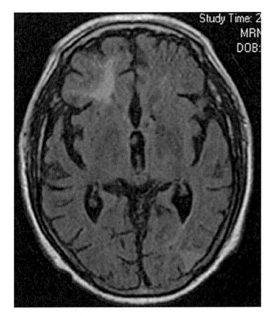

Fig. 21.10. Fluid attenuated inversion recovery (FLAIR) magnetic resonance image showing a right anterior borderzone infarction and left posterior borderzone infarction in a 92-year-old man who showed somnolence, abulia and mild right hemiparesis. Neuropsychological tests performed 10 days after symptom onset showed frontal executive dysfunction and transcortical sensory aphasia.

hemisphere, mood disturbances such as apathy or euphoria may also develop (Hashiguchi *et al.*, 2000). Sometimes the anterior borderzones are affected bilaterally, which results in akinetic mutism and apathy as well as focal neurological deficit such as paraparesis mimicking spinal lesion, quadriplegia or triplegia, or bladder disturbance (Ringelstein *et al.*, 1983a,b; Bogousslavsky and Regli 1986, 1992).

The posterior type located in parietotemporoccipital triangle produces Wernicke type of aphasia, hemispatial neglect, anosognosia, transcortical sensory aphasia, cortical hemihypesthesia, sensorimotor hemiparesis or hemianopia (Ringelstein *et al.*, 1983a, b; Bogousslavsky and Regli 1986, 1992).

Behavioral and neuropsychological findings in chronic hypoperfusion

The relation between chronic ischemia and cognitive functions in humans is not completely understood, but several reports have suggested that cognitive impairments can be associated with a chronic cerebral hypoperfusion state caused by a variety of medical conditions (Lass *et al.*, 1999; Zuccala *et al.*, 2001; Antonelli Incalzi *et al.*, 2003). For instance, cognitive

impairment is common among elderly people with systolic hypotension caused by heart failure (Zuccala *et al.*, 2001). A significant decline was observed in all cognitive domains except for attention and executive function between 1 and 5 years after coronary artery bypass grafting (Selnes *et al.*, 2001). Patients with chronic obstructive pulmonary disease showed cognitive decline of frontal type with worsening hypoxemia (Antonelli Incalzi *et al.*, 2003). It has been reported that the correction of a chronic cerebral hypoperfusion state can lead to recovery of mental decline (Tsuda *et al.*, 1994; Tatemichi *et al.*, 1995).

Cognitive impairment associated with chronic hypoperfusion is not as distinctive as that in anterior or posterior type of borderzone infarction (Roman 2004). It is characterized by slow onset and gradual progression. The periventricular white matter, basal ganglia (Pullicino *et al.*, 1993), and hippocampus (Crystal *et al.*, 1993) are susceptible to chronic ischemic hypoperfusive states. Therefore, interruption of prefrontal–basal ganglia circuits or hippocampal damage may explain the cognitive decline in these patients.

Dementia associated with stroke of subcortical location
Behavioral and neuropsychological features in basal ganglia lesions
Caudate infarction

Patients with infarcts in the territory of the lateral lenticulostriate arteries show motor and neuropsychological deficits whereas those with infarcts in the territory of the anterior lenticulostriate arteries have relatively mild neuropsychological deficits (Kumral *et al.*, 1999).

Caudate infarction often results in abnormal behavior and cognitive impairment (Mendez *et al.*, 1989; Caplan *et al.*, 1990; Kumral *et al.*, 1999) (Fig. 21.11). Hemichorea (Kawamura *et al.*, 1988) can occur, but happens less often. Abnormal behaviors associated with caudate infarction include abulia, apathy, blunting of response and lack of initiative (Mendez *et al.*, 1989; Caplan *et al.*, 1990; Kumral *et al.*, 1999). The mechanism of abulia can be explained by interruption of the limbic–frontal connection (Caplan *et al.*, 1990). Agitation, anxiety and talkativeness or disinhibition can also occur (Richfield *et al.*, 1987; Caplan *et al.*, 1990). Mendez *et al.* (1989) reported that dorsolateral caudate involvement may

311

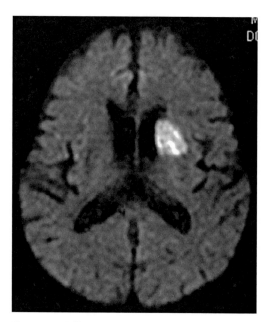

Fig. 21.11. Diffusion-weighted magnetic resonance imaging showing a left caudate infarction in an 80-year-old man who presented with abulia, lack of spontaneity and apathy. Neuropsychological tests, performed 10 days later, revealed frontal executive dysfunction, naming difficulty and mild memory impairment with retrieval defect type.

Lentiform nucleus infarction

Unilateral lentiform nucleus infarction (putamen and globus pallidus) commonly cause movement disorders such as dystonia but rarely cause neurobehavioral disorders such as abulia or disinhibition (Bhatia and Marsden 1994). It has also been reported that speech disturbance, obsessive–compulsive disorder and auditory hallucinations may occur in these patients (Maraganore *et al.*, 1991; Laplane *et al.*, 1992). Laplane *et al.* (1992) considered that these psychiatric disorders in globus pallidal lesions could be related to disturbances in the circuit linking the frontal associative cortex and the basal ganglia.

Capsular genu lesions

Cognitive impairment in capsular genu infarction (Fig. 21.12) is characterized by fluctuating alertness, inattention, memory loss, apathy, abulia and psychomotor retardation (Tatemichi *et al.*, 1992a). Several reports have shown that amnesia was the major presenting feature (Kooistra and Heilman 1988; Lai *et al.*, 1990; Terao *et al.*, 1991; Chukwudelunzu *et al.*, 2001) but other reports showed that pure abulia

cause decreased spontaneous verbal and motor activities and ventromedial lesions may result in disinhibited, inappropriate and impulsive behavior.

The common cognitive impairment is memory disturbance, with retrieval defect and aphasia (Mendez *et al.*, 1989; Caplan *et al.*, 1990; Kumral *et al.*, 1999). Patients with left caudate lesions have verbal amnesia, while patients with right caudate lesions show visual amnesia (Kumral *et al.*, 1999). Neuropsychological tests in caudate lesions show decreased free recall of episodic and semantic items, with good recognition memories scores (Mendez *et al.*, 1989). These abnormalities have been explained by the disconnection of the caudate from the frontal lobe (Pozzilli *et al.*, 1987; Kumral *et al.*, 1999). A variety of aphasia such as transcortical motor aphasia, characterized by semantic and verbal paraphasias and perseverations without comprehension impairment, occurs in patients with a left caudate lesion (Alexander *et al.*, 1987; Mendez *et al.*, 1989; Caplan *et al.*, 1990; Kumral *et al.*, 1999). Alexander *et al.* (1987) argued that acute disconnection of linguistic pathways between anterior and posterior speech areas, which are connected with the caudate nucleus, may yield aphasia.

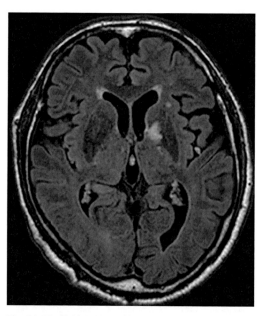

Fig. 21.12. Fluid-attenuated inversion recovery (FLAIR) magnetic resonance imaging showing a left genu portion of the internal capsule including the globus pallidum in a 79-year-old man who presented with memory impairment and behavioral changes such as abulia and apathy. Neuropsychological tests, performed 30 days later, revealed frontal executive dysfunction, naming difficulty and verbal memory impairment.

without other neurological deficits can occur (Yamanaka et al., 1996). The most prominent findings in capsular genu infarctions have been reported to be faciolingual and motor deficits as a result of the disruption of corticopontine and corticobulbar fibers (Bogousslavsky and Regli 1990), but other series have showed that pyramidal and corticobulbar tracts were minimally involved (Tatemichi et al., 1992a). Essential features of cognitive impairment in capsular genu infarct are similar, with the clinical features found in polar (Bogousslavsky et al., 1986) or paramedian thalamic infarction (Guberman and Stuss 1983).

The mechanism for cognitive impairments associated with genu infarctions seems to involve interruption of the inferior (Kooistra and Heilman 1988) and anterior (Tatemichi et al., 1992b) thalamic peduncles. The ventral amygdalofugal pathway sends fibers to the dorsomedial nucleus of thalamus via inferior thalamic peduncles (Klingler and Gloor 1960), and the efferent pathway of dorsomedial nucleus projects to the prefrontal cortex also through inferior thalamic peduncles (Krettek and Price 1977). Infarction of inferior thalamic peduncles that course in the vicinity of the genu of the internal capsule seemingly disconnect dorsal medial thalamus from amygdalae and the frontal cortex. Anterior thalamic peduncles convey reciprocal connections between the dorsomedial nucleus and the cingulate gyrus, as well as the prefrontal and orbitofrontal cortex (Nieuwenhuys et al., 1988). Functional brain imaging showed a focal hypoperfusion in ipsilateral inferior and medial frontal cortex (Tatemichi et al., 1992b; Yamanaka et al., 1996) and hypometabolic activity in the temporal cortex ipsilateral to the capsular lesion (Chukwudelunzu et al., 2001).

Behavioral and neuropsychological findings in thalamic lesions

Tuberothalamic arterial territory infarction

Cognitive and behavioral abnormalities after tuberothalamic artery infarction are anterograde amnesia, apathy and frontal executive dysfunction (Fig. 21.13). However, symptoms may differ depending on the hemisphere involved. Patients with left-sided lesions have transcortical aphasia, verbal and visual memory impairment and acalculia; patients with right-sided lesions show hemispatial neglect, visual memory impairment and disturbed visuospatial processing (Bogousslavsky et al., 1986).

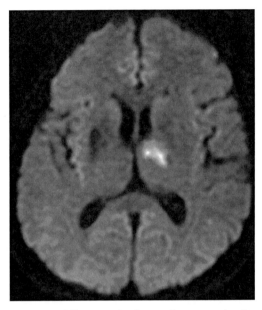

Fig. 21.13. Diffusion-weighted magnetic resonance imaging shows a right anterior thalamic infarct involving the anterior nucleus and mamillothalamic fasciculus in a 63-year-old man who developed anterograde amnesia and abulia.

Memory disturbance associated with thalamic infarction is usually described as "diencephalic amnesia" (von Cramon et al., 1985; Graff-Radford et al., 1990). The pattern of memory loss in patients with a thalamic lesion resembles that seen after lesions in the medial temporal area (Aggleton and Saunders 1997). The neuropsychological findings in patients with thalamic lesions are characterized by deficits of free recall and recognition (van der Werf et al., 2000, 2003a) but some studies suggest that the memory impairment is a retrieval deficit, that is, recognition better than recall (Ghika-Schmid and Bogousslavsky 2000; Carrera and Bogousslavsky 2006). Another feature that has been described in amnesia related to tuberothalamic infarction is "palipsychism." Ghika-Schmid and Bogousslavsky (2000) reported that most patients with tuberothalamic infarction had palipsychism which is the superimposition of temporally unrelated information during cognitive activities, with ongoing parallel simultaneous processing in more than one domain. It has also been reported that bizarre confabulations can occur, which are similar to those found after medial frontal lobe lesions (Benson et al., 1996).

The anatomical basis of diencephalic amnesia remains unclear, but it has been reported that hippocampal-related neural structures such as the mamillothalamic tract and anterior thalamic nuclei are critical to memory function (Graff-Radford *et al.*, 1990). Many reports have emphasized that the mamillothalamic tract is responsible for anterograde amnesia. According to van der Werf *et al.* (2000), the mamillothalamic tract was affected in 24 of 25 patients with diencephalic amnestic syndrome, whereas 11 of 13 patients with no or mild memory impairments despite thalamic lesions had an intact mamillothalamic tract. They argued that lesioning of the mamillothalamic tract is the best predictor of the occurrence of an amnestic syndrome.

As noted above, patients with thalamic lesions but intact mamillothalamic tracts usually have no amnesia or, if present, show mild amnesia. In these patients, frontal cortical dysfunction may explain the nature of the memory disorder, which shows evidence of frontal-type memory problems including impaired spatial working memory, increased forgetting rates, poor prospective memory and inadequate elaborative encoding as well as frontal disinhibition (Daum and Ackermann 1994).

Other than amnesia, neurobehavioral symptoms associated with tuberothalamic infarctions are apathy, abulia, perseveration and, less often, disinhibition (Ghika-Schmid and Bogousslavsky 2000; van der Werf *et al.*, 2000; Linek *et al.*, 2005). Ghika-Schmid and Bogousslavsky (2000) stressed the importance of severe perseverative behavior, which is apparent in thinking, spontaneous speech, memory and executive tasks. Other abnormalities associated with tuberothalamic artery infarction include aphasia, especially transcortical motor aphasia; fantastic paraphasia; neologism (Carrera and Bogousslavsky 2006); neglect and topographic disorientation, especially after right-sided lesions (Bogousslavsky *et al.*, 1986); hypophonia; dysarthria; and ipsilateral ptosis (Ghika-Schmid and Bogousslavsky 2000; Kim *et al.*, 2005).

Paramedian artery territory infarction

The essential features of an infarction in the territory of the paramedian artery (Fig. 21.14) are clinical evidence of arousal disturbance, memory impairment and vertical gaze palsy combined with impairment in attention span, orientation, intellect and visual perception (Castaigne *et al.*, 1981; Graff-Radford *et al.*, 1985; Bogousslavsky *et al.*, 1986, 1988; Chung *et al.*, 1996; Schmahmann 2003). Bilateral paramedian thalamic infarction can occur, since both thalamic regions are occasionally supplied from a common trunk on one side (Graff-Radford *et al.*, 1985).

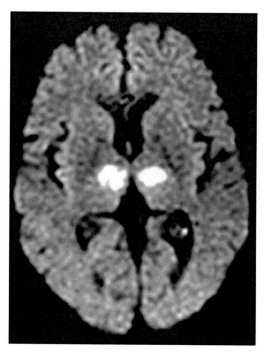

Fig. 21.14. Diffusion-weighted magnetic resonance imaging shows bilateral paramedian infarction in a 67-year-old woman who presented with altered mentality, and rapid stupor. One day later, she became alert but showed persistent abulia, apathy and severe amnesia as well as vertical gaze palsy.

Paramedian artery territory infarction may cause alterations in consciousness ranging from somnolence to coma (Weidauer *et al.*, 2004). Consciousness usually fluctuates and improves, but prolonged coma may result if the lesion extends into the midbrain tegmentum (Chung *et al.*, 1996). Approximately 50% of patients with bilateral lesions have persistent impairment of vigilance (Weidauer *et al.*, 2004). The initial stupor and subsequent hypersomnia is attributable to bilateral lesions in the intralaminar nuclei, which are part of rostral extension of the midbrain reticular activating system (Guberman and Stuss 1983).

Anterograde amnesia frequently develops, but patients with paramedian thalamic infarction are known to present with less-severe amnesia than those with tuberothalamic infarction (Carrera *et al.*, 2004). The memory disturbance after paramedian thalamic infarction has been reported to be associated with damage to the intralaminar or dorsomedial nuclei of the thalamus. However, there is controversy as to whether damage to these nuclei can give rise to anterograde amnesia (Carrera and Bogousslavsky 2006). For instance, patients with a lesion affecting the intralaminar nuclei present with discrete amnesia but accompanied by severe distractibility, suggesting that the intralaminar nuclei are probably not memory structures per se (Mennemeier *et al.*, 1992). Rather, coexisting damage to the anterior and dorsomedial nuclei may result in the most severe amnesia (Perren *et al.*, 2005). Therefore, memory disturbances associated with paramedian thalamic infarction could be explained by frontal dysfunction resulting from damage to dorsomedial and intralaminar nuclei (van der Werf *et al.*, 2000). Other behavioral abnormalities observed in paramedian thalamic infarctions are utilization behavior (Eslinger *et al.*, 1991) and Kluver–Bucy syndrome, especially after bilateral paramedian artery infarction (Muller *et al.*, 1999).

Inferolateral artery territory infarction

Ataxia and hypesthesia are the most common symptoms after inferolateral territory infarct (Bogousslavsky *et al.*, 1988), but behavioral changes and cognitive impairment can occur (Carrera and Bogousslavsky 2006). Patients with these lesion occasionally show executive dysfunction, including in planning, initiation and regulation of goal-directed behavior (van der Werf *et al.*, 2003b), or aphasia (Botez and Barbeau 1971).

Dementia associated with small-vessel ischemic disease
Anatomy of cerebral small vessels

The penetrating small arteries of the brain are unique. The vessels forming the terminal branches from the major cerebral arteries divide and ramify in the pia mater to cortical and deep penetrating branches. The deep penetrating branches arise from the main artery penetrating into white matter to the depth of 3 or 4 cm perpendicularly. They are thin and long, lacking communications, thus constituting many independent small vascular systems. Unlike the main arterioles, the deep penetrating branches extend into the small lumen, thus making them sensitive to systemic hypertension (Fisher 1965).

Small-vessel pathology and its radiologic manifestations

There are several major pathophysiologic mechanisms underlying small-vessel disease pathology. By far the most common lesion associated with small-vessel disease is lipohyalinosis or small-artery arteriosclerosis (Fig. 21.15), predominantly affecting the small arteries

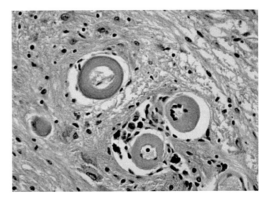

Fig. 21.15. Lipohyalinosis. Small vessels become thickened, and normal wall components are replaced by a homogeneous, glassy (hyaline) substance, composed of collagen and other proteins.

and arterioles. The major cause of lipohyalinosis is hypertension. It encourages thickening of the small arterioles, by replacing normal structures with hyaline substances, thus decreasing perfusion through arteriole lumen narrowing. This results in proliferation of smooth muscle fiber with segmental fibrinoid degeneration (Fisher 1965).

The second most common lesion is atheromatous disease in intracranial branching small vessels. This results either in lacunar infarction from microatheroma from a plaque originating in the orifice of a branch, proliferating into the orifice or extending into a branch from the parent artery (so-called junctional plaque) or in microemboli. The lesion caused by this mechanism is not located in a deep brain area but rather in the base of the infarct in touch with the orifice of the branch artery (Chung and Caplan 2007). Those changes are not always related to hypertension and are more prevalent in Asians, Africans, females and those with diabetes mellitus.

A third lesion type results from a hemodynamic mechanism related to large-vessel stenosis without small-vessel disease. The brain areas supplied by these small vessels lack collaterals, resulting in ischemic infarct when the parent vessel is compromised, for example MCA stenosis results in lenticulostriate artery territorial infarct. This is also called internal borderzone or watershed infarction. Other suggested mechanisms are cardioembolic, vasospasm, vasculitis, lupus anticoagulant and genetical, in CADASIL (cerebral autosomal dominant arteriopathy with subcortical infarcts and leukoencephalopathy). These small-vessel pathologies manifest radiologically as either lacunes or ischemic white matter changes in brain MRI. More specifically, lacunar infarction refers

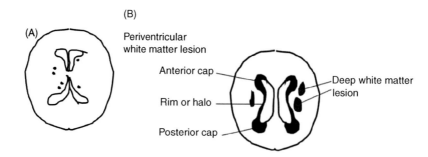

Fig. 21.16. (A) Lacunar states in basal ganglia and thalamus. (B) Periventricular white matter and deep white matter.

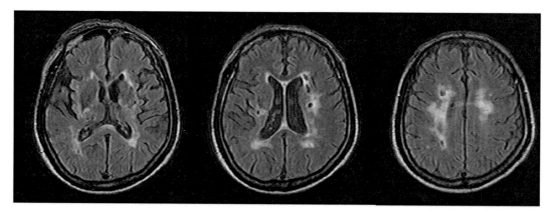

Fig. 21.17. Subcortical vascular dementia with predominantly lacunar changes.

to a condition of small infarctions less than 15 mm in size resulting from occlusion of one single, deep penetrating artery (Fisher 1965).

These lesions are frequently located in deep gray nuclei (basal ganglia and thalamus), pons and white matter of the centrum semiovale. Ischemic white matter changes (leukoaraiosis) in cerebral white matter is primarily incomplete ischemic demyelination of the subcortical white matter of the hemispheres (Babikian and Ropper 1987). It consists of periventricular white matter (anterior cap, rim or halo and posterior cap) and deep white matter lesions (Fig. 21.16).

Overview of subcortical vascular dementia

Small-vessel disease dementia, SVaD, refers to the dementia resulting from ischemic lesions caused by small-vessel disease (Roman 1993a–c).

There are two types of SVaD syndrome: one is dementia associated with predominant subcortical ischemic lacunes in deep nuclei (basal ganglia or thalamus) or internal capsule, known as the lacunar type of SVaD, and the other is dementia associated with predominant ischemic changes in white matter,

which is known as the white matter type of SVaD or Binswanger's disease (subcortical arteriosclerotic encephalopathy) (Erkinjuntti et al., 2000) (Fig. 21.17 and 21.18).

Lacunar state and Bingswanger's disease commonly occur together because the underlying pathology involves the lenticulostriate and the penetrating subcortical arterioles of the hemispheric white matter simultaneously (Fig. 21.19). This may explain why patients with lacunar strokes are more likely to have white matter changes (Hijdra et al., 1990) and to develop dementia (Tatemichi et al., 1993) than those with other stroke subtypes.

Cognitive impairments in SVaD are related to ischemic interruption of frontal cortical circuits (Cummings 1993) or disruption of cholinergic pathways that traverse the subcortical white matter (Bocti et al., 2005).

Cognitive changes of SVaD largely overlap with AD. Furthermore, some studies suggest that pure VaD is not common and patients with SVaD might have comorbidity of AD. However, there are differences in the profile of cognitive deficits between patients

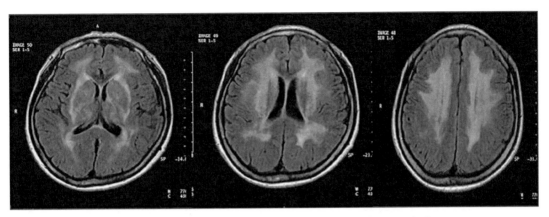

Fig. 21.18. Subcortical vascular dementia with predominantly white matter changes or Binswanger's disease.

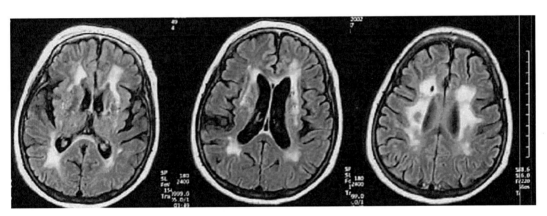

Fig. 21.19. Subcortical vascular dementia with both mixed lacunar and white matter changes.

with AD and SVaD. Executive functions, planning and sequencing, speed of mental processing, performance on unstructured tasks and attention tend to be disproportionately impaired in SVaD. Memory impairment in AD is mediated by temporal areas; consequently, performance is poor in both recall and recognition. However, memory deficits in SVaD are more related to inattention through frontal executive dysfunction, leading to a retrieval defect pattern that is worse in recall but better on recognition and cued recall (Desmond *et al.*, 1999). The traditional cognitive screening test, the Mini-Mental State Examination (MMSE), is biased toward detection of memory and language disturbance and, therefore, may not be sensitive in detecting the early presence of executive dysfunctions in SVaD (Dubois *et al.*, 2000).

Frontal involvement even in the early stage of SVaD also explains the fact that behavioral abnormalities in SVaD differ from those in AD. That is, patients with SVaD are more likely to show depression,

agitation and anxiety than those with AD. Therefore, it is important to recognize behavioral manifestation in SVaD for early detection of these diseases.

Neurological aspects of subcortical vascular dementia

Patients with lacunar states often have a history of abrupt onset and sometimes stepwise deterioration, as in MID. They tend to have more extensive medical histories of hypertension, and a greater likelihood of focal neurologic symptoms and signs compared with those with Binswanger's type of SVaD (Stuss and Cummings 1990). Unlike most of the other vascular dementias, Binswanger's disease often has an insidious onset with no significant lateralizing symptoms, and it may sometimes be mistaken for a degenerative disorder at the beginning of the disease process (Pantoni *et al.*, 1996).

Once the disease has progressed, neurological manifestations of two groups do not differ. The neurological deficits associated with the two groups of SVaD can be divided into corticobulbar, corticospinal and extrapyramidal dysfunctions. Corticobulbar dysfunctions include central facial palsy, dysarthria and dysphagia. In addition to these symptoms, emotional lability or pathological laughing or crying with jaw jerk can occur, especially when the corticobulbar tracts are affected bilaterally. Corticospinal involvement manifests as motor weakness, asymmetrically increased deep tendon reflexes, and extensor plantar responses. When ischemic insult involves the extrapyramidal system, vascular parkinsonism occurs, which includes bradykinesia and rigidity, as well as small stepped gait (marche à petits pas), decreased arm swing, stooped posture, multistep turning, festination and shuffling during walking (Roman 1987). Finally glabellar, snout, rooting and grasp reflexes of frontal releasing signs are often present.

Neuropsychological aspect of subcortical vascular dementia

Frontal executive function, attention and speed

The subcortical syndrome characterized by prominent dysexecutive syndrome, bradyphrenia and mild memory deficits of retrieval is the primary clinical manifestation of SVaD (Desmond et al., 1999). Of the frontal subcortical circuit, the anterior cingulate circuit and the dorsolateral prefrontal circuit play major roles in manifestation of SVaD symptoms (Cummings 1983; Cummings and Benson 1993).

The impairment in executive function reflects the deficits in a number of cognitive functions, including attention or short-term memory (working memory), ability to plan a prospective action and behavioral monitoring, and is responsible for a functional disability in everyday complex actions (Baddeley 1986; Mega and Cummings 1994; Damasio 1998).

Patients with SVaD have significantly greater perseveration during tasks that assess set-shifting than during semantic testing (Lamar et al., 1997). A recurrent perseveration is believed to be the result of left temporal and parietal lobe pathologies and is associated with poor memory and language function, while a stuck-in-set perseveration is caused by frontosubcortical pathologies and is associated with the failure in mental set-shifting (Eslinger and Grattan 1993). Unstructured tasks that require executive abilities, such as behavioral initiation, are also useful assessments. Other neuropsychological investigations suggest that deficits of frontal function can be identified

before the onset of memory or other cognitive disturbances in patients with small-vessel disease and ischemic injury to deep hemispheric gray and white matter structures. These findings suggest that changes in frontal functions occur well before the onset of memory problems in SVaD and this is a potential key to identifying patients at risk for developing VaD (Boone et al., 1992).

Memory and visuospatial function

Short-term memory, as estimated by Digit Span, has consistently been reported to be similarly affected in SVaD and AD (Looi and Sachder 1999). The comparison of qualitative memory aspects in SVaD and AD have shown that both groups perform poorly on free recall of memory test. When free recall and recognition abilities are compared, patients with SVaD show better recognition memory than free recall, while those with AD show lesser efficacy on cued recall and impaired recognition than those with SVaD (Looi and Sachder 1999; Tierney et al., 2001). This pattern is considered a retrieval defect pattern of memory, where patients are helped by semantic cues. Use of cued recall and recognition tasks significantly enhances the ability to discriminate SVaD from AD (Lafosse et al., 1997). Better performances on recognition than recall also suggest that the underlying mechanisms of memory deficits in SVaD are problems of psychomotor slowing and retrieval more than storage problems. Visuospatial functions are reported to be better in SVaD than in AD, but overall specificity and positive predictive values are low (Schmidtke and Hüll 2002).

Language function

Language has not been extensively studied in SVaD. Language tasks requiring semantics, including complex syntax comprehension and picture naming, are impaired in both AD and SVaD, but single-word repetition, oral reading of words and sentences and fluency output is relatively spared in SVaD (Vuorinen et al., 2000). On confrontation naming, patients with SVaD are better on tests of naming, indicating preservation of semantic knowlege (Tierney et al., 2001; Baillon et al., 2003), but those with SVaD manifest more perseveration in naming than those with AD (Cannatà et al., 2002).

Neuropsychiatric aspects of SVaD subcortical vascular dementia

There are more profound behavioral and affect changes in SVaD than in AD in most reports. Using the Neuropsychiatric Inventory (NPI) to explore behavior, those with cortical VaD and SVaD had higher mean composite NPI scores in all domains than those with AD (Aharon-Peretz *et al.*, 2000; Fuh *et al.*, 2005). Their behavioral changes are characterized by depression, personality change, emotional bluntness and psychomotor retardation. Subsequent studies also report that depression and anxiety are more common in SVaD than in AD (Padovani *et al.*, 1995). Even when recognizing emotion, those with SVaD performed significantly worse than those with Alzheimer type dementia on the emotion recognition task even when the cognitive status of each group did not differ (Shimokawa *et al.*, 2000).

Vascular mild cognitive impairment

The term vascular cognitive impairment (VCI) was first proposed as an umbrella term to emphasize the preventability of vascular-related cognitive dysfunction (Bowler and Hachinski, 1995) (see also Ch. 11). It comprises all types of vascular-related events. To minimize confusion related to the concept of MCI and for criteria utilized with mildly impaired groups, the term vascular MCI (V-MCI) is now being used for the group of patients with MCI of vascular origin. An alternative term is vascular cognitive impairment no dementia, VCIND (Rockwood *et al.*, 1999). The most widely used diagnostic criteria of V-MCI is that of the Canadian Study of Health and Aging (Rockwood, 1999). The importance of V-MCI is that it is the most prevalent form of vascular-related cognitive disorder among those aged 65 to 84 years (Rockwood 1999).

Furthermore, the clinical importance of V-MCI might be even higher than that of the degenerative types of MCI since modifying the vascular risk factors and drug treatment could prevent the progression of V-MCI to vascular dementia. Nonetheless, diagnostic criteria and the clinical and imaging characteristics of V-MCI have not been well defined. The most widely used diagnostic criteria for V-MCI may be the criteria of VCIND proposed by Canadian Study of Health and Aging (Standardization of the Diagnosis of Dementia in the Canadian study of health and aging) (Rockwood *et al.*, 1999). However, these criteria include patients with multiple or single territory infarction and showing diverse clinical features according to the involved vessels, whereas the vascular cognitive impairment associated with small-vessel disease can be relatively homogeneous in terms of both lesion location and clinical manifestations.

A search of PubMed with two key words, "subcortical vascular" and "MCI" gave a total of 11 articles, of which only six were relevant to the topic of V-MCI associated with subcortical small-vessel disease (Frisoni *et al.*, 2002; Meyer *et al.*, 2002; de Mendonca *et al.*, 2005; Galluzzi *et al.*, 2005; Zanetti *et al.*, 2006; Bombois *et al.*, 2007). Of the six papers (Table 21.1), only two provided relatively detailed criteria for subject recruitment: one paper was a cross-sectional study involving only 29 patients (Galluzzi *et al.*, 2005) and the other was a longitudinal study involving 29 patients (Frisoni *et al.*, 2002).

These studies have focused on neuropsychological features and have not looked at whether the patients with V-MCI defined with their criteria differ from other groups with dementia or MCI in terms of MRI or PET findings. Our group has conducted studies involving patients with MCI associated with small-vessel disease, which we call subcortical vascular MCI (svMCI; Seo *et al.*, 2008a,b). Diagnoses of svMCI were based on the following criteria modified from those proposed by Petersen *et al.* (1999): (1) subjective cognitive complaints by the patient or the caregiver; (2) normal general cognitive function as measured by a score on the Mini-Mental State Examination (MMSE) above the 16th percentile of age- and sex-matched norms; (3) normal activities of daily living as judged by both an interview with a clinician and the standardized ADL scale; (4) objective cognitive decline on standardized neuropsychological tests; (5) presence of focal neurological signs suggestive of stroke; (6) significant small-vessel ischemic changes without territory infarction on T2-weighted or fluid attenuated inversion recovery (FLAIR) images defined as periventricular white matter high signal (caps or rim) longer than 10 mm, and deep white matter high signal consistent with extensive white matter lesion or diffusely confluent lesion ≥ 25 mm in maximum diameter. Compared with patients with SVaD, those with svMCI were worse in all cognitive domains apart from recognition of Rey figures, alternating hand movement and Luria loop, where the two groups showed comparable performances (Seo *et al.*, 2008a). In another study (Seo *et al.*, 2008b), we compared neuropsychological performances between patients with svMCI and those with amnestic MCI (aMCI), showing that patients with svMCI performed less well in frontal executive function and the Rey copy task than patients with aMCI, whereas the opposite was true for memory, which is consistent with the previous reports (Galluzzi *et al.*, 2005).

319

Table 21.1. Reported articles in subcortical vascular mild cognitive impairment

Authors	Subjects	Types of study	Results	Diagnostic criteria
Meyer et al. (2002)	10 svMCI	Longitudinal (3.72 ± 2.94 years)	During 3.72 ± 2.94 years of follow-up of normal subjects, 12 of 291 developed subcortical small-vessel dementia; of these, 10 patients had prodromal MCI	Modified Petersen's criteria + focal neurological sign + small-vessel features (detailed description of small-vessel features was not given)
Frisoni et al. (2002)	29 svMCI	Longitudinal (32 ± 8 months)	29 patients with V-MCI showed a poor performance on frontal tests and impairment of balance and gait; of those followed for at least 40 months, 50% with V-MCI died	Modified Petersen's criteria + modified criteria for SVaD from Erkinjuntti et al. (2000)
Galluzzi et al. (2005)	29 svMCI	Cross-sectional	Letter fluency, digit span forward, EPS, stance and gait, and irritability were best prediction of svMCI	Modified Petersen's criteria + modified criteria for SVaD from Erkinjuntti et al. (2000)
Mendonca et al. (2005)	15 svMCI	Cross-sectional	Of 40 with MCI, 15 were found to have subcortical vascular features	Modified Petersen's criteria + Hachinski ischemic score + small-vessel features (detailed description of small-vessel features was not given)
Zanetti et al. (2006)	34 with mcd-MCI	Longitudinal (3 years)	Of 34 with mcd-MCI, 9 evolved to SVaD	Multiple domain MCI + ischemic changes shown by CT (detailed description of small-vessel features was not given)
Bombois et al. (2007)	170 consecutive MCI patients	Cross-sectional	Of 170 MCI, subcortical hyperintensities were found in 157	NA

Notes:
svMCI, subcortical vascular mild cognitive impairment; mcd, minimal cerebral dysfunction; SVaD, subcortical vascular dementia; NA, not available.

These patients were also compared in terms cortical atrophy pattern using three-dimensional volumetric images for cortical thickness analysis across the entire brain (Seo et al., 2008a). As presented in Fig. 20.20, compared with healthy controls, patients with svMCI showed cortical thinning in inferior frontal and orbitofrontal gyri, anterior cingulate, insula, superior temporal gyrus and lingual gyrus, while cortical thinning in patients with SVaD involved all these areas plus dorsolateral prefrontal and temporal cortices. These findings suggest that a hierarchy exists between svMCI and SVaD and that svMCI defined according to our criteria is a transitional stage between healthy controls and SVaD. Another imaging study using [^{18}F]-fluorodeoxyglucose positron emission tomography showed that svMCI is distinct from aMCI in terms of glucose metabolism (Seo et al., 2008b).

Acknowledgement
This study was supported by a research grant from Healthcare Biotechnology, Ministry of Health and Welfare, and by a grant from the Korea Health 21 RandD Project, Ministry of Health and Welfare, Republic of Korea (A050079).

Appendix
National Institutes of Neurological Disorders and Stroke and the Association Internationale pour la Recherche et l'Enseignement en Neurosciences (NINDS-AIREN) criteria for vascular dementia

Probable criteria
1. Dementia. Impairment of memory and > 2 cognitive domains
2. Cerebrovascular disease:
   - focal signs on neurologic examination (hemiparesis, lower facial weakness, Babinski's sign, sensory deficit, hemianopia, and dysarthria)
   - evidence of relevant cerebrovascular disease by brain imaging: large vessel infarcts, single strategically placed infarction, multiple basal ganglia and white matter lacunes (WMLs), extensive WMLs or combinations thereof
3. A relationship between the above disorders indicated by the presence of ≥ 1 of the following:
   - onset of dementia within 3 months after a recognized stroke
   - abrupt deterioration in cognitive functions
   - fluctuating, stepwise progression of cognitive deficits
4. Clinical features consistent with the diagnosis of probable vascular dementia:

- early presence of a gait disturbance, history of unsteadiness of frequent, unprovoked falls, early urinary incontinence, pseudobulbar palsy, personality and mood changes

Possible

1. Dementia with focal neurologic signs but without neuroimaging confirmation of the definite cerebrovascular disease, or
2. Dementia with focal signs but without a clear temporal relationship between dementia and stroke
3. Dementia and focal signs but with a subtle onset and variable course of cognitive deficits

Adapted from Roman et al. (1993a–c). Reproduced with permission.

State of California Alzheimer's Disease Diagnostic and Treatment Centers (ADDTC) criteria for vascular dementia (ischemic vascular disease; IVD)

Probable

A. Dementia and evidence of two or more ischemic strokes on the basis of the history, neurologic signs and/or findings on neuroimaging studies (CT scan or T_1-weighted MRI study)
B. The diagnosis of probable IVD is supported by:
   1. Evidence of multiple infarctions in brain regions known to affect cognition
   2. A history of transient ischemic attacks
   3. A history of vascular risk factors (e.g. hypertension, heart disease, diabetes mellitus)
   4. Elevated Hachinski Ischemic Scale score

Possible
Dementia and one or more of the following:

A. A single stroke without documented temporal relationship to the onset of dementia, or
B. Binswanger's syndrome (without multiple strokes), including all of the following:
   1. Early-onset urinary incontinence or gait disturbance not otherwise explained
   2. Vascular risk factors
   3. Extensive white matter changes on neuroimaging studies

Definite
Diagnosis requires histopathologic examination of the brain, as well as:

A. Clinical evidence of dementia
B. Pathologic confirmation of multiple infarcts, some outside of the cerebellum

Mixed dementia
In the presence of one or more other systemic or brain disorders thought to be causally related to the dementia

Adapted from Chui et al. (1992). Reproduced with permission.

Diagnostic and Statistical Manual of Mental Disorders, 4th edn (DSM-IV) diagnostic criteria for vascular dementia

A. The development of multiple cognitive deficits manifested by both:
   1. Memory impairment (impaired ability to learn new information or to recall previously learned information).
   2. One (or more) of the following cognitive disturbances:
      (a) aphasia (language disturbance)
      (b) apraxia (impaired ability to carry out motor activities despite intact motor function)
      (c) agnosia (failure to recognize or identify objects despite intact sensory function)
      (d) disturbance in executive functioning (planning, organizing, sequencing, abstracting)
B. The cognitive deficits in criteria A1 and A2 each cause significant impairment in social or occupational functioning and represent a significant decline from a previous level of functioning.
C. Focal neurologic signs and symptoms (e.g. exaggeration of deep tendon reflexes, extensor plantar response, pseudobulbar palsy, gait abnormalities, weakness of an extremity) or laboratory evidence indicative of cerebrovascular disease (e.g. multiple infarctions involving cortex and underlying white matter) that are judged to be etiologically related to the disturbance
D. The deficits do not occur exclusively during the course of a delirium.

Reprinted with permission from American Psychiatric Association (1994).

Hachinski Ischemic Scale for vascular dementia

Characteristic	Score[a]
Abrupt onset	2
Stepwise progression	1
Fluctuating course	2
Nocturnal confusion	1
Relative preservation of personality	1
Depression	1
Somatic complaints	1
Emotional incontinence	1
History of hypertension	1
History of strokes	2
Evidence of associated atherosclerosis	1

Characteristic	Score[a]
Focal neurologic symptoms	2
Focal neurologic signs	2

Notes:
[a] A score of ≤ 4 suggests Alzheimer's disease; a score ≥ 7 suggests vascular dementia.
Source: Adapted from Hachinski et al. (1975). Reproduced with permission.

International Classification of Disease-10 (ICD-10) research criteria for vascular dementia

G1. Evidence of dementia of specified level of severity, as set out under the general criteria of dementia

G2. Unequal distribution of deficits in higher cognitive functions, with some affected and others relatively spared. Thus memory may be quite markedly affected while thinking, reasoning, and information processing may show only mild decline

G3. There is evidence for focal brain damage, manifest as at least one of the following: unilateral spastic weakness of the limbs, unilaterally increased tendon reflexes, an extensor plantar response, pseudobulbar palsy

G4. There is evidence from the history, examination, or tests of significant cerebrovascular disease, which may reasonably be judged to be etiologically related to the dementia (history of stroke, evidence of cerebral infarction)

From World Health Organization (1993), Reproduced with permission.

References

Absher JR, Cummings JL (1995). Neurobehavioral examination of frontal lobe functions. *Aphasiology* 9:181–92.

Aggleton JP, Saunders RC (1997). The relationships between temporal lobe and diencephalic structures implicated in anterograde amnesia. *Memory*: 5:49–71.

Aharon-Peretz J, Kliot D, Tomer R (2000). Behavioral differences between white matter lacunar dementia and Alzheimer's disease: a comparison on the neuropsychiatric inventory. *Dement Geriatr Cogn Disord* 11(5):294–8.

Albert MA (1973). A simple test of visual neglect. *Neurology* 23:658–64.

Albert ML, Soffer D, Silverberg R, Reches A (1979). The anatomic basis of visual agnosia. *Neurology* 29(6):876–9.

Aldrich MS, Alessi AG, Beck RW, Gilman S (1987). Cortical blindness: etiology, diagnosis, and prognosis. *Ann Neurol* 21(2):149–58.

Alexander MP, Naeser MA, Palumbo CL (1987). Correlation of subcortical CT lesion sites and aphasia profiles. *Brain* 110:961–91.

Alexander MP, Hiltbrunner B, Fischer RS (1989). Distributed anatomy of transcortical sensory aphasia. *Arch Neurol* 46(8):885–92.

American Psychiatric Association (1994). *Diagnostic and Statistical Manual of Mental Disorders*, 4th edn. Washington, DC: American Psychiatric Association.

Andersen G, Vestergaard K, Riis JY, Ingeman-Nielsen M (1996). Intellectual impairment in the first year following stroke, compared to an age-matched population sample. *Cerebrovasc Dis* 6:363–9.

Andrew J, Nathan PW (1964). Lesion on the anterior frontal lobes and disturbances of micturition and defaecation. *Brain* 87:233–62.

Antonelli Incalzi R, Marra C, Giordano A et al. (2003). Cognitive impairment in chronic obstructive pulmonary disease: A neuropsychological and spect study. *J Neurol* 250(3):325–32.

Babikian V, Ropper AH (1987). Binswanger's disease: a review. *Stroke* 18(1):2–12.

Babinski J (1914). Contribusion a l'etude des troubles mentaux dans l'hemiplegie organique cerebrale (anosognosie). *Rev Neurol* 27:845–7.

Baddeley A (1986). *Working Memory*. New York: Oxford University Press.

Baillon S, Muhommad S, Marudkar M et al. (2003). Neuropsychological performance in Alzheimer's disease and vascular dementia: comparisons in a memory clinic population. *Int J Geriatr Psychiatry* 18:602–8.

Benson DF, Cummings JL (1982). Angular gyrus syndrome simulating Alzheimer's disease. *Arch Neurol* 39(10):616–20.

Benson DF, Marsden CD, Meadows JC (1974). The amnesic syndrome of posterior cerebral artery occlusion. *Acta Neurol Scand* 50(2):133–45.

Benson DF (1988). Classical syndromes of aphasia. In *Handbook of Neuropsychology*, vol.1, eds. Boller F, Grafman J. Amsterdam: Elsevier Science, 267–280.

Benson DF, Djenderedjian A, Miller BL et al. (1996). Neural basis of confabulation. *Neurology* 46:1239–43.

Benton AL, Varney NR, Hamsher KD (1978). Visuospatial judgment. A clinical test. *Arch Neurol* 35(6):364–7.

Benton AL, Tranel D (1993). Visuoperceptual, visuospatial, and visuoconstructive disorders. In *Clinical Neuropsychology* 3rd edn, eds. Heilman KM and Valenstein E. New York: Academic Press, 165–213.

Beschin N, Robertson IH (1997). Personal versus extrapersonal neglect: a group study of their dissociation using a reliable clinical test. *Cortex* 33(2):379–84.

Bhatia KP, Marsden CD (1994). The behavioural and motor consequences of focal lesions of the basal ganglia in man. *Brain* **117** (Pt 4):859–76.

Bocti C, Swartz RH, Gao FQ *et al.* (2005). A new visual rating scale to assess strategic white matter hyperintensities within cholinergic pathways in dementia. *Stroke* **36**:2126–31.

Bogousslavsky J, Regli F (1986). Unilateral watershed cerebral infarcts. *Neurology* **36**(3):373–7.

Bogousslavsky J, Regli F (1990). Capsular genu syndrome. *Neurology* **40**:1499–502.

Bogousslavsky J, Regli F (1992). Centrum ovale infarcts: subcortical infarction in the superficial territory of the middle cerebral artery. *Neurology* **42**(10):1992–8.

Bogousslavsky J, Regli F, Assal G (1986). The syndrome of unilateral tuberothalamic artery territory infarction. *Stroke* **17**:434–41.

Bogousslavsky J, Regli F, Uske A (1988). Thalamic infarcts: clinical syndromes, etiology, and prognosis. *Neurology* **38**(6):837–48.

Bombois S, Debette S, Delbeuck X *et al.* (2007). Prevalence of subcortical vascular lesions and association with executive function in mild cognitive impairment subtypes. *Stroke* **38**(9):2595–7.

Boone KB, Miller BL, Lesser IM *et al.* (1992). Neuropsychological correlates of white-matter lesions in healthy elderly subjects: a threshold effect. *Arch Neurol* **49**:549–54.

Botez MI, Barbeau A (1971). Role of subcortical structures, and particularly of the thalamus, in the mechanisms of speech and language. A review. *Int J Neurol* **8**:300–20.

Bowler JV, Hachinski V (1995). Vascular cognitive impairment: a new approach to vascular dementia. *Baillières Clin Neurol* **4**(2):357–76.

Broca P (1977). Remarks on the seat of the faculty of articulate speech, followed by the report of a case of aphemia (loss of speech). In *Neurologic Classics in Modern Translation*, eds. Rottenberg DA, Hochberg FH. New York: Hafner Press, 136–49.

Brust JC, Behrens MM (1977). "Release hallucinations" as the major symptom of posterior cerebral artery occlusion: a report of 2 cases. *Ann Neurol* **2**(5):432–6.

Brust J, Sawada T, Kazui S (2001). Anterior cerebral artery. In *Stroke Syndrome*, 2nd edn, eds. Bogousslavsky J, Caplan L. Cambridge, UK: Cambridge University Press, 439–60.

Cannatà. AP, Alberoni M, Franceschi M, Mariani C (2002). Frontal impairment in subcortical ischemic vascular dementia in comparison to Alzheimer's disease. *Dement Geriatr Cogn Disord* **13**:101–11.

Caplan LR, Schmahmann JD, Kase CS *et al.* (1990). Caudate infarcts. *Arch Neurol* **47**:133–43.

Carrera E, Bogousslavsky J (2006). The thalamus and behavior: effects of anatomically distinct strokes. *Neurology* **66**:1817–23.

Carrera E, Michel P, Bogousslavsky J (2004). Anteromedian, central, and posterolateral infarcts of the thalamus: three variant types. *Stroke* **35**:2826–31.

Castaigne P, Lhermitte F, Buge A *et al.* (1981). Paramedian thalamic and midbrain infarct: clinical and neuropathological study. *Ann Neurol* **10**:127–48.

Chui HC, Victoroff, JI, Margolin D *et al.* (1992). Criteria for the diagnosis of ischemic vascular dementia proposed by the State of California Alzheimer's Disease Diagnostic and Treatment Centers. *Neurology* **42**:473–80.

Chukwudelunzu FE, Meschia JF, Graff-Radford NR, Lucas JA (2001). Extensive metabolic and neuropsychological abnormalities associated with discrete infarction of the genu of the internal capsule. *J Neurol Neurosurg Psychiatry* **71**(5):658–62.

Chung CS, Caplan LR, Han W *et al.* (1996). Thalamic haemorrhage. *Brain* **119**(Pt 6):1873–86.

Chung CS, Caplan LR (2007). Stroke and other neurovascular disorders. In *Textbook of Clinical Neurology*, 3rd edn, ed. Goetz GC. Phildelphia, PA: Saunders, 1019–45.

Critchley M (1951). Types of visual perseveration: "paliopsia" and "illusory visual spread". *Brain* **74**(3):267–99.

Crystal HA, Dickson DW, Sliwinski MJ *et al.* (1993). Pathological markers associated with normal aging and dementia in the elderly. *Ann Neurol* **34**:566–73.

Cummings JL (1993). Frontal-subcortical circuits and human behavior. *Arch Neurol* **50**(8):873–80.

Cummings JL, Benson DF (1983). *Dementia: A Clinical Approach*. Boston, MA: Butterworth.

Damasio H (1981). Cerebral localization of the aphasias. In *Acquired Aphasia*, ed. Sarno MT. Orlando, FL: Academic Press, 27–55.

Damasio AR (1998). The somatic marker hypothesis and the possible functions of the prefrontal cortex In *The Prefrontal Cortex. Executive and Cognitive Functions*, eds. Roberts AC, Robbins TW, Weiskrantz L. New York: Oxford University Press, 36–50.

Damasio AR, Anderson SW (2003). The frontal lobes. In *Clinical Neuropsychology*, 4th edn, eds. Heilman KM, Valenstein E. New York: Oxford University Press, 404–46.

Damasio H, Damasio AR (1983). The localization of lesions in conduction aphasia. In *Localization and Neuroimaging in Neuropsychology*, ed. Kertesz A. Orlando, FL: Academic Press, 231–43.

Damasio A, Yamada T, Damasio H, Corbett J, McKee J (1980). Central achromatopsia: behavioral, anatomic, and physiologic aspects. *Neurology* **30**(10):1064–71.

Damasio AR, Damasio H, van Hoesen GW (1982). Prosopagnosia: anatomic basis and behavioral mechanisms. *Neurology* **32**(4):331–41.

Daum I, Ackermann H (1994). Frontal-type memory impairment associated with thalamic damage. *Int J Neurosci* **77**(3–4):187–98.

De Groot JC, de Leeuw FE, Oudkerk M *et al.* (2000). Cerebral white matter lesions and cognitive function: the Rotterdam Scan Study. *Ann Neurol* **47**:145–51.

de Mendonça A, Ribeiro F, Guerreiro M, Palma T, Garcia C (2005). Clinical significance of subcortical vascular disease in patients with mild cognitive impairment. *Eur J Neurol* **12**(2):125–30.

Desmond DW, Erkinjuntti T, Sano M *et al.* (1999). The cognitive syndrome of vascular dementia: implications for clinical trials. *Alzheimer Dis Assoc Disord* **13**(Suppl 3):S21–9.

De Renzi E, Zambolin A, Crisi G (1987). The pattern of neuropsychological impairment associated with left posterior cerebral artery infarcts. *Brain* **110**(Pt 5): 1099–116.

De Reuck J, Sieben G, De Coster W, van der Eecken H (1981). Stroke pattern and topography of cerebral infarcts. A clinicopathological study. *Eur Neurol* **20**(5):411–15.

Devinsky O (1992). Aphasia. In *Behavioral Neurology 100 Maxims*. St. Louis MO: Mosby Year Book, 88–130.

Dong MJ, Peng B, Lin XT *et al.* (2007). The prevalence of dementia in the People's Republic of China: a systematic analysis of 1980–2004 studies. *Age Ageing* **36**(6):619–24.

Dubois B, Slachevsky A, Litvan I, Pillon B (2000). The FAB: a frontal assessment battery at bedside. *Neurology* **55**(11):1621–6.

Erkinjuntti T (1987). Types of multi-infarct dementia. *Acta Neurol Scand* **75**(6):391–9.

Erkinjuntti T, Sawada T, Whitehouse PJ (1999). The Osaka Conference on Vascular Dementia 1998. *Alzheimer Dis Assoc Disord* **13**(Suppl 3):S1–3.

Erkinjuntti T, Inzitari D, Pantoni L *et al.* (2000). Research criteria for subcortical vascular dementia in clinical trials. *J Neural Transm Suppl* **59**:23–30.

Eslinger PJ, Grattan LM (1993). Frontal lobe and frontal-striatal substrates for different forms of human cognitive flexibility. *Neuropsychologia* **31**(1):17–28.

Eslinger PJ, Warner GC, Grattan LM, Easton JD (1991). "Frontal lobe" utilization behavior associated with paramedian thalamic infarction. *Neurology* **41**(3):450–2.

Farah MJ (2003). Disoders of visual-spatial perception and cognition. In *Clinical Neuropsychology*. 4th edn, eds. Heilman KM, Valenstein E. New York: Oxford University Press, 146–60.

Fisher, CM (1965). Lacunes: small deep cerebral infarcts. *Neurology* **15**:774–84.

Fisher CM (1982). Disorientation for place. *Arch Neurol* **39**(1):33–6.

Fisher CM (1986). The posterior cerebral artery syndrome. *Can J Neurol Sci* **13**(3):232–9.

Freedman M, Alexander MP, Naeser MA (1984). Anatomic basis of transcortical motor aphasia. *Neurology* **34**(4): 409–17.

Frisoni GB, Galluzzi S, Bresciani L, Zanetti O, Geroldi C (2002). Mild cognitive impairment with subcortical vascular features: clinical characteristics and outcome. *J Neurol* **249**:1423–32.

Fuh JL, Wang SJ, Cummings JL (2005). Neuropsychiatric profiles in patients with Alzheimer's disease and vascular dementia. *J Neurol Neurosurg Psychiatry* **76**(10):1337–41.

Galluzzi S, Sheu CF, Zanetti O, Frisoni GB (2005). Distinctive clinical features of mild cognitive impairment with subcortical cerebrovascular disease. *Dement Geriatr Cogn Disord* **19**(4):196–203. [Epub 2005 Jan 25.]

Gazzaniga MS, Ivry RB, Mangun GR (2002). Emotion. In *Cognitive Neuroscience: The Biology of the Mind* 2nd edn, eds. Gazzaniga MS, Ivry RB, Mangun GR. New York: WW Norton, 537–76.

Gerstmann J (1940). Syndrome of finger agnosia, disorientation for right and left, agraphia and acalculia. *Arch Neurol Psychiatry* **44**:398–408.

Geschwind N (1965a). Disconnexion syndromes in animals and man. I. *Brain* **88**(2):237–94.

Geschwind N (1965b). Disconnexion syndromes in animals and man. II. *Brain* **88**(3):585–644.

Geschwind N, Fusillo M (1966). Color-naming defects in association with alexia. *Arch Neurol* **15**(2):137–46.

Ghika-Schmid F, Bogousslavsky J (2000). The acute behavioral syndrome of anterior thalamic infarction: a prospective study of 12 cases. *Ann Neurol* **48**(2):220–7.

Graff-Radford NR, Damasio H, Yamada T, Eslinger PJ, Damasio AR (1985). Nonhaemorrhagic thalamic infarction. Clinical, neuropsychological and electrophysiological findings in four anatomical groups defined by computerized tomography. *Brain* **108**(Pt 2):485–516.

Graff-Radford NR, Tranel D, van Hoesen GW, Brandt JP (1990). Diencephalic amnesia. *Brain* **113**(Pt 1):1–25.

Guberman A, Stuss D (1983). The syndrome of bilateral paramedian thalamic infarction. *Neurology* **33**(5):540–6.

Hachinski VC, Iliff LD, Zilkha E *et al.* (1975). Cerebral blood flow in dementia. *Arch Neurol* **32**(9):632–7.

Hahm DS, Kang Y, Cheong SS, Na DL (2001). A compulsive collecting behavior following an A. com aneurysmal rupture. *Neurology* **56**(3):398–400.

Halligan PW, Cockburn J, Wilson BA (1991). The behavioural assessment of visual neglect. *Neuropsychol Rehab* **1**:5–32.

Hashiguchi S, Mine H, Ide M, Kawachi Y (2000). Watersged infarction associated with dementia and cerebral atrophy. *Psychiatry Clin Neurosci* **54**(2):163–8.

Hecaen H, de Ajuriaguerra J (1954). Balint's syndrome (psychic paralysis of visual fixation) and its minor forms. *Brain* 77(3):373–400.

Heilman KM, Bowers D, Coslett HB, Whelan H, Watson RT (1985). Directional hypokinesia: prolonged reaction times for leftward movements in patients with right hemisphere lesions and neglect. *Neurology* 35(6):855–9.

Heilman KM, Rothi LJ, Valenstein E (1982). Two forms of ideomotor apraxia. *Neurology* 32(4):342–6.

Heilman KM, Rothi LJG (2003a). Apraxia. In *Clinical Neuropsychology*, 4th edn, eds. Heilman KM, Valenstein E. New York: Oxford University Press, 215–35.

Heilman KM, Rothi LJG (2003b). Neglect and related disorders. In *Clinical Neuropsychology*, 4th edn, eds. Heilman KM, Valenstein E. New York: Oxford University Press, 296–346.

Heilman KM, van den Abell T (1979). Right hemispheric dominance for mediating cerebral activation. *Neuropsychologia* 17(3–4):315–21.

Heilman KM, van den Abell T (1980). Right hemisphere dominance for attention: the mechanism underlying hemispheric asymmetries of inattention (neglect). *Neurology* 30(3):327–30.

Heilman KM, Watson RT (1991). Intentional motor disorders. In *Frontal Lobe Function and Dysfunction*, eds. Levin HS, Eisenberg HM, Benton AL. New York: Oxford University Press, 199–213.

Hillis AE, Newhart M, Heidler J et al. (2005). Anatomy of spatial attention: insights from perfusion imaging and hemispatial neglect in acute stroke. *J Neurosci* 25:3161–7.

Hijdra A, Verbeeten B Jr., Verhulst JAPM (1990). Relation of leukoaraiosis to lesion type in stroke patients. *Stroke* 21:890–4.

Kanwisher N, McDermott J, Chun MM (1997). The fusiform face area: a module in human extrastriate cortex specialized for face perception. *J Neurosci* 17(11):4302–11.

Karnath HO, Fruhmann Berger M, Kuker W, Rorden C (2004). The anatomy of spatial neglect based on voxelwise statistical analysis: a study of 140 patients. *Cereb Cortex* 14:1164–72.

Karnath HO, Zopf R, Johannsen L et al. (2005). Normalized perfusion MRI to identify common areas of dysfunction: patients with basal ganglia neglect. *Brain* 128:2462–9.

Karussis D, Leker RR, Abramsky O (2000). Cognitive dysfunction following thalamic stroke: a study of 16 cases and review of the literature. *J Neurol Sci* 172:25–9.

Kawamura M, Hirayama K, Hasegawa K, Takahashi N, Yamaura A (1987). Alexia with agraphia of kanji (Japanese morphograms). *J Neurol Neurosurg Psychiatry* 50(9):1125–9.

Kawamura M, Takahashi N, Hirayama K (1988). Hemichorea and its denial in a case of caudate

infarction diagnosed by magnetic resonance imaging. *J Neurol Neurosurg Psychiatry* 51:590–1.

Kertesz A, Sheppard A, MacKenzie R (1982). Localization in transcortical sensory aphasia. *Arch Neurol* 39(8):475–8.

Kertesz A, Nicholson I, Cancelliere A, Kassa K, Black SE (1985). Motor impersistence: a right hemisphere syndrome. *Neurology* 35(5):662–6.

Kim EJ, Lee DK, Kang DH et al. (2005). Ipsilateral ptosis associated with anterior thalamic infarction. *Cerebrovasc Dis* 20:410–11.

Kim JS, Choi-Kwon S (2000). Poststroke depression and emotional incontinence: correlation with lesion location. *Neurology* 54(9):1805–10.

Klingler J, Gloor P (1960). The connections of the amygdala and of the anterior temporal cortex in the human brain. *J Comp Neurol* 115:333–69.

Kokmen E, Whisnant JP, O'Fallon WN, Chu CP, Beard CM (1996). Dementia after ischemic stroke: a population-based study in Rochester, Minnesota (1960–1984). *Neurology* 46:154–9.

Kolb B, Whishaw IQ (2003). Disconnection syndromes. In *Fundamentals of Human Neuropsychology*, 5th edn, eds. Kolb B, Whishaw IQ. New York: Worth, 426–46.

Kooistra CA, Heilman KM (1988). Memory loss from a subcortical white matter infarct. *J Neurol Neurosurg Psychiatry* 51:866–9.

Krettek JE, Price JL (1977). The cortical projections of the mediodorsal nucleus and adjacent thalamic nuclei in the rat. *J Comp Neurol* 171:157–91.

Kumral E, Evyapan D, Balkir K (1999). Acute caudate vascular lesions. *Stroke* 30(1):100–8.

Kwon JC, Lee HJ, Chin J et al. (2002). Hanja alexia with agraphia after left posterior inferior temporal lobe infarction: a case study. *J Korean Med Sci* 17(1):91–5.

Lafosse JM, Reed BR, Mungas D et al. (1997). Fluency and memory differences between ischemic vascular dementia and Alzheimer's disease. *Neuropsychology* 11(4):514–22.

Lai C, Okada Y, Sadoshima S et al. (1990). A case of left internal capsular infarction with auditory hallucination and peculiar amnesia and dysgraphia. *No To Shinkei* 42:873–77.

Lamar M, Podell K, Carew TG et al. (1997). Perseverative behavior in Alzheimer's disease and subcortical ischemic vascular dementia. *Neuropsychology* 11(4):523–34.

Lance JW (1976). Simple formed hallucinations confined to the area of a specific visual field defect. *Brain* 99(4):719–34.

Laplane D, Attal N, Sauron B, de Billy A, Dubois B (1992). Lesions of basal ganglia due to disulfiram neurotoxicity. *J Neurol Neurosurg Psychiatry* 55(10):925–9.

Lass P, Buscombe JR, Harber M, Davenport A, Hilson AJ (1999). Cognitive impairment in patients with renal

325

failure is associated with multiple-infarct dementia. *Clin Nucl Med* **24**:561–5.

Lee DY, Lee JH, Ju YS *et al.* (2002). The prevalence of dementia in older people in an urban population of Korea: the Seoul study. *J Am Geriatr Soc* **50**(7):1233–9.

Lhermitte F (1983). "Utilization behaviour" and its relation to lesions of the frontal lobes. *Brain* **106**(Pt 2):237–55.

Lhermitte F, Pillon B, Serdaru M (1986). Human autonomy and the frontal lobes. Part I: imitation and utilization behavior: a neuropsychological study of 75 patients. *Ann Neurol* **19**(4):326–34.

Linek V, Sonka K, Bauer J (2005). Dysexecutive syndrome following anterior thalamic ischemia in the dominant hemisphere. *J Neurol Sci* **229–230**:117–20.

Looi JC, Sachdev PS (1999). Differentiation of vascular dementia from AD on neuropsychological tests. *Neurology* **53**(4):670–8.

Luders H, Lesser RP, Hahn J *et al.* (1991). Basal temporal language area *Brain* **114**(Pt 2):743–54.

Maraganore DM, Harding AE, Marsden CD (1991). A clinical and genetic study of familial Parkinson's disease. *Mov Disord* **6**(3):205–11.

Marshall JC, Halligan PW (1993). Visuo-spatial neglect: a new copying test to assess perceptual parsing. *J Neurol* **240**:37–40.

Meador KJ, Watson RT, Bowers D, Heilman KM (1986). Hypometria with hemispatial and limb motor neglect. *Brain* **109**(Pt 2):293–305.

Mega MS, Cummings JL (1994). Frontal subcortical circuits and neuropsychiatric disorders. *J Neuropsychiatry Clin Neurosci* **6**:358–70.

Mendez MF, Adams NL, Lewandowsky K (1989). Neurobehavioral changes associated with caudate lesions. *Neurology* **39**:349–54.

Mennemeier M, Fennell E, Valenstein E, Heilman KM (1992). Contributions of the left intralaminar and medial thalamic nuclei to memory. Comparisons and report of a case. *Arch Neurol* **49**(10):1050–8.

Mesulam MM, Waxman SG, Geschwind N, Sabin TD (1976). Acute confusional states with right middle cerebral artery infarctions. *J Neurol Neurosurg Psychiatry* **39**(1):84–9.

Mesulam MM, van Hoesen GW, Pandya DN, Geschwind N (1977). Limbic and sensory connections of the inferior parietal lobule (area PG) in the rhesus monkey: a study with a new method for horseradish peroxidase histochemistry. *Brain Res* **136**(3):393–414.

Meyer JS, Xu G, Thornby J, Chowdhury MH, Quach M (2002). Is mild cognitive impairment prodromal for vascular dementia like Alzheimer's disease? *Stroke* **33**(8):1981–5.

Mori E, Yamadori A (1987). Acute confusional state and acute agitated delirium. Occurrence after infarction in the right middle cerebral artery territory. *Arch Neurol* **44**(11):1139–43.

Moroney JT, Bagiella E, Desmond DW *et al.* (1997). Meta-analysis of the Hachinski Ischemic Score in pathologically verified dementias. *Neurology* **49**:1096–105.

Mort DJ, Malhotra P, Mannan SK *et al.* (2003). The anatomy of visual neglect. *Brain* **126**:1986–97.

Muller A, Baumgartner RW, Rohrenbach C, Regard M (1999). Persistent Kluver–Bucy syndrome after bilateral thalamic infarction. *Neuropsychiatry Neuropsychol Behav Neurol* **12**(2):136–9.

Na DL, Adair JC, Williamson DJ *et al.* (1998). Dissociation of sensory-attentional from motor-intentional neglect. *J Neurol Neurosurg Psychiatry* **64**(3):331–8.

Nieuwenhuys R, Voogd J, van Huijzen C (1988). *The Human Central Nervous System: A Synopsis and Atlas.* New York: Springer-Verlag.

Ogden JA (1985). Anterior–posterior interhemispheric differences in the loci of lesions producing visual hemineglect. *Brain Cogn* **4**:59–75.

Padovani A, Di Piero V, Bragoni M *et al.* (1995). Patterns of neuropsychological impairment in mild dementia: a comparison between Alzheimer's disease and multi-infarct dementia. *Acta Neurol Scand* **92**(6):433–42.

Pantoni L, Garcia JH, Brown GG (1996). Vascular pathology in three cases of progressive cognitive deterioration. *J Neurol Sci* **135**:131–9.

Park KC, Jeong Y, Hwa Lee B *et al.* (2005). Left hemispatial visual neglect associated with a combined right occipital and splenial lesion: another disconnection syndrome, *Neurocase* **11**(5):310–18.

Park KC, Lee BH, Kim EJ *et al.* (2006). Deafferentation-disconnection neglect induced by posterior cerebral artery infarction. *Neurology* **66**(1):56–61.

Pasquier F, Leys D (1997). Why are stroke patients prone to develop dementia? *J Neurol* **244**(3):135–42.

Perren F, Clarke S, Bogousslavsky J (2005). The syndrome of combined polar and paramedian thalamic infarction. *Arch Neurol* **62**:1212–16.

Petersen RC (2000). Aging, mild cognitive impairment, and Alzheimer's disease. *Neurol Clin* **18**:789–806.

Petersen RC, Smith GE, Waring SC *et al.* (1999). Mild cognitive impairment: clinical characterization and outcome. *Arch Neurol* **56**:303–8.

Piercy MF, Hecaen H, de Ajuriaguerra J (1960). Constructional apraxia associated with unilateral cerebral lesions. *Brain* **83**:225–42.

Poppel E, Held R, Frost D (1973). Residual visual function after brain wounds involving the central visual pathways in man. *Nature* **243**(5405):295–6.

Pozzilli C, Passafiume D, Bastianello S, D'Antona R, Lenzi GL (1987). Remote effects of caudate hemorrhage: a clinical and functional study. *Cortex* **23**:341–9.

Pullicino PM, Caplan LR, Hommel M (1993). *Advances in Neurology*, Vol. 62: *Cerebral Small Artery Disease*. New York: Raven Press.

Rasquin SMC, Lodder J, Visser PJ Lousberg R, Verhey FRJ (2004). Predictive accuracy of MCI sybtypes for Alzheimer's disease and vascualar dementia in subjects with mild cognitive impairment; a 2 year follow-up study. *Dementi Geriatr Cogn Disord* **19**:113–19.

Richfield EK, Twyman R, Berent S (1987). Neurological syndrome following bilateral damage to the head of the caudate nuclei. *Ann Neurol* **22**:768–71.

Ringelstein EB, Zeumer H, Angelou D (1983a). The pathogenesis of strokes from internal carotid artery occlusion. Diagnostic and therapeutic implications. *Stroke* **14**(6):867–75.

Ringelstein EB, Berg-Dammer E, Zeumer H (1983b). The so-called atheromatous pseudoocclusion of the internal carotid artery. A diagnostic and therapeutical challenge. *Neuroradiology* **25**(3):147–55.

Rockwood K, Bowler J, Erkinjuntti T, Hachinski V, Wallin A (1999). Subtypes of vascular dementia. *Alzheimer Dis Assoc Disord* **13**(Suppl 3):S59–65.

Roman GC (1987). Senile dementia of the Bingswanger type: a vascular form of dementia in the elderly. *JAMA* **258**:1782–8.

Roman GC (2004). Brain hypoperfusion: a critical factor in vascular dementia. *Neurol Res* **26**:454–8.

Roman GC, Tatemichi TK, Erkinjuntti T *et al.* (1993a). Vascular dementia: diagnostic criteria for research studies. Report of the NINDS–AIREN International Workshop. *Neurology* **31**:269–82.

Roman GC, Tatemichi TK, Erkinjuntti T *et al.* (1993b). Vascular dementia: diagnostic criteria for research studies. Report of the NINDS–AIREN International Workshop. *Neurology* **43**: 250–60.

Roman GC, Tatemichi TK, Erkinjuntti T *et al.* (1993c). Vascular dementia: diagnostic criteria for research studies – Report of the NINDS–AIREN International Workshop. *Neurology* **43**:1609–11.

Ropper AH, Brown RH, Brown RJ (2005). Disorders of speech and language. *Adams and Victor's Principles of Neurology*, 8th edn, Ch. 23. New York: McGraw-Hill, 413–32.

Ross ED (1981). The aprosodias. Functional–anatomic organization of the affective components of language in the right hemisphere. *Arch Neurol* **38**(9):561–9.

Sandson J, Albert ML (1987). Perseveration in behavioral neurology. *Neurology* **37**(11):1736–41.

Seo SW, Ahn J, Yoon U *et al.*, (2008a). Cortical thinning in vascular mild cognitive impairment and vascular dementia of subcortical type. *J Neuroimaging* in press.

Seo SW, Cho SS, Park A, Chin J, Na DL (2008b). Subcortical vascular versus amnestic mild cognitive impairment: comparison of cerebral glucose metabolism. *J Neuroimaging* in press.

Schmahmann JD (2003). Vascular syndromes of the thalamus. *Stroke* **34**:2264–78.

Schmidtke K. Hüll M (2002). Neuropsychological differentiation of small vessel disease, Alzheimer's disease and mixed dementia. *J Neurol Sci* **17–22**:203–4.

Selnes OA, Royall RM, Grega MA *et al.* (2001). Cognitive changes 5 years after coronary artery bypass grafting: is there evidence of late decline? *Arch Neurol* **58**(4): 598–604.

Seo SW, Jung K, You H *et al.* (2007). Dominant limb motor impersistence associated with callosal disconnection. *Neurology* **68**(11):862–4.

Serra Catafau J, Rubio F, Peres Serra J (1992). Peduncular hallucinosis associated with posterior thalamic infarction. *J Neurol* **239**(2):89–90.

Shimokawa A, Yatomi N, Anamizu S *et al.* (2000). Comprehension of emotions: comparison between Alzheimer type and vascular type dementias. *Dement Geriatr Cogn Disord* **11**(5):268–74.

Soma Y, Sugishita M, Kitamura K, Maruyama S, Imanaga H (1989). Lexical agraphia in the Japanese language. Pure agraphia for Kanji due to left posteroinferior temporal lesions. *Brain* **112**(Pt 6):1549–61.

Starkstein SE, Robinson RG (1991). The role of the frontal lobes in affective disorder following stroke. In *Frontal Lobe Function and Dysfunction*, eds. Levin HS, Eisenberg HM, Benton AL. New York: Oxford University Press, 288–303.

Starkstein SE, Robinson RG, Price TR (1987). Comparison of cortical and subcortical lesions in the production of poststroke mood disorders. *Brain* **110**(Pt 4):1045–59.

Stuss DT, Cummings JL (1990). Subcortical vascular dementias. In *Subcortical Dementia*, ed. Cummings JL. New York: Oxford University Press, 145–63.

Tatemichi TK, Foulkes MA, Mohr JP *et al.* (1990). Dementia in stroke survivors in the Stroke Data Bank cohort. Prevalence, incidence, risk factors, and computed tomographic findings. *Stroke* **21**(6):858–66.

Tatemichi TK, Desmond DW, Prohovnik I *et al.* (1992a). Confusion and memory loss from capsular genu infarction: a thalamocortical disconnection syndrome? *Neurology* **42**:1966–79.

Tatemichi TK, Steinke W, Duncan C *et al.* (1992b). Paramedian thalamopeduncular infarction: clinical syndromes and magnetic resonance imaging. *Ann Neurol* **32**(2):162–71.

Tatemichi TK, Desmond DW, Paik M *et al.* (1993). Clinical determinants of dementia related to stroke. *Ann Neurol* **33**:568–75.

Tatemichi TK, Paik M, Bagiella E *et al.* (1994). Risk of dementia after stroke in a hospitalized cohort: results of a longitudinal study. *Neurology* **44**:1885–91.

Tatemichi TK, Desmond DW, Prohovnik I, Eidelberg D (1995). Dementia associated with bilateral carotid occlusions: neuropsychological and haemodynamic course after extracranial to intracranial bypass surgery *J Neurol Neurosurg Psychiatry* **58**(5):633–6.

Terao Y, Bandou M, Nagura H *et al.* (1991). Persistent amnestic syndrome due to infarction of the genu of the left internal capsule. *Rinsho Shinkeigaku* **31**:1002–6.

Tierney MC, Black SE, Szalai JP *et al.* (2001). Recognition memory and verbal fluency differentiate probable Alzheimer disease from subcortical ischemic vascular dementia. *Arch Neurol* **58**(10):1654–9.

Tranel D (1994). "Acquired sociopathy": the development of sociopathic behavior following focal brain damage. *Prog Exp Pers Psychopathol Res* 285–311.

Tsuda Y, Yamada K, Hayakawa T *et al.* (1994). Cortical blood flow and cognition after extracranial–intracranial bypass in a patient with severe carotid occlusive lesions. *Acta Neurochir (Wien)* **129**(3–4):198–204.

Tucker DM, Watson RT, Heilman KM (1977). Discrimination and evocation of affectively intoned speech in patients with right parietal disease. *Neurology* **27**(10):947–50.

Ungerleider LG, Mishkin M (1982). Two cortical visual systems. In *Analysis of Visual Behavior*, eds. Ingle DJ, Goodale MA, Mansfield RJW. Cambridge, MA: MIT Press, 549–86.

Vallar G, Bottini G, Paulesu E (2003). Neglect syndromes: the role of the parietal cortex. *Adv Neurol* **93**:293–319.

van der Werf YD, Witter MP, Uylings HB, Jolles J (2000). Neuropsychology of infarctions in the thalamus: a review. *Neuropsychologia* **38**(5):613–27.

van der Werf YD, Jolles J, Witter MP, Uylings HB (2003a). Contributions of thalamic nuclei to declarative memory functioning. *Cortex* **39**:1047–62.

van der Werf YD, Scheltens P, Lindeboom J *et al.* (2003b). Deficits of memory, executive functioning and attention following infarction in the thalamus; a study of 22 cases with localised lesions. *Neuropsychologia* **41**:1330–44.

von Cramon DY, Hebel N, Schuri U (1985). A contribution to the anatomical basis of thalamic amnesia. *Brain* **108**(Pt 4):993–1008.

Vuorinen E, Laine M, Rinne J (2000). Common pattern of language impairment in vascular dementia and in Alzheimer disease. *Alzheimer Dis Assoc Disord* **14**(2):81–6.

Weidauer S, Nichtweiss M, Zanella FE, Lanfermann H (2004). Assessment of paramedian thalamic infarcts: MR imaging, clinical features and prognosis. *Eur Radiol* **14**(9):1615–26.

Wernicke E (1874). *Der Aphasische Symptomenkomplex.* Breslau: Cohn and Weigart.

World Health Organization (1993). *International Classification of Disease (ICD-10): Classification of Mental and Behavioral Disorders. Diagnostic Criteria for Research.* Geneva: World Health Organization.

Yamanaka K, Fukuyama H, Kimura J (1996). Abulia from unilateral capsular genu infarction: report of two cases. *J Neurol Sci* **143**:181–4.

Yanagihara T (2002). Vascular dementia in Japan. *Ann N Y Acad Sci* **977**:24–8.

Zangwill OL (1979). Two cases of crossed aphasia in dextrals. *Neuropsychologia* **17**(2):167.

Zanetti M, Ballabio C, Abbate C *et al.* (2006). Mild cognitive impairment subtypes and vascular dementia in community-dwelling elderly people: a 3-year follow-up study *J Am Geriatr Soc* **54**(4):580–6.

Zhang ZX, Zahner GE, Román GC *et al.* (2005). Dementia subtypes in China: prevalence in Beijing, Xian, Shanghai, and Chengdu. *Arch Neurol* **62**(3):447–53.

Zuccala G, Onder G, Pedone C (2001). For the GIFA-ONLUS Study Group. Hypotension and cognitive impairment: selective association in patients with hearing failure. *Neurology* **57**(11):1986–92.

Chapter 22

CADASIL: a genetic model of arteriolar degeneration, white matter injury and dementia in later life

Stephen Salloway, Thea Brennan-Krohn, Stephen Correia, Michelle Mellion and Suzanne delaMonte

Introduction

Cerebral microvascular disease, as seen on magnetic resonance imaging (MRI) is common in the elderly (de Leeuw *et al.*, 2000) and there is growing evidence that it makes a major contribution to cognitive impairment and dementia in the elderly, especially in the presence of fibrillar amyloid and tau pathology (Bennett *et al.*, 1992, 1994; Snowdon, 1997; Snowdon *et al.*, 2000; White *et al.*, 2002) Understanding the unique impact of cerebral microvascular disease on cognition in the elderly is challenging because the base rate of Alzheimer's disease (AD) is high in this age group (Alzheimer's Association, 2007) making it difficult to reliably exclude patients with concomitant AD (Jellinger, 2002).

The CADASIL syndrome (cerebral autosomal dominant arteriopathy with subcortical infarcts and leukoencephalopathy) provides a valuable model for studying the pathogenesis of microvascular disease and the specific impact of subcortical vascular white matter injury on cognitive function. CADASIL is a genetic disorder characterized by progression of subcortical arteriolar degeneration and white matter lesions, with the development of white matter changes and clinical symptoms in early to mid adulthood, well before the onset of significant Alzheimer's pathology. Subcortical vascular dementia occurs in later stages of the illness, with a general correspondence between the severity of white matter lesions on MRI and the extent of cognitive deficits (Amberla *et al.*, 2004). Moreover, the cognitive profile of CADASIL overlaps considerably with that of sporadic ischemic vascular disease in the elderly but differs from that of patients with AD (Charlton *et al.*, 2006). Taken together, these observations provide support for the consideration of CADASIL as a useful model of sporadic ischemic vascular disease in the elderly. Further, much has been learned about mutations in the *Notch3* gene and notch signaling, providing a model for exploring the molecular pathogenesis of other forms of microvascular disease in the elderly.

CADASIL

CADASIL is a genetic, adult-onset neurologic disorder characterized by recurrent subcortical strokes, which result in vascular dementia generally in the absence of vascular risk factors. The responsible gene has been identified as *Notch3* on chromosome 19p131–13.2 (Joutel *et al.*, 1996). The phenomenon of a family with small vessel disease with no risk factors and vascular dementia was first described by van Bogaert in 1955 (cited in Bousser and Tournier-Lasserve, 2001). Since that time, reports of this familial cerebral arteriopathy have appeared in the literature under different eponyms, such as hereditary multi-infarct dementia, chronic familial vascular encephalopathy and familial Binswanger's syndrome (Salloway and Desbiens, 2004). It was not until 1993, that Joutel *et al.* (1993) coined the term CADASIL to accurately describe this systemic arteriopathy according to its main clinical and MRI features.

Epidemiology and vascular risk factors

The true prevalence of CADASIL is not yet known. Families affected by CADASIL have been reported throughout the world, and though awareness of the disorder is increasing, the condition remains underdiagnosed. Dong *et al.* (2003) screened 218 consecutive patients presenting with lacunar stroke for CADASIL mutations in exons 3–6 of the *Notch3* gene and found a single mutation, giving a frequency of 0.05%. However, when the screening group was narrowed to patients with both lacunar stroke and

The Behavioral Neurology of Dementia, eds. Bruce L. Miller and Bradley F. Boeve. Published by Cambridge University Press.
© Cambridge University Press 2009.

leukoaraiosis, frequency increased to 2.0% for those with disease onset at 65 years and 11.1% for those with disease onset at 50 years. CADASIL is not strongly associated with vascular risk factors such as hypertension (Desmond *et al.*, 1999) and neither white matter hyperintensities (WMH) nor lacunar infarction are significantly associated with blood pressure or glucose control in group analyses (Viswanathan *et al.*, 2006).

Clinical features

CADASIL is characterized by five main clinical features: ischemic stroke; WMHs and lacunar infarcts, identified by MRI; migraine; mood disturbances and dementia. Figure 22.1 shows the typical age of onset and progression of symptoms in CADASIL (Singhal *et al.*, 2004). The clinical presentation of CADASIL varies widely both among and within families (Dichgans *et al.*, 1998), and no significant correlations between genotype and phenotype have yet been found. The disorder usually becomes evident in young to middle adulthood with migraine or an ischemic event. The mean age of symptom onset is approximately 37($\pm$13) years (Dichgans *et al.*, 1998; Desmond *et al.*, 1999). The mean disease duration is approximately 20 years and the mean age of death approximately 65($\pm$10) years (Chabriat *et al.*, 1995; Dichgans *et al.*, 1998; Desmond *et al.*, 1999). The mean age of death appears to be 5–10 years higher in women than in men (Dichgans *et al.*, 1998; Opherk *et al.*, 2004). Functional disability is rare before the age of 40, but increases rapidly with age. Half of all patients aged 45–54 years are significantly disabled, and 38% of patients aged 55–64 years are unable to walk without assistance. Patients become bedridden at a median age of approximately 64, and

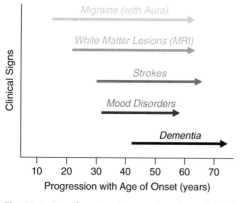

Progression of Symptoms in CADASIL

Fig. 22.1. Age of onset and progression of core clinical features of CADASIL.

by the time of death nearly 80% are completely dependent (Dichgans *et al.*, 1998; Opherk *et al.*, 2004).

Migraine

Migraine with aura is a common early symptom, affecting 40–60% of patients with CADASIL; the mean age of onset is 28.3 ($\pm$11.7) years (Desmond *et al.*, 1999) but the onset of migraine has been reported in patients as young as 6 years (Vahedi *et al.*, 2004). The auras are predominantly visual and sensory, and most are indistinguishable from typical migraine with aura. However, there is a higher frequency of basilar, hemiplegic and prolonged aura in this population. Hemiplegia may occur during a headache episode and the *Notch3* gene is located in close proximity to the gene for familial hemiplegic migraine on chromosome 19 (Salloway and Desbiens, 2004). The frequency of attacks is variable and can range from one attack in a lifetime to several per month. Although white matter lesions are fairly common among patients with migraine, the pattern is usually milder in severity (Agostoni and Rigamonti, 2007), and the frequency of migraine with or without aura in patients with sporadic subcortical ischemic vascular disease is unclear. CADASIL provides an important window for exploring the mechanisms underlying the interface of migraine and cerebral ischemia.

Ischemic episodes

Ischemic stroke can begin anywhere from a person's thirties to their sixties; it affects 85% of patients with CADASIL and is the most common initial presentation (Bousser and Tournier-Lasserve, 2001). Clinically, patients present with classic lacunar syndromes that produce sensory or motor symptoms. However, some ischemic events will be clinically silent or produce mild and vague symptoms of dizziness, fatigue or confusion. Ischemic events usually recur, with an accumulation of deficits eventually leading to a classical stepwise decline, with gait difficulties, pseudobulbar palsy, urinary incontinence and a dementia syndrome with frontal lobe features (Leim *et al.*, 2007). Ischemic events tend to have the greatest clinical impact in the fifties to seventies, with increasing evidence that disability in CADASIL is closely tied to the number and size of lacunar infarctions and hypodense lesions on T_1-weighted MRI. Ischemic episodes usually occur earlier in CADASIL than in sporadic forms of subcortical vascular disease, with evidence of neurological resilience early in the course but classical stepwise deterioration late in the illness.

Psychiatric disturbance

Psychiatric disturbances are also evident in CADASIL, but behavioral symptoms are not well characterized. Families frequently note symptoms of irritability, mild depression and a decline in motivation and speed of responding as the first signs of the illness (Dichgans et al., 1998; Thomas et al., 2002; Leyhe et al., 2005). More significant mood disturbance affects approximately 20% of patients (Chabriat et al., 1995; Dichgans et al., 1998; Desmond et al., 1999). Mood lability may be seen, with depression alternating with mania (Bousser and Tournier-Lasserve, 2001) and panic attacks, schizophrenia and personality changes have been reported (Chabriat et al., 1995; Lagas and Juvonen, 2001; Thomas et al., 2002; Leyhe et al., 2005). Pathological affect, apathy and disinhibition may occur in later stages.

Cognitive impairment

Cognitive impairment generally occurs in the domains of attention, processing speed, executive functioning and inefficient learning and retrieval of new information. Deficits are particularly evident on tasks requiring cognitive set-shifting, response inhibition, working memory, verbal fluency and abstract concept formation (Taillia et al., 1998; Yousry et al., 1999; Amberla et al., 2004; Peters et al., 2004a, 2005). Visuospatial impairments have been reported less frequently (e.g. Taillia et al., 1998; Yousry et al., 1999). Verbal fluency was found to be consistently impaired in CADASIL and Binswanger's disease, with greater levels of impairment than AD (Charlton et al., 2006). Episodic memory is generally well preserved until late in the illness (Amberla et al., 2004) and tends to be characterized by encoding and retrieval deficits rather than a storage deficit. Overall, the cognitive deficits elicited by formal neuropsychological assessment align well with the subjective complaints of patients in the early stages of the illness, which tend to focus on reduced mental efficiency and poor recall. The cognitive deficits worsen with age (Peters et al., 2004a) and with the presence of infarction (Amberla et al., 2004), and demented and non-demented patients with CADASIL differ mainly by the severity rather than the pattern of cognitive deficits (Peters et al., 2005). A review of some key studies of cognitive functioning in CADASIL, with a focus on studies with the largest samples, follows.

Amberla et al. (2004) found that patients with genetically confirmed CADASIL but no clinical evidence of transient ischemic attack, stroke or dementia performed more poorly than controls on tests of immediate memory, working memory and executive functions. The authors interpreted this as evidence of incipient cognitive impairment in CADASIL even before the onset of clinical ischemic symptoms.

Peters et al. (2005) reported on 65 patients with CADASIL and 30 control individuals matched for age, gender and education. CADASIL subjects demonstrated pronounced deficits on measures of attention and psychomotor processing speed (e.g. Stroop interference condition, Trails B, and a composite score from performance on Symbol-Digit, digit-span backward and digit cancellation tasks). The pattern of cognitive test performance was similar in CADASIL subjects who scored below the cutoff for dementia on the Mattis Dementia Rating Scale (i.e. ≤ 123 versus > 123) ($n = 9$) and those who scored above it ($n = 56$), but deficits were far more pronounced among the latter group. Moreover, CADASIL subjects over 45 years of age performed significantly more poorly than controls on more tests than those under 45 years.

Peters et al. (2004b) also examined the 2-year progression of symptoms in 80 CADASIL individuals – the largest systematically studied cohort to date. Deficits were greatest on tests of mental processing speed (Trails A); executive functioning, with impairments in rapid cognitive set-switching (Trails B); and ability to inhibit a prepotent response in favor of an alternative response (Stroop Interference Task). Language functions and episodic memory were generally well preserved over the follow-up period. Cognitive test performance and variability were inversely correlated with age. There was a significant correlation between cognitive test performance and measures of functional disability and stroke.

The foregoing review indicates that the cognitive features of CADASIL tend to coalesce around the cognitive domains of complex attention, processing speed and executive functioning. These deficits likely arise because of a partial or, in the presence of lacunar infarction, complete disconnection. These same cognitive domains are the most consistently affected in sporadic subcortical ischemic vascular disease (Gunning-Dixon and Raz, 2003; Desmond, 2004) and disconnection is thought to underlie these deficits as well (Roman, 1987). However, there is evidence that hippocampal atrophy is a key factor in the development of the dementia syndrome in patients with subcortical lacunar infarctions (Fein *et al.*, 2000). The role of the hippocampus in the development of dementia in CADASIL is uncertain. In a preliminary study, our group showed no difference in hippocampal volume between a group of eight non-demented CADASIL patients and 10 age-matched controls (Patel *et al.*, 2007). However, O'Sullivan and colleagues (2007) recently demonstrated that hippocampal volume is an independent predictor of cognitive performance in CADASIL.

Magnetic resonance imaging features

Widespread diffuse WMHs, indicating leukoencephalopathy, on T_2-weighted MRI and T_1-weighted hypodensities are the imaging hallmarks of CADASIL (Fig. 22.2). The WMHs usually appear as punctate or nodular signals between the ages of 20 and 30 years (van den Boom *et al.*, 2003a), although individuals under 20 have not been extensively studied. Almost all gene-positive individuals will have evidence of WMH after age 30 (van den Boom *et al.*, 2003a). Over time, the WMHs become diffuse, symmetric and involve all

of the white matter. Cerebral microbleeds are also common in CADASIL, occurring in approximately one-third of individuals (Lesnik Oberstein *et al.*, 2001; Dichgans, 2002; Viswanathan *et al.*, 2006). Intracerebral hemorrhage has been less frequently reported (Maclean *et al.*, 2005; Choi *et al.*, 2006; Werbrouck and de Bleecker, 2006) and may be related to the number of cerebral microbleeds (Choi *et al.*, 2006) and anticoagulant treatment (Werbrouck and de Bleecker, 2006).

The WMHs occur most prominently in the centrum semiovale, frontal, temporal and periventricular white matter (Auer *et al.*, 2001). They are also found in the internal and external capsules; corpus callosum; subcortical arcuate fibers; brainstem, particularly the pons and cerebellum; and in subcortical gray matter structures, including the caudate and lentiform nuclei and the thalamus (Chabriat *et al.*, 1998, 1999a; Yousry *et al.*, 1999; Auer *et al.*, 2001; O'Sullivan *et al.*, 2001). Orbitofrontal and occipital white matter are relatively spared. Lacunar infarcts tend to have a similar distribution (Yousry *et al.*, 1999) but are somewhat less frequent in parietal, occipital and infratentorial regions (van den Boom *et al.*, 2002).

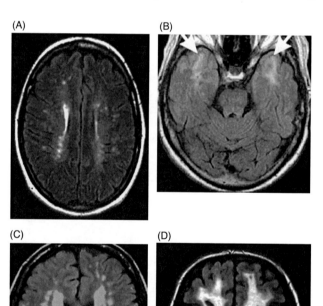

(A) (B) (C) (D)

Fig. 22.2. White matter hyperintensities on axial fluid-attenuated inversion recovery (FLAIR) magnetic resonance images in CADASIL. (A) A 25-year-old mutation carrier with no symptoms. (B) A 45-year old with very early cognitive symptoms. Arrows show white matter hyperintensities in the anterior temporal lobes. (C) A 58-year old with executive dysfunction and moderate areas of confluent white matter hyperintensities in the periventricular and deep white matter. (D) A 65-year old with dementia and extensive white matter hyperintensities with multiple lacunar infarctions.

Microbleeds occur in CADASIL, particularly with increasing age (Lesnik Oberstein et al., 2001; Dichgans, 2002), occurring most commonly in the thalamus, basal ganglia and brainstem (Lesnik Oberstein et al., 2001; Viswanathan et al., 2006): a distribution that contrasts with that of WMH and lacunes (Viswanathan et al., 2006). They have been shown to be associated with elevated systolic blood pressure, a history of hypertension, poor glucose control (indicated by glycosylated hemoglobin levels) and the volume of WMH and lacunar infarction (Viswanathan et al., 2006).

The regional distribution of MRI lesions in CADASIL corresponds with the cerebral angioarchitecture (van den Boom et al., 2003b). The lesions are thought to arise from disruption of normal cerebral hemodynamics (van den Boom et al., 2003b) resulting from the degradation of the smooth muscle layer, particularly in deep penetrating small arteries (Chabriat et al., 1999a; Auer et al., 2001). There is a positive correlation between age and both T_1- and T_2-weighted lesion load (Chabriat et al., 1999a; Opherk et al., 2006; Peters et al., 2006). Opherk et al. (2006) demonstrated a strong modifying effect of genetic factors on the MRI lesion volume in CADASIL. However, prior studies failed to find an association between the specific genetic abnormalities and MRI lesion load (Dichgans et al., 1999; Singhal et al., 2004). The discrepant results could reflect differences in the way that the genetic information was analyzed.

The MRI features of CADASIL overlap considerably, with the more common sporadic form of subcortical ischemic vascular changes related to hypertensive arteriosclerosis (Davous, 1998). However, certain MRI features may help to differentiate the groups, particularly the presence of anterior temporal WMH, and extension of WMH into the cortical U-fibers (Auer et al., 2001). Patients with CADASIL also tend to have greater WMH involvement in the superior frontal white matter (Auer et al., 2001) and in the external capsule and corpus callosum (O'Sullivan et al., 2001; Markus et al., 2002), although these regions are less specific for CADASIL. Identification of WMH in the anterior temporal lobe and in the external capsule may also help to differentiate CADASIL from multiple sclerosis (O'Riordan et al., 2002), a common misdiagnosis in CADASIL (Trojano and Paolicelli, 2001).

MRI studies in CADASIL have generally found associations between white matter lesion load and extent of functional and cognitive impairment. In a sample of 75 patients, Chabriat et al. (1999b) found that dementia only occurred in the presence of high-grade WMHs. Using semi-automated techniques, Dichgans et al. (1999) studied a group of 64 patients with CADASIL and found that both lacunar infarct and WMH volumes were significantly correlated with measures of functional disability and were inversely correlated with overall cognitive function based on the Mini-Mental State Examination (MMSE). Liem et al. (2007) demonstrated that lacunar lesion load is more predictive of cognitive dysfunction than either WMH or microbleeds. In contrast to these studies, a few reports in the literature with smaller groups of patients have failed to demonstrate an association between MRI lesions and extent of disability or cognitive impairment (e.g. Taillia et al., 1998; Trojano et al., 1998; Scheid et al., 2006).

Peters et al. (2006) showed that the progression of WMH over time may be a less sensitive predictor of decline than loss of brain volume. They demonstrated significant loss of brain volume over a 2-year follow-up in a group of 76 patients with CADASIL. Age and hypertension were significant predictors of volume loss over the follow-up period but T_2-weighted lesion load at baseline was not. Volume loss over the follow-up period was significantly associated with declines on clinical measures of stroke-related disability and on a structured dementia interview, but only a statistical trend was found for the association with the Mattis Dementia Rating Scale. Change in volume identified in T_2-weighted images was not significantly correlated with change in any of these clinical measures. This study highlights the potential for brain volume measurements as a predictor of decline in CADASIL.

Studies in CADASIL using MRI are limited by the sensitivity of conventional T_2-weighted techniques to subtle white matter injury that nonetheless contributes to cognitive impairment (Filippi and Grossman, 2002). Diffusion-tensor imaging (DTI) is more sensitive to disruption of white matter integrity than conventional MRI methods (Moseley, 2002). This technique provides indirect information about the structural integrity of white matter based on measurement of the magnitude and orientation of water diffusion in tissue (Malloy et al., 2007). Higher levels of diffusivity and lower levels of diffusion directional coherence (anisotropy) are interpreted as evidence of decreased white matter integrity. Diffusion-tensor imaging is an excellent technique for studying the full spectrum of white matter change in CADASIL.

333

Diffusion-tensor imaging studies in CADASIL have consistently found declines in white matter integrity compared with controls in both lesioned and normal-appearing white matter (NAWM) on T_2-weighted imaging and in certain subcortical gray matter structures. These DTI changes correlate significantly with measures of disability and cognitive function. For example, Chabriat et al. (1999b) found DTI changes in NAWM in patients with CADASIL compared with controls and these changes correlated significantly with a rating of disability but not with a global cognitive screening measure. O'Sullivan et al. (2004) showed higher diffusivity in NAWM of non-demented patients with CADASIL compared with controls and these changes correlated with declines in executive function.

Changes in DTI have also been found in subcortical gray matter structures in CADASIL, including the thalamus, putamen and globus pallidus (Molko et al., 2001; O'Sullivan et al., 2004), and increased diffusivity in the thalamus correlates with executive dysfunction (O'Sullivan et al., 2004) and with performance on the MMSE (Molko et al., 2001). O'Sullivan et al. (2005) showed that executive function and verbal memory were associated with a distinct regional pattern of white matter changes in CADASIL: executive functions were correlated with decreased white matter integrity in distributed frontal white matter regions and in the cingulum bundle, whereas verbal memory ability was associated with DTI changes in the striatum only. Controlling for WMH volume did not appreciably alter the results, highlighting the importance on cognitive functioning of subtle changes in white matter integrity that are not visible on T_2-weighted MRI. Diffusion-tensor imaging is also sensitive to the progression of white matter injury in CADASIL. Molko et al. (2002) found that, compared with controls, patients with CADASIL had increased diffusivity in the entire brain image after 29 months and the change was associated with increased disability. A more recent larger study also showed that increased diffusivity over a 2-year period was a significant predictor of worsening disability and cognitive decline in CADASIL but T_2-weighted lesion volume was not (Holtmannspotter et al., 2005).

The foregoing studies involved analysis of images of scalar DTI parameters of diffusivity and anisotropy. These parameters consider the magnitude of diffusion in each image voxel. Using DTI tractography allows an alternative way to visualize DTI data that incorporates both the magnitude and direction of greatest diffusion. Tractography visualizations provide a computer-generated representation of the three-dimensional topography of white matter architecture. We recently demonstrated the utility of quantitative DTI tractography in which measurements of the fiber models are used as markers of the structural integrity of specific fiber bundles. (Fig. 22.3) (Correia et al., 2008).

Pathology

CADASIL is associated with degeneration of small and medium-sized arterioles in subcortical white and gray matter. Figure 22.4 shows characteristic gross and microscopic brain changes in postmortem CADASIL. Granular material accumulates in the walls of the arterial smooth muscle layer, and the presence of granular osmophilic material (GOM) adjacent to the basement membrane of the smooth muscle cells of cerebral arterioles on electron microscopy has become a hallmark pathological feature. As the disease progresses, GOM increases and cytoarchitectural changes include detachment of cells, with increasing space between the endothelium and the vascular smooth muscle cells (VSMCs) and disruption of the elastin and smooth muscle actin layers. Destruction of VSMCs may also cause decreased secretion of vascular endothelial growth factor (VEGF) and loss of vascular permeability (Ruchoux and Maurage, 1998; Brulin et al., 2002). In arterioles, endothelial cells are swollen, leading to loss of tight junctions (Ruchoux and Maurage, 1998). There is severe adventitial fibrosis from the site of the penetrating artery at the cortical surface to the distal end, transforming the vessel into an "earthen pipe" (Okeda et al., 2002). Over time, there is dilatation of the perivascular spaces, which appear as areas of signal hyperintensity on T_2-weighted MRI. The subcortical white matter shows rarefaction, demyelination and gliosis – more extensive but qualitatively similar to that seen in Binswanger's disease. The progressive white matter injury is likely related to impairments in flow, reactivity and autoregulation through the subcortical arterioles. However, we have recently demonstrated impairments in notch signaling in glial cells as well, suggesting that CADASIL is also a disease of the glia in subcortical white matter (Brennan-Krohn et al., 2007). Large-vessel infarctions are rarely seen. Lacunar infarction is common and occurs primarily in subcortical white and gray matter structures, though lacunar infarction also involves the brainstem. Autopsy examination of patients in

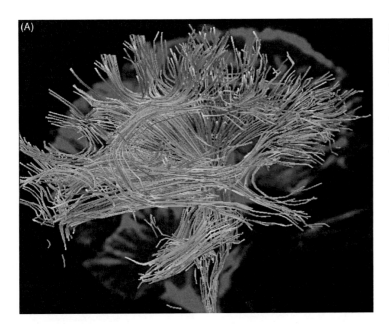

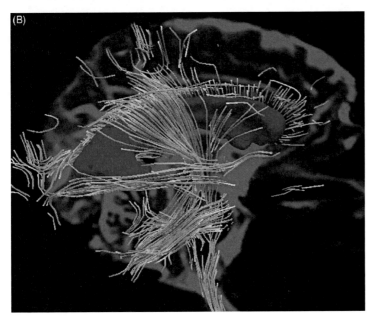

Fig. 22.3. Diffusion-tensor imaging using streamtube models in normal elderly and CADASIL. (A) Whole-brain streamtube model (sagittal view) for a 72-year-old healthy volunteer. (B) Whole-brain streamtube model of a 60-year-old patient with CADASIL and mild dementia. Note the marked decrease in streamtube density in the patient with CADASIL. Streamtube models are superimposed on non-diffusion encoded T$_2$-weighted magnetic resonance images; the lateral ventricles are portrayed in blue.

their sixties who had late-stage disease reveals good preservation of the cortical ribbon, with widespread gliosis and demyelination of the subcortical white matter studded by numerous small holes in the white matter, which may represent areas where subcortical arterioles have dropped out.

The actual cause of ischemic events and lacunar infarction in CADASIL is not clear as CADASIL is not typically associated with hyalinosis, arteriosclerosis, luminal narrowing, atherothrombosis or amyloid angiopathy. Fragility and fragmentation of the vessel wall is the likely cause of microhemorrhage in later stages of the illness. As mentioned above, late-stage disease is associated with cerebral atrophy, and apoptotic changes have recently been reported in the cerebral cortex in postmortem tissue (Viswanathan *et al.*, 2006). Fibrillar amyloid or tau pathology has only been reported in a single case but we have observed

335

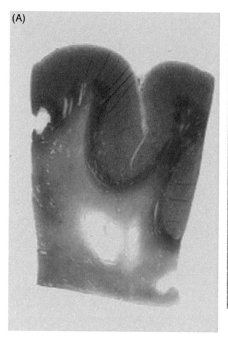

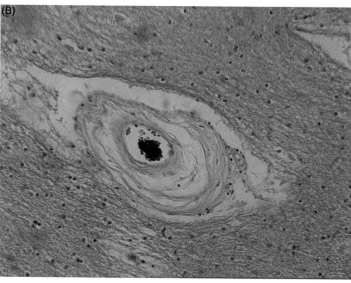

Fig. 22.4. Gross and microscopic changes in postmortem CADASIL brain. (A) Luxol fast blue, hematoxylin and eosin stain of the frontal lobe showing cavitary necrosis in the deep white matter with relative preservation of the subcortical U-fibers and normal thickness of the cortical ribbon. (B) Light microscopic hematoxylin and eosin stain of a subcortical arteriole demonstrating mural fibrosis and disintegration of the smooth muscle layer, dilatation of the perivascular space, and pallor of the surrounding white matter.

an additional case of stage III Braak neurofibrillary pathology without amyloid plaques (unpublished data). Arteriolar changes are also observed in other organs such as the skin but symptoms related to vasculopathy in other organ systems, peripheral nerve and muscle are rarely reported (Prakash *et al.*, 2002).

Animal models of CADASIL

Postnatal *Notch3* brain expression in mice is limited to vascular VSMCs within the walls of small to medium penetrating arteries, the same vessels predominantly damaged in CADASIL (Prakash *et al.*, 2002). A mouse with an R142C *Notch3* knock-in (corresponding to the common human CADASIL mutation R141C) did not show a CADASIL-like phenotype (Lundkvist *et al.*, 2005). In 2003, however, a group of French researchers reported their creation of a transgenic mouse in which VSMCs expressed a full-length human Notch3 protein carrying the R90C change in low levels. By 10 months of age, the mice showed disruption of normal VSMC anchorage to the extracellular matrix of adjacent cells, VSMC cytoskeleton changes and initial signs of VSMC degeneration. By contrast, Notch3 accumulation and GOM deposits did not appear until 14–16

months. (The mice did not develop brain parenchyma lesions or clinical symptoms.) The authors concluded that VSMC degeneration is not initiated by the build-up of Notch3 or GOM but perhaps by the disruption of VSMC anchorage (Ruchoux *et al.*, 2003). They subsequently found that transgenic mice that had begun to exhibit cystoskeletal changes and disruption of adhesion of VSMCs to neighboring cells, but not accumulation of Notch3 and GOM, had impairment in pressure-induced contraction and flow-induced dilatation in isolated arteries; in other words, mechano-transduction (but not response to vasoactive agents) was impaired at an early stage in the disease, prior to Notch3 and GOM accumulation (Dubroca *et al.*, 2005). Mice at this early stage already showed impairment in reactivity to vasodilator stimuli and in cerebral blood flow autoregulation (Lacombe *et al.*, 2005).

Genetic aspects of Binswanger's disease

White matter hyperintensities as seen in Binswanger's disease have been shown to be strongly heritable (Carmelli *et al.*, 1998; Atwood *et al.*, 2004; Turner *et al.*, 2004). However, only limited work has been

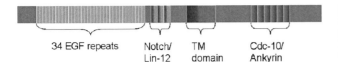

34 EGF repeats   Notch/   TM   Cdc-10/
                  Lin-12   domain Ankyrin

done on the specific genes that confer this risk apart from those known to impart general risk for hypertension, and even less work has been directed at the identification of genes that mediate the impact of vascular pathology on brain parenchyma (Leblanc *et al.*, 2006). Sierra *et al.* (2002) found that, among 60 hypertensive patients (age 50–60 years) with white matter lesions, 64% had the DD genotype of the gene for angiotensin-converting enzyme compared with 22% of those without white matter lesions. In a large community-based sample of adults aged 44–75 years, Schmidt *et al.* (2000) found that diastolic blood pressure and the LL genotype of the gene *PON1*, encoding paraoxinase, predicted the 3-year progression of white matter lesions. The association between apolipoprotein E genotype (*APOE*) and white matter lesions has been mixed, with some studies showing that allele type imparts a risk for white matter lesions (Skoog, 1997; Bronge *et al.*, 1999) and others showing no association (Barber *et al.*, 1999; Sawada *et al.*, 2000). These mixed results could be partially explained by a finding from the population-based Rotterdam study suggesting that individuals with the *APOE* ε4 allele have increased risk for white matter lesions if they also have hypertension (de Leeuw *et al.*, 2004).

CADASIL genetics

Much more is known about the molecular genetics of the disease-causing mutations in CADASIL. Positional cloning and linkage analysis was used to locate the responsible gene on chromosome 19p13.1–13.2. Transmission of CADASIL *Notch3* mutations is autosomal dominant with 100% penetrance. *Notch 3* is a large gene comprising 33 exons that is ubiquitously found in human adult tissues, but its expression is restricted to vascular smooth muscle cells (Fig. 22.5). The gene encodes a transmembrane protein of 2321 amino acid residues (Joutel *et al.*, 1996). The function of Notch3 is to maintain cell–cell interaction or communication between vascular smooth muscle cells and arterial endothelial cells, thus maintaining arterial vessel homeostasis by promoting smooth muscle survival (Shawber and Kitajewski, 2004). The Notch3 proteins are large, single-pass, transmembrane receptors. There is an extracellular domain that contains

34 tandem epidermal growth factor (EGF)-like repeats, three cyteine-rich Notch/Lin12 repeats, a single transmembrane domain and an intracellular domain. Each EGF repeat contains six conserved cysteine residues, which form three disulfide bonds, and almost all disease-causing mutations result from a missense mutation leading to a loss or gain of a cysteine residue in the EGF repeats encoded by the first 23 exons. The change in cysteine results in an odd number of cysteine residues and to disruption of disulfide pairing. (Even the rare mutations that do not involve a cysteine directly may affect the location and function of neighboring cysteine residues [Mazzei *et al.*, 2004].)

There is considerable phenotypic heterogeneity among family members with the same mutation, suggesting involvement of environmental and other genetic factors in phenotypic expression. Significant relationships between genotype and phenotype have proven elusive. In a study of 127 CADASIL subjects from 65 families with 17 different mutations, no correlation was found between mutation and presence or age of onset of stroke, migraine, dementia, dependency or MRI lesion load, nor did particular families show specific phenotypes (Singhal *et al.*, 2004). Figure 22.6 shows an example of phenotypic variability in terms of extent of WMHs and clinical course between two members of the same family with the same Notch3 CADASIL mutation. Nevertheless, a few observations of specific genotype–phenotype correlations have been reported. The C117F mutation appears to be associated with a lower age at death and the C174Y mutation with a lower age at onset for stroke, immobilization and death (Opherk *et al.* 2004). A Colombian family with the C455R mutation showed unusually early onset of stroke (median age 31 years; range 19–40) (Arboleda-Velasquez *et al.*, 2002) and the R153C mutation has been identified as a risk factor for cerebral microbleeds in CADASIL (Lesnik Oberstein *et al.*, 2001). A Japanese family with the S180C mutation had an unusual phenotype characterized by hallucinations and delusions and a decrease in the mean age at onset of stroke in each of three generations.

Notch is processed in a similar manner to cleavage of the amyloid precursor protein, and inhibition of presenilin/γ-secretase also inhibits Notch. The Notch intracellular domain consists of several distinct units: a

337

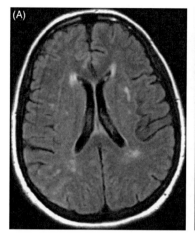 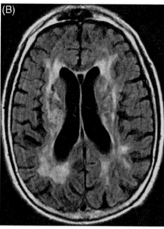

Fig. 22.6. Phenotypic heterogeneity in a CADASIL family. (A) Axial fluid-attenuated inversion recovery (FLAIR) non-contrast magnetic resonance image (MRI) of 55-year-old woman with mild subcortical white matter hyperintensities (leukoencephalopathy). She has had mild headaches but no significant cognitive, mood or motor symptoms. (B) Axial FLAIR non-contrast MRI of the brother of the patient in (A). Note the higher degree of leukoencephalopathy with multiple subcortical lacunar infarcts, as well as moderate cerebral atrophy and ventricular enlargement. This patient developed depression and recurrent ischemic episodes beginning at age 50, dementia at age 53 and died at age 55. The clinical course was complicated by alcohol abuse.

RAM domain is followed by a nuclear localization sequence, six ankyrin repeats (ANK) and a PEST domain, which is apparently involved in Notch receptor turnover (Weinmaster, 1997; Baron, 2003; Bianchi *et al.*, 2006). Notch receptors bind DSL ligands (*delta* and *serrate/jagged* in *Drosophila* and vertebrates, *Lag-2* in *Caenorhabditis elegans*). Like the Notch receptors, the ligands are single-pass transmembrane proteins with multiple EGFs in their extracellular domains (Weinmaster, 1997). In the Golgi apparatus, the full-length Notch3 protein is proteolytically cleaved by furine convertase into a 210 kDa extracellular fragment and a 97 kDa transmembrane and intracellular fragment (site 1 or S1 cleavage) (Joutel *et al.*, 2000). The two fragments are non-covalently linked and transported to the plasma membrane as a heterodimeric receptor (Louvi *et al.*, 2006). Upon ligand binding, S2 cleavage occurs at an extracellular site, allowing presenilin/γ-secretase-dependent S3 cleavage in the intramembrane domain and subsequent release of the soluble intracellular domain (NIc). This is then transferred to the nucleus, where it binds via the RAM domain and ANK repeats to the transcription factor RBP-Jk/CBF1 and converts it from a transcription repressor to a transcription activator (Baron, 2003; Bianchi *et al.*, 2006).

Molecular effects of mutations in CADASIL

Despite the thorough characterization of CADASIL-related *Notch3* mutations, the pathophysiological mechanisms by which the mutations cause the vascular, histological and clinical effects of the disease are very poorly understood. The two main hypotheses for the pathogenesis of the disease are (1) accumulation of Notch3 protein products and GOM in the VSMCs, or (2) impaired signaling. Studies have variously supported and refuted both of these proposals.

The distribution pattern of *Notch3* mutations suggests that the mutations exert a gain-of-function effect because they are located in areas of high sequence diversity among *Notch* orthologs (Donahue and Kosik, 2004). These areas can tolerate significant diversity, presumably including that caused by CADASIL mutations, without a loss of function. Sites coding for signaling processes are, by comparison, usually highly conserved and suffer from loss-of-function mutations, so the findings of this study do not support a signaling deficit (Donahue and Kosik, 2004). Furthermore, the 210 kDa extracellular fragment of the protein has been found to accumulate at the cytoplasmic membrane of cerebral VSMCs. Because production of Notch3 does not appear to be increased, the accumulation is probably caused by impaired clearance of the ectodomain from the cell surface, most likely as a result of improper oligomerization of the mutant protein fragment owing to a change in the tertiary structure or aggregation state of Notch3 (Arboleda-Velasquez *et al.*, 2005). Murine Notch3 cell lines with an R142C mutation (corresponding to the prevalent human mutation R141C) exhibited normal signaling but impaired processing, trafficking and localization of Notch3 (Karlstrom *et al.*, 2002). (However, later attempts to make a mouse model of CADASIL with this particular mutation were not successful, so its validity as a model of human disease is unclear [Lundkvist *et al.*, 2005].) CADASIL-like mutations engineered into *Notch3* in rats may cause a decrease in the ratio of receptor fragments to full-length protein but do not appear to affect signaling

(Haritunians *et al.*, 2002, 2005). Three-dimensional homology models of the first six EGF-like domains have suggested that some of the mutations would cause protein misfolding, perhaps leading also to homo- or heterodimeric intermolecular cross-linkage as a result of the uneven number of cysteine residues (Dichgans *et al.*, 2000).

Two studies have found signaling impairment caused by mutations in the ligand-binding domain but not by mutations in EGF 2–5, the area of highest mutation density (Joutel *et al.*, 2004; Peters *et al.*, 2004b). However, in one of the studies, the mutant receptors, although targeted to the cell surface, showed a decreased ratio of cleaved receptor fragments to full-length protein (Peters *et al.*, 2004b), which is in accord with the findings of impaired trafficking and localization by Karlström *et al.* (2002) above. The finding that VSMC impairment precedes the onset of GOM and Notch3 accumulation in a mouse model of CADASIL seems to support a signaling hypothesis over an accumulation hypothesis (Ruchoux *et al.*, 2003; Dubroca *et al.*, 2005; Lacombe *et al.*, 2005).

Differential diagnosis
Patients with CADASIL may initially be misdiagnosed with multiple sclerosis, cerebral vasculitis or Binswanger's disease, and it is not uncommon for patients to be treated for multiple sclerosis for an extended period before the diagnosis of CADASIL is made. Familial hemiplegic migraine, another rare autosomal dominant disorder, can resemble CADASIL clinically, especially among younger patients. It involves attacks of migraine with aura associated with transient hemiplegia, and, in about 20% of cases, permanent cerebellar signs including nystagmus and ataxia. It is associated with mutations in the *CACNA1A* calcium channel gene, located near *Notch3* (Carrera *et al.*, 2001). The differential diagnosis also includes mitochondrial encephalopathies such as MELAS (mitochondrial encephalopathy, lactic acidosis, and stroke-like episodes) and leukodystrophies such as metachromatic leukodystrophy, which shows diffuse white matter changes and can begin in adults (Koga *et al.*, 1995).

Genetic testing
The diagnosis of CADASIL can be made by utilizing genetic analysis, MRI and skin biopsy. Genetic analysis of the entire *Notch3* gene is highly sensitive and specific for detection of disease-causing mutations.

The cost of the testing may be a concern, and analysis of a single exon can be done in patients with a known family mutation at a greatly reduced cost. Identification of arteriolar changes on electron microscopy from a skin biopsy can aid in diagnosis, but the sensitivity of this method is limited by samples yielding few skin arterioles and variability in rater experience in interpreting the specimen. Adding Notch3 antibody stains to skin specimens can significantly improve sensitivity and specificity but the Notch3 antibody is not widely available.

Treatment and management
The diagnosis of CADASIL usually generates a great deal of fear and apprehension about the future. It is important that these fears be aired and addressed and patients and families be provided with support and education to understand the disorder and the likely clinical course. Lifestyle modifications and stress management are essential for establishing a predictable daily routine that supports the highest level of functioning for the patient. Employment responsibilities must be adjusted to match the patient's changing capabilities. Patients and families have many questions about what to say to other family members about the illness, especially children, and deciding who should be tested. Some have questions about family planning. Asymptomatic minor children should not be tested until they reach majority status and can independently weigh the risks and benefits of testing. Asymptomatic adults who are considering testing should meet with a neurologist, genetics counselor and a psychologist familiar with the disorder in a genetic-testing protocol similar to that used in Huntington's disease.

Specific treatments for patients with CADASIL are not currently available. Antiplatelet agents are recommended for empirical prevention of strokes, but they have not been tested in CADASIL patients. Low-dose enteric coated aspirin can be used for patients early in the disease, with use of standard doses of antiplatelet agents in patients who have experienced one or more ischemic events. Combining antiplatelet agents is not recommended. Warfarin and tissue plasminogen activator should be avoided because of increased risk of hemorrhage. Homocysteine should be checked and elevated levels treated. Prophylactic medications should be used for patients with frequent migraine headaches, with limited use of non-steroidal anti-inflammatory agents and butalbital–caffeine medications as abortive therapy. Triptans should be avoided because of a small increased risk of vasoconstriction and stroke. Headache treatment with acetezolamide has been beneficial in anectodal reports. Irritability and depression are common early symptoms that usually respond well to standard antidepressant medications. Cholinesterase inhibitors have shown some efficacy in improving cognition in vascular dementia trials and may be used empirically in CADASIL patients with cognitive impairment. A recent placebo-controlled trial of donepezil in patients with CADASIL and cognitive impairment demonstrated improvement on some executive function tests in the patients who received donepezil (Dichgans et al., 2008). L-arginine has been suggested for empiric use in CADASIL because of studies showing reduced infarct volume in some experimental stroke models and increased vasoreactivity in CADASIL patients (Willmot et al., 2005). Enthusiasm is limited by an increased death rate in a post-myocardial infarction trial with L-arginine (Schulman et al., 2006). Future CADASIL treatments will employ genetic modification and neuroprotective strategies based on advances in understanding the pathophysiology and mechanism of arteriolar degeneration and white matter injury.

Summary

CADASIL provides an important model for understanding the pathophysiology of subcortical arteriolar degeneration and its impact on white matter integrity, and subsequent effect on cognition and disability in the elderly in the absence of concomitant amyloid and tau pathology. The phenotypic presentation of the cognitive and neuroimaging features of CADASIL and Binswanger's disease is similar despite differences in the underlying vasculopathy. Overall, the cognitive dysfunction in CADASIL parallels the deficits in processing speed, attention and executive function that characterize Binswanger's disease. However, younger CADASIL patients appear better able to tolerate a higher burden of WMH. The extent of lacunar infarctions and cortical, and possibly hippocampal, atrophy play an important role in the dementia syndrome in both disorders. Though the exact mechanism linking Notch3 mutations and degeneration of vascular smooth muscle cells is not yet known, much has been learned about Notch signaling, and it is hoped that these insights will help to motivate a search to elucidate the genetics and pathogenesis of subcortical ischemic vascular disease in the elderly.

References

Agostoni, E. and Rigamonti, A. (2007) Migraine and cerebrovascular disease. Neurol Sci, 28(Suppl 2), S156–60.

Alzheimer's Association (2007) Alzheimer's Disease Facts and Figures. Chicago, IL: Alzheimer's Association.

Amberla, K., Waljas, M., Tuominen, S. et al. (2004) Insidious cognitive decline in CADASIL. Stroke, 35, 1598–602.

Arboleda-Velasquez, J. F., Lopera, F., Lopez, E. et al. (2002) C455R Notch3 mutation in a Colombian CADASIL kindred with early onset of stroke. Neurology, 59, 277–9.

Arboleda-Velasquez, J. F., Rampal, R., Fung, E. et al. (2005) CADASIL mutations impair Notch3 glycosylation by Fringe. Hum Mol Genet, 14, 1631–9.

Atwood, L. D., Wolf, P. A., Heard-Costa, N. L. et al. (2004) Genetic variation in white matter hyperintensity volume in the Framingham Study. Stroke, 35, 1609–13.

Auer, D. P., Putz, B., Gossl, C. et al. (2001) Differential lesion patterns in CADASIL and sporadic subcortical arteriosclerotic encephalopathy: MR imaging study with statistical parametric group comparison. Radiology, 218, 443–51.

Barber, R., Gholkar, A., Scheltens, P. et al. (1999) Apolipoprotein E epsilon4 allele, temporal lobe atrophy, and white matter lesions in late-life dementias. Arch Neurol, 56, 961–5.

Baron, M. (2003) An overview of the Notch signalling pathway. Semin Cell Dev Biol, 14, 113–19.

Bennett, D. A., Gilley, D. W., Wilson, R. S., Huckman, M. S. and Fox, J. H. (1992) Clinical correlates of high signal lesions on magnetic resonance imaging in Alzheimer's disease. J Neurol, 239, 186–90.

Bennett, D. A., Gilley, D. W., Lee, S. and Cochran, E. J. (1994) White matter changes: neurobehavioral manifestations of Binswanger's disease and clinical correlates in Alzheimer's disease. Dementia, 5, 148–52.

Bianchi, S., Dotti, M. T. and Federico, A. (2006) Physiology and pathology of notch signalling system. J Cell Physiol, 207, 300–8.

Bousser, M. and Tournier-Lasserve, E. (2001) Cerebral autosomal dominant arteriopathy with subcortical infarcts and leukoencephalopathy: from stroke to vessel wall physiology. J Neurol Neurosurg Psychiatry, 70, 285–7.

Brennan-Krohn, T., Dong, M., Rivera, E., Salloway, S. and De La Monte, S. (2007) CADASIL: molecular analysis of aberrant gene expression in the brain. In Annual Meeting of the American Academy of Neurology, abstract PO7.119.

Bronge, L., Fernaeus, S., Blomberg, M. et al. (1999) White matter lesions in Alzheimer patients are influenced by apoliprotein E genotype. Dement Geriatr Cogn Disord, 10, 89–96.

Brulin, P., Godfraind, C., Leteurtre, E. and Ruchoux, M. M. (2002) Morphometric analysis of ultrastructural vascular changes in CADASIL: analysis of 50 skin biopsy specimens and pathogenic implications. *Acta Neuropathol (Berl)*, **104**, 241–8.

Carmelli, D., Decarli, C., Swan, G. E. *et al.* (1998) Evidence for genetic variance in white matter hyperintensity volume in normal elderly male twins. *Stroke*, **29**, 1177–81.

Carrera, P., Stenirri, S., Ferrari, M. and Battistini, S. (2001) Familial hemiplegic migraine: a ion channel disorder. *Brain Res Bull*, **56**, 239–41.

Chabriat, H., Bousser, M. G. and Pappata, S. (1995) Cerebral autosomal dominant arteriopathy with subcortical infarcts and leukoencephalopathy: a positron emission tomography study in two affected family members. *Stroke*, **26**, 1729–30.

Chabriat, H., Levy, C., Taillia, H. *et al.* (1998) Patterns of MRI lesions in CADASIL. *Neurology*, **51**, 452–7.

Chabriat, H., Mrissa, R., Levy, C. *et al.* (1999a) Brain stem MRI signal abnormalities in CADASIL. *Stroke*, **30**, 457–9.

Chabriat, H., Pappata, S., Poupon, C. *et al.* (1999b) Clinical severity in CADASIL related to ultrastructural damage in white matter: in vivo study with diffusion tensor MRI. *Stroke*, **30**, 2637–43.

Charlton, R. A., Morris, R. G., Nitkunan, A. and Markus, H. S. (2006) The cognitive profiles of CADASIL and sporadic small vessel disease. *Neurology*, **66**, 1523–6.

Choi, J. C., Kang, S. Y., Kang, J. H. and Park, J. K. (2006) Intracerebral hemorrhages in CADASIL. *Neurology*, **67**, 2042–4.

Correia, S., Lee, S. Y., Voorn, T. *et al.* (2008) Quantitative tractography metrics of white matter integrity in diffusion-tensor MRI. *Neuroimage*, **42**, 568–81.

Davous, P. (1998) Cadasil: a review with proposed diagnostic criteria. *Eur J Neurol*, **5**, 219–33.

De Leeuw, F. E., de Groot, J. C. and Breteler, M. M. B. (2000) White matter changes: frequency and risk factors. In Pantoni, L., Intzitari, D. and Wallin, A. (eds.) *The Matter of White Matter: Clinical and Pathophysiological Aspects of White Matter Disease Related to Cognitive Decline and Vascular Dementia*. Utrecht: Academic Pharmaceutical Productions, pp. 19–33.

De Leeuw, F. E., Richard, F., de Groot, J. C. *et al.* (2004) Interaction between hypertension, apoE, and cerebral white matter lesions. *Stroke*, **35**, 1057–60.

Desmond, D. W. (2004) The neuropsychology of vascular cognitive impairment: is there a specific cognitive deficit? *J Neurol Sci*, **226**, 3–7.

Desmond, D. W., Moroney, J. T., Lynch, T. *et al.* (1999) The natural history of CADASIL: a pooled analysis of previously published cases. *Stroke*, **30**, 1230–3.

Dichgans, M. (2002) Cerebral autosomal dominant arteriopathy with subcortical infarcts and leukoencephalopathy: phenotypic and mutational spectrum. *J Neurol Sci*, **203–204**, 77–80.

Dichgans, M., Mayer, M., Uttner, I. *et al.* (1998) The phenotypic spectrum of CADASIL: clinical findings in 102 cases. *Ann Neurol*, **44**, 731–9.

Dichgans, M., Filippi, M., Bruning, R. *et al.* (1999) Quantitative MRI in CADASIL: correlation with disability and cognitive performance. *Neurology*, **52**, 1361–7.

Dichgans, M., Ludwig, H., Muller-Hocker, J., Messerschmidt, A. and Gasser, T. (2000) Small in-frame deletions and missense mutations in CADASIL: 3D models predict misfolding of Notch3 EGF-like repeat domains. *Eur J Hum Genet*, **8**, 280–5.

Dichgans, M., Markus, H., Salloway, S. *et al.* (2008) Donepezil in patients with subcortical vascular impairment: a randomized, double-blind trial in CADASIL. *Lancet Neurol*, **7**, 310–18.

Donahue, C. P. and Kosik, K. S. (2004) Distribution pattern of Notch3 mutations suggests a gain-of-function mechanism for CADASIL. *Genomics*, **83**, 59–65.

Dong, Y., Hassan, A., Zhang, Z. *et al.* (2003) Yield of screening for CADASIL mutations in lacunar stroke and leukoaraiosis. *Stroke*, **34**, 203–5.

Dubroca, C., Lacombe, P., Domenga, V. *et al.* (2005) Impaired vascular mechanotransduction in a transgenic mouse model of CADASIL arteriopathy. *Stroke*, **36**, 113–17.

Fein, G., Di Sclafani, V., Tanabe, J. *et al.* (2000) Hippocampal and cortical atrophy predict dementia in subcortical ischemic vascular disease. *Neurology*, **55**, 1626–35.

Filippi, M. and Grossman, R. I. (2002) MRI techniques to monitor MS evolution: the present and the future. *Neurology*, **58**, 1147–53.

Gunning-Dixon, F. M. and Raz, N. (2003) Neuroanatomical correlates of selected executive functions in middle-aged and older adults: a prospective MRI study. *Neuropsychologia*, **41**, 1929–41.

Haritunians, T., Boulter, J., Hicks, C. *et al.* (2002) CADASIL Notch3 mutant proteins localize to the cell surface and bind ligand. *Circ Res*, **90**, 506–8.

Haritunians, T., Chow, T., De Lange, R. P. *et al.* (2005) Functional analysis of a recurrent missense mutation in Notch3 in CADASIL. *J Neurol Neurosurg Psychiatry*, **76**, 1242–8.

Holtmannspotter, M., Peters, N., Opherk, C. *et al.* (2005) Diffusion magnetic resonance histograms as a surrogate marker and predictor of disease progression in CADASIL: a two-year follow-up study. *Stroke*, **36**, 2559–65.

Jellinger, K. A. (2002) The pathology of ischemic-vascular dementia: an update. *J Neurol Sci*, **203–204**, 153–7.

Joutel, A., Bousser, M. G., Biousse, V. *et al.* (1993) A gene for familial hemiplegic migraine maps to chromosome 19. *Nat Genet*, **5**, 40–5.

341

Joutel, A., Corpechot, C., Ducros, A. *et al.* (1996) *Notch3* mutations in CADASIL, a hereditary adult-onset condition causing stroke and dementia. *Nature*, **383**, 707–10.

Joutel, A., Andreux, F., Gaulis, S. *et al.* (2000) The ectodomain of the Notch3 receptor accumulates within the cerebrovasculature of CADASIL patients. *J Clin Invest*, **105**, 597–605.

Joutel, A., Monet, M., Domenga, V., Riant, F. and Tournier-Lasserve, E. (2004) Pathogenic mutations associated with cerebral autosomal dominant arteriopathy with subcortical infarcts and leukoencephalopathy differently affect Jagged1 binding and Notch3 activity via the RBP/JK signaling pathway. *Am J Hum Genet*, **74**, 338–47.

Karlström, H., Beatus, P., Dannaeus, K. *et al.* (2002) A CADASIL-mutated Notch 3 receptor exhibits impaired intracellular trafficking and maturation but normal ligand-induced signaling. *Proc Natl Acad Sci USA*, **99**, 17119–24.

Koga, S. J., Hodges, M., Markin, C. and Gorman, P. (1995) MELAS syndrome. *West J Med*, **163**, 379–81.

Lacombe, P., Oligo, C., Domenga, V., Tournier-Lasserve, E. and Joutel, A. (2005) Impaired cerebral vasoreactivity in a transgenic mouse model of cerebral autosomal dominant arteriopathy with subcortical infarcts and leukoencephalopathy arteriopathy. *Stroke*, **36**, 1053–8.

Lagas, P. A. and Juvonen, V. (2001) Schizophrenia in a patient with cerebral autosomally dominant arteriopathy with subcortical infarcts and leucoencephalopathy (CADASIL disease). *Nord J Psychiatry*, **55**, 41–2.

Leblanc, G. G., Meschia, J. F., Stuss, D. T. and Hachinski, V. (2006) Genetics of vascular cognitive impairment: the opportunity and the challenges. *Stroke*, **37**, 248–55.

Lesnik Oberstein, S. A., van den Boom, R., van Buchem, M. A. *et al.* (2001) Cerebral microbleeds in CADASIL. *Neurology*, **57**, 1066–70.

Leyhe, T., Wiendl, H., Buchkremer, G. and Wormstall, H. (2005) CADASIL: underdiagnosed in psychiatric patients? *Acta Psychiatr Scand*, **111**, 392–6; discussion 396–7.

Liem, M. K., van der Grond, J., Haan, J. *et al.* (2007) Lacunar infarcts are the main correlate with cognitive dysfunction in CADASIL. *Stroke*, **38**, 923–8.

Louvi, A., Arboleda-Velasquez, J. F. and Artavanis-Tsakonas, S. (2006) CADASIL: a critical look at a Notch disease. *Dev Neurosci*, **28**, 5–12.

Lundkvist, J., Zhu, S., Hansson, E. M. *et al.* (2005) Mice carrying a R142C Notch 3 knock-in mutation do not develop a CADASIL-like phenotype. *Genesis*, **41**, 13–22.

Maclean, A. V., Woods, R., Alderson, L. M. *et al.* (2005) Spontaneous lobar haemorrhage in CADASIL. *J Neurol Neurosurg Psychiatry*, **76**, 456–7.

Malloy, P., Correia, S., Stebbins, G. and Laidlaw, D. H. (2007) Neuroimaging of white matter in aging and dementia. *Clin Neuropsychol*, **21**, 73–109.

Markus, H. S., Martin, R. J., Simpson, M. A. *et al.* (2002) Diagnostic strategies in CADASIL. *Neurology*, **59**, 1134–8.

Mazzei, R., Conforti, F. L., Lanza, P. L. *et al.* (2004) A novel *Notch3* gene mutation not involving a cysteine residue in an Italian family with CADASIL. *Neurology*, **63**, 561–4.

Molko, N., Pappata, S., Mangin, J. F. *et al.* (2001) Diffusion tensor imaging study of subcortical gray matter in cadasil. *Stroke*, **32**, 2049–54.

Molko, N., Cohen, L., Mangin, J. F. *et al.* (2002) Visualizing the neural bases of a disconnection syndrome with diffusion tensor imaging. *J Cogn Neurosci*, **14**, 629–36.

Moseley, M. (2002) Diffusion tensor imaging and aging: a review. *NMR Biomed*, **15**, 553–60.

O'Riordan, S., Nor, A. M. and Hutchinson, M. (2002) CADASIL imitating multiple sclerosis: the importance of MRI markers. *Mult Scler*, **8**, 430–2.

O'Sullivan, M., Jones, D. K., Summers, P. E. *et al.* (2001) Evidence for cortical "disconnection" as a mechanism of age-related cognitive decline. *Neurology*, **57**, 632–8.

O'Sullivan, M., Morris, R. G., Huckstep, B. *et al.* (2004) Diffusion tensor MRI correlates with executive dysfunction in patients with ischaemic leukoaraiosis. *J Neurol Neurosurg Psychiatry*, **75**, 441–7.

O'Sullivan, M., Barrick, T. R., Morris, R. G., Clark, C. A. and Markus, H. S. (2005) Damage within a network of white matter regions underlies executive dysfunction in CADASIL. *Neurology*, **65**, 1584–90.

O'Sullivan, M., Ngo, E., Viswanathan, A. *et al.* (2007) Hippocampal volume is an independent predictor of cognitive performance in CADASIL. *Neurobiol Aging*, e-pub ahead of print.

Okeda, R., Arima, K. and Kawai, M. (2002) Arterial changes in cerebral autosomal dominant arteriopathy with subcortical infarcts and leukoencephalopathy (CADASIL) in relation to pathogenesis of diffuse myelin loss of cerebral white matter: examination of cerebral medullary arteries by reconstruction of serial sections of an autopsy case. *Stroke*, **33**, 2565–9.

Opherk, C., Peters, N., Herzog, J., Luedtke, R. and Dichgans, M. (2004) Long-term prognosis and causes of death in CADASIL: a retrospective study in 411 patients. *Brain*, **127**: 2533–9.

Opherk, C., Peters, N., Holtmannspotter, M. *et al.* (2006) Heritability of MRI lesion volume in CADASIL: evidence for genetic modifiers. *Stroke*, **37**, 2684–9.

Patel, K., Correia, S., Foley, J. *et al.* (2007) Cognitive impairment, hippocampal volume, and white matter integrity in CADASIL. In *35th Annual Meeting of the International Neuropsychological Society*, abstract 95.

Peters, N., Herzog, J., Opherk, C. and Dichgans, M. (2004a) A two-year clinical follow-up study in 80 CADASIL subjects: progression patterns and implications for clinical trials. *Stroke*, **35**, 1603–8.

Peters, N., Opherk, C., Zacherle, S. *et al.* (2004b) CADASIL-associated *Notch3* mutations have differential effects both on ligand binding and ligand-induced Notch3 receptor signaling through RBP-Jk. *Exp Cell Res*, **299**, 454–64.

Peters, N., Opherk, C., Danek, A. *et al.* (2005) The pattern of cognitive performance in CADASIL: a monogenic condition leading to subcortical ischemic vascular dementia. *Am J Psychiatry*, **162**, 2078–85.

Peters, N., Holtmannspotter, M., Opherk, C. *et al.* (2006) Brain volume changes in CADASIL: a serial MRI study in pure subcortical ischemic vascular disease. *Neurology*, **66**, 1517–22.

Prakash, N., Hansson, E., Betsholtz, C., Mitsiadis, T. and Lendahl, U. (2002) Mouse Notch 3 expression in the pre- and postnatal brain: relationship to the stroke and dementia syndrome CADASIL. *Exp Cell Res*, **278**, 31–44.

Roman, G. C. (1987) Senile dementia of the Binswanger type. A vascular form of dementia in the elderly. *JAMA*, **258**, 1782–8.

Ruchoux, M. M. and Maurage, C. A. (1998) Endothelial changes in muscle and skin biopsies in patients with CADASIL. *Neuropathol Appl Neurobiol*, **24**, 60–5.

Ruchoux, M. M., Domenga, V., Brulin, P. *et al.* (2003) Transgenic mice expressing mutant Notch3 develop vascular alterations characteristic of cerebral autosomal dominant arteriopathy with subcortical infarcts and leukoencephalopathy. *Am J Pathol*, **162**, 329–42.

Salloway, S. and Desbiens, S. (2004) CADASIL and other genetic causes of stroke and vascular dementia. In Paul, R., Cohen, R., Ott, B. and Salloway, S. (eds.) *Vascular Dementia: Cerebrovascular Mechanisms and Clinical Management*. Totowa, NJ, Humana Press, pp. 87–98.

Sawada, H., Udaka, F., Izumi, Y. *et al.* (2000) Cerebral white matter lesions are not associated with *ApoE* genotype but with age and female sex in Alzheimer's disease. *J Neurol Neurosurg Psychiatry*, **68**, 653–6.

Scheid, R., Preul, C., Lincke, T. *et al.* (2006) Correlation of cognitive status, MRI- and SPECT-imaging in CADASIL patients. *Eur J Neurol*, **13**, 363–70.

Schmidt, R., Schmidt, H., Fazekas, F. *et al.* (2000) MRI cerebral white matter lesions and paraoxonase *PON1* polymorphisms: three-year follow-up of the Austrian stroke prevention study. *Arterioscler Thromb Vasc Biol*, **20**, 1811–16.

Schulman, S. P., Becker, L. C., Kass, D. A. *et al.* (2006) L-Arginine therapy in acute myocardial infarction: the Vascular Interaction with Age in Myocardial Infarction (VINTAGE MI) randomized clinical trial. *JAMA*, **295**, 58–64.

Shawber, C. J. and Kitajewski, J. (2004) Notch function in the vasculature: insights from zebrafish, mouse and man. *Bioessays*, **26**, 225–34.

Sierra, C., de la Sierra, A., Mercader, J. *et al.* (2002) Silent cerebral white matter lesions in middle-aged essential hypertensive patients. *J Hypertens*, **20**, 519–24.

Singhal, S., Bevan, S., Barrick, T., Rich, P. and Markus, H. S. (2004) The influence of genetic and cardiovascular risk factors on the CADASIL phenotype. *Brain*, **127**, 2031–8.

Skoog, I. (1997) The relationship between blood pressure and dementia: a review. *Biomed Pharmacother*, **51**, 367–75.

Snowdon, D. A. (1997) Aging and Alzheimer's disease: lessons from the Nun Study. *Gerontologist*, **37**, 150–6.

Snowdon, D. A., Greiner, L. H. and Markesbery, W. R. (2000) Linguistic ability in early life and the neuropathology of Alzheimer's disease and cerebrovascular disease. Findings from the Nun Study. *Ann N Y Acad Sci*, **903**, 34–8.

Taillia, H., Chabriat, H., Kurtz, A. *et al.* (1998) Cognitive alterations in non-demented CADASIL patients. *Cerebrovasc Dis*, **8**, 97–101.

Thomas, N., Mathews, T. and Loganathan, A. (2002) Cadasil: presenting as a mood disorder. *Scott Med J*, **47**, 36–7.

Trojano, M. and Paolicelli, D. (2001) The differential diagnosis of multiple sclerosis: classification and clinical features of relapsing and progressive neurological syndromes. *Neurol Sci*, **22**(Suppl 2), S98–102.

Trojano, L., Ragno, M., Manca, A. and Caruso, G. (1998) A kindred affected by cerebral autosomal dominant arteriopathy with subcortical infarcts and leukoencephalopathy (CADASIL). A 2-year neuropsychological follow-up. *J Neurol*, **245**, 217–22.

Turner, S. T., Jack, C. R., Fornage, M. *et al.* (2004) Heritability of leukoaraiosis in hypertensive sibships. *Hypertension*, **43**, 483–7.

Vahedi, K., Chabriat, H., Levy, C. *et al.* (2004) Migraine with aura and brain magnetic resonance imaging abnormalities in patients with CADASIL. *Arch Neurol*, **61**, 1237–40.

van den Boom, R., Lesnik Oberstein, S. A., van Duinen, S. G. *et al.* (2002) Subcortical lacunar lesions: an MR imaging finding in patients with cerebral autosomal dominant arteriopathy with subcortical infarcts and leukoencephalopathy. *Radiology*, **224**, 791–6.

van den Boom, R., Lesnik Oberstein, S. A., Ferrari, M. D., Haan, J. and van Buchem, M. A. (2003a) Cerebral autosomal dominant arteriopathy with subcortical infarcts and leukoencephalopathy: MR imaging findings at different ages: 3rd–6th decades. *Radiology*, **229**, 683–90.

van den Boom, R., Lesnik Oberstein, S. A., Spilt, A. *et al.* (2003b) Cerebral hemodynamics and white matter hyperintensities in CADASIL. *J Cereb Blood Flow Metab*, **23**, 599–604.

Viswanathan, A., Gray, F., Bousser, M. G., Baudrimont, M. and Chabriat, H. (2006) Cortical neuronal apoptosis in CADASIL. *Stroke*, **37**, 2690–5.

Weinmaster, G. (1997) The ins and outs of notch signaling. *Mol Cell Neurosci*, **9**, 91–102.

Werbrouck, B. F. and de Bleecker, J. L. (2006) Intracerebral haemorrhage in CADASIL. A case report. *Acta Neurol Belg*, **106**, 219–21.

White, L., Petrovitch, H., Hardman, J. *et al.* (2002) Cerebrovascular pathology and dementia in autopsied Honolulu-Asia Aging Study participants. *Ann N Y Acad Sci*, **977**, 9–23.

Willmot, M., Gray, L., Gibson, C., Murphy, S. and Bath, P. M. (2005) A systematic review of nitric oxide donors and L-arginine in experimental stroke; effects on infarct size and cerebral blood flow. *Nitric Oxide*, **12**, 141–9.

Yousry, T. A., Seelos, K., Mayer, M. *et al.* (1999) Characteristic MR lesion pattern and correlation of T_1 and T_2 lesion volume with neurologic and neuropsychological findings in cerebral autosomal dominant arteriopathy with subcortical infarcts and leukoencephalopathy (CADASIL). *Am J Neuroradiol*, **20**, 91–100.

Rapidly progressive dementias
Prion disorders and other rapidly progressive dementias

Michael D. Geschwind, Aissa Haman and Indre V. Viskontas

Introduction

Because most dementias develop slowly, rapidly progressing dementias (RPDs) present a unique challenge to neurologists. Assessment of patients with an RPD often requires consideration of diagnoses that only marginally overlap with those for slowly progressing dementias. With the possible exceptions of dementia with Lewy bodies (DLB) and corticobasal degeneration (CBD), the disorders that commonly lead to slowly progressive adult dementia, such as Alzheimer's disease (AD) and frontotemporal dementia (FTD), rarely present as RPDs.[1-3]

Since the start of the twenty-first century, our group has assessed more than 975 individuals with RPD, many of whom were referred with a suspected diagnosis of Creutzfeldt–Jakob disease (CJD). A recent review of these data show that 54% were diagnosed with prion disease (37% probable or definite sporadic, 15% genetic and 2% acquired), 28% had an undetermined diagnosis (insufficient records, although most met criteria for possible CJD[4]), and, most importantly, 18% were shown to have other non-prion conditions, many of which were treatable. The diagnostic breakdown of these non-prion RPDs was 26% neurodegenerative, 15% autoimmune, 11% infectious, 11% psychiatric, 9% miscellaneous other, while 28% were still undetermined, often leukoencephalopathies or encephalopathies of unknown etiology (unpublished data). Differentiating prion disease from other causes of RPDs is paramount; therefore, we will begin our discussion of RPDs by focusing initially on prion disease, the prototypical RPD.

Prion diseases

As is the case for many rare medical conditions, prion disease nomenclature can be confusing. The original

description of the disease is attributed to Alfons Jakob, who noted that his five RPD cases were nearly identical to a case described by Hans Creutzfeldt in 1920.[5-7] In the years following, the disease was called Jakob's disease or Jakob–Creutzfeldt disease until Clarence J. Gibbs, a prominent researcher in the field, started using the term Creutzfeldt–Jakob disease because the acronym was closer to his own initials.[8] As descriptions of prion disease have become more refined, it is now clear that several of Jakob's original cases and the case described by Creutzfeldt did not have the disease that we now call Creutzfeldt–Jakob disease (CJD).[9]

The most common form of human prion disease, sporadic CJD (sCJD), seems to occur spontaneously, and the cause remains unknown. Sporadic CJD accounts for about 85% of human prion disease cases. Genetic forms account for 10–15% and acquired cases account for less than 1%. In most Western countries, prion diseases occur at a rate of 1–2 per million per year. In a study of prion disease mortality from 1999 to 2002 in nine European countries, in addition to Canada and Australia, mortality rates were 1.67 per million for all forms of prion disease and 1.39 per million for sCJD specifically.[10]

Sporadic Creutzfeldt–Jakob disease
Demographics

The reported median survival time of sCJD is about 4 months with a mean of about 5 to 8 months: the vast majority (85–90%) of patients die within a year of disease onset.[11-13] In our cohort, we have found that the mean survival time for our cases is close to 1 year (unpublished data), much longer than the reported mean in the literature. This discrepancy in mean survival rate likely results from the difficulty in determining when the first symptom appeared. We conduct extensive patient and family interviews, in addition to reviewing all medical records. This labor-intensive approach generally yields earlier first symptom discovery than that in the patient's medical records.[14]

Diagnosis

When assessing a patient with an RPD, particularly one who shows prominent motor and/or cerebellar dysfunction, sCJD should be considered. The most commonly used clinical criteria for sCJD are the World Health Organization (WHO) criteria, revised in 1998, and the older Masters *et al.* (1979) criteria.[15,16] Both sets include three categories of diagnostic certainty: definite, probable or possible. Presently, a definite diagnosis can only be made from pathology, either biopsy or autopsy, demonstrating the presence of the disease-causing form of the prion protein.[17] A lack of specificity plagues the Master's criteria, as many patients with neurodegenerative conditions other than prion disease, such as CBD, DLB, progressive supranuclear palsy (PSP), and multiple system atrophy (MSA), typically fulfill these criteria. While the WHO criteria are more specific and have been widely accepted, they too have significant shortcomings. For example, WHO criteria include akinetic mutism, which only occurs at the very end-stage of prion disease, too late for any potential treatment to be effective. They also combine cerebellar and visual symptoms as "visual/cerebellar," yet the neuroanatomy and circuitry of cerebellar and visual symptomatology are distinct and there is no evidence that these two symptoms co-occur. The same can be said for combined pyramidal/extrapyramidal symptoms – they are distinct anatomically and do not necessarily occur together. Similarly, as we describe below, the 14-3-3 protein and the electroencephalograph (EEG) scan (included in WHO probable diagnostic criteria) both lack sensitivity and specificity, dangerously missing treatable disorders while missing many cases of CJD. These criteria are problematic because they fail to capture many of the early symptoms of the disease and, instead, focus on symptoms and signs that generally appear later in the disease course. For example, akinetic mutism and the characteristic EEG often are not observed until the late stages of the illness. In contrast, early signs of the illness, such as behavioral changes or aphasia, are not included in these criteria.[14]

We identified the first symptom in 114 sCJD subjects referred to our center and found that the most common symptoms were cognitive (39% of patients), followed by cerebellar (21%), behavioral (20%), constitutional (20%), sensory (11%), motor (9%) and visual (7%). Three of the categories of symptoms we found to be most common – behavioral, constitutional and sensory symptoms (e.g. headache, malaise, vertigo)[14] – are not included in current diagnostic criteria.[15,16]

Putative biomarkers

Ancillary tests used in the WHO criteria, EEG and 14-3-3, have variable utility in the diagnosis of sCJD. Early in the disease, EEG measures may show focal slowing. Later in the disease, periodic sharp-wave complexes (1–2 Hz periodic sharp waves, epileptiform discharges or triphasic waves), which are either focal or diffuse, may appear. Because these EEG changes occur as the disease progresses, several serial EEGs are often needed. The sensitivity and specificity of these changes for CJD have varied greatly in the literature, with sensitivity varying between 50% and 66% and specificity from 74 to 91% among pathology-proven subjects.[13,18–20] Other conditions with similar EEG findings that may mimic CJD include hepatic encephalopathy, Hashimoto's encephalopathy and late stages of other neurodegenerative diseases such as AD and DLB.[2,21,22] In the proper clinical context and when other conditions with overlapping EEG findings have been excluded, EEG should have high specificity for CJD.

In addition to EEG, surrogate protein markers in cerebrospinal fluid (CSF) have also shown some efficacy in distinguishing CJD from other conditions, although their utility is controversial.[23–28] The reported sensitivity and specificity of 14-3-3 protein in CJD has ranged considerably in the literature, and each successive large study appears to show declining sensitivity and specificity,[2,19,26,29] calling into question the utility of this protein as a biomarker for sCJD. Among pathology-proven cases, the reported sensitivity has varied from 47%[30,28] to 100%,[23,31] with most larger studies reporting in the mid to high 80th percentile.[13,19,26,32] The 14-3-3 protein comes in seven isoforms, five of which (beta, gamma, epsilon, eta, and zeta) are found in the brain. Most 14-3-3 studies in CJD have examined the beta isoform; however, one report suggested that the gamma isoform has higher specificity for CJD.[33]

Proteins other than 14-3-3 that have also been considered as surrogate markers for CJD include total tau, neuron-specific enolase, S-100 and β-amyloid 42 (low levels). Numerous studies have shown quite variable results with all of these CSF proteins in the diagnosis of CJD. Cutoffs for tau levels as a marker

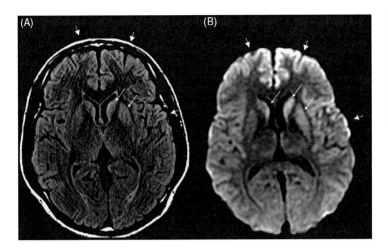

Fig. 23.1. Axial Fluid-attenuated inversion recovery (FLAIR) (A) and diffusion-weighted (B) magnetic resonance imaging of the brain of a patient with sporadic Creutzfeldt–Jakob disease. Note the hyperintensities in the striatum (caudate heads [arrows] and putamen [arrows]) and frontal cortical gyri (cortical ribboning: arrowheads). Note there is also subtle right putamen and medial and posterior thalamus hyperintensity.

for CJD have been 1000, 1200 and 1300 pg/ml, with > 1200 or > 1300 pg/ml being the most common among studies.[26,34,35] One large study suggests that these CSF proteins have higher sensitivity in more rapidly progressive disease,[26] consistent with the idea that these markers are probably just markers of rapid neuronal injury and may lack true specificity for CJD.[28] It is essential for the clinician to know that several conditions may clinically mimic CJD and can also have a positive protein 14-3-3, making it necessary to rule out these other conditions.[27,28,36]

In a recent evaluation of an RPD cohort referred to our center (150 with sCJD and 47 with non-prion RPD), we found that 14-3-3 has a sensitivity of 48% and a specificity of only 66%. The EEG had a sensitivity of less than 45% by the time patients were referred. The sensitivity of the EEG increased to approximately 50% when patients were followed prospectively during their entire disease course.[30] In this cohort, preliminary data suggest that two other surrogate biomarkers for sCJD, total tau and neuron-specific enolase may have somewhat higher sensitivity and specificity for CJD than either 14-3-3 or EEG, although this finding needs to be explored further. We feel these latter CSF biomarkers, like 14-3-3, are merely signs of rapid neuronal injury and are not specific for prion disease. They are, therefore, of questionable diagnostic utility. Development of an antemortem, prion-specific test is needed.[37–40]

Diagnosis with magnetic resonance imaging

Diffusion-weighted imaging (DWI) and fluid-attenuated inversion recovery (FLAIR) magnetic resonance imaging (MRI) have high sensitivity (≈92%) and specificity

(≈95%) for CJD. Hyperintensity is most commonly seen in the cerebral cortex but it may also be found in the basal ganglia (caudate and putamen) and the thalamus.[41,42] These abnormalities may be symmetric or asymmetric.[43,44] Figure 23.1 shows typical DWI and FLAIR sequences of a patient with sCJD.

At the University of California at San Francisco (UCSF), we have modified the WHO revised criteria by separating visual and cerebellar symptoms, adding a category of other focal cortical symptoms (such as aphasia, neglect, acalculia or apraxia) and replacing the 14-3-3 test with a brain MRI consistent with sCJD (Table 23.1).[4] We are continuing to develop these criteria by monitoring their specificity and by striving for the earliest possible diagnosis while maintaining high specificity.

Brain biopsy

While brain biopsy remains the only way to make a definitive antemortem diagnosis of CJD, it can be problematic from an infection control standpoint as prion proteins are not removed by standard surgical sterilization methods,[45] creating a risk of transmission to operating room personnel. Our own unpublished data suggest that brain biopsy has 86% sensitivity for diagnosis (MD Geschwind, unpublished data).

Direct detection of the PrP^{Sc} isoform of prion protein

To date there is no test available for antemortem diagnosis of prion diseases; autopsy analysis of central nervous system (CNS) tissue (or lymphatic tissues) is required for assessment of the disease in affected humans and animals. Using immunohistochemistry, pathologists can detect the most common changes

Table 23.1. Various criteria for probable sporadic Creutzfeldt-Jakob disease

UCSF criteria	WHO European criteria[a]	Masters' criteria
1. Rapid cognitive decline 2. 2 of the following 6 symptoms: • myoclonus • pyramidal/extrapyrimidal symptoms • visual • cerebellar • akinetic mutism • focal cortical sign (e.g. neglect, aphasia, acalculia, apraxia) 3. Typical EEG and/or MRI	1. Progressive dementia 2. 2 of the following 4 symptoms: • myoclonus • pyramidal/extrapyrimidal symptoms • visual/cerebellar • akinetic mutism 3. Typical EEG 4. Routine investigations should not suggest an alternative diagnosis	1. Progressive dementia 2. 1 of the following: • myoclonus • pyramidal symptoms • extrapyramidal symptoms • cerebellar symptoms • typical EEG

Notes:
UCSF, University of California at San Francisco; WHO, World Health Organization; EEG, electroencephalography; MRI, magnetic resonance imaging.
[a]WHO revised criteria allow EEG or CSF 14-3-3 protein and < 2 year duration to death.
Sources: World Health Organization (1998),[15] Masters *et al.* (1979).[16]

that characterize prion disease, such as astrocytic gliosis, neuronal loss and vacuolation, paralleled by accumulation in certain regions of the brain of an abnormal isoform, PrP^{Sc}, of the ubiquitous cellular prion protein PrP^C.[17] A number of tests are commercially available for the immunodetection of PrP^{Sc}; most share a common platform of an enzyme-linked immunosorbent assay in which antibodies against PrP can capture and detect PrP^{Sc}. Many tests exploit the resistance to proteolytic digestion of PrP^{Sc} and utilize specific proteolytic enzymes for the digestion of brain homogenates from suspected cases.[46,47] Among these tests, the conformation-dependent immunoassay offers a major advantage of detecting immunochemical differences between PrP^C and PrP^{Sc} without the need for proteases to remove PrP^C. The conformation-dependent immunoassay is being developed to detect PrP^{Sc} in blood and other bodily fluids.[37–39]

The protein misfolding cyclic amplification reaction is a method for multiplying prions. In principle, it is similar to using the polymerase chain reaction to multiply DNA. This methodology can increase PrP^{Sc} levels from a sample more than one-million-fold,[48] and possibly more.[40] This assay has been reported to detect prions in blood of experimentally infected hamsters.[49] One problem with this assay is that it may actually create PrP^{Sc} de novo from PrP^C.[50]

Other disorders commonly mistaken for sporadic Creutzfeldt–Jakob disease

Atypical rapid forms of other more common neurodegenerative diseases are often misdiagnosed as prion disease, particularly AD and atypical parkinsonian dementias, such as CBD and DLB. Paraneoplastic (e.g. Anti-Hu, CV2 and MaTa) and non-paraneoplastic (e.g. anti-voltage-gated potassium channel, anti-glutamic acid decarboxylase and Hashimoto's encephalopathy) autoimmune conditions may also mimic CJD.[2,22,51–54] Vasculitis may clinically resemble sCJD, although the MRI can help to differentiate them (Table 23.2). Cancers, such as intravascular lymphoma, primary CNS lymphoma (PCNSL) or gliomatosis cerebri can present like sCJD; however, brain MRI easily differentiates these neoplastic conditions from prion disease.[55–59] Subacute infections, such as subacute sclerosing panencephalitis from German measles or rubella, can look somewhat like CJD, particularly variantCJD (vCJD) in a young person. Lyme disease and human immunodeficiency virus (HIV) should probably always be ruled out when considering CJD. Toxins, such as bismuth (found in some antidiarrheal agents), when taken in large quantities can cause a CJD-like clinical picture, with ataxia, myoclonus and encephalopathy.[60,61] Thiamine deficiency causing Wernicke's encephalopathy is readily treatable and should always be considered.[53] These diseases are discussed in more detail in the section below on other rapidly progressing dementias.

Prion disease mechanics

For many years, prion diseases were mistakenly thought to be caused by "slow viruses," in part through the transmissibility of the diseases and the long incubation period between exposure and symptom onset.[62,63] Challenging this notion is the finding

Table 23.2. Typical magnetic resonance imaging findings in some forms of rapidly progressive dementia

Finding	Possible causes
Cortical gray matter T_2-weighted hyperintensity[a]	CJD, paraneoplastic disease, Hashimoto's encephalopathy, antibody-mediated disease (e.g. VGKC), sarcoid, mitochondrial disease
Subcortical white matter T_2-weighted hyperintensity	Vascular, HIV, PML, lymphoma, paraneoplastic disorder, Hashimoto's encephalopathy, multiple sclerosis/ADEM8, Lyme encephalopathy, toxic metabolic disorder, leukodystrophies, sarcoid, mitochondrial disease
Cortical restricted diffusion	Vascular, seizures, CJD
Striatal or thalamic restricted diffusion	Vascular, seizures, CJD, thiamine deficiency, central pontine myelinolysis, *Bartonella* infection
Basal ganglia/thalamic T_2-weighted hyperintensity	CJD, lymphoma, paraneoplastic (anti-CV2/CRMP5), NIBD, thiamine deficiency, *Bartonella* infection, Wilson's disease
Contrast enhancing	Primary or metastatic cancer, lymphoma, sarcoid, multiple sclerosis, vasculitis
Vascular distribution	Multi-infarct dementia, vasculitis, intravascular lymphoma
Hemorrhage	Primary or metastatic cancer, vasculitis, fungal (e.g. aspergillosis), CAA
Meningeal enhancement	Infectious (fungal, spirochaetal, mycobacterial), neoplastic meningitis, sarcoid, Wegener's granulosis, Behçet's disease
Medial temporal lobe T_2-weighted hyperintensity	CJD, HSV encephalitis, paraneoplastic disorder, antibody-mediated disease (e.g. VGKC), Hashimoto's encephalopathy

Notes:
ADEM, acute disseminated encephalomyelitis; CJD, Creutzfeldt–Jakob disease; NIBD, neurofilament inclusion body disease; PML, progressive mulitfocal leukoencephalopathy; CAA, cerebral amyloid angiopathy; VGKC, anti-voltage-gated potassium channel; HIV, human immunodeficiency virus; HSV, herpes simplex virus.
[a]ADEM can involve gray matter as well as white matter.

that the infectious agent does not contain nucleic acid, which is a necessary component of viruses. Furthermore, treatments that are known to eliminate viruses and other microorganisms proved ineffective in the prevention of disease transmission from one organism to another, while treatments that denature or destroy proteins prevented transmission. Taken together, these findings strongly suggested that the disease agent is a protein.[64,65] In 1997, Stanley B. Prusiner received the Nobel Prize in Medicine and Physiology for his discovery that the prion protein is indeed the culprit.

In humans, the endogenous cellular form of the prion protein (PrP^C) is encoded by the gene *PRNP* located on the short arm of chromosome 20, which encodes a protein of 254 amino acid residues.[66,67] The mature PrP^C protein is attached to the outer cell membrane by a glycosylphosphatidylinositol anchor,[68–70] but transmembrane forms of PrP^C have also been identified.[71–73]

In prion diseases, PrP^C changes its conformation into an abnormally shaped, disease-causing form of PrP called the prion, or PrP^{Sc} (where Sc stands for scrapie, the prion disease in sheep and goats). The normal form contains three α-helixes (spirals) and little β-sheet (flat) structures, whereas PrP^{Sc} has less α-helical content and mostly β-sheet structure.[74,75]

The process by which PrP^{Sc} is made from PrP^C is incompletely understood. It is likely that when PrP^C comes into contact with PrP^{Sc}, the latter protein induces the former to take on its shape.[76] There may also be other proteins or molecules involved in the conformational change in vivo.[77–79]

Function of the normal prion protein

Several lines of *PRNP* knockout mice have been developed; these mice cannot be infected with, nor can they replicate, prions, providing convincing evidence that the presence of PrP^C is a necessary condition for the development of prion disease.[80–83] Knockout mice are clinically asymptomatic, but they develop peripheral nerve demyelination,[84] an increased susceptibility to ischemic brain injury,[85] altered sleep and circadian rhythms[86,87] and altered hippocampal neuropathology and physiology, including deficits in hippocampal-dependent spatial learning and hippocampal synaptic plasticity.[88,89] Mice or cell lines lacking PrP^C are also more susceptible to oxidative stress. Prion PrP^C also protects neurons during hypoxic–ischemic injury.[85,90–95] For an excellent review on PrP^C knockout mice, see Weissmann *et al.*[96]

The primary function of PrP^C may be neuroprotective, either alone or in concert with other proteins.

349

Evidence for this view is found in the demonstration that PrP^C is upregulated after cerebral ischemia, and overproduction of PrP^C seems to be protective in an ischemia mouse model.[97] In addition, PrP^C may play a role in neuronal excitability,[98] neuritigenesis,[95,99,100] and signal transduction.[85]

Genetic markers for Creutzfeldt–Jakob disease

Codon 129 in *PRNP* is polymorphic, encoding methionine (M) or valine (V), such that an individual can be MM, VV or MV. Homozygosity at codon 129 is associated with increased risk for developing prion disease, with greatest risk in persons with codon 129 MM, followed by VV and then MV.[101–103] In addition to affecting an individual's susceptibility to developing prion disease, the codon 129 polymorphism can play a role in how a prion disease presents clinically and pathologically.[102,104]

In a study of 300 pathology-proven sCJD subjects, investigators subdivided sCJD molecularly into approximately six different forms (or variants) based on the patient's *PRNP* codon 129 polymorphism (MM, MV or VV) and on their prion type (type 1 or 2).[102,104] Seventy percent of their patients had type 1 PrP^{Sc} and had at least one methionine allele (MM or MV; most were MM). These patients presented as classic sCJD, with a rapidly progressive dementia, early and prominent myoclonus and a classic EEG.[20] Twenty-five percent of patients had a specific, distinct neuropathology called kuru plaques, with significant ataxia, and were type 2 with at least one valine allele (MV2 or VV2). The MM2 variant was associated with either a thalamic form (MM2-T) or a dementing cortical form (MM2-C) of sCJD. Lastly, a rare form VV, less than 1% of their cases, was described, with a progressive dementia, lack of classic EEG and severe cortical and basal ganglia pathology, sparing the cerebellum and brainstem.[102] Unfortunately, even within an individual, different prion types can be found in different brain regions,[105] suggesting that subdividing patients into categories based on prion types may not be as useful as initially believed.

Other prion diseases

Sporadic fatal insomnia

A rare form of prion disease that presents clinically and pathologically similarly to fatal familial insomnia is sporadic fatal insomnia. Symptoms include thalamic symptoms, particularly insomnia and dysautonomia, and cerebellar ataxia. Upon pathology, patients show thalamic and olivary pathology.[106–108]

Genetic prion diseases

Genetic prion diseases have been divided into three forms based on their clinical and pathological presentation: familial CJD (fCJD), Gerstmann–Sträussler–Scheinker disease (GSS) and fatal familial insomnia. More than 30 mutations and at least three polymorphisms in the prion gene have been identified[109] and new mutations continue to be found. In most cases, *PRNP* mutations are autosomal dominant with complete penetrance.[109] Clinically, fCJD typically presents either identically to sCJD, as a rapidly progressive dementia with motor features, or it can present as a more slowly progressing dementia.

Typical presentation for GSS is either as a parkinsonian or an ataxic disease, progressing over years, although a rare spastic form of GSS has also been reported.[110] Five mutations, at codons 102, 105, 117, 145, 198 and 217, in the open reading frame of the prion gene have been associated with GSS.[110] The mean age of onset is approximately 47 years, with average survival approximately 57 months.[111] Most (75%) patients survive more than 2 years.[12] Fatal familial insomnia is caused by a *PRNP* mutation at codon 178, changing an aspartate to an asparagine (D178N), and the presence of methionine at codon 129 on the same allele. The amino acid (methionine or valine) encoded by codon 129 on the normal allele greatly affects disease presentation. Disease duration is variable but usually lasts 1 to 2, or even more years, although sometimes the disease can be more rapidly progressive. Symptoms involve the sleep–wake cycle, dysautonomia and motor dysfunction. Anatomically, fatal familial insomnia predominantly involves the thalamus and adjacent structures, resulting in dysautonomia, altered sleep–wake cycles and circadian rhythms.[112] Paradoxically, many (60%) patients with genetic prion disease do not report a known family history of the disease, although closer review often uncovers a family history of AD or Parkinson's disease that was likely misdiagnosed.[113] Since many patients do not have a positive family history, some clinicians prefer the term genetic, rather than familial, CJD.[12]

Variant Creutzfeldt–Jakob disease

In 1995, a new form of human prion disease called variant CJD (vCJD) was identified in the UK and shortly thereafter was linked to consumption of meat from cows with bovine spongiform encephalopathy (BSE).[114–117] Since the early 1990s, more than 200 cases of vCJD have been identified in 11 countries, with the vast majority in the UK and France.[118] The clinical features of vCJD are similar to those of sCJD, with some exceptions. Patients with vCJD tend to be younger than patients with sCJD (mean age 28 years), with an age range of 12–74 years.[119] Early in the illness, patients usually experience profound psychiatric symptoms, which most commonly take the form of depression or, less often, a schizophrenia-like psychosis. This psychiatric prodrome is often the only symptom for at least 6 months before the onset of other neurological features.[120] Patients frequently have painful paresthesias, which are usually persistent but may also be transient. Motor features typically include ataxia, chorea, myoclonus and/or dystonia.[121] Cognitive impairment is an early feature.[122] The classic EEG changes seen in sCJD are rarely seen in vCJD and then only in late stages.[123] Brain MRI in vCJD typically shows more hyperintensity in the pulvinar than the anterior putamen on T_2-weighted MRI sequences (the pulvinar sign), a feature that often distinguishes it from sCJD and other forms of prion disease,[124–126] although sCJD,[127] incident CJD[128] and other RPDs, such as paraneoplastic limbic encephalitis and Bartonella encephalopathy,[129,130] can rarely also have this MRI feature. As in sCJD, by the time of death, patients become completely immobile and mute and they usually succumb to aspiration pneumonia.

The characteristic neuropathological profile of vCJD includes, in both the cerebellum and cerebrum, numerous kuru-type amyloid "florid" plaques of high concentrations of PrP^{Sc} surrounded by vacuoles to give a "flower" appearance. The PrP^{Sc} type in vCJD is called type 2b; it has a different ratio of glycosylated forms than type 2a sCJD PrP^{Sc}.[102,117,131] In vCJD, the prion appears to be present at very high levels in the lymphoreticular system. Antemortem pathological diagnosis of vCJD can be made by tonsillar or brain biopsy. Postmortem, the prion is found throughout the lymphoreticular system and the CNS.[117,132–134] Why vCJD tends to occur in younger patients has not been fully explained, but it may be that BSE prions are more readily acquired across the gastrointestinal track when inflammation is present. As children have a higher incidence of gastritis than adults, they may be more susceptible to consumed BSE prions.[135,136]

As of November 2007, four patients have acquired vCJD via blood transfusion from patients with vCJD who had donated blood prior to the onset of symptoms.[137–140] Although all patients so far with clinical vCJD have been codon 129 MM, data from transgenic mice models suggest that persons with MV and VV may be susceptible to vCJD, particularly via human to human transmission, such as by blood donation.[141,142] Although the incidence of vCJD has declined over recent years, it is not known if an increase will occur in the future. It is possible that many individuals, particularly those who are codon 129 MV or VV, are latently infected with vCJD and may have much longer incubation times than those who have already presented with the disease.[137,143]

Treatment of prion disease

Many compounds have been used successfully to remove prions or inhibit their formation in vitro. Such compounds include quinoline derivatives,[144–146] antibiotics such as doxycycline and tetracycline,[147] Congo red and its analogs[148] and various "chemical chaperones."[149,150] Several of these compounds and others have been effective in preventing or delaying disease onset in vivo when mixed with the prions prior to inoculation or given before or at the time of prion inoculation.[147,151–154] In most mice models, there are usually only a few days between the first clear signs of neurologic disease and death or incapacity. By the time an animal develops symptoms, the disease is so fulminant that no treatment will likely have efficacy. Therefore, in animal models of prion disease, investigators often start potential treatment at the midpoint of incubation. While several compounds have prevented disease before or at the time of inoculation,[155] no treatment has cured animals when given later in the incubation period and only a few compounds have delayed disease onset.[156]

As of 2007, the only two drugs are in formal treatment trials for prion disease: oral quinacrine and oral doxycycline. Quinacrine is a quinoline derivative used orally for many decades to treat malaria. Quinacrine binds readily to PrP^C and appears to prevent conversion of PrP^C to PrP^{Sc},[146] possibly by binding to the C-terminal helix of PrP^C.[157] Quinacrine appears to work via the former mechanism, though the mechanism is far from clear.[146] In in-vitro models of prion disease, quinacrine eliminates prions[144,158] and may even allow recovery of some cellular functions.[159] Two prion studies in mice with oral quinacrine, however, showed no benefit in survival.[146,160]

Because quinacrine has been used in medicine orally for decades and crosses the blood–brain barrier, compassionate treatment was begun in humans with prion disease.[146,161–163] To better answer whether quinacrine is efficacious in human prion disease, two formal studies were initiated in humans, one in the UK (PRION1 by the Medical Research Council) and another in the USA, at our center (UCSF; CJD Quinacrine Treatment Study).[155] The UK trial enrolled patients with all forms of human prion disease and was essentially an unblinded, observational study. The UCSF study is a randomized, double-blinded placebo-controlled (delayed treatment start) study of quinacrine in sCJD with the primary outcome being survival from start of treatment (the trial is funded by the US National Institutes of Health and can be seen at www.clinicaltrials.gov or http://memory.ucsf.edu). Tetracyclines, such as doxycycline, may also have anti-prion activity, possibly through interaction with PrP^{Sc} or PrP^{Sc} fibrils.[146,147] A randomized, double-blinded, placebo-controlled human treatment trial with oral doxycycline began in 2007 in Italy and similar trials are planned to begin in France and Germany.

Many papers have shown that antibodies or single-chain fragments of antibodies can eliminate prions in cell culture,[164–167] but getting antibodies into the brain in sufficient amounts may be a difficult hurdle to overcome.[168] Vaccination against PrP^{C} has also been studied and may be helpful in preventing infection, particularly after known exposure.[166,169–174] With all of these immunological methods, however, it is not yet clear what deleterious effects may occur in humans from blocking the normal function of PrP^{C}.[175] Removal of PrP^{C} from neurons in prion-infected, symptomatic adult mice appears to allow some recovery of function and reverse some of the pathological features of prion disease, such as vacuolation.[176] This form of genetic manipulation is not feasible presently in humans.

Other rapidly progressing dementias
Non-prion neurodegenerative diseases
There are several non-prion neurodegenerative diseases that can, in rare cases, present as rapidly progressing dementias. These include AD, DLB, FTD with amytrophic lateral sclerosis (FTD-ALS), CBD and PSP.[14] Several cases of AD presenting as adult-onset RPD have been reported in conjunction with cerebral amyloid angiopathy.[177–179] Figure 23.2 shows a T$_1$-weighted MRI of a patient with cerebral amyloid angiopathy. Indicative of the rare but persistent occurrences of rapid presentations of these diseases, a large German study of 413 autopsied suspected cases of CJD found that 7% had AD and 3% had

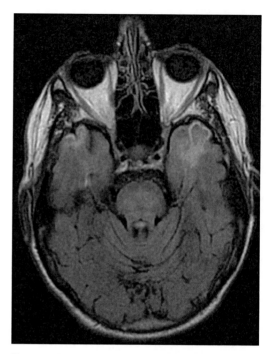

Fig. 23.2. Magnetic resonance T$_1$-weighted sequences of the brain in a patient with cerebral amyloid angiopathy. Note the cortical and patchy subcortical white matter hyperintensities in bilateral temporal lobes.

DLB. Myoclonus and extrapyramidal signs had occurred in more than 70% of the DLB and more than 50% of the AD patients, suggesting that these symptoms, although part of WHO criteria,[15] do not always help to distinguish CJD from these two disorders.[1] Similarly, in a French study of 465 patients with suspected CJD, the two most frequent non-CJD pathologic diagnoses were AD and DLB.[180]

Since the "parkinsonian dementias," namely DLB and the FTD spectrum disorders including PSP, CBD and FTD, are discussed in more detail in other chapters of this book, they will only be briefly described here. Dementia with Lewy bodies is a progressive dementia often associated with fluctuations in cognitive function, persistent well-formed visual hallucinations and/or parkinsonism.[181] Duration of DLB is often shorter than for many other neurodegenerative dementias; patients generally survive for only about 3 years,[182] although death within 1 year of diagnosis can occur. Although FTD generally shows a faster course than AD, it is rarely rapidly progressive. Patients usually present with a frontal syndrome, including behavioral, personality and cognitive changes occurring over years, followed by dementia.

Fifteen percent or more of patients with FTD develop ALS and these patients typically die within 1.4 years after diagnosis.[183–186] Corticobasal degeneration is a clinically and pathologically heterogeneous atypical parkinsonian dementia often confused clinically with AD, PSP or FTD.[187–191] Rapidly progressing CBD can also be confused with CJD,[192,193] though the FLAIR and DWI MRI abnormalities seen in CJD are not found in CBD.[41] As in CJD, patients with PSP develop dementia, akinetic-rigid parkinsonism (symmetric bradykinesia and axial rigidity), postural instability, swallowing and speech problems, and often progress to a hypokinetic, mute state.[194–199] Abnormalities of eye movements, particularly slowed velocity of saccades progressing to supranuclear gaze palsy, are hallmarks of the PSP syndrome.[195,200,201] Importantly, our CJD group has been referred many RPD cases thought to be caused by prion disease but they were merely exacerbations of more common non-prion neurodegenerative diseases as a result of concurrent infection or metabolic perturbation.

Autoimmune encephalopathies (paraneoplastic and non-paraneoplastic)

One of the most common causes of RPD at our center are autoimmune encephalopathies and related conditions. When first reported in the literature, these autoimmune-related RPDs were all thought to be paraneoplastic; caused by the cross-reaction of antibodies or other components of immune system, activated by the presence of a cancer, with antigens of the nervous system. Since the initial discovery of these conditions, however, many cases have been reported in which no tumor has been identified. In patients without a known cancer diagnosis, other indicators of a paraneoplastic etiology can include subacute development of multifocal neurologic symptoms, CSF evidence of inflammation (e.g. pleiocytosis, elevated IgG index or oligoclonal bands), elevated systemic tumor markers (e.g. cancer-associated antigen [CEA], carcinoembryonic antigen 125 [CA-125], prostrate-specific antigen [PSA]), a family history of cancer, unexplained anorexia or weight loss, a history of cancer risk factors or the presence of certain paraneoplastic antibodies in the serum and/or CSF. In this section, we will discuss both paraneoplastic and non-paraneoplastic autoimmune encephalopathies.

Paraneoplastic neurologic disorders can present as a rapidly progressive limbic encephalopathy, often a form of RPD. These encephalopathies may be focal or diffuse with other neurological involvement, such as cerebellar, ocular or peripheral symptoms. The most common symptoms are a subacute amnestic syndrome, presenting as problems with short-term anterograde memory or more variable retrograde amnesia. Depression, personality changes, anxiety and emotional lability often precede the cognitive dysfunction. Seizures are common.[202–205] Some cancers are more likely to show progressive limbic encephalopathy than others, such as small cell lung cancer (75% of cases), germ-cell tumors (ovarian or testicular), thymoma, Hodgkin's lymphoma and breast cancer.[202,203] The most common antibodies associated with progressive limbic encephalopathy are anti-Hu (ANNA-1) (in 50% of those with small cell lung cancer), anti-Ma2 (an antineuronal antibody also called anti-Ta; antigen is Ma2), CV2 (Anti-CMRP-5), Yo (PCA-1) and anti-neuropil.[202,206–208] Patients with limbic encephalopathy and thymoma (often anti-CV2 or anti-VGKC antibodies) can have significant neurologic improvement following tumor removal and treatment.[209] Many patients often have more than one antibody. These antibodies may better predict the cancer than the neurological syndrome.[210]

Although little is known concerning the mechanism of non-paraneoplastic immune-mediated encephalopathies, recent research has uncovered a greater understanding of several of these conditions, such as syndromes caused by anti-voltage-gated potassium channels (VGKC) antibodies and by anti-neuropil antibodies.[204,206,211] Recent data suggest that autoimmune encephalopathies associated with extracellular antigens (e.g. anti-VGKC, neuropil, and N-methyl-D-aspartate [NMDA] antibodies) are often very responsive to immunomodulatory therapy, whereas those associated with intracellular antigens, such as the classic paraneoplastic syndromes (e.g. Anti-Hu, Yo, Ri, Ma, amphiphysin) are less responsive to treatment.[205,212] Novel antibodies against components of the CNS are continually being identified.[206,213] If an autoimmune-mediated encephalopathy or RPD syndrome is strongly suspected, owing to prominent limbic encephalopathy, T_2-weighted limbic hyperintensity on MRI, CSF findings, serological findings, concurrent or family history of autoimmune disorders, one should have a low threshold for sending serum and CSF to a laboratory that specializes in identifying such antibodies.

Another treatable autoimmune disorder presenting as an RPD is Hashimoto's encephalopathy.[214] This syndrome is rare, but likely underdiagnosed, and is associated with chronic lymphocytic Hashimoto's thyroiditis.[54,215–218] This condition is often considered in a patient with encephalopathy and either elevated anti-thyroperoxidase or anti-thyroglobulin antibodies without any other cause identified for the neurological condition. Earliest signs include depression, personality changes or psychosis, progressing into a cognitive decline associated with myoclonus, ataxia, pyramidal and extrapyramidal signs, stroke-like episodes, altered levels of consciousness, confusion and/or seizures. Hallucinations or other psychoses are common.[22,54,215,218] Compared with CJD, Hashimoto's encephalopathy is more frequently associated with seizures and tends to have a more fluctuating course.[22] The disease is more common in women (85%) than in men, though this relationship with gender remains to be explored.[22] Patients may be euthyroid, hypothyroid and even hyperthyroid, although the diagnosis cannot be made until a patient is euthyroid.[22] When patients are euthyroid, elevated levels of either anti-thyroglobulin or anti-thyroperoxidase and neurologic and psychiatric symptoms without evidence of other known etiology suggest Hashimoto's encephalopathy. The etiology of Hashimoto's encephalopathy may involve the presence of a shared antigen in the brain and thyroid.[54,215,218,219] Most (90%) patients respond favorably to immunosuppression, which is typically administered via an initial high dose of steroids followed by a long, slow taper.[21,215,217,218,220,221] As these anti-thyroid antibodies are not believed to cause this condition directly, several other names have been used, including non-vasculitic autoimmune meningo-encephalitis and steroid-responsive encephalopathy associated with autoimmune thyroiditis.[218,221] Until more is known about the etiology of this condition, many prefer the term Hashimoto's encephalopathy.[216] Sarcoid, another RPD that is treated with immunosuppression, is a systemic illness of unknown etiology characterized by the formation of non-necrotizing granulomas. Few (5%) patients with sarcoidosis show CNS involvement, but those that do can be mistaken for RPD. For definitive diagnosis, tissue biopsy is required. One must first exclude other granulomatous diseases, particularly tuberculosis, before starting immunosuppression.[222]

Vascular disease

Large-vessel occlusions, multiple diffuse infarcts or even single strokes, such as in the thalamus or anterior corpus callosum, or certain frontal lobe regions, can result in an RPD.[223,224] Encephalopathy can result from global cerebral ischemia produced by micro-angiopathic thromboses in thrombotic thrombocytopenic purpura or by hyperviscosity syndromes from blood dyscrasias, such as polycythemia, or gammopathies, such as Waldenstrom's macroglobulinemia. These conditions can be distinguished from RPD through the abnormalities seen on brain MRI, indicating the presence of strokes and/or hemorrhage involving both the white or gray matter.[59,225,226] In addition, body imaging for systemic involvement may also help.[227] If primary CNS vasculitis is suspected, cerebral angiogram or brain and meningeal brain biopsy of the affected area may be required. Intravascular lymphoma can mimic CNS vasculitis on angiogram; if this condition is suspected (based on an elevated serum lactate dehydrogenase or MRI findings), then one should avoid the angiogram and proceed directly to biopsy.[56,228]

Infectious diseases

Dementia can be a presenting feature of acquired immunodeficiency syndrome (AIDS),[229] and eventually occurs in 25% of patients with the disease. Therefore, HIV testing should accompany every evaluation of patients with RPDs. AIDS-dementia complex, HIV encephalopathy or HIV-associated dementia is a neurological complication of AIDS, and it typically occurs in the later stages of HIV infection.[230] This condition has diminished since the introduction of highly active antiretroviral therapy. Some patients, however, develop RPD during seroconversion or immune reconstitution.[231] Use of methamphetamine or cocaine in the context of HIV infection can cause an accelerated course of HIV dementia.[232]

Subacute and chronic opportunistic infections associated with HIV and other immunocompromised states may also present as RPD. While cryptococcal and JC virus infections typically present with meningitis or progressive focal neurologic deficits, respectively, they may present as subacute dementia syndromes.[233] Infection of the CNS with mycobacteria can present as an RPD, but with meningoencephalitis.[234] Many undiagnosed RPDs may actually result from infectious organisms that are not yet detectable using standard microbiological techniques.[28,234–236] Figure 23.3 shows a FLAIR MRI of a patient referred with a CJD diagnosis but in whom we identified enteroviral meningoencephalitis. (For an excellent review on diagnosis and etiology of encephalitis see Glaser et al. [2006].[235])

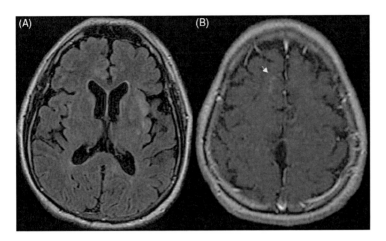

Fig. 23.3. Meningoencephalitis. (A) Axial Fluid-attenuated inversion recovery (FLAIR) magnetic resonance sequences of the brain in a patient with enteroviral meningoencephalitis. Note the hyperintensities involving both gray and white matter in anterior cingulate and left insula. (B) On axial T_2-weighted sequence, note the region of contrast enhancement in the right superior frontal lobe (arrow).

Spirochaete infections are rare but worth considering because they are easily treatable. Every evaluation of an RPD, or any dementia for that matter, should include a test for CNS infection with *Treponema pallidum* neurosyphilis. Though usually presenting late in the disease, cognitive dysfunction is the most common neurological syndrome of syphilis.[236] The CSF in neurosyphilis usually shows a pleiocytosis and an elevated protein.[236] Lyme disease is caused by a systemic infection of the spirochaete *Borrelia burgdorferi*, transmitted via a tick bite. Neurological manifestations can include cranial nerve palsy, meningitis, polyradiculopathy, depression, psychosis and dementia.[237] While uncommon, it has been reported to present as RPD.[238]

The virus that causes measles can result in the chronic CNS infection subacute sclerosing panencephalitis. This typically occurs in children, particularly from countries in which measles is still common.[239] Patients develop progressive dementia, seizures (focal and/or generalized), myoclonus, ataxia, rigidity and visual disturbances. Late in the disease, patients are unresponsive, with spastic quadriparesis, brisk deep tendon reflexes and positive Babinski signs. An EEG may show periodic slow-wave complexes, with associated sharp waves every 3–10 seconds that are synchronous with myoclonus. When elevated antibody titers to the measles virus in the blood and CSF are found, a definitive diagnosis may be made.[240]

An infection by the bacterium *Triopheryma whippelii*, which causes Whipple's disease, can present as a neuropsychiatric syndrome that although typically insidious is capable of progressing rapidly over months. In most patients, the infection presents as a malabsorption syndrome, with diarrhea, abdominal pain, weight loss, arthralgias, wasting, fever and lymphadenopathy; but gastrointestinal symptoms may be absent in as many as 15%. Few (~5%) patients show neurologic symptoms at first presentation, though CNS involvement may occur in up to 45% throughout the course of the infection.[241] When there is CNS involvement, dementia or cognitive impairments are frequent symptoms (> 71% of cases),[241–243] as is ataxia.[244] When dementia, ophthalmoplegia, and myoclonus are seen concomitantly, this condition is highly likely. This triad of symptoms occurs in approximately 10% of cases. Oculomasticatory myorrythmia is virtually pathognomic.[241] Most commonly, CNS Whipple's infection can be mistaken for CBD or PSP.[188] Diagnosis of Whipple's disease is made by identification of inclusions staining with periodic acid–Schiff stain, *T. whipellii* in foamy macrophages on jejunal biopsy or by *T. whipellii* polymerase chain reaction detection in CSF or jejunal biopsy. Although very rare, Whipple's disease is important to recognize as it is readily treatable with antibiotics.[241,243,245,246]

Malignancies

Many malignancies presenting as RPDs are readily identified by brain MRI with contrast, although several of them, including PCNSL and intravascular lymphoma, are more difficult to diagnose. Primary CNS lymphoma is an extranodal form of non-Hodgkin's lymphoma, usually presenting with symptoms of intracranial mass lesions, such as headaches, seizures, and focal neurological deficits. It may also present as an RPD.[247] A diffusely infiltrating PCNSL, sometimes called lymphomatosis cerebri, also occurs.[57] Other symptoms of PCNSL include personality changes, irritability, memory loss, lethargy, confusion, disorientation, psychosis, dysphasia, ataxia, gait disorder and myoclonus.[57,58,247,248] Unfortunately, definitive diagnosis often requires brain biopsy, though in cases of ocular involvement, diagnosis can sometimes be made by vitrectomy. Prior to biopsy, it is best to avoid using corticosteroids because steroids can cause tumor cell necrosis, temporarily shrinking the tumor but interfering with tissue diagnosis.[59,249] Prognosis is poor, with patients surviving only a median of 4 months or fewer without treatment, 12–18 months with whole-brain radiation therapy (WBRT) alone, and 40 or more months with a combination of aggressive chemotherapy and radiotherapy. Chemotherapy includes high-dose systemic methotrexate. Patients over 60 have a higher risk of neurotoxicity, presenting as an RPD with ataxia and incontinence around 1 year after WBRT. Therefore, WBRT is not recommended in older patients.[249]

Intravascular lymphoma is caused by the proliferation of clonal lymphocytes within blood vessels, with relative sparing of parenchyma, and can occur in the CNS.[250] When in the CNS, it can present as an acute or subacute dementia, often with transient ischemic attacks or strokes. Systemic symptoms (e.g. fever and weight loss) can occur. Typically, the tumor cells are angiotropic large B cell lymphoma or other activated or transformed lymphocytes. Laboratory findings can include elevated erythrocyte sedimentation rate, serum lactate dehydrogenase, CSF pleiocytosis and increased protein.[251,252] Prognosis is usually poor, particularly if not treated early. Similarly to PCNSL, the combination of chemo- and radiotherapy yields better results than radiotherapy alone.[250,252,253]

Toxic-metabolic conditions

Vitamin deficiencies, endocrinologic disturbances and adult presentations of inborn errors of metabolism can also cause RPDs. Vitamin deficiencies can lead to cognitive impairment, as well as other neurologic deficits. Niacin deficiency causes "the three Ds" – dermatitis, diarrhea and dementia. Diagnosis is usually based on clinical suspicion, as treatment simply involves 40–250 mg/day niacin, but it can be made definitively by the presence of nicotinic acid metabolites in the urine. Symptoms generally resolve rapidly with treatment.[254,255] Vitamin B_1 (thiamine) deficiency can lead to Wernicke's encephalopathy, common symptoms of which include ophthalmoparesis (with vertical and/or horizontal nystagmus),

ataxia and memory loss. Hyperintensities in DWI can be seen in mammillary bodies and dorsomedial nucleus of the thalamus. Pathologically, these areas often show hemorrhagic necrosis. The thalamic involvement on DWI MRI can overlap with CJD[41,256–258] and Bartonella encephalopathy.[129] Again, because this condition is usually reversible with treatment, all patients with dementia should be screened for vitamin B_{12} deficiency.

Adults presenting with RPD may have metabolic disorders that typically afflict children.[30] Such adult-onset metabolic diseases generally also show weakness, spasticity and ataxia, and possibly rapid cognitive decline. When gastrointestinal disturbance, fluctuating course, an unexplained pain syndrome and/or worsening after use of new medicines is seen, porphyria should be considered.

Patients with Kuf's disease, a rare autosomal recessive adult form of neuronal ceroid lipofuscinoses, develop a progressive encephalopathy resulting from an accumulation of acid-phosphate-staining ceroid and lipofuscins. The disease typically presents in early adulthood and has been classified into two types: patients with type A present with a progressive myoclonic epilepsy, while type B patients present with psychosis progressing to dementia.[259]

Exposure to heavy metals, such as arsenic, mercury, aluminum, lithium and lead, can lead to cognitive decline, particularly if the exposure is acute. Most cases of acute exposure, however, result in florid encephalopathies that progress over hours to days, not weeks to months as is typical of RPDs. Miners with manganese toxicity may have parkinsonism, but typically not dementia.[53]

Overdoses of bismuth (often via products such as Pepto-bismol) can cause a syndrome mimicking CJD. Symptoms include apathy, mild ataxia and headaches, progressing to myoclonus, dysarthria, severe confusion, hallucinations (auditory and visual), seizures and, in severe cases, death.[60,260–262] Blood levels of bismuth greater than 50 μg are generally considered toxic.[60,262] While prolonged bismuth intoxication can lead to permanent tremors, in most cases the condition is reversible.[60,260] Diagnosis is usually made following a careful history.

Non-organic (psychiatric) causes of rapidly progressing dementia

Finally, when all neurological possibilities have been ruled out, psychological causes should be considered.

Box 23.1 Ten pearls for diagnosis of rapidly progressing dementia

1. Don't forget the basics (e.g. calcium, magnesium, phosphate, thyroid-stimulating hormone, medications)
2. Most patients with RPD are elderly with a metabolic or infectious perturbation, although many have an underlying neurodegenerative disease, such as AD.
3. The most frequent CJD misdiagnoses are other more common neurodegenerative diseases, such as AD, DLB, FTD and CBD, often with prominent extrapyramidal or behavioral features.
4. Consider possible autoimmune etiologies, including paraneoplastic and non-paraneoplastic antibody-mediated conditions. Consider Hashimoto's encephalopathy (a diagnosis of exclusion)!
5. An appropriate MRI should be with contrast and contain adequate DWI and apparent diffusion coefficient sequences to assess for restricted diffusion
6. Most with CJD have DWI hyperintensity in cerebral cortex, "cortical ribboning" and/or striatal/thalamic hyperintensity; these findings are often missed in radiology reports. Read your own images.
7. Lumbar puncture is necessary when diagnosis is not clear; CSF "biomarkers" (14–3–3, neuron-specific endase and tau) are not diagnostic but may suggest rapid neuronal injury. Do not forget IgG index and oligoclonal bands for autoimmune conditions.
8. CJD is the great mimicker – early in the course, it can look like many conditions.
9. EEG only shows classic CJD findings (paroxysmal EEG discharges) in 50–70% of those with sCJD.
10. When in doubt, admit for more thorough, expeditious work-up.

Depression can cause pseudodementia, and cognitive impairments appearing on neuropsychological testing may result from apathy. Some atypical psychiatric disorders, particularly disorders of personality, conversion, psychosis and malingering can lead to symptoms of dementia.[263] In these cases, ruling out potentially treatable or organic disorders is paramount. Muddying the waters, many neurodegenerative disorders including CJD, DLB and CBD can present with psychiatric features.[14,120,121,264–266]

Summary

A structured approach to the evaluation of an RPD is critical for quick diagnosis (Box 23.1). Most often, elderly patients presenting with RPD are suffering from delirium caused by a urinary infection or pneumonia. Once the simplest causes have been excluded, a systematic approach in which each category of etiology is considered in turn is most effective. Admitting the patient may be desirable as numerous tests are necessary. A body CT scan with and without contrast is particularly helpful in diagnosing sarcoid, malignancies and paraneoplastic conditions. In some cases, a brain biopsy may be necessary, though of course only considered as a last resort. When prion disease is in the differential, precautions must be taken in the operating room and when handling brain tissue.

References

1. Tschampa, H. J., M. Neumann, I. Zerr *et al.* Patients with Alzheimer's disease and dementia with Lewy bodies mistaken for Creutzfeldt–Jakob disease. *J Neurol Neurosurg Psychiatry*, 2001; **71**(1): 33–9.

2. Poser, S., B. Mollenhauer, A. Kraubeta *et al.* How to improve the clinical diagnosis of Creutzfeldt–Jakob Disease. *Brain*, 1999; **122**(Pt 12): 2345–51.

3. Olichney, J. M., D. Galasko, D. P. Salmon *et al.* Cognitive decline is faster in Lewy body variant than in Alzheimer's disease. *Neurology*, 1998; **51**(2): 351–7.

4. Geschwind, M. D., A. Haman, and B. L. Miller. Rapidly progressive dementia. *Neurol Clin*, 2007; **25**(3): 783–807.

5. Creutzfeldt, H. G. On a particular focal disease of the central nervous system (preliminary communication), 1920. *Alzheimer Dis Assoc Disord*, 1989; **3**(1–2): 3–25.

6. Jakob, A. Concerning a disorder of the central nervous system clinically resembling multiple sclerosis with remarkable anatomic findings (spastic pseudosclerosis). Report of a fourth case. *Alzheimer Dis Assoc Disord*, 1989; **3**(1–2): 26–45.

7. Katscher, F. It's Jakob's disease, not Creutzfeldt's. *Nature*, 1998; **393**(6680): 11.

8. Gibbs, C. J. Jr. Spongiform encephalopathies – slow, latent, and temperate virus infections – in retrospect In *Prion Diseases of Humans and Animals*, S. B. Prusiner, eds., J. Collinge, J. Powell and B. Anderton. London: Ellis Horwood, 1992, pp. 53–62.

9. Masters, C. L. Creutzfeldt–Jakob disease: its origins. *Alzheimer Dis Assoc Disord*, 1989; **3**(1–2): 46–51.

10. Ladogana, A., M. Puopolo, E. A. Croes *et al.* Mortality from Creutzfeldt–Jakob disease and related disorders in Europe, Australia, and Canada. *Neurology*, 2005; **64**(9): 1586–91.

11. Brown, P., C. J. Gibbs, Jr., P. Rodgers-Johnson *et al.* Human spongiform encephalopathy: the National

357

Institutes of Health series of 300 cases of experimentally transmitted disease. *Ann Neurol*, 1994; **35**(5): 513–29.

12. Pocchiari, M., M. Puopolo, E. A. Croes *et al.* Predictors of survival in sporadic Creutzfeldt–Jakob disease and other human transmissible spongiform encephalopathies. *Brain*, 2004; **127**(10): 2348–59.

13. Collins, S. J., P. Sanchez-Juan, C. L. Masters *et al.* Determinants of diagnostic investigation sensitivities across the clinical spectrum of sporadic Creutzfeldt–Jakob disease. *Brain*, 2006; **129**(Pt 9): 2278–87.

14. Rabinovici, G. D., P. N. Wang, J. Levin *et al.* First symptom in sporadic Creutzfeldt–Jakob disease. *Neurology*, 2006; **66**(2): 286–7.

15. World Health Organization. *Emerging and Other Communicable Diseases, Surveillance and Control: Global Surveillance, Diagnosis and Therapy of Human Transmissible Spongiform Encephalopathies.* Geneva: World Health Organization, 1998.

16. Masters, C. L., J. O. Harris, D. C. Gajdusek *et al.* Creutzfeldt–Jakob disease: patterns of worldwide occurrence and the significance of familial and sporadic clustering. *Ann Neurol*, 1979; **5**(2): 177–88.

17. Kretzschmar, H. A., J. W. Ironside, S. J. DeArmond *et al.* Diagnostic criteria for sporadic Creutzfeldt–Jakob disease. *Arch Neurol*, 1996; **53**(9): 913–20.

18. Pals, P., B. Van Everbroeck, R. Sciot *et al.* A retrospective study of Creutzfeldt–Jakob disease in Belgium. *Eur J Epidemiol*, 1999; **15**(6): 517–19.

19. Zerr, I., M. Pocchiari, S. Collins *et al.* Analysis of EEG and CSF 14-3-3 proteins as aids to the diagnosis of Creutzfeldt–Jakob disease. *Neurology*, 2000; **55**(6): 811–15.

20. Steinhoff, B. J., I. Zerr, M. Glatting *et al.* Diagnostic value of periodic complexes in Creutzfeldt–Jakob disease. *Ann Neurol*, 2004; **56**(5): 702–8.

21. Henchey, R., J. Cibula, W. Helveston *et al.* Electroencephalographic findings in Hashimoto's encephalopathy. *Neurology*, 1995; **45**(5): 977–81.

22. Seipelt, M., I. Zerr, R. Nau *et al.* Hashimoto's encephalitis as a differential diagnosis of Creutzfeldt–Jakob disease. *J Neurol Neurosurg Psychiatry*, 1999; **66**(2): 172–6.

23. Hsich, G., K. Kenney, C. J. Gibbs *et al.* The 14-3-3 brain protein in cerebrospinal fluid as a marker for transmissible spongiform encephalopathies. *N Engl J Med*, 1996; **335**(13): 924–30.

24. Otto, M. and J. Wiltfang. Differential diagnosis of neurodegenerative diseases with special emphasis on Creutzfeldt–Jakob disease. *Restor Neurol Neurosci*, 2003; **21**(3–4): 191–209.

25. Van Everbroeck, B., S. Quoilin, J. Boons *et al.* A prospective study of CSF markers in 250 patients with possible Creutzfeldt–Jakob disease. *J Neurol Neurosurg Psychiatry*, 2003; **74**(9): 1210–14.

26. Sanchez-Juan, P., A. Green, A. Ladogana *et al.* CSF tests in the differential diagnosis of Creutzfeldt–Jakob disease. *Neurology*, 2006; **67**(4): 637–43.

27. Chapman, T., D. W. McKeel, Jr., and J. C. Morris. Misleading results with the 14-3-3 assay for the diagnosis of Creutzfeldt–Jakob disease. *Neurology*, 2000; **55**(9): 1396–7.

28. Geschwind, M. D., J. Martindale, D. Miller *et al.* Challenging the clinical utility of the 14-3-3 protein for the diagnosis of sporadic Creutzfeldt–Jakob disease. *Arch Neurol*, 2003; **60**(6): 813–16.

29. Zerr, I., M. Bodemer, O. Gefeller *et al.* Detection of 14-3-3 protein in the cerebrospinal fluid supports the diagnosis of Creutzfeldt–Jakob disease. *Ann Neurol*, 1998; **43**(1): 32–40.

30. Geschwind, M. D., A. Haman, C. Torres-Chae. *et al.* CSF findings in a large United States sporadic CJD cohort. In *Proceedings of the Annual Conference of the American Academy of Neurology*, Boston, 2007, A142.

31. Lemstra, A. W., M. T. van Meegan, J. P. Vreyling *et al.* 14-3-3 testing in diagnosing Creutzfeldt–Jakob disease. *Neurology*, 2000; **55**: 514–16.

32. Beaudry, P., P. Cohen, J. P. Brandel *et al.* 14-3-3 Protein, neuron-specific enolase, and S-100 protein in cerebrospinal fluid of patients with Creutzfeldt–Jakob disease. *Dement Geriatr Cogn Disord*, 1999; **10**(1): 40–6.

33. Van Everbroeck, B. R. J., J. Boons and P. Cras, 14-3-3 {gamma}-isoform detection distinguishes sporadic Creutzfeldt–Jakob disease from other dementias. *J Neurol Neurosurg Psychiatry*, 2005; **76**(1): 100–2.

34. Otto, M., J. Wiltfang, L. Cepek *et al.* Tau protein and 14-3-3 protein in the differential diagnosis of Creutzfeldt–Jakob disease. *Neurology*, 2002; **58**(2): 192–7.

35. Van Everbroeck, B., A. Green, E. Vanmechelen *et al.* Phosphorylated tau in cerebrospinal fluid as a marker for Creutzfeldt–Jakob disease. *J Neurol Neurosurg Psychiatry*, 2002; **73**(1): 79–81.

36. Huang, N., S. K. Marie, J. A. Livramento *et al.* 14-3-3 protein in the CSF of patients with rapidly progressive dementia. *Neurology*, 2003; **61**(3): 354–7.

37. Safar, J., H. Wille, V. Itri *et al.* Eight prion strains have PrP(Sc) molecules with different conformations. *Nat Med*, 1998; **4**(10): 1157–65.

38. Safar, J. G., M. D. Geschwind, C. Deering *et al.* Diagnosis of human prion disease. *Proc Natl Acad Sci USA*, 2005; **102**(9): 3501–6.

39. Safar, J. G., H. Wille, M. D. Geschwind *et al.* Human prions and plasma lipoproteins. *Proc Natl Acad Sci USA*, 2006; **103**: 11312–17.

40. Saa, P., J. Castilla, and C. Soto. Ultra-efficient replication of infectious prions by automated protein misfolding cyclic amplification. *J Biol Chem*, 2006; **281**(46): 35245–52.

41. Young, G. S., M. D. Geschwind, N. J. Fischbein *et al.* Diffusion-weighted and fluid-attenuated inversion

recovery imaging in Creutzfeldt–Jakob disease: high sensitivity and specificity for diagnosis. *Am J Neuroradiol*, 2005; **26**(6): 1551–62.

42. Shiga, Y., K. Miyazawa, S. Sato *et al.* Diffusion-weighted MRI abnormalities as an early diagnostic marker for Creutzfeldt–Jakob disease. *Neurology*, 2004; I**63**: 443–9.

43. Bavis, J., P. Reynolds, C. Tegeler *et al.* Asymmetric neuroimaging in Creutzfeldt–Jakob disease: a ruse. *J Neuroimaging*, 2003; **13**(4): 376–79.

44. Cambier, D. M., K. Kantarci, G. A. Worrell *et al.* Lateralized and focal clinical, EEG, and FLAIR MRI abnormalities in Creutzfeldt–Jakob disease. *Clin Neurophysiol*, 2003; **114**(9): 1724–8.

45. Peretz, D., S. Supattapone, K. Giles *et al.* Inactivation of prions by acidic sodium dodecyl sulfate. *J Virol*, 2006; **80**(1): 322–31.

46. Muller, W. E., J. L. Laplanche, H. Ushijima *et al.* Novel approaches in diagnosis and therapy of Creutzfeldt–Jakob disease. *Mech Ageing Dev*, 2000; **116**(2–3): 193–218.

47. Serban, D., A. Taraboulos, S. J. DeArmond *et al.* Rapid detection of Creutzfeldt–Jakob disease and scrapie prion proteins. *Neurology*, 1990; **40**(1): 110–17.

48. Soto, C., G. P. Saborio, and L. Anderes. Cyclic amplification of protein misfolding: application to prion-related disorders and beyond. *Trends Neurosci*, 2002; **25**(8): 390–4.

49. Castilla, J., P. Saa, C. Soto. Detection of prions in blood. *Nat Med*, 2005; **11**(9): 982–5.

50. Castilla, J., R. Nonno, N. Fernández-Borges *et al.* FC7.4 de novo generation of prions in a cell-free system. In *Prion2007*. Edinburgh, UK: NeuroPrion, 2007, p. 16.

51. Chang, C. C., S. D. Eggers, J. K. Johnson *et al.* Anti-GAD antibody cerebellar ataxia mimicking Creutzfeldt–Jakob disease. *Clin Neurol Neurosurg*, 2007; **109**: 54–7.

52. Saiz, A., F. Graus, J. Dalmau *et al.* Detection of 14-3-3 brain protein in the cerebrospinal fluid of patients with paraneoplastic neurological disorders. *Ann Neurol*, 1999; **46**: 774–7.

53. Geschwind, M. D. and C. Jay. Assessment of rapidly progressive dementias. Concise review related to Chapter 362: Alzheimer's Disease and Other Primary Dementias. In *Harrison's Textbook of Internal Medicine*, eds. E. Braunwald, A. S. Fauci, D. L. Kaspar *et al.* New York: McGraw Hill, 2003. [Online supplement.] McGraw Hill.

54. Ghika-Schmid, F., J. Ghika, F. Regli *et al.* Hashimoto's myoclonic encephalopathy: an underdiagnosed treatable condition? *Mov Disord*, 1996; **11**(5): 555–62.

55. Slee, M., P. Pretorius, O. Ansorge *et al.* Parkinsonism and dementia due to gliomatosis cerebri mimicking sporadic Creutzfeldt–Jakob disease (CJD). *J Neurol Neurosurg Psychiatry*, 2006; **77**(2): 283–4.

56. Heinrich, A., S. Vogelgesang, M. Kirsch *et al.* Intravascular lymphomatosis presenting as rapidly progressive dementia. *Eur Neurol*, 2005; **54**(1): 55–8.

57. Bakshi, R., J. C. Mazziotta, P. S. Mischel *et al.* Lymphomatosis cerebri presenting as a rapidly progressive dementia: clinical, neuroimaging and pathologic findings. *Dement Geriatr Cogn Disord*, 1999; **10**(2): 152–7.

58. Carlson, B. A., Rapidly progressive dementia caused by nonenhancing primary lymphoma of the central nervous system. *Am J Neuroradiol*, 1996; **17**(9): 1695–7.

59. Josephson, S. A., A. M. Papanastassiou, M. S. Berger *et al.* The diagnostic utility of brain biopsy procedures in patients with rapidly deteriorating neurological conditions or dementia. *J Neurosurg*, 2007; **106**(1): 72–5.

60. Jungreis, A. C. and H. H. Schaumburg. Encephalopathy from abuse of bismuth subsalicylate (Pepto-Bismol). *Neurology*, 1993; **43**(6): 1265.

61. Teepker 2002 #6458 to add.

62. Gajdusek, D. C. Unconventional viruses and the origin and disappearance of kuru. *Science*, 1977; **197**(4307): 943–60.

63. Brown, P., R. G. Rohwer and D. C. Gajdusek, Newer data on the inactivation of scrapie virus or Creutzfeldt–Jakob disease virus in brain tissue. *J Infect Dis*, 1986; **153**(6): 1145–8.

64. Prusiner, S. B. Novel proteinaceous infectious particles cause scrapie. *Science*, 1982; **216**(4542): 136–44.

65. Gajdusek, D. C., C. J. Gibbs, Jr., D. M. Asher *et al.* Precautions in medical care of, and in handling materials from, patients with transmissible virus dementia (Creutzfeldt–Jakob disease). *N Engl J Med*, 1977; **297**(23): 1253–8.

66. Oesch, B., D. Westaway, M. Walchli *et al.* A cellular gene encodes scrapie PrP 27–30 protein. *Cell*, 1985; **40**(4): 735–46.

67. Basler, K., B. Oesch, M. Scott *et al.* Scrapie and cellular PrP isoforms are encoded by the same chromosomal gene. *Cell*, 1986; **46**(3): 417–28.

68. Taraboulos, A., K. Jendroska, D. Serban *et al.* Regional mapping of prion proteins in brain. *Proc Natl Acad Sci USA*, 1992; **89**(16): 7620–4.

69. Borchelt, D. R., M. Rogers, N. Stahl *et al.* Release of the cellular prion protein from cultured cells after loss of its glycoinositol phospholipid anchor. *Glycobiology*, 1993; **3**(4): 319–29.

70. Borchelt, D. R., A. Taraboulos and S. B. Prusiner. Evidence for synthesis of scrapie prion proteins in the endocytic pathway. *J Biol Chem*, 1992; **267**(23): 16188–99.

71. Hegde, R. S., P. Tremblay, D. Groth *et al.* Transmissible and genetic prion diseases share a common pathway of neurodegeneration. *Nature*, 1999; **402**(6763): 822–6.

72. Hegde, R. S., J. A. Mastrianni, M. R. Scott *et al.* A transmembrane form of the prion protein in neurodegenerative disease. *Science*, 1998; **279**(5352): 827–34.

359

73. Hay, B., S. B. Prusiner, and V. R. Lingappa. Evidence for a secretory form of the cellular prion protein. *Biochemistry*, 1987; **26**(25): 8110–15.

74. Prusiner, S. B. Shattuck lecture: neurodegenerative diseases and prions. *N Engl J Med*, 2001; **344**(20): 1516–26.

75. Prusiner, S. B. The prion diseases. *Brain Pathol*, 1998; **8**(3): 499–513.

76. Prusiner, S. B. Prions. *Proc Natl Acad Sci USA*, 1998; **95**(23): 13363–83.

77. Deleault, N. R., R. W. Lucassen and S. Supattapone. RNA molecules stimulate prion protein conversion. *Nature*, 2003; **425**(6959): 717–20.

78. Wong, C., L. W. Xiong, M. Horiuchi *et al.* Sulfated glycans and elevated temperature stimulate PrP(Sc)-dependent cell-free formation of protease-resistant prion protein. *Embo J*, 2001; **20**(3): 377–86.

79. Telling, G. C., M. Scott, J. Mastrianni *et al.* Prion propagation in mice expressing human and chimeric PrP transgenes implicates the interaction of cellular PrP with another protein. *Cell*, 1995; **83**(1): 79–90.

80. Bueler, H., A. Aguzzi, A. Sailer *et al.* Mice devoid of PrP are resistant to scrapie. *Cell*, 1993; **73**(7): 1339–47.

81. Prusiner, S. B., D. Groth, A. Serban *et al.* Ablation of the prion protein (PrP) gene in mice prevents scrapie and facilitates production of anti-PrP antibodies. *Proc Natl Acad Sci USA*, 1993; **90**(22): 10608–12.

82. Katamine, S., N. Nishida, T. Sugimoto *et al.* Impaired motor coordination in mice lacking prion protein. *Cell Mol Neurobiol*, 1998; **18**(6): 731–42.

83. Sailer, A., H. Bueler, M. Fischer *et al.* No propagation of prions in mice devoid of PrP. *Cell*, 1994; **77**(7): 967–8.

84. Nishida, N., P. Tremblay, T. Sugimoto *et al.* A mouse prion protein transgene rescues mice deficient for the prion protein gene from purkinje cell degeneration and demyelination. *Lab Invest*, 1999; **79**(6): 689–97.

85. Spudich, A., R. Frigg, E. Kilic *et al.* Aggravation of ischemic brain injury by prion protein deficiency: role of ERK-1/-2 and STAT-1. *Neurobiol Dis*, 2005; **20**(2): 442–9.

86. Tobler, I., S. E. Gaus, T. Deboer *et al.* Altered circadian activity rhythms and sleep in mice devoid of prion protein. *Nature*, 1996; **380**(6575): 639–42.

87. Tobler, I., T. Deboer, and M. Fischer. Sleep and sleep regulation in normal and prion protein-deficient mice. *J Neurosci*, 1997; **17**(5): 1869–79.

88. Criado, J. R., M. Sanchez-Alavez, B. Conti *et al.* Mice devoid of prion protein have cognitive deficits that are rescued by reconstitution of PrP in neurons. *Neurobiol Dis*, 2005; **19**(1–2): 255–65.

89. Colling, S. B., M. Khana, J. Collinge *et al.* Mossy fibre reorganization in the hippocampus of prion protein null mice. *Brain Res*, 1997; **755**(1): 28–35.

90. Brown, D. R., R. S. Nicholas, and L. Canevari. Lack of prion protein expression results in a neuronal phenotype sensitive to stress. *J Neurosci Res*, 2002; **67**(2): 211–24.

91. Miele, G., M. Jeffrey, D. Turnbull *et al.* Ablation of cellular prion protein expression affects mitochondrial numbers and morphology. *Biochem Biophys Res Commun*, 2002; **291**(2): 372–7.

92. Klamt, F., F. Dal-Pizzol, M. J. Conte da Frota *et al.* Imbalance of antioxidant defense in mice lacking cellular prion protein. *Free Radic Biol Med*, 2001; **30**(10): 1137–44.

93. Wong, B. S., T. Liu, R. Li *et al.* Increased levels of oxidative stress markers detected in the brains of mice devoid of prion protein. *J Neurochem*, 2001; **76**(2): 565–72.

94. Weise, J., R. Sandau, S. Schwarting *et al.* Deletion of cellular prion protein results in reduced Akt activation, enhanced postischemic caspase-3 activation, and exacerbation of ischemic brain injury. *Stroke*, 2006; **37**(5): 1296–300.

95. Kuwahara, C., A. M. Takeuchi, T. Nishimura *et al.* Prions prevent neuronal cell-line death. *Nature*, 1999; **400**(6741): 225–6.

96. Weissmann, C. and E. Flechsig. PrP knock-out and PrP transgenic mice in prion research. *Br Med Bull*, 2003; **66**: 43–60.

97. Shyu, W. C., S. Z. Lin, M. F. Chiang *et al.* Overexpression of PrPC by adenovirus-mediated gene targeting reduces ischemic injury in a stroke rat model. *J Neurosci*, 2005; **25**(39): 8967–77.

98. Mallucci, G. R., S. Ratte, E. A. Asante *et al.* Post-natal knockout of prion protein alters hippocampal CA1 properties, but does not result in neurodegeneration. *Embo J*, 2002; **21**(3): 202–10.

99. Santuccione, A., V. Sytnyk, I. Leshchyns'ka *et al.* Prion protein recruits its neuronal receptor NCAM to lipid rafts to activate p59fyn and to enhance neurite outgrowth. *J Cell Biol*, 2005; **169**(2): 341–54.

100. Kanaani, J., S. B. Prusiner, J. Diacovo *et al.* Recombinant prion protein induces rapid polarization and development of synapses in embryonic rat hippocampal neurons in vitro. *J Neurochem*, 2005; **95**(5): 1373–86.

101. Palmer, M. S., A. J. Dryden, J. T. Hughes *et al.* Homozygous prion protein genotype predisposes to sporadic Creutzfeldt–Jakob disease. *Nature*, 1991; **352**(6333): 340–2.

102. Parchi, P., A. Giese, S. Capellari *et al.* Classification of sporadic Creutzfeldt–Jakob disease based on molecular and phenotypic analysis of 300 subjects. *Ann Neurol*, 1999; **46**(2): 224–33.

103. Laplanche, J. L., N. Delasnerie-Laupretre, J. P. Brandel *et al.* Molecular genetics of prion diseases in France. French Research Group on Epidemiology of Human Spongiform Encephalopathies. *Neurology*, 1994; **44**(12): 2347–51.

104. Parchi, P., R. Castellani, S. Capellari *et al.* Molecular basis of phenotypic variability in sporadic Creutzfeldt–Jakob disease. *Ann Neurol*, 1996; **39**(6): 767–78.

105. Polymenidou, M., K. Stoeck, M. Glatzel *et al.* Coexistence of multiple PrPSc types in individuals with Creutzfeldt–Jakob disease. *Lancet Neurol*, 2005; **4**(12): 805–14.

106. Mastrianni, J. A., R. Nixon, R. Layzer *et al.* Prion protein conformation in a patient with sporadic fatal insomnia. *N Engl J Med*, 1999; **340**(21): 1630–8.

107. Parchi, P., S. Capellari, S. Chin *et al.* A subtype of sporadic prion disease mimicking fatal familial insomnia. *Neurology*, 1999; **52**(9): 1757–63.

108. Watts, J. C., A. Balachandran, and D. Westaway. The expanding universe of prion diseases. *PLoS Pathol*, 2006; **2**(3): e26.

109. Kong, Q. K., W. K. Surewicz, R. B. Petersen *et al.* Inherited prion diseases. In *Prion Biology and Disease*, ed. S. B. Prusiner. Cold Spring Harbor: Cold Spring Harbor Laboratory Press, 2004, pp. 673–776.

110. Ghetti, B., S. R. Dlouhy, G. Giaccone *et al.* Gerstmann–Straussler–Scheinker disease and the Indiana kindred. *Brain Pathol*, 1995; **5**(1): 61–75.

111. Kovacs, G. G., G. Trabattoni, J. A. Hainfellner *et al.* Mutations of the prion protein gene phenotypic spectrum. *J Neurol*, 2002; **249**(11): 1567–82.

112. Gambetti, P., P. Parchi, and S. G. Chen. Hereditary Creutzfeldt–Jakob disease and fatal familial insomnia. *Clin Lab Med*, 2003; **23**: 43–64.

113. Will, R. G., A. Alperovitch, S. Poser *et al.* Descriptive epidemiology of Creutzfeldt–Jakob disease in six European countries, 1993–1995. EU Collaborative Study Group for CJD. *Ann Neurol*, 1998; **43**(6): 763–7.

114. Bruce, M. E., R. G. Will, J. W. Ironside *et al.* Transmissions to mice indicate that "new variant" CJD is caused by the BSE agent. *Nature*, 1997; **389**(6650): 498–501.

115. Hill, A. F., M. Desbruslais, S. Joiner *et al.* The same prion strain causes vCJD and BSE. *Nature*, 1997; **389**(6650): 448–50, 526.

116. Scott, M. R., R. Will, J. Ironside *et al.* Compelling transgenetic evidence for transmission of bovine spongiform encephalopathy prions to humans. *Proc Natl Acad Sci USA*, 1999; **96**(26): 15137–42.

117. Will, R. G., J. W. Ironside, M. Zeidler *et al.* A new variant of Creutzfeldt–Jakob disease in the UK. *Lancet*, 1996; **347**(9006): 921–5.

118. UK National CJD Surveillance Unit. *vCJD Cases Worldwide.* Edinburgh: Western General Hospital, 2007.

119. Lorains, J. W., C. Henry, D. A. Agbamu *et al.* Variant Creutzfeldt–Jakob disease in an elderly patient. *Lancet*, 2001; **357**(9265): 1339–40.

120. Zeidler, M., E. C. Johnstone, R. W. Bamber *et al.* New variant Creutzfeldt–Jakob disease: psychiatric features. *Lancet*, 1997; **350**(9082): 908–10.

121. Will, R. G., M. Zeidler, G. E. Stewart *et al.* Diagnosis of new variant Creutzfeldt–Jakob disease. *Ann Neurol*, 2000; **47**(5): 575–82.

122. Kapur, N., P. Abbott, A. Lowman *et al.* The neuropsychological profile associated with variant Creutzfeldt–Jakob disease. *Brain*, 2003; **126**(Pt 12): 2693–702.

123. Binelli, S., P. Agazzi, G. Giaccone *et al.* Periodic electroencephalogram complexes in a patient with variant Creutzfeldt–Jakob disease. *Ann Neurol*, 2006; **59**(2): 423–7.

124. Zeidler, M., R. J. Sellar, D. A. Collie *et al.* The pulvinar sign on magnetic resonance imaging in variant Creutzfeldt–Jakob disease. *Lancet*, 2000; **355**(9213): 1412–18.

125. Collie, D. A., R. J. Sellar, M. Zeidler *et al.* MRI of Creutzfeldt–Jakob disease: imaging features and recommended MRI protocol. *Clinical Radiology*, 2001; **56**(9): 726–39.

126. Collie, D. A., D. M. Summers, R. J. Sellar *et al.* Diagnosing variant Creutzfeldt–Jakob disease with the pulvinar sign: MR imaging findings in 86 neuropathologically confirmed cases. *Am J Neuroradiol*, 2003; **24**(8): 1560–9.

127. Petzold, G. C., I. Westner, G. Bohner *et al.* False-positive pulvinar sign on MRI in sporadic Creutzfeldt–Jakob disease. *Neurology*, 2004; **62**(7): 1235–6.

128. Wakisaka, Y., N. Santa, K. Doh-ura *et al.* Increased asymmetric pulvinar magnetic resonance imaging signals in Creutzfeldt–Jakob disease with florid plaques following a cadaveric dura mater graft. *Neuropathology*, 2006; **26**(1): 82–8.

129. Singhal, A. B., M. C. Newstein, R. Budzik *et al.* Diffusion-weighted magnetic resonance imaging abnormalities in *Bartonella* encephalopathy. *J Neuroimaging*, 2003; **13**(1): 79–82.

130. Mihara, M., S. Sugase, K. Konaka *et al.* The "pulvinar sign" in a case of paraneoplastic limbic encephalitis associated with non-Hodgkin's lymphoma. *J Neurol Neurosurg Psychiatry*, 2005; **76**(6): 882–4.

131. Will, R. Variant Creutzfeldt–Jakob disease. *Folia Neuropathol*, 2004; **42**(Suppl A): 77–83.

132. Hill, A. F., M. Zeidler, J. Ironside *et al.* Diagnosis of new variant Creutzfeldt–Jakob disease by tonsil biopsy. *Lancet*, 1997; **349**(9045): 99–100.

133. Hill, A. F., R. J. Butterworth, S. Joiner *et al.* Investigation of variant Creutzfeldt–Jakob disease and other human prion diseases with tonsil biopsy samples. *Lancet*, 1999; **353**(9148): 183–9.

134. Hilton, D. A., A. C. Ghani, L. Conyers *et al.* Prevalence of lymphoreticular prion protein accumulation in UK tissue samples. *J Pathol*, 2004; **203**(3): 733–9.

135. Heikenwalder, M., N. Zeller, H. Seeger *et al.* Chronic lymphocytic inflammation specifies the organ tropism of prions. *Science*, 2005; **307**(5712): 1107–10.

136. Seeger, H., M. Heikenwalder, N. Zeller *et al.* Coincident scrapie infection and nephritis lead to urinary prion excretion. *Science*, 2005; **310**(5746): 324–6.

137. Peden, A. H., M. W. Head, D. L. Ritchie *et al.* Preclinical vCJD after blood transfusion in a PRNP codon 129 heterozygous patient. *Lancet*, 2004; **364**(9433): 527–9.

138. Llewelyn, C. A., P. E. Hewitt, R. S. Knight *et al.* Possible transmission of variant Creutzfeldt–Jakob disease by blood transfusion. *Lancet*, 2004; **363**(9407): 417–21.

139. UK Health Protection Agency. *Variant CJD and Blood Products*. London: Health Protection Agency, 2007.

140. Wroe, S. J., S. Pal, D. Siddique *et al.* Clinical presentation and pre-mortem diagnosis of variant Creutzfeldt–Jakob disease associated with blood transfusion: a case report. *Lancet*, 2006; **368**(9552): 2061–7.

141. Bishop, M. T., P. Hart, L. Aitchison *et al.* Predicting susceptibility and incubation time of human-to-human transmission of vCJD. *Lancet Neurol*, 2006; **5**(5): 393–8.

142. Aguzzi, A. and M. Glatzel. vCJD tissue distribution and transmission by transfusion: a worst-case scenario coming true? *Lancet*, 2004; **363**(9407): 411–12.

143. Ironside, J. W., M. T. Bishop, K. Connolly *et al.* Variant Creutzfeldt–Jakob disease: prion protein genotype analysis of positive appendix tissue samples from a retrospective prevalence study. *BMJ*, 2006; **332**(7551): 1186–8.

144. Korth, C., B. C. H. May, F. E. Cohen *et al.* Acridine and phenothiazine derivatives as pharmacoptherapeutics for prion disease. *Proc Natl Acad Sci USA*, 2001; **98**(17): 9836–41.

145. Murakami-Kubo, I., K. Doh-Ura, K. Ishikawa *et al.* Quinoline derivatives are therapeutic candidates for transmissible spongiform encephalopathies. *J Virol*, 2004; **78**(3): 1281–8.

146. Barret, A., F. Tagliavini, G. Forloni *et al.* Evaluation of quinacrine treatment for prion diseases. *J Virol*, 2003; **77**(15): 8462–9.

147. Forloni, G., S. Iussich, T. Awan *et al.* Tetracyclines affect prion infectivity. *Proc Natl Acad Sci USA*, 2002; **99**(16): 10849–54.

148. Sellarajah, S., T. Lekishvili, C. Bowring *et al.* Synthesis of analogues of Congo red and evaluation of their anti-prion activity. *J Med Chem*, 2004; **47**(22): 5515–34.

149. Tatzelt, J., S. B. Prusiner and W. J. Welch. Chemical chaperones interfere with the formation of scrapie prion protein. *Embo J*, 1996; **15**(23): 6363–73.

150. Georgieva, D., D. Schwark, M. von Bergen *et al.* Interactions of recombinant prions with compounds of therapeutical significance. *Biochem Biophys Res Commun*, 2006; **344**(2): 463–70.

151. Priola, S. A., A. Raines, and W. S. Caughey. Porphyrin and phthalocyanine antiscrapie compounds. *Science*, 2000; **287**: 1503–6.

152. Tagliavini, F., R. A. McArthur, B. Canciani *et al.* Effectiveness of anthracycline against experimental prion disease in Syrian hamsters. *Science*, 1997; **276**: 1119–22.

153. Ehlers, B. and H. Diringer. Dextran sulphate 500 delays and prevents mouse scrapie by impairment of agent replication in spleen. *J Gen Virol*, 1984; **65**: 1325–30.

154. Kimberlin, R. H. and C. A. Walker. The antiviral compound HPA-23 can prevent scrapie when administered at the time of infection. *Arch Virol*, 1983; **78**: 9–18.

155. Korth, C. and P. J. Peters. Emerging pharmacotherapies for Creutzfeldt–Jakob disease. *Arch Neurol*, 2006; **63**(4): 497–501.

156. Doh-ura, K., K. Ishikawa, I. Murakami-Kubo *et al.* Treatment of transmissible spongiform encephalopathy by intraventricular drug infusion in animal models. *J Virol*, 2004; **78**(10): 4999–5006.

157. Vogtherr, M., S. Grimme, B. Elshorst *et al.* Antimalarial drug quinacrine binds to C-terminal helix of cellular prion protein. *J Med Chem*, 2003; **46**(17): 3563–4.

158. Doh-Ura, K., T. Iwaki, and B. Caughey. Lysosomotropic agents and cysteine protease inhibitors inhibit scrapie-associated prion protein accumulation. *J Virol*, 2000; **74**(10): 4894–7.

159. Sandberg, M. K., P. Wallen, M. A. Wikstrom *et al.* Scrapie-infected GTI-1 cells show impaired function of voltage-gated N-type calcium channels (Ca(v) 2.2) which is ameliorated by quinacrine treatment. *Neurobiol Dis*, 2004; **15**(1): 143–51.

160. Collins, S. J., V. Lewis, M. Brazier *et al.* Quinacrine does not prolong survival in a murine Creutzfeldt–Jakob disease model. *Ann Neurol*, 2002; **52**(4): 503–6.

161. Scoazec, J. Y., P. Krolak-Salmon, O. Casez *et al.* Quinacrine-induced cytolytic hepatitis in sporadic Creutzfeldt–Jakob disease. *Ann Neurol*, 2003; **53**(4): 546–7.

162. Nakajima, M., T. Yamada, T. Kusuhara *et al.* Results of quinacrine administration to patients with Creutzfeldt–Jakob disease. *Dement Geriatr Cogn Disord*, 2004; **17**(3): 158–63.

163. Haik, S., J. P. Brandel, D. Salomon *et al.* Compassionate use of quinacrine in Creutzfeldt–Jakob disease fails to show significant effects. *Neurology*, 2004; **63**(12): 2413–15.

164. Heppner, F. L., C. Musahl, I. Arrighi *et al.* Prevention of scrapie pathogenesis by transgenic expression of

anti-prion protein antibodies. *Science*, 2001; **294** (5540): 178–82.

165. Peretz, D., R. A. Williamson, G. Legname *et al.* A change in the conformation of prions accompanies the emergence of a new prion strain. *Neuron*, 2002; **34**(6): 921–32.

166. Pankiewicz, J., F. Prelli, M. S. Sy *et al.* Clearance and prevention of prion infection in cell culture by anti-PrP antibodies. *Eur J Neurosci*, 2006; **23**(10): 2635–47.

167. Donofrio, G., F. L. Heppner, M. Polymenidou *et al.* Paracrine inhibition of prion propagation by anti-PrP single-chain Fv miniantibodies. *J Virol*, 2005; **79**(13): 8330–8.

168. Love, R. Antibodies effective against scrapie infection, report European researchers. *Lancet*, 2001; **358**(9284): 816.

169. Goni, F., E. Knudsen, F. Schreiber *et al.* Mucosal vaccination delays or prevents prion infection via an oral route. *Neuroscience*, 2005; **133**(2): 413–21.

170. Bade, S., M. Baier, T. Boetel *et al.* Intranasal immunization of Balb/c mice against prion protein attenuates orally acquired transmissible spongiform encephalopathy. *Vaccine*, 2006; **24**(9): 1242–53.

171. Sigurdsson, E. M., M. S. Sy, R. Li *et al.* Anti-prion antibodies for prophylaxis following prion exposure in mice. *Neurosci Lett*, 2003; **336**(3): 185–7.

172. Magri, G., M. Clerici, P. Dall'Ara *et al.* Decrease in pathology and progression of scrapie after immunisation with synthetic prion protein peptides in hamsters. *Vaccine*, 2005; **23**(22): 2862–8.

173. White, A. R., P. Enever, M. Tayebi *et al.* Monoclonal antibodies inhibit prion replication and delay the development of prion disease. *Nature*, 2003; **422**(6927): 80–3.

174. Sadowski, M., J. Pankiewicz, H. Scholtzova *et al.* Targeting prion amyloid deposits in vivo. *J Neuropathol Exp Neurol*, 2004; **63**(7): 775–84.

175. Heppner, F. L. and A. Aguzzi. Recent developments in prion immunotherapy. *Curr Opin Immunol*, 2004; **16**(5): 594–8.

176. Mallucci, G. R., M. D. White, M. Farmer *et al.* Targeting cellular prion protein reverses early cognitive deficits and neurophysiological dysfunction in prion-infected mice. *Neuron*, 2007; **53**(3): 325–35.

177. Lopez, O., D. Claassen and F. Boller. Alzheimer's disease, cerebral amyloid angiopathy, and dementia of acute onset. *Aging (Milan)*, 1991; **3**(2): 171–5.

178. Barcikowska, M., B. Mirecka, W. Papierz *et al.* [A case of Alzheimer's disease simulating Creutzfeldt–Jakob disease.] *Neurol Neurochir Pol*, 1992; **26**(5): 703–10.

179. Caselli, R. J., M. E. Couce, D. Osborne *et al.* From slowly progressive amnesic syndrome to rapidly progressive Alzheimer disease. *Alzheimer Dis Assoc Disord*, 1998; **12**(3): 251–3.

180. Haik, S., J. P. Brandel, V. Sazdovitch *et al.* Dementia with Lewy bodies in a neuropathologic series of suspected Creutzfeldt–Jakob disease. *Neurology*, 2000; **55**(9): 1401–4.

181. McKeith, I. G., D. Galasko, K. Kosaka *et al.* Consensus guidelines for the clinical and pathologic diagnosis of dementia with Lewy bodies (DLB): report of the Consortium on DLB International Workshop. *Neurology*, 1996; **47**(5): 1113–24.

182. Walker, Z., R. Allen, S. Shergill *et al.* Three years survival in patients with a clinical diagnosis of dementia with Lewy bodies. *Int J Geriatr Psychiatry*, 2000; **15**(3): 267–73.

183. Mitsuyama, Y. Presenile dementia with motor neuron disease. *Dementia*, 1993; **4**(3–4): 137–42.

184. Nasreddine, Z. S., M. Loginov, L. N. Clark *et al.* From genotype to phenotype: a clinical pathological, and biochemical investigation of frontotemporal dementia and parkinsonism (FTDP-17) caused by the P301L tau mutation. *Ann Neurol*, 1999; **45**(6): 704–15.

185. Levy, M. L., B. L. Miller, J. L. Cummings *et al.* Alzheimer disease and frontotemporal dementias. Behavioral distinctions. *Arch Neurol*, 1996; **53**(7): 687–90.

186. Rosen, H. J., J. Lengenfelder and B. Miller. Frontotemporal dementia. *Neurol Clin*, 2000; **18**(4): 979–92.

187. Schneider, J. A., R. L. Watts, M. Gearing *et al.* Corticobasal degeneration: neuropathologic and clinical heterogeneity. *Neurology*, 1997; **48**(4): 959–69.

188. Litvan, I., Y. Agid, C. Goetz *et al.* Accuracy of the clinical diagnosis of corticobasal degeneration: a clinicopathologic study. *Neurology*, 1997; **48**(1): 119–25.

189. Gimenez-Roldan, S., D. Mateo, C. Benito *et al.* Progressive supranuclear palsy and corticobasal ganglionic degeneration: differentiation by clinical features and neuroimaging techniques. *J Neural Transm Suppl*, 1994; **42**: 79–90.

190. Mathuranath, P. S., J. H. Xuereb, T. Bak *et al.* Corticobasal ganglionic degeneration and/or frontotemporal dementia? A report of two overlap cases and review of literature. *J Neurol Neurosurg Psychiatry*, 2000; **68**(3): 304–12.

191. Kertesz, A., P. Martinez-Lage, W. Davidson *et al.* The corticobasal degeneration syndrome overlaps progressive aphasia and frontotemporal dementia. *Neurology*, 2000; **55**(9): 1368–75.

192. Kleiner-Fisman, G., C. Bergeron and A. E. Lang. Presentation of Creutzfeldt–Jakob disease as acute corticobasal degeneration syndrome. *Mov Disord*, 2004; **19**(8): 948–9.

193. Avanzino, L., L. Marinelli, A. Buccolieri *et al.* Creutzfeldt–Jakob disease presenting as corticobasal degeneration: a neurophysiological study. *Neurol Sci*, 2006; **27**(2): 118–21.

363

194. Grafman, J., I. Litvan and M. Stark. Neuropsychological features of progressive supranuclear palsy. *Brain Cogn*, 1995; **28**(3): 311–20.

195. Litvan, I., Y. Agid, D. Calne *et al.* Clinical research criteria for the diagnosis of progressive supranuclear palsy (Steele–Richardson–Olszewski syndrome): report of the NINDS–SPSP International Workshop. *Neurology*, 1996; **47**(1): 1–9.

196. Litvan, I., Y. Agid, J. Jankovic *et al.* Accuracy of clinical criteria for the diagnosis of progressive supranuclear palsy (Steele–Richardson–Olszewski syndrome). *Neurology*, 1996; **46**(4): 922–30.

197. Litvan, I., M. S. Mega, J. L. Cummings *et al.* Neuropsychiatric aspects of progressive supranuclear palsy. *Neurology*, 1996; **47**(5): 1184–9.

198. Yagishita, A. and M. Oda. Progressive supranuclear palsy: MRI and pathological findings. *Neuroradiology*, 1996; **38**(Suppl 1): S60–6.

199. Leigh, R. J. and D. S. Zee *Contemporary Neurology Series, 55*: The Neurology of Eye Movements, 3rd edn. New York: Oxford University Press, 1999, pp. x, 646.

200. Josephs, K. A., Y. Tsuboi and D. W. Dickson. Creutzfeldt–Jakob disease presenting as progressive supranuclear palsy. *Eur J Neurol*, 2004; **11**(5): 343–6.

201. Boxer, A. L., M. D. Geschwind, N. Belfor *et al.* Patterns of brain atrophy that differentiate corticobasal degeneration syndrome from progressive supranuclear palsy. *Arch Neurol*, 2006; **63**(1): 81–6.

202. Dropcho, E. J. Paraneoplastic diseases of the nervous system. *Curr Treat Options Neurol*, 1999; **1**(5): 417–27.

203. Gultekin, S. H., M. R. Rosenfeld, R. Voltz *et al.* Paraneoplastic limbic encephalitis: neurological symptoms, immunological findings and tumour association in 50 patients. *Brain*, 2000; **123**(Pt 7): 1481–94.

204. Vernino, S., M. D. Geschwind and B. Boeve. Autoimmune encephalopathies. *Neurologist*, 2007; **13**(3): 140–7.

205. Bien, C. G. Limbic encephalitis: extension of the diagnostic armamentarium. *J Neurol Neurosurg Psychiatry*, 2007; **78**(4): 332–3.

206. Ances, B. M., R. Vitaliani, R. A. Taylor *et al.* Treatment-responsive limbic encephalitis identified by neuropil antibodies: MRI and PET correlates. *Brain*, 2005; **128**(Pt 8): 1764–77.

207. Rosenfeld, M. R., J. G. Eichen, D. F. Wade *et al.* Molecular and clinical diversity in paraneoplastic immunity to Ma proteins. *Ann Neurol*, 2001; **50**(3): 339–48.

208. Dalmau, J., F. Graus, A. Villarejo *et al.* Clinical analysis of anti-Ma2-associated encephalitis. *Brain*, 2004; **127**(Pt 8): 1831–44.

209. Antoine, J. C., J. Honnorat, C. T. Anterion *et al.* Limbic encephalitis and immunological perturbations in two

210. Pittock, S. J., T. J. Kryzer and V. A. Lennon. Paraneoplastic antibodies coexist and predict cancer, not neurological syndrome. *Ann Neurol*, 2004; **56**(5): 715–19.

211. Vincent, A., B. Lang and K. A. Kleopa. Autoimmune channelopathies and related neurological disorders. *Neuron*, 2006; **52**(1): 123–38.

212. Bataller, L., K. A. Kleopa, G. F. Wu *et al.* Autoimmune limbic encephalitis in 39 patients: immunophenotypes and outcomes. *J Neurol Neurosurg Psychiatry*, 2007; **78**(4): 381–5.

213. Tuzun, E. and J. Dalmau. Limbic encephalitis and variants: classification, diagnosis and treatment. *Neurologist*, 2007; **13**(5): 261–71.

214. Brain, L., E. H. Jellinek and K. Ball. Hashimoto's disease and encephalopathy. *Lancet*, 1966; **2**(7462): 512–14.

215. Kothbauer-Margreiter, I., M. Sturzenegger, J. Komor *et al.* Encephalopathy associated with Hashimoto thyroiditis: diagnosis and treatment. *J Neurol*, 1996; **243**(8): 585–93.

216. Chong, J. Y. and L. P. Rowland. What's in a NAIM? Hashimoto encephalopathy, steroid-responsive encephalopathy associated with autoimmune thyroiditis, or nonvasculitic autoimmune meningoencephalitis? *Arch Neurol*, 2006; **63**(2): 175–6.

217. Chong, J. Y., L. P. Rowland and R. D. Utiger. Hashimoto encephalopathy: syndrome or myth? *Arch Neurol*, 2003; **60**(2): 164–71.

218. Castillo, P., B. Woodruff, R. Caselli *et al.* Steroid-responsive encephalopathy associated with autoimmune thyroiditis. *Arch Neurol*, 2006; **63**(2): 197–202.

219. Shein, M., A. Apter, Z. Dickerman *et al.* Encephalopathy in compensated Hashimoto thyroiditis: a clinical expression of autoimmune cerebral vasculitis. *Brain Dev*, 1986; **8**(1): 60–4.

220. Peschen-Rosin, R., M. Schabet and J. Dichgans. Manifestation of Hashimoto's encephalopathy years before onset of thyroid disease. *Eur Neurol*, 1999; **41**(2): 79–84.

221. Josephs, K. A., F. A. Rubino and D. W. Dickson. Nonvasculitic autoimmune inflammatory meningoencephalitis. *Neuropathology*, 2004; **24**(2): 149–52.

222. Schielke, E., C. Nolte, W. Muller *et al.* Sarcoidosis presenting as rapidly progressive dementia: clinical and neuropathological evaluation. *J Neurol*, 2001; **248**(6): 522–4.

223. Rabinstein, A. A., J. G. Romano, A. M. Forteza *et al.* Rapidly progressive dementia due to bilateral internal carotid artery occlusion with infarction of the total

length of the corpus callosum. *J Neuroimaging*, 2004; **14**(2): 176–9.

224. Auchus, A. P., C. P. Chen, S. N. Sodagar *et al.* Single stroke dementia: insights from 12 cases in Singapore. *J Neurol Sci*, 2002; **203–204**: 85–9.

225. Schaefer, P. W. Diffusion-weighted imaging as a problem-solving tool in the evaluation of patients with acute strokelike syndromes. *Top Magn Reson Imaging*, 2000; **11**(5): 300–9.

226. Anderson, S. C., C. P. Shah and F. R. Murtagh. Congested deep subcortical veins as a sign of dural venous thrombosis: MR and CT correlations. *J Comput Assist Tomogr*, 1987; **11**(6): 1059–61.

227. Wynne, P. J., D. S. Younger, A. Khandji *et al.* Radiographic features of central nervous system vasculitis. *Neurol Clin*, 1997; **15**(4): 779–804.

228. Menendez Calderon, M. J., M. E. Segui Riesco, M. Arguelles *et al.* [Intravascular lymphomatosis. *A report of three cases.] Ann Med Intern*, 2005; **22**(1): 31–4.

229. Navia, B. A. and R. W. Price. The acquired immunodeficiency syndrome: dementia as the presenting sole manifestation of human immunodeficiency virus infection. *Arch Neurol*, 1987; **44**: 65–9.

230. Brew, B. J. AIDS dementia complex. *Neurol Clin*, 1999; **17**(4): 861–81.

231. Wallace, M. R., J. A. Nelson, J. A. McCutchan *et al.* Symptomatic HIV seroconverting illness is associated with more rapid neurological impairment. *Sex Transm Infect*, 2001; **77**(3): 199–201.

232. Nath, A., W. F. Maragos, M. J. Avison *et al.* Acceleration of HIV dementia with methamphetamine and cocaine. *J Neurovirol*, 2001; **7**(1): 66–71.

233. Ala, T. A., R. C. Doss and C. J. Sullivan. Reversible dementia: a case of cryptococcal meningitis masquerading as Alzheimer's disease. *J Alzheimers Dis*, 2004; **6**(5): 503–8.

234. Heckman, G. A., C. Hawkins, A. Morris *et al.* Rapidly progressive dementia due to *Mycobacterium neoaurum* meningoencephalitis. *Emerg Infect Dis*, 2004; **10**(5): 924–7.

235. Glaser, C. A., S. Honarmand, L. J. Anderson *et al.* Beyond viruses: clinical profiles and etiologies associated with encephalitis. *Clin Infect Dis*, 2006; **43**(12): 1565–77.

236. Timmermans, M. and J. Carr. Neurosyphilis in the modern era. *J Neurol Neurosurg Psychiatry*, 2004; **75**(12): 1727–30.

237. Kaplan, R. F. and L. Jones-Woodward. Lyme encephalopathy: a neuropsychological perspective. *Semin Neurol*, 1997; **17**(1): 31–7.

238. Waniek, C., I. Prohovnik, M. A. Kaufman *et al.* Rapidly progressive frontal-type dementia associated with Lyme disease. *J Neuropsychiatry Clin Neurosci*, 1995; **7**(3): 345–7.

239. Kouyoumdjian, J. A. [Subacute sclerosing panencephalitis in an adult: report of a case.] *Arq Neuropsiquiatr*, 1985; **43**(3): 312–15.

240. Espay, A. J. and A. E. Lang. Infectious etiologies of movement disorders. In *Principles of Neurologic Infectious Diseases*, ed. K. L. Roos. New York: McGraw-Hill, 2005, pp. 383–408.

241. Anderson, M. Neurology of Whipple's disease. *J Neurol Neurosurg Psychiatry*, 2000; **68**(1): 2–5.

242. Durand, D. V., C. Lecomte, P. Cathebras *et al.* Whipple disease. Clinical review of 52 cases. The SNFMI Research Group on Whipple Disease. Societe Nationale Francaise de Medecine Interne. *Medicine (Baltimore)*, 1997; **76**(3): 170–84.

243. Louis, E. D., T. Lynch, P. Kaufmann *et al.* Diagnostic guidelines in central nervous system Whipple's disease. *Ann Neurol*, 1996; **40**(4): 561–8.

244. Matthews, B. R., L. K. Jones, D. A. Saad *et al.* Cerebellar ataxia and central nervous system whipple disease. *Arch Neurol*, 2005; **62**(4): 618–20.

245. Singer, R. Diagnosis and treatment of Whipple's disease. *Drugs*, 1998; **55**(5): 699–704.

246. Ramzan, N. N., E. Loftus, Jr., L. J. Burgart *et al.* Diagnosis and monitoring of Whipple disease by polymerase chain reaction. *Ann Intern Med*, 1997; **126**(7): 520–7.

247. Bataille, B., V. Delwail, E. Menet *et al.* Primary intracerebral malignant lymphoma: report of 248 cases. *J Neurosurg*, 2000; **92**(2): 261–6.

248. Rollins, K. E., B. K. Kleinschmidt-DeMasters, J. R. Corboy *et al.* Lymphomatosis cerebri as a cause of white matter dementia. *Human Pathology*, 2005; **36**(3): 282–90.

249. Batchelor, T. and J. S. Loeffler. Primary CNS lymphoma. *J Clin Oncol*, 2006; **24**(8): 1281–8.

250. Zuckerman, D., R. Seliem and E. Hochberg. Intravascular lymphoma: the oncologist's "great imitator." *Oncologist*, 2006; **11**(5): 496–502.

251. Chapin, J. E., L. E. Davis, M. Kornfeld *et al.* Neurologic manifestations of intravascular lymphomatosis. *Acta Neurol Scand*, 1995; **91**(6): 494–9.

252. Vieren, M., R. Sciot and W. Robberecht. Intravascular lymphomatosis of the brain: a diagnostic problem. *Clin Neurol Neurosurg*, 1999; **101**(1): 33–6.

253. Fetell, M. R. Lymphomas. In *Merrit's Textbook of Neurology*, 9th edn, ed. L. Rowland. Baltimore, MD: Williams & Wilkins, 1995, pp. 351–9.

254. Kinsella, L. J. and D. E. Riley. Nutritional deficiencies and syndromes associated with alcoholism. In *Textbook of Clinical Neurology*, ed. C. Goetz. St. Louis, MO: Saunders, 2003, pp. 973–94.

255. Kertesz, S. G. Pellagra in 2 homeless men. *Mayo Clin Proc*, 2001; **76**(3): 315–18.

256. Chu, K., D. W. Kang, H. J. Kim *et al*. Diffusion-weighted imaging abnormalities in Wernicke encephalopathy: reversible cytotoxic edema? *Arch Neurol*, 2002; **59**(1): 123–7.

257. Unlu, E., B. Cakir and T. Asil. MRI findings of Wernicke encephalopathy revisited due to hunger strike. *Eur J Radiol*, 2006; **57**(1): 43–53.

258. Halavaara, J., A. Brander, J. Lyytinen *et al*. Wernicke's encephalopathy: is diffusion-weighted MRI useful? *Neuroradiology*, 2003; **45**(8): 519–23.

259. Hinkebein, J. H. and C. D. Callahan. The neuropsychology of Kuf's disease: a case of atypical early onset dementia. *Arch Clin Neuropsychol*, 1997; **12**(1): 81–9.

260. Gorbach, S. L. Bismuth therapy in gastrointestinal diseases. *Gastroenterology*, 1990; **99**(3): 863–75.

261. Gordon, M. F., R. I. Abrams, D. B. Rubin *et al*. Bismuth toxicity. *Neurology*, 1994; **44**(12): 2418.

262. Benet, L. Z. Safety and pharmacokinetics: colloidal bismuth subcitrate. *Scand J Gastroenterol Suppl*, 1991; **185**: 29–35.

263. Hampel, H., C. Berger and N. Muller. A case of Ganser's state presenting as a dementia syndrome. *Psychopathology*, 1996; **29**(4): 236–41.

264. Wall, C. A., T. A. Rummans, A. J. Aksamit *et al*. Psychiatric manifestations of Creutzfeldt–Jakob disease: a 25-year analysis. *J Neuropsychiatry Clin Neurosci*, 2005; **17**(4): 489–95.

265. Barber, R., A. Panikkar and I. G. McKeith. Dementia with Lewy bodies: diagnosis and management. *Int J Geriatr Psychiatry*, 2001; **16**(Suppl 1): S12–18.

266. Litvan, I., J. L. Cummings and M. Mega. Neuropsychiatric features of corticobasal degeneration. *J Neurol, Neurosurg Psychiatry*, 1998; **65**(5): 717–21.

Chapter 24

Delirium masquerading as dementia

S. Andrew Josephson

Delirium is one of the first mental disorders to be described in the ancient literature. Nearly 2500 years ago, Hippocrates detailed a syndrome of acute, fluctuating confusion that we would today term delirium.[1] Unfortunately, this common disorder remains largely unrecognized and understudied in modern times, even by neurologists and psychiatrists, despite its staggering morbidity and costs to society.

Delirium is a relatively distinct clinical entity, and its recognition is an important step in the work-up of suspected dementia, especially given the tendency of delirium to be caused by potentially reversible disorders. Review of the literature on delirium is complicated by multiple synonyms for this condition including "acute confusional state," "encephalopathy", "acute brain failure" and "postoperative or intensive care unit (ICU) psychosis."[2]

Definitions of delirium used for clinical descriptions as well as for research have varied widely. At the core of these descriptions lies an impairment of cognition across multiple domains, particularly attention, that has an acute onset and fluctuating course. This definition would seem to delineate delirium from the more chronic dementias, but these boundaries can be blurred when the delirium is long standing or when the features of a dementia resemble delirium such as is often found in patients with dementia with Lewy bodies (DLB)[2,3] or late-stage dementias. The most widely used formal research criteria for delirium is found in the *Diagnostic and Statistical Manual of Mental Disorders* (DSM-IV-TR) and is shown in Box 24.1.[3]

Epidemiology, morbidity and costs associated with delirium

A number of relatively small studies give some rough but surprisingly wide-ranging estimates as to the epidemiology of delirium in various settings although large-scale, population-based and descriptive data are still needed in order to fully define the scope of this important problem.

Delirium occurs in 14–56% of hospitalized patients, with the higher end of this estimate quoted for "frail" elderly patients and for patients following hip repair.[4–6] Postoperative delirium occurs conservatively in two million persons each year in the USA and is more common with increasing severity of illness.[7] Elderly patients in the ICU deserve special mention, as nearly one-third were found to be delirious upon admission in one study and nearly 85% experienced delirium at some time prior to discharge.[8] Elderly patients in the ICU who needed mechanical ventilation and survived their initial illness had an incidence of delirium of 80% in a prospective cohort.[9] These estimates illustrate the high frequency of this cognitive syndrome, especially in severely ill hospitalized elderly patients, a population expected to grow in the coming decades with advances in life expectancy and the aging of the "baby boomer" generation.

Prior cognitive dysfunction serves as an important risk factor for delirium; therefore, patients with pre-existing dementia are at particularly high risk for developing delirium both as outpatients and while in the hospital for any reason. This patient group, with dementia who then experience a superimposed delirium, has been reported on in only a limited basis in the literature. A recent review found the prevalence of delirium superimposed on dementia to range from 22 to 89% in hospitalized and community populations aged 65 and older.[10] These same authors published data from a 3-year cross-sectional retrospective cohort of 76 000 patients in a managed care database, using ICD-9 codes[11] and chart review, and found that 13% of over 7000 patients with dementia also experienced delirium at some point during the study period.[12]

Delirium has been viewed in the past as merely a transient condition with a benign prognosis. However, recent work suggests significant short-term and

The Behavioral Neurology of Dementia, eds. Bruce L. Miller and Bradley F. Boeve. Published by Cambridge University Press.
© Cambridge University Press 2009.

Box 24.1 *Diagnostic and Statistical Manual of Mental Disorders* (DSM-IV-TR) criteria for the diagnosis of delirium

(a) Disturbance of consciousness (that is, reduced clarity of awareness of the environment, with reduced ability to focus, sustain, or shift attention)

(b) A change in cognition (such as memory deficit, disorientation, language disturbance) or the development of a perceptual disturbance that is not better accounted for by a pre-existing established or evolving dementia

(c) The disturbance developed over a short period of time (usually hours to days) and tends to fluctuate during the course of the day

(d) Where the delirium is due to a general medical condition – there is evidence from the history, physical examination, or laboratory findings that the disturbance is caused by the direct physiological consequences of a general medical condition

Where the delirium is due to substance intoxication – there is evidence from the history, physical examination, or laboratory findings of either 1 or 2:

1. The symptoms in criteria (a) and (b) developed during substance intoxication

2. Medication use – etiologically related to the disturbance

Where the delirium is due to substance withdrawal – there is evidence from the history, physical examination, or laboratory findings that the symptoms in criteria (a) and (b) developed during or shortly after the withdrawal syndrome

Where delirium is due to multiple etiologies – there is evidence from the history, physical examination, or laboratory findings that the delirium has more than one etiology (for example, more than one etiological general medical condition, a general medical condition plus substance intoxication, or medication side effects)

(e) Delirium not otherwise specified – this category should be used to diagnose a delirium that does not meet criteria for any of the specific types of delirium described. Examples include a clinical presentation of delirium that is suspected to be due to a general medical condition or substance use but for which there is insufficient evidence to establish a specific etiology, or where delirium is due to causes not listed (for example, sensory deprivation)

Source: Reprinted with permission from the *Diagnostic and Statistical Manual of Mental Disorders*, 4th edn Text Revision (Copyright 2000). American Psychiatric Association.[3]

long-term morbidity in patients with delirium, including prolonged hospitalization and poor recovery from surgery.[13] Delirious patients are more likely to be discharged to a nursing home from an inpatient hospitalization than their age-matched counterparts.[14] Delirium's association with increased length of stay has been shown to lead to increased healthcare costs, which likely average over 2 billion dollars a year in the USA alone, making delirium an extremely important economic healthcare concern.[9,15,16]

Delirium leads to increased hospital mortality, and death as an outcome ranges from 25 to 33% in delirious inpatients. One problem with these mortality data is that it has been difficult to demonstrate if delirium serves simply as a marker for more severe medical illness.[4] One study of delirium in ICU patients on a ventilator showed a higher 6-month mortality compared with controls after adjustments for age, severity of illness, comorbid conditions and sedative use.[9]

A comprehensive understanding of the morbidity of delirium is hampered by the high rate of non-detection by clinicians, which approaches one-third of all delirium cases in the hospital.[2,5] The lack of recognition of delirium can be tracked back to the limited education on this topic in medical school and postgraduate teaching programs. Additionally, there is continued misperception of delirium as a normal and benign response to illness or hospitalization in the elderly. Similarly, some clinicians only recognize delirium in its most agitated and severe form, missing those patients in whom delirium presents with decreased alertness or more mild cognitive symptoms.

Clinical characteristics of delirium

Delirium is characterized by the acute onset of a cognitive disturbance that fluctuates, often in a typical pattern that leads to worsening in the evening, commonly termed "sundowning." The cognitive hallmark of delirium is lack of attention, although all cognitive domains including memory, orientation, visuospatial, language and executive function can be affected. Common associated symptoms present in some delirious patients include hallucinations or delusions, altered sleep–wake cycle, changes in affect and autonomic symptoms including tachycardia and blood pressure instability. These associated features are not present in all patients with delirium and, therefore, are not required in the definition of this entity.

Traditionally, patients with delirium have been classified into hyperactive and hypoactive subtypes, with some also describing a "mixed" intermediate subtype. Alcohol and benzodiazepine withdrawal syndromes are the classic prototype for the hyperactive subtype, with prominent agitation, hallucinations, autonomic instability, and hyperarousal.[17] The hypoactive subtype, where patients present with decreased alertness with prominent apathy and psychomotor slowing, is easily missed by clinicians and has a wide range of etiologies including the classic example of narcotic or sedative administration.[5]

The distinction between these subtypes is likely artificial. Delirium more accurately represents a spectrum of behavioral syndromes ranging from hypoactivity to hyperactivity, often changing seamlessly within seconds in an individual patient. However, where a patient with delirium will fall within this spectrum of activity is partially dependent on the etiology of the delirium. It is important for clinicians to recognize this spectrum of delirium's diverse clinical presentations. The hypoactive subtype is more commonly missed, in part because some clinicians view delirium only as the classic delirium tremens-associated agitated, hyperactive state that includes hallucinations and altered sleep–wake cycle.[9,18]

Following resolution of an episode of delirium, patients may or may not return to their previous cognitive baseline. This area needs prospective research using modern neuropsychological and neuroimaging techniques to define any permanent injury occurring as the result of delirium. To what degree patients recall events that occurred during their episode of delirium has not been well studied. Anecdotally, some patients are amnesic for the delirium episode while others remember the episode as a frightening event, occasionally re-experiencing the unpleasant episode in a manner similar to patients with post-traumatic stress disorder.[16]

Risk factors for delirium

Primary prevention of delirum will require the identification of patients at risk for this disorder. Ultimately, large population-based studies will be needed to identify these risk factors more fully, but smaller studies since the early 1990s have identified baseline patient characteristics as well as in-hospital interventions that are associated with an increased risk of developing delirium.

The two most consistently identified risk factors for delirium are increasing age and baseline cognitive dysfunction.[8,19–21] The absence of rigorous baseline neuropsychological testing of patients makes it difficult to determine if these two risk factors are truly independent or if the cohort of patients with increasing age in these various studies had pre-existing cognitive dysfunction.

Clearly, baseline cognitive deficits seem to serve as a risk factor for delirium. The mechanism for this risk may relate either to decreased metabolic cerebral "reserve" or to the pathophysiology of an underlying degenerative illness such as Alzheimer's disease or DLB. One study of a prospective cohort of 120 patients over 65 years in the ICU showed that patients with a previous diagnosis of dementia were 40% more likely to develop delirium after adjustment for baseline functional status, severity of illness and invasiveness of in-hospital procedures.[8] A recent *Cochrane Database Review* concluded that 45% of patients with a Mini-Mental State Examination (MMSE) score less than 24 developed delirium in the hospital.[5] Other patient risk factors that have been identified in various studies include baseline vision and hearing impairment, baseline functional impairment, a previous episode of delirium, and pre-admission use of sedatives or narcotics.[19,20,22]

Factors that are associated with delirium in hospitals include dehydration, malnutrition, sleep deprivation, sensory deprivation, bladder catheterization, physical restraints, adding more than three new medications, an abnormal serum sodium and both fever and hypothermia.[2,19,22] Given the high incidence of delirium in the postoperative setting, some studies have attempted to examine surgical and anesthetic characteristics that place these patients at increased risk for delirium. Non-cardiac thoracic surgeries as well as cardiac revascularization procedures with a long duration of cardiopulmonary bypass have been identified as higher risk for development of postoperative delirium.[20,23] Interestingly, both postoperative use of pain medications and inadequate treatment of pain postoperatively have been identified as risk factors for the development of delirium.[2,20] A study of anesthesia type showed no difference in rates of delirium between epidural and general anesthesia for knee replacement in a group of patients with a mean age near 70 years.[24]

Three separate studies from the 1990s, each including 100–250 patients, have attempted to develop a scoring system to calculate the risk for developing delirium in patients admitted to the hospital, and each has shown increasing risk with a higher number of patient or hospital-acquired risk factors.[21,22,25] It would be valuable to develop a widely accepted scoring system to assess risk prior to hospital admission or surgery so that appropriate environmental, nursing and perhaps medication interventions could be put in place for higher risk groups in order to prevent the development of delirium.

Etiologies of delirium

The first step in evaluating a patient with delirium is distinguishing it from a more chronic degenerative condition. Dementia with Lewy bodies can masquerade as delirium owing to its fluctuating course, high incidence of hallucinations and disordered sleep–wake cycle. A careful history of the time course of the illness is imperative to make the separation between dementia and delirium. However, because degenerative diseases place the patient at higher risk for delirium, it is likely that many patients will have both conditions, complicating the clinical assessment.

The etiology of delirium is often multifactorial and the factors that can contribute to or cause delirium are varied, making an exhaustive, all-inclusive list difficult. Nonetheless, some general categories of causes for delirium can be identified. Clearly, patients experiencing the same insults have varied responses; for example, only a minority exposed to an anticholinergic medication become delirious. These different responses to similar exposures are likely explained by a multitude of patient characteristics, including baseline intactness of the cholinergic system, metabolic influences upon drug metabolism and the patient's baseline cognitive state. Consequently, the emergence of delirium in a patient offers critical insights into pre-existing medical factors.

A wide range of medications can lead to delirium, and some estimates suggest that medications cause up to one-third of that seen.[17] The most common classes of medication that lead to delirium include those with anticholinergic properties, narcotics and benzodiazepines. Nearly any medication can lead to delirium in the right patient at the right dose; therefore, a careful analysis of medications and the time course of their initiation in relation to the onset of the delirium are key steps in the evaluation of the delirious patient.

Illicit drugs and toxins are another common etiology of delirium. In addition to more traditional street drugs, inhalants and poisons, the recent increase in the use of so-called "club" drugs such as methylenedioxymethamphetamine (MDMA, ecstasy),

gamma-hydroxybutyrate (GHB), and the PCP-like agent ketamine have led to young persons presenting to various emergency-room settings in a delirious state.[26] Withdrawal from alcohol or sedatives including benzodiazepines continues to precipitate a delirium that is usually hyperactive in nature and characterized by hallucinations and autonomic instability.

Infections are another common cause of delirium. In particular, infections of the central nervous system itself, including encephalitis and meningitis, must be considered in a patient with a new onset of confusion. However, systemic illnesses, such as a urinary tract infection, sepsis or pneumonia, are the most common precipitants for delirium.[27] It is unclear why seemingly trivial systemic infections trigger delirium in susceptible patients, but pro-inflammatory cytokines may have some role through their effects on central nervous system tissues and function.

Various metabolic derangements increase the risk for delirium, especially in patients with advanced age or baseline cognitive impairment. Hypoxia, hypoglycemia, renal or liver dysfunction, vitamin deficiencies, electrolyte disturbances, anemia of any cause and endocrinopathies including thyroid derangements all have been described as causing delirium.[1] Initial laboratory evaluation of a patient with delirium should focus on these etiologies.

Vascular disease is often overlooked in reviews of delirium. However, despite traditional teaching to the contrary, acute stroke-precipitated confusional states are common. A recent small study found that the presence of a hemorrhagic stroke subtype and the presence of pre-stroke anticholinergic medications were risk factors for delirium in acute stroke.[28] It is rare to see a single small lesion, aside from injury in the anteromedial thalamus, account for a clinical presentation of delirium.[29] Commonly, acute stroke places patients in an environment where delirium is more likely to develop, both through sensory overload and unfamiliarity and through increased risk for infections and electrolyte disturbances while in the inpatient setting.

Other disorders that must be considered in the patient with unexplained delirium include non-convulsive status epilepticus, central nervous system vasculitis and large space-occupying lesions in the brain. As discussed below, the utility of imaging and electroencephalography (EEG) in the work-up of delirium to look for these etiologies is unknown.

Finally, a terminal end-of-life delirium has been described that has been given many names, including "terminal restlessness"; notably, this delirium may be caused by the usual etiologies of delirium and, given its effect on quality of end-of-life care, should be investigated and treated aggressively when appropriate.[30]

The pathophysiology of delirium

The pathophysiology of delirium is poorly understood. Neuroanatomically, a disorder characterized by an attentional deficit provides limited localizing value. Attention has a diffuse anatomy in the central nervous system and includes thalamic and bihemispheric projections, especially to the frontal lobes.[31] Some have proposed, based upon studies of acute stroke-precipitated inattention from right middle cerebral artery territory infarcts, a separate attentional cerebral localization that is more focal in the right parietal lobe.[31] Regardless, the attentional deficit that is the hallmark of delirium is more often the final common pathway of various diffuse cerebral processes rather than the result of a focal lesion.

Some evidence exists for a cholinergic deficiency as a cause for certain types of delirium.[32,33] Anticholinergic medications can precipitate delirium, and some studies have correlated the level of serum anticholinergic compounds with the severity of delirium.[32] In addition, cholinergic deficiency is common in DLB, a condition that can mimic delirium; patients with DLB often respond remarkably well to cholinesterase inhibitors.[35] Based upon these studies and the important role of acetylcholine in focus and attention, cholinesterase inhibitors offer hope for the treatment of delirium.[34] Yet, there has been little work in this area to date.

The explanation for increasing incidence of delirium with age still remains unexplained despite many theories. In one small study, regional cerebral blood flow as measured by xenon computed tomography (CT) was found to be reduced in delirious patients. Age may be a risk factor for delirium owing to decreased cerebral blood flow or decreased "reserve" with increasing age as a result of progressive atherosclerosis of large arteries.[36] The elderly have more cormorbid baseline factors that could lead to delirium, including functional hearing and visual loss and a greater burden of structural brain disease such as small-vessel ischemic disease, making them particularly at risk for a diffuse metabolic insult to the hemispheres.[16] Finally, the metabolism and pharmacokinetics of medications change in the elderly, leading to differential susceptibility to compounds that do not lead to delirium in younger patients.

The diagnosis and evaluation of the delirious patient

History

Recognition of patients with delirium continues to be a difficult task, and up to one-third of patients suffering from delirium are not identified.[2] The evaluation should begin with a careful history. As the patient will have diminished reliability as a historian, often a collateral source is needed. The classic acute onset and fluctuating nature of a cognitive disturbance characterized by lack of attention is important in making the diagnosis. Other associated features are variably present, including hallucinations, altered sleep-wake cycle, myoclonus or tremor and autonomic instability.

The two most important elements of the history include establishing the patient's baseline level of cognitive functioning and reviewing all current medications. With regards to the history, premorbid cognitive difficulties must be identified by the clinician, both because pre-existing cognitive dysfunction serves as an important risk factor for delirium and because some neurodegenerative disorders, most notably DLB, may present with a chronic delirium.[19] Baseline cognitive function is determined by reviewing outpatient records and through an interview of a collateral source, such as a spouse. A collateral source can help to facilitate more formal assessment of cognitive function using established tools such as the modified Blessed Dementia Rating Scale.[37,38] Medication lists need to be reviewed in full, with particular attention to recent medication additions including prescribed, over-the-counter and herbal products. As nearly one-third of all cases of delirium may be induced by medications, establishing the time course of addition of medications in comparison with the onset of cognitive changes is key.[17]

Since systemic infections are a common etiology of delirium, special attention needs to be paid in the history to any symptoms of infection. Presence of changes in urinary symptoms, cough, shortness of breath and fever should be assessed in all patients with delirium and further explored through the physical examination, laboratory tests and, potentially, with imaging studies.

Physical examination

The general physical examination of the delirious patient should focus on ruling out signs of infection and assessing volume status, as systemic infection and dehydration have each been identified as causes of delirium.[19] Examination of the head and neck should include screening for meningismus as well as using jugular venous pulsations to assess volume status. The pulmonary examination should be directed toward searching for signs of pneumonia or fluid overload. Cardiac examination should pay close attention to murmurs, as endocarditis with associated sepsis may lead to a delirium.

The mental status portion of the neurologic evaluation is discussed below. The remainder of the neurological examination should focus mainly on identifying signs of parkinsonism and assessing for focal abnormalities. Parkinsonism is present most commonly in idiopathic Parkinson's disease and, in the delirious patient population, DLB. Both of these conditions predispose the patient to delirium via the underlying condition and through the use of dopaminergic medications in treatment.

Focal weakness or numbness may be indicative of a new stroke. While traditionally ischemic stroke is not thought of as a common etiology for delirium, small thalamic infarctions, as well as perhaps non-dominant cortical infarctions, may present with acute delirium.[29] In addition, a patient with baseline cognitive dysfunction and advancing age may become delirious after a stroke owing to decreased mobility, infection or aspiration.

Mental status examination

The mental status examination serves as the key element of the neurologic examination leading to a diagnosis of delirium. The rest of the examination detailed above is then directed mainly towards elucidating an etiology for the delirium in order to guide treatment. The patient's level of alertness can easily be assessed at the bedside, recalling that the spectrum of clinical presentations of delirium includes patients with increased as well as decreased levels of alertness.

Much can be gained from informally assessing the individual during the history portion of the examination. Disorganized thinking is common in patients with delirium, and it is often manifested through tangential conversation and a fragmented flow of ideas.

Inattention serves as a core feature of delirium and can be assessed at the bedside by asking the patient to repeat digits forward. In this task, patients are given successively longer series of numbers, from 2 to 9 digits, and asked to repeat them back to the examiner. A maximum forward digit span of less than five almost certainly indicates inattention unless some other language or hearing barrier exists. Other key

features of delirium include deficits in copying, anomia for low-frequency items and problems with complex commands.

A MMSE can be easily administered and may be helpful in patients with delirium, especially in quantifying orientation. Many of the tasks on the MMSE assess attention and are vulnerable to delirium, such as spelling "world" backwards and serial subtraction by 7 or 3. Although not practical in all patients, more detailed neuropsychological testing of multiple cognitive domains in these patients is an important area of research in order to delineate more fully the cognitive deficits that are present in delirious patients.

Established scales to diagnose delirium

Numerous groups have attempted to define methods to diagnose delirium that are simple to administer and are easily scored. These tests have been studied, in general, through comparisons with formal application of criteria from the *Diagnostic and Statistical Manual of Mental Disorders*[3] or the *International Classification of Diseases*.[11] All of these scales, therefore, even when proven to be sensitive and specific, can only be as accurate as these "gold standard" criteria for capturing the spectrum of delirious patients. Indeed, these current DSM and ICD criteria are limited in their scope. Scales that have been examined for the diagnosis of delirium include the Confusion Assessment Method (CAM), the Organic Brain Syndrome Scale, the Delirium Rating Scale, the Nursing Delirium Screening Scale (Nu-DESC), the MMSE and the portable Mental State Questionnaire.[5,39]

Perhaps the most widely studied, and most commonly used, of these scales is the CAM.[40] Developed in the late 1980s, this scale includes at its core four cardinal features of delirium: (1) acute onset and fluctuating course, (2) inattention, (3) disorganized thinking, and (4) altered level of consciousness. To make the diagnosis of delirium using the CAM, a patient must have evidence of the first two features and one of the last two features, as shown in Box 24.2. This scale has a high sensitivity and specificity for the diagnosis of delirium when compared with DSM and can be abstracted retrospectively reasonably well through chart review.[4] However, the CAM has yet to be validated or shown to be reliable using large population-based techniques.

Historically, delirium in patients in the ICU has been overlooked, yet the presence of delirium leads to a poor prognosis for patients in this setting.[9] A version of the CAM adapted for mainly non-verbal

Evidence of Features 1 and 2 is required plus one of features 3 and 4

Feature 1: Acute Onset and Fluctuating Course
This feature is usually obtained from a family member or nurse and is shown by positive responses to the following questions: Is there evidence of an acute change in mental status from the patient's baseline? Did the (abnormal) behavior fluctuate during the day (that is, tend to come and go, or increase and decrease in severity)?

Feature 2: Inattention
This feature is shown by a positive response to the following questions: Did the patient have difficulty focusing attention, for example, being easily distractible, or having difficulty keeping track of what was being said?

Feature 3: Disorganized Thinking
This feature is shown by a positive response to the following question: Was the patient's thinking disorganized or incoherent, such as rambling or irrelevant conversation, unclear or illogical flow of ideas, or unpredictable switching from subject to subject?

Feature 4: Altered Level of Consciousness
This feature is shown by any answer other than "alert" to the following question: Overall, how would you rate this patient's level of consciousness? (alert [normal], vigilant [hyperalert], lethargic [drowsy, easily aroused], stupor [difficult to arouse], or coma [unarousable])

Note: Reproduced with permission from the American College of Physicians.[40]

patients in the ICU has been used by some ICU staff to increase recognition of delirium.[18] Recently, combination of this CAM-ICU scale with the Richmond Agitation Sedation Scale (RASS) has been used in a prospective study of ventilated patients in an attempt to recognize more cases of delirium and distinguish these patients from those with coma.[9] Other groups have focused on developing simple delirium-screening checklists that can be applied by nurses in the ICU, essentially creating an important other vital sign to be monitored regularly in the intensive care unit.[41]

Laboratory assessment for the delirious patient

There are no established guidelines to aid the clinician in determining an appropriate laboratory work-up for the delirious patient. A complete blood count and metabolic panel, including measurement of electrolytes and assessment of renal and liver function is essential in all patients. This initial screen can evaluate for the presence of an elevated white count, anemia, electrolyte disturbances and liver or kidney dysfunction, all of which are known causes of delirium. Given the high rate of systemic infection in elderly patients leading to delirium, obtaining a urinalysis and chest radiograph in these patients as part of the initial work-up is worthwhile.[16] Table 24.1 has a suggested work-up of a patient with delirium. After an initial

screening, more rigorous testing should be performed if the etiology of the delirium remains unclear. Other laboratory tests, including blood cultures, ammonia, erythrocyte sedimentation rate, cerebral spinal fluid examination, EEG and infectious or autoimmune serologies, should be guided by the clinical picture as well as by the initial evaluation and laboratory work-up. Partial complex status must be ruled out with EEG in every patient with delirium without a clear etiology.

There are no clear data as to the yield of brain imaging in delirious patients. Most clinicians will proceed to imaging quickly if the initial laboratory work-up is unrevealing. A non-contrast head CT can exclude intracerebral hemorrhage and many large space-occupying lesions. Magnetic resonance imaging (MRI) of the brain with gadolinium can definitively exclude most cases of acute stroke and allow for assessment of structural changes consistent with neurodegenerative disease, toxic exposures and encephalitis. Therefore, MRI is likely the test of choice if brain imaging is to be performed on patients with delirium, but this technique may be limited by the patient's inability to remain still for long periods of time as well as cost.

Management of delirium

Management of the patient with delirium involves both addressing symptoms of the disorder and identifying

Table 24.1. Initial evaluation of a patient with delirium

	Components
Initial evaluation	History with special attention to all medications (including over-the-counter items)
	Physical examination
	Complete blood count
	Electrolyte panel including calcium, magnesium, phosphorus
	Liver function tests including albumin, urine analysis and culture
	Chest radiograph
	Electrocardiogram
Further evaluation guided by initial evaluation	Brain imaging with magnetic resonance with diffusion and gadolinium (preferred) or computed tomography
	Serum ammonia
	Erythrocyte sedimentation rate
	Blood cultures
	Lumbar puncture (if suspicion of meningitis, should be performed initially)
	Electroencephalograph (if high suspicion of status epilepticus, should be performed initially)
	Autoimmune and infectious serologies

and treating the underlying etiology. Tapering or discontinuing likely offending medications is the first step in management of a delirious patient, given the high incidence of medication-induced or medication-exacerbated delirium.

Environmental and structural interventions can be extremely effective in managing the delirious patient, especially in those who develop delirium after admission to the hospital or ICU. Inouye and colleagues[40] published a study of a multicomponent intervention designed to reduce and treat delirium in over 850 patients 70 years and older admitted to a general medical ward. These patients were matched (not randomized) to either an intervention unit or a standard care unit in the hospital. A variety of nursing methods were used to assess and treat various factors that may contribute to delirium, including cognitive impairment (through increasing orientation reminders and cognitive stimulation), sleep deprivation (by instituting unit-wide noise reduction and environmental improvement at night), immobility (through early and frequent mobilization), visual impairment (by making available

visual aids and adaptive equipment), hearing impairment (through providing amplifying devices and communication techniques) and dehydration (by instituting aggressive volume repletion). The study demonstrated good adherence to this regimen in the intervention group. The patients in the intervention group demonstrated a decreased incidence of delirium as well as a decreased number of days with delirium. Elements of this protocol are inexpensive and quite easy to employ in most hospital or nursing home settings.

Other studies have shown a decreased incidence of delirium with staff education programs or through early involvement of geriatrics or psychiatry consultations.[6,43,44] None of these intervention studies has demonstrated a drastic decrease in delirium rates in the hospital, suggesting that while these measures may be effective in preventing some cases of delirium, primary prevention is likely the key to this illness.[42]

Medications are often administered to treat agitation in patients with a hyperactive delirium. This strategy seems to be superior to physical restraints for delirious patients as the latter tends to increase confusion and agitation in these already impaired patients. Both benzodiazepines and antipsychotic drugs have been used for this purpose, and little evidence exists to guide the choice of one over the other. Benzodiazepines are clearly the proper choice of these two classes of agent in cases of alcohol or sedative withdrawal. Antipsychotic choice has been guided by small studies that have examined the use of typical versus atypical antipsychotic agents, with mixed results.[45–47] This last issue has become more complicated with recent US Food and Drug Administration (FDA) warnings regarding apparent increased mortality in elderly individuals exposed to atypical antipsychotic drugs.[48]

Other medications that may prove to be effective in the future in treatment of delirium include drugs targeting an acetylcholine deficit, such as cholinesterase inhibitors, as well as stimulant medications for those with a more hypoactive delirium.[34,49,50]

Future directions

The field of delirium remains, some 2500 years after its initial description, largely understudied compared with diseases with much lower prevalence. The opportunities for future research in this area are enormous and have been mentioned throughout the course of this chapter.

Detailed clinical descriptions of delirium using careful modern cognitive techniques and neuropsychological testing are needed in order to fully define the spectrum of this disease and distinguish it from other cognitive disorders, including the neurodegenerative diseases. Large population-based studies are needed to ascertain the prevalence of this disorder and determine risk factors for delirium. Eventually, patients preparing for elective hospitalization or surgery may be able to be stratified for risk of development of delirium, and high-risk patients could be counseled as to this risk and perhaps given specialized intraoperative or in-hospital care to detect and treat this disorder. This type of primary prevention program is likely the key to significantly reducing the incidence of this disease.

Imaging data including MRI as well as functional and perfusion studies are sorely lacking in patients with a history of delirium or in those who are actively delirious. These imaging data may provide important information towards elucidating the pathophysiology of delirium. Genetic data involving patients with delirium are also lacking; many of the differential responses to medication that can cause a delirium may be a result of polymorphisms in the P450 system or other drug metabolism pathways.

Finally, the field of delirium remains desperately in need of novel therapeutic approaches, which must be tested in double-blind random-controlled trials. It is only through these types of research approach that this very common and costly medical problem can eventually be adequately addressed.

References

1. Lipowski JL. *Delirum: Acute Confusional States.* New York: Oxford University Press, 1990.

2. Meagher DJ. Delirium: optimising management. *BMJ* 2001;**322**(7279):144–149.

3. American Psychiatric Association. *Diagnostic and Statistical Manual of Mental Disorders.* 4th edn, text revision. Washington DC: American Psychiatric Press, 2000.

4. Inouye SK, Leo-Summers L, Zhang Y *et al.* A chart-based method for identification of delirium: validation compared with interviewer ratings using the confusion assessment method. *J Am Geriatr Soc* 2005;**53**(2):312–318.

5. Britton A, Russell R. Multidisciplinary team interventions for delirium in patients with chronic cognitive impairment. *Cochrane Database Syst Rev* 2004;(2):CD000395.

6. Marcantonio ER, Flacker JM, Wright RJ, Resnick NM. Reducing delirium after hip fracture: a randomized trial. *J Am Geriatr Soc* 2001;**49**(5):516–522.

7. Rizzo JA, Bogardus ST, Jr Leo-Summers L *et al.* Multicomponent targeted intervention to prevent delirium in hospitalized older patients: what is the economic value? *Med Care* 2001;**39**(7):740–752.

8. McNicoll L, Pisani MA, Zhang Y *et al.* Delirium in the intensive care unit: occurrence and clinical course in older patients. *J Am Geriatr Soc* 2003;**51**(5):591–598.

9. Ely EW, Shintani A, Truman B *et al.* Delirium as a predictor of mortality in mechanically ventilated patients in the intensive care unit. *JAMA* 2004; **291**(14):1753–1762.

10. Fick DM, Agostini JV, Inouye SK. Delirium superimposed on dementia: a systematic review. *J Am Geriatr Soc* 2002;**50**(10):1723–1732.

11. World Health Organization. *International Classification of Disease (ICD-10): Classification of Mental and Behavioral Disorders. Diagnostic Criteria for Research.* Geneva: World Health Organization, 1993.

12. Fick DM, Kolanowski AM, Waller JL, Inouye SK. Delirium superimposed on dementia in a community-dwelling managed care population: a 3-year retrospective study of occurrence, costs, and utilization. *J Gerontol A Biol Sci Med Sci* 2005;**60**(6):748–753.

13. Jackson JC, Gordon SM, Hart RP, Hopkins RO, Ely EW. The association between delirium and cognitive decline: a review of the empirical literature. *Neuropsychol Rev* 2004;**14**(2):87–98.

14. Inouye SK, Rushing JT, Foreman MD, Palmer RM, Pompei P. Does delirium contribute to poor hospital outcomes? A three-site epidemiologic study. *J Gen Intern Med* 1998;**13**(4):234–242.

15. Ely EW, Gautam S, Margolin R *et al.* The impact of delirium in the intensive care unit on hospital length of stay. *Intensive Care Med* 2001;**27**(12):1892–1900.

16. Jacobson SA. Delirium in the elderly. *Psychiatr Clin North Am* 1997;**20**(1):91–110.

17. Alagiakrishnan K, Wiens CA. An approach to drug induced delirium in the elderly. *Postgrad Med J* 2004; **80**(945):388–393.

18. Ely EW, Inouye SK, Bernard GR *et al.* Delirium in mechanically ventilated patients: validity and reliability of the confusion assessment method for the intensive care unit (CAM-ICU). *JAMA* 2001;**286**(21):2703–2710.

19. Inouye SK. Predisposing and precipitating factors for delirium in hospitalized older patients. *Dement Geriatr Cogn Disord* 1999;**10**(5):393–400.

20. Amador LF, Goodwin JS. Postoperative delirium in the older patient. *J Am Coll Surg* 2005;**200**(5):767–773.

21. Inouye SK, Viscoli CM, Horwitz RI, Hurst LD, Tinetti ME. A predictive model for delirium in hospitalized elderly medical patients based on admission characteristics. *Ann Intern Med* 1993; **119**(6):474–481.

22. Francis J, Martin D, Kapoor WN. A prospective study of delirium in hospitalized elderly. *JAMA* 1990; **263**(8):1097–1101.

23. Rolfson DB, McElhaney JE, Rockwood K et al. Incidence and risk factors for delirium and other adverse outcomes in older adults after coronary artery bypass graft surgery. *Can J Cardiol* 1999;**15**(7):771–776.

24. Williams-Russo P, Sharrock NE, Mattis S, Szatrowski TP, Charlson ME. Cognitive effects after epidural vs general anesthesia in older adults. A randomized trial. *JAMA* 1995;**274**(1):44–50.

25. Inouye SK, Charpentier PA. Precipitating factors for delirium in hospitalized elderly persons. Predictive model and interrelationship with baseline vulnerability. *JAMA* 1996;**275**(11):852–857.

26. Smith KM, Larive LL, Romanelli F. Club drugs: methylenedioxymethamphetamine, flunitrazepam, ketamine hydrochloride, and gamma-hydroxybutyrate. *Am J Health Syst Pharm* 2002;**59**(11):1067–1076.

27. Manepalli J, Grossberg GT, Mueller C. Prevalence of delirium and urinary tract infection in a psychogeriatric unit. *J Geriatr Psychiatry Neurol* 1990;**3**(4):198–202.

28. Caeiro L, Ferro JM, Claro MI et al. Delirium in acute stroke: a preliminary study of the role of anticholinergic medications. *Eur J Neurol* 2004;**11**(10):699–704.

29. Mori E, Yamadori A. Acute confusional state and acute agitated delirium. Occurrence after infarction in the right middle cerebral artery territory. *Arch Neurol* 1987;**44**(11):1139–1143.

30. Jackson KC, Lipman AG. Drug therapy for delirium in terminally ill patients. *Cochrane Database Syst Rev* 2004(2):CD004770.

31. Filley CM. The neuroanatomy of attention. *Semin Speech Lang* 2002;**23**(2):89–98.

32. Trzepacz PT. Update on the neuropathogenesis of delirium. *Dement Geriatr Cogn Disord* 1999;**10**(5):330–334.

33. Trzepacz PT. Is there a final common neural pathway in delirium? Focus on acetylcholine and dopamine. *Semin Clin Neuropsychiatry* 2000;**5**(2):132–148.

34. Wengel SP, Roccaforte WH, Burke WJ. Donepezil improves symptoms of delirium in dementia: implications for future research. *J Geriatr Psychiatry Neurol* 1998;**11**(3):159–161.

35. Duda JE. Pathology and neurotransmitter abnormalities of dementia with Lewy bodies. *Dement Geriatr Cogn Disord* 2004;**17**(Suppl 1):3–14.

36. Yokota H, Ogawa S, Kurokawa A, Yamamoto Y. Regional cerebral blood flow in delirium patients. *Psychiatry Clin Neurosci* 2003;**57**(3):337–339.

37. Blessed G, Tomlinson BE, Roth M. The association between quantitative measures of dementia and of senile change in the cerebral grey matter of elderly subjects. *Br J Psychiatry* 1968;**114**(512):797–811.

38. Uhlmann RF, Larson EB, Buchner DM. Correlations of Mini-Mental State and modified Dementia Rating Scale to measures of transitional health status in dementia. *J Gerontol* 1987;**42**(1):33–36.

39. Gaudreau JD, Gagnon P, Harel F, Tremblay A, Roy MA. Fast, systematic, and continuous delirium assessment in hospitalized patients: the nursing delirium screening scale. *J Pain Symptom Manage* 2005;**29**(4):368–375.

40. Inouye SK, van Dyck CH, Alessi CA et al. Clarifying confusion: the confusion assessment method. A new method for detection of delirium. *Ann Intern Med* 1990;**113**(12):941–948.

41. Bergeron N, Dubois MJ, Dumont M, Dial S, Skrobik Y. Intensive Care Delirium Screening Checklist: evaluation of a new screening tool. *Intensive Care Med* 2001;**27**(5):859–864.

42. Inouye SK, Bogardus ST, Jr., Charpentier PA et al. A multicomponent intervention to prevent delirium in hospitalized older patients. *N Engl J Med* 1999;**340**(9):669–676.

43. Lundstrom M, Edlund A, Karlsson S et al. A multifactorial intervention program reduces the duration of delirium, length of hospitalization, and mortality in delirious patients. *J Am Geriatr Soc* 2005;**53**(4):622–628.

44. Cole MG, Primeau FJ, Bailey RF et al. Systematic intervention for elderly inpatients with delirium: a randomized trial. *Cmaj* 1994;**151**(7):965–970.

45. Han CS, Kim YK. A double-blind trial of risperidone and haloperidol for the treatment of delirium. *Psychosomatics* 2004;**45**(4):297–301.

46. Kim KY, Bader GM, Kotlyar V, Gropper D. Treatment of delirium in older adults with quetiapine. *J Geriatr Psychiatry Neurol* 2003;**16**(1):29–31.

47. Skrobik YK, Bergeron N, Dumont M, Gottfried SB. Olanzapine vs haloperidol: treating delirium in a critical care setting. *Intensive Care Med* 2004;**30**(3):444–449.

48. Kuehn BM. FDA warns antipsychotic drugs may be risky for elderly. *JAMA* 2005;**293**(20):2462.

49. Gagnon B, Low G, Schreier G. Methylphenidate hydrochloride improves cognitive function in patients with advanced cancer and hypoactive delirium: a prospective clinical study. *J Psychiatry Neurosci* 2005;**30**(2):100–107.

50. Moretti R, Torre P, Antonello RM, Cattaruzza T, Cazzato G. Cholinesterase inhibition as a possible therapy for delirium in vascular dementia: a controlled, open 24-month study of 246 patients. *Am J Alzheimers Dis Other Demen* 2004;**19**(6):333–339.

Chapter 25

Paraneoplastic disorders of the memory and cognition

Luis Bataller and Josep Dalmau

Introduction

Once considered rare, paraneoplastic disorders (PND) of the brain are becoming increasingly recognized as a cause of higher cortical dysfunction (cognition, memory, attention, affection and behavior) and disruption of sleep and level of consciousness (Gultekin *et al.*, 2000; Ances *et al.*, 2005). Symptoms may be limited to these cortical functions or develop in association with syndromes of the brainstem, cerebellum, dorsal root ganglia and peripheral nerves. Although the term PND can be applied to a number of non-metastatic neurologic complications of cancer, most PND are immune mediated and this chapter will focus on these disorders.

It has been suggested that approximately 1:10 000 cancer patients develop PND, although there are no data supporting such a low incidence (Darnell and Posner 2003). Our experience in a single institution suggests a higher frequency: closer to 1:500–1:1000 with an even higher incidence reported for particular cancer populations such as small cell lung cancer (SCLC, ∼5%) and thymoma (∼30%) (Elrington *et al.*, 1991; Muller-Hermelink and Marx 2000). For PND affecting memory and cognition, the incidence can only be estimated for patients with paraneoplastic limbic encephalitis (PLE), at approximately 1:2000–1:3000.

Cancer-related dementia

The occurrence of dementia in patients with cancer and inflammatory infiltrates of the brain was initially reported by Brierley and colleagues in 1960. They described three patients with progressive dementia and "subacute encephalitis of later adult life, mainly affecting the limbic areas"; two of the patients had evidence of cancer (one confirmed at autopsy) but the authors considered "most unlikely that this finding

was in any way related to the encephalitis although its occurrence should be noted." In 1968, Corsellis and colleagues coined the term "limbic encephalitis" to describe one patient with severe short-term memory loss and two patients with memory loss and dementia in association with bronchial carcinoma; in all three patients the neuropathological findings consisted of both inflammatory and degenerative changes concentrated in the temporal parts of the limbic gray matter. The same authors reviewed the extant literature, identifying eight other cases with dominant clinical and pathological involvement of the limbic system, and established for the first time a relationship between systemic cancer and dementia or memory deficits.

Once the relationship between cancer and memory or cognitive dysfunction was established, three pathogenic hypotheses were advanced: (1) a degeneration (not further defined) of the nervous system in which inflammatory infiltrates were a secondary "reaction to the tissue breakdown", (2) a viral infection, and (3) an immune-mediated response against the nervous system, which is the currently accepted hypothesis.

Immune-mediated mechanisms

There are several immunological and pathological findings that support an immune-mediated pathogenesis for most PND of memory and cognition. They include (1) detection of antibodies in serum or cerebrospinal fluid (CSF) to specific neuronal proteins usually expressed by the underlying tumor (onconeuronal antigens) (Table 25.1); (2) absence of these antibodies in similar disorders without a cancer association; (3) presence of inflammatory abnormalities in the CSF, including lymphocytic pleocytosis, increased protein concentration, oligoclonal bands and intrathecal synthesis of IgG or specific onconeuronal antibodies; and (4) presence of infiltrates of B cells and predominantly T cells in the involved areas of the central nervous system (CNS), where the T cells are usually composed of CD4 and CD8 cells and

Table 25.1. Immunological associations in paraneoplastic disorders of the memory and cognition

Antibodies	Tumor	Associated syndromes
Antibodies to intracellular neuronal antigens		
Hu	SCLC	Encephalomyelitis, sensory neuronopathy
CV2/CRMP5	SCLC, thymoma	Encephalomyelitis, chorea, uveitis, sensorimotor neuropathy
Ma2	Testis, non-SCLC, other	Limbic, hypothalamic and upper brainstem encephalitis
Amphiphysin	SCLC, breast	Stiff-person syndrome
Ri	Breast, gynecological, SCLC	Opsoclonus–myoclonus–ataxia of the adult, brainstem encephalitis, cerebellar degeneration
Antibodies to neuronal cell membrane antigens		
VGKC	Thymoma, SCLC, non-SCLC	Hyponatremia, peripheral nerve hyperexcitability, Morvan's syndrome; mild or absent CSF abnormalities
Novel neuropil antibodies (to NMDA, AMPA receptors)	Teratoma, thymoma	Severe psychiatric symptoms, central hypoventilation

Notes:
SCLC, small cell lung cancer; CSF, cerebrospinal fluid; VGKC, voltage-gated potassium channel; CRMP, collapsin response-mediator protein; NMDA, *N*-methyl-D-aspartate; AMPA, alpha-amino-3-hydroxy-5-methyl-4-isoxazolepropionic acid.

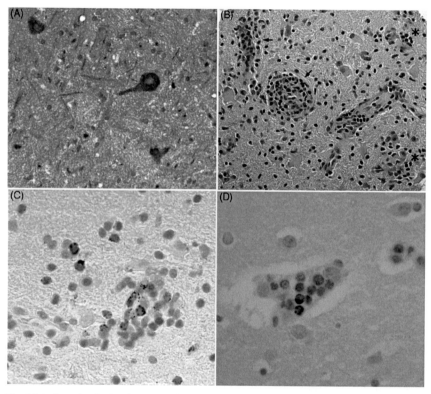

Fig. 25.1. Deposits of IgG and presence of cytotoxic T cells in the biopsy of brain of a patient with paraneoplastic limbic encephalitis. (A) Deposits of IgG in neurons (brown staining). (B) Perivascular (arrows) and interstitial (asterisks) infiltrates of mononuclear cells; most of the cells in the perivascular space were B cells, and most of the cells in the interstitial space were T cells (not shown). (C) Interstitial T cells expressing T cell intracellular antigen 1 (TIA-1; a marker of activated cytotoxic T cells). (D) A small neuronophagic group of T cells expressing granzyme B.

cluster around neurons undergoing degeneration (neuronophagic nodules) (Jean *et al.*, 1994).

These CNS-infiltrating T cells often express cytotoxic proteolytic enzymes (T cell intracellular antigen [TIA]-positive cells) and may be accompanied by deposits of paraneoplastic antibodies predominantly in the areas more heavily infiltrated by T cells (Fig. 25.1) (Bernal *et al.*, 2002). The specificity of the

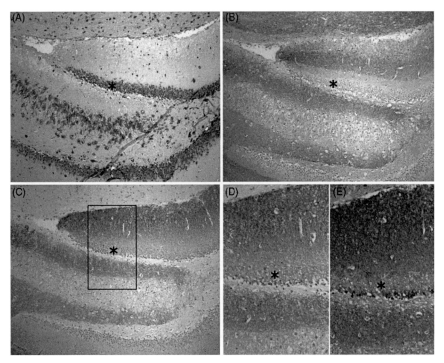

Fig. 25.2. Antibodies to intracellular and cell-membrane antigens in patients with limbic encephalitis. (A) Sagittal section of rat hippocampus immunolabeled with anti-Hu antibodies. (B,C) Consecutive sections of hippocampus immunolabeled with Kv 1.2 antibodies to voltage-gated potassium channels (B) and a novel neuropil antibody (C). (D) The area in the rectangle in (C) at higher magnification. (E) Reactivity of another neuropil antibody in a consecutive section of the same region. Note the difference between (A) and (B–E); the anti-Hu antibody (A) reacts with intracellular antigens (Hu) while the other antibodies react with areas of the neuropil that are rich in dendrites and synapses but spare the neuronal cell bodies. In all panels, the asterisks are placed in the same region (neurons of the dentate gyrus) to allow comparison between reactivities. Sections counterstained with hematoxylin.

T cells for onconeuronal antigens has been demonstrated using peripheral blood and tumor cells lines or fibroblasts engineered to express the onconeuronal antigens (Albert *et al.*, 1998; Tanaka *et al.*, 1999). Although it is clear that the CNS-infiltrating T cells contribute to the neuronal degeneration and to the neurologic disease, an anti-tumor effect is less evident. The fact that many patients with PND have a detectable tumor or eventually have tumor progression suggests that the paraneoplastic anti-tumor response is not sustained enough to destroy the tumor efficiently or control its growth (Bataller and Dalmau 2004). Overall, considering all patients with paraneoplastic antibodies to intracellular antigens (i.e. Hu, CV2/CRMP5 [collapsin response-mediator protein 5], amphiphysin), which are the ones associated with cytotoxic T cell immunity, approximately 10% of patients survive their tumor and neurologic deficits, 50% die as a result of the neurologic disease, and 40% die as a result of tumor progression (Rojas *et al.*, 2000; Graus *et al.*, 2001; Sillevis *et al.*, 2002; Dalmau *et al.*, 2004).

In contrast to the PND associated with immunity against intracellular antigens, recent studies have described several disorders associated with antibodies reacting with neuronal cell membrane antigens predominantly expressed in the neuropil of hippocampus and, sometimes, cerebellum (Fig. 25.2). These disorders usually involve the limbic system and may occur as paraneoplastic or non-paraneoplastic syndromes. The best characterized antibodies of this group are those to *N*-methyl-D-aspartate (NMDA) receptor (Dalmau *et al.*, 2008) and the voltage-gated potassium channels (VGKC; Kv1.1, Kv1.2 and Kv1.6) (Vincent *et al.*, 2004). Other novel neuropil antibodies to diverse cell membrane antigens different from VGKC have been isolated (Ances *et al.*, 2005). Because these antibodies have only recently been reported and because the clinical outcome of these patients is better than those associated with antibodies to intracellular antigens, there are no pathological studies to confirm the presence of inflammatory infiltrates, or the presence of cytotoxic T cells in the brain of these patients.

379

Table 25.2. Causes of delirium and cognitive dysfunction in cancer patients

	Causes
Direct involvement of the CNS by tumor[a]	Primary brain tumor, brain metastasis, neoplastic meningitis
Cerebrovascular disease[a]	Disseminated intravascular coagulation, non-bacterial thrombotic endocarditis, arteritis, venous occlusion, tumor hemorrhage
Infections	Bacterial, viral, fungal, parasitic infections
Metabolic and endocrine disorders	Organ failure (liver, kidney, lung), hypovolemic shock, electrolyte imbalance, endocrine dysfunction (adrenal, thyroid)
Nutritional deficiencies	Thiamine, cobalamin, niacin
Chemotherapy	Many chemotherapies can cause delirium: ifosfamide, methotrexate, 5-fluoruracil, asparaginase, cis-platinum, vincristine, procarbazine, among others
Radiation therapy	Acute or early-delayed neurotoxicity (headache, confusion, decrease of attention, hypersomnia), late-delayed neurotoxicity[b] (dementia)
Surgery	Transient postoperative delirium
Drugs	Corticosteroids, opioids, sedatives

Notes:
[a]These disorders frequently result in persistent cognitive deficits.
[b]Includes radiation necrosis, progressive cerebral atrophy and hydrocephalus, which frequently evolve to dementia.

There are no animal models for any PND of memory and cognition associated with antibodies to either intracellular antigens or cell membrane antigens.

Symptom presentation and diagnosis

Cancer patients often develop confusion, delirium and cognitive dysfunction. In a cancer hospital, these symptoms and decline of level of consciousness were the second most common reason for neurologic consultation after pain (Posner 1995). Table 25.2 shows the mechanisms more frequently involved, including direct invasion of the nervous system by the tumor or metastasis, and an extensive list of non-metastatic complications. However, PND is rarely diagnosed in this setting because these disorders usually present before the presence of a cancer is known. Therefore, rather than oncologists or neuro-oncologists, the physicians that more frequently first encounter these patients are primary care physicians or neurologists.

The symptom presentation of PND is usually subacute and the disorder rapidly evolves in weeks or a few months to cause severe deficits that are often irreversible. An important concern for the physician is early recognition of the disorder, because prompt treatment of the tumor and immunosuppression may favorably affect the neurologic outcome (Keime-Guibert et al., 1999; Dalmau et al., 2004), particularly when the limbic system is involved and the immune response associates with neuropil antibodies (Gultekin et al., 2000; Ances et al., 2005). Overall, the diagnosis of PND is usually based on the recognition of the neurologic syndrome, the demonstration of the associated cancer and the identification of paraneoplastic antibodies (Graus et al., 2004).

Recognition of the neurologic syndrome

Limbic encephalitis in adults and opsoclonus–myoclonus in children are the two main PND that affect memory and cognition, and each has characteristic clinical features that allow their prompt recognition. Another PND that may cause depression of level of consciousness, seizures, memory deficits or dementia is paraneoplastic encephalomyelitis (Dalmau et al., 1992). In this disorder, the multifocal or diffuse inflammatory abnormalities result in diverse syndromes that are also frequent in patients without cancer and, therefore, requires a more extensive differential diagnosis (Graus et al., 2004).

Clinical and laboratory tests that support a paraneoplastic cause of a disorder of memory or cognition include (1) the subacute development of symptoms, (2) the presence of associated symptoms or syndromes that are frequently paraneoplastic (i.e. dorsal root ganglionopathy, opsoclonus, subacute ataxia), (3) the concomitant occurrence of systemic paraneoplastic features (i.e. unintentional loss of weight, hypertrophic osteoarthropathy or clubbing, inappropriate secretion of antidiuretic hormone [SIADH]), (4) the presence of CSF inflammatory abnormalities, (4) the detection

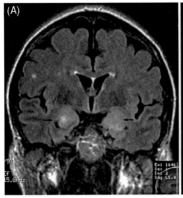 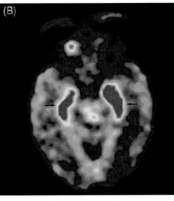

Fig. 25.3. Paraneoplastic limbic encephalitis. (A) Fluid-attenuated inversion recovery (FLAIR) magnetic resonance in coronal section, showing bilateral hyperintense signal abnormalities (arrows) in the medial region of the temporal lobes. (B) Fluorodeoxyglucose (FDG) positron emission tomography of the same patient showing an axial section at the level of the hippocampi; note the intense FDG hyperactivity indicated with the arrows.

of T_2-weighted or fluid-attenuated inversion recovery (FLAIR) magnetic resonance imaging (MRI) abnormalities selectively involving the hippocampi, and (5) the demonstration of $[^{18}F]$-fluorodeoxyglucose (FDG) positron emission tomography (PET) hyperactivity selectively involving the medial aspect of the temporal lobes in the absence of epileptic activity (Fig. 25.3) (Ances *et al.*, 2005; Kassubek *et al.*, 2001).

Associated cancer

Because PND usually develop at early stages of cancer, the tumor (or its recurrence) may be difficult to demonstrate. In most instances, the tumor is revealed by computed tomography (CT) of the chest, abdomen and pelvis. Whole-body FDG-PET is very useful in demonstrating occult primary tumors or small metastatic lesions, which may be more accessible for biopsy than the primary neoplasm (Linke *et al.*, 2004; Younes-Mhenni *et al.*, 2004). Despite the high sensitivity of FDG-PET in demonstrating PND-associated tumors, there are instances where the tumor escapes detection by all tests, including PET (Dalmau *et al.*, 1999). In addition, FDG-PET may lead to false-positive results. The interpretation of FDG-PET findings is facilitated when the type of neurologic syndrome and associated antibodies are considered; for example, detection of FDG-PET hyperactivity in the colon of a young man with anti-Ma2-associated limbic encephalitis likely represents a false-positive finding or an unrelated neoplasm (the usual neoplasm being in the testis in 90% of patients) (Voltz *et al.*, 1999).

In addition to radiologic or metabolic imaging, serum cancer markers such as carcinoembryonic antigen, Ca-125, CA-15.3, or prostate-specific antigen (PSA) are helpful. If no tumor is detected, close oncologic surveillance should be undertaken in patients

with a typical PND (i.e. limbic encephalitis) with or without paraneoplastic antibodies, and in patients with any neurologic disorder associated with paraneoplastic antibodies. A common practice is cancer screening every 6 months for at least 5 years; in 90% of patients, the tumor is demonstrated within the first year of PND symptom presentation (Graus *et al.*, 2004; Younes-Mhenni *et al.*, 2004). Patients whose cancer is in remission and who develop PND should be examined for tumor recurrence.

Paraneoplastic antibodies

The term "paraneoplastic antibodies" is applied to antibodies that serve as markers of the paraneoplastic origin of a neurological syndrome. Several concepts are important when testing for paraneoplastic antibodies. First, antibodies are present in approximately 60% of patients with PND of the CNS; therefore, the absence of antibodies does not rule out that a syndrome could be paraneoplastic (Alamowitch *et al.*, 1997). Second, paraneoplastic antibodies may be identified (usually at low titer) in the serum of a variable proportion of patients with cancer but without PND (i.e. anti-Hu and anti-CV2/CRMP5 in 20% and 10% of patients with SCLC, respectively) (Graus *et al.*, 1997; Bataller *et al.*, 2004). Third, detection of intrathecal synthesis of antibodies is a strong indicator that the associated neurological syndrome is paraneoplastic.

Based on the location of the antigen, the antibodies associated with PND of memory and cognition can be largely grouped in two categories: antibodies to intraneuronal antigens and antibodies to cell membrane antigens, the latter including antibodies to VGKC and "novel neuropil antibodies" such as the NMDA receptor and the alpha-amino-3-hydroxy-5-methyl-4-isoxazolepropionic acid (AMPA) receptor, among others (Ances *et al.*, 2005; Dalmau *et al.*, 2008; Lai *et al.*, 2008). This classification

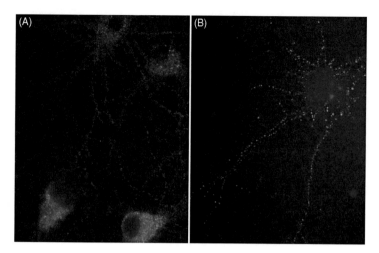

Fig. 25.4. Immunolabeling of cell membrane and processes of cultured hippocampal neurons. (A) Immunolabeling of cultured neurons with Kv1.2 antibodies (green) to voltage-gated potassium channels and immunolabeling produced by serum of a patient with paraneoplastic limbic encephalitis associated with carcinoma of the thymus and a novel neuropil antibody (antigen unknown; red). (B) Immunolabeling of a neuron with antibodies from a patient with ovarian teratoma and multifocal encephalitis (green); the autoantigen is EFA6A, a protein that interacts on the cell surface with members of the "two-pore potassium channel" family.

has implications for treatment and prognosis (as discussed below).

Antibodies to intraneuronal antigens

Antibodies to intraneuronal antigens that are relevant for syndromes of memory and cognition include those for Hu, Ma2, CV2/CRMP5 and amphiphysin. These four antigens and the corresponding antibodies have been well characterized by different laboratories and reported in large series of patients with PND. Detection of any of these antibodies strongly supports the diagnosis of PND even if no tumor is found at initial evaluation (Graus *et al.*, 2004). Some antibodies are more syndrome specific than others; for example anti-Ma2 antibodies almost always associate with limbic or upper brainstem dysfunction (Dalmau *et al.*, 2004), while anti-Hu or anti-CV2/CRMP5 antibodies associate with a much wider spectrum of symptoms (Graus *et al.*, 2001; Yu *et al.*, 2001).

Antibodies to cell membrane antigens

Antibodies to cell membrane antigens, include VGKC and novel neuropil antibodies. Antibodies to VGKC immunohistochemically react with the neuropil of hippocampus and cerebellum (Vincent *et al.*, 2004). In clinical practice, these antibodies are detected by radioimmunoassay and are usually associated with non-PLE, neuromyotonia and a syndrome that combines peripheral nerve hyperexcitability, autonomic and sleep disorders and cognitive dysfunction (Morvan's syndrome). However, VGKC antibodies have also been identified in patients with PLE; therefore, detection of these antibodies does not exclude the need to search for a tumor. The tumors more frequently involved are thymoma and, rarely, lung cancer (Liguori *et al.*, 2001; Pozo-Rosich *et al.*, 2003).

In addition to VGKC antibodies, there is a large and heterogeneous group of antibodies directed against cell membrane antigens that are enriched in the neuronal processes of the hippocampus and cerebellum (Fig. 25.4) (Ances *et al.*, 2005). These antibodies, including those to the NMDA and AMPA receptors and others not characterized, are difficult to detect with conventional immunohistochemical or immunoblot techniques and are usually demonstrated with modified immunohistochemical techniques. As experience of these is limited, it is unclear whether similar antibodies may occur in patients with non-paraneoplastic limbic encephalitis. The identity of most antigens is unknown, but the patterns of antibody reactivity with the hippocampus is so characteristic (Fig. 25.2) that their detection should prompt the search for tumors of the thymus or ovarian teratoma, and they predict neurologic response to treatment of the tumor and IgG-depleting strategies (Ances *et al.*, 2005; Vitaliani *et al.*, 2005).

Diagnostic criteria for paraneoplastic disorders

The three sources of information discussed above (type of neurologic syndrome, detection of cancer and presence or absence of paraneoplastic antibodies) have been used to define general guidelines for the diagnosis of PND (Table 25.3) (Graus *et al.*, 2004). These criteria are also applicable to PND of the memory and cognition taking in consideration that

Table 25.3. Diagnostic criteria for paraneoplastic neurological syndromes

Criteria	
Definite	1. A classical syndrome[a] and cancer
	2. A non-classical syndrome that resolves or significantly improves after cancer treatment
	3. A non-classical syndrome with paraneoplastic antibodies (well characterized or not)[b] and cancer
	4. A neurologic syndrome (classical or not) with well-characterized antibodies, and no detected cancer
Possible	1. A classical syndrome, no paraneoplastic antibodies and no cancer, but at high risk to have an underlying tumor
	2. A neurologic syndrome (classical or not) with partially characterized paraneoplastic antibodies and no detected cancer
	3. A non-classical syndrome with cancer, but without paraneoplastic antibodies

Notes:
PND, paraneoplastic disorder.
[a]The two classical PND syndromes of memory and cognition are limbic encephalitis in adults and opsoclonus–myoclonus in children.
[b]Well-characterized PND antibodies include those to the antigens Hu, CV2/CRMP5, amphiphysin and Ma2. Other well-characterized PND antibodies (anti-Yo, anti-Ri) infrequently associate with PND with dominant memory and cognitive dysfunction (Yo), or are extremely infrequent (Ri).
Source: Reproduced from Graus *et al.* (2004) with permission of the BMJ Publishing Group.

the antibodies to the neuropil and cell membrane antigens, although pathogenically interesting, need further validation to be considered as well-characterized paraneoplastic antibodies. Disorders associated with these antibodies, as occur with anti-VGKC antibodies, should be considered as "possible PND" and be carefully evaluated for alternative non-cancer, related, immune-mediated disorders.

Paraneoplastic limbic encephalitis

Paraneoplastic limbic encephalitis is characterized by the rapid development of short-term memory deficits, irritability, depression, sleep dysfunction, confusion, seizures or hallucinations (Bakheit *et al.*, 1990; Gultekin *et al.*, 2000). In general, the short-term memory deficits are striking and dominate the clinical picture, but they can be obscured by seizures or prominent psychiatric symptoms, resulting in diagnostic delays. One study of 50 patients found that 46% had an acute confusional state, 14% cognitive decline and 42% psychiatric symptoms (Gultekin *et al.*, 2000). Another study of 24 patients found that 92% had cognitive dysfunction and 50% psychiatric symptoms (Lawn *et al.*, 2003). Although rigorous neuropsychological evaluations were not provided in any of these studies, there have been frequent case reports of patients with severe cognitive decline and dementia (Corsellis *et al.*, 1968; Fujii *et al.*, 2001). This is not surprising considering that PLE can be the presentation of a multifocal encephalitis that may involve cerebral cortex and basal ganglia among other areas of the neuraxis (encephalomyelitis) (Dalmau *et al.*, 1992; Graus *et al.*, 2001).

Seizures occur in approximately 60% of patients with PLE. Temporal lobe or psychomotor seizures (40%), generalized seizures (24%) or a combination of seizure types (36%) were identified in a study of 50 patients (Gultekin *et al.*, 2000). One of our patients had orgasmic epilepsy as the presentation of PLE (Fadul *et al.*, 2005). Epilepsia partialis continua can be the presentation of paraneoplastic multifocal cortical encephalitis, which in some patients also involves the medial temporal lobes, causing limbic dysfunction (Shavit *et al.*, 1999; Mut *et al.*, 2005).

Although electroencephalography (EEG) has limited specificity for PLE, it is useful in assessing whether the changes in the level of consciousness or behavior are related to temporal lobe seizures or non-convulsive status epilepticus. In the study of Gultekin *et al.* (2000), 45% of the patients had epileptic activity; a more recent study by Lawn *et al.* (2003) demonstrated focal or generalized slowing with or without epileptic activity, maximal in the temporal lobes, in all patients studied.

Brain MRI usually shows uni- or bilateral FLAIR and T_2-weighted medial temporal lobe hyperintensities that infrequently enhance with contrast. As the disorder evolves, repeat MRI studies usually show progressive loss of volume of the hippocampal gyri, with persistence of T_2-weighted and FLAIR abnormalities, and decreased enhancement (Fig. 25.5) (Dirr *et al.*, 1990; Lawn *et al.*, 2003). In patients without seizures and a normal MRI, the FDG-PET may help to demonstrate temporal lobe hyperactivity, likely caused by focal inflammatory infiltrates (Fig. 25.3) (Scheid *et al.*, 2004). A recent study showed that brain MRI and FDG-PET complemented each other in

(A)

Paraneoplastic limbic encephalitis

(B)

Non-paraneoplastic limbic encephalitis

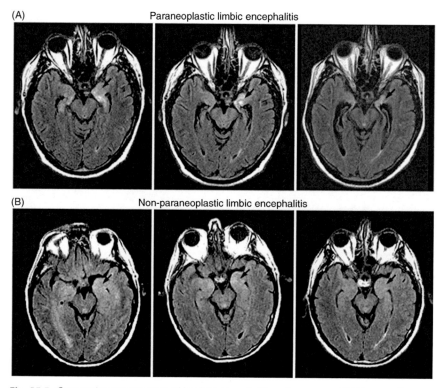

Fig. 25.5. Comparative outcome assessed by Fluid-attenuated inversion recovery (FLAIR) magnetic resonance imaging in a patient with paraneoplastic limbic encephalitis (PLE) and a patient with non-paraneoplastic limbic encephalitis. (A) FLAIR sequences obtained over 14 months in a patient with PLE associated with carcinoma of the thyroid gland and with a paraneoplastic antibody against intracellular onconeuronal antigens. (B) FLAIR sequences obtained over 16 months in a patient with non-PLE and Sjögren's syndrome. The patient with PLE (A) had progressive neurologic deterioration, with severe memory deficits and brainstem and cerebellar dysfunction, which eventually caused his death. The patient with Sjögren's syndrome (B) had remarkable recovery of his memory deficits despite persistence of the FLAIR MRI abnormalities. Note the progressive atrophy developing in the hippocampi (arrows) of the patient with PLE (A) compared with no significant atrophic changes in the patient in (B).

demonstrating temporal lobe abnormalities, and in some cases the PET findings correlated with the neurologic symptoms (Ances *et al.*, 2005). Despite the sensitivity of these techniques, there were patients whose MRI and FDG-PET scans were normal.

The CSF is abnormal in 80% of patients with PLE. It typically shows moderate lymphocytic pleocytosis (white blood cells: < 200 cells/μl), increased protein concentration (often < 2 g/l), elevated IgG index or oligoclonal bands.

The pathological substrate of PLE is an inflammatory infiltrate of mononuclear cells, which predominantly involves the medial temporal lobes, amygdala, cingulum and orbitofrontal regions (Fig. 25.1) (Corsellis *et al.*, 1968; Bakheit *et al.*, 1990). Although the clinical and radiological features may suggest a disorder restricted to the limbic system, the inflammatory infiltrates are rarely confined to this system (Gultekin *et al.*, 2000). These infiltrates are composed of B cells and CD4

T cells in a perivascular distribution, and CD4 and CD8 T cells forming neuronophagic nodules. As a result, there is neuronal loss, reactive gliosis and microglial proliferation. Although these findings are not specific for paraneoplastic disease, they are common to all PLE associated with antibodies to intracellular antigens (Voltz *et al.*, 1999; Bernal *et al.*, 2002; Muehlschlegel *et al.*, 2005).

In general, the diagnosis of PLE is suggested by the clinical picture along with the EEG, CSF and neuroimaging findings (Gultekin *et al.*, 2000; Lawn *et al.*, 2003). However, none of these allows a definitive identification of the paraneoplastic etiology of the disorder, and the differential diagnosis is extensive (Table 25.4) (Scheid *et al.*, 2005; Stubgen 1998). These limitations emphasize the importance of testing for paraneoplastic antibodies, which are found in the serum or CSF of 60–70% of patients with PLE. There are several antibodies that associate with a similar

Table 25.4. Differential diagnosis of limbic encephalopathy

Disorder	Distinctive features or tests
Disorders that selectively involve the limbic system	
Herpes simplex (HSV) encephalitis	HSV DNA in CSF (sensitivity 94%, specificity 98%)
Paraneoplastic limbic encephalitis	Paraneoplastic antibodies detectable in serum and CSF of 60% of the patients (see subtypes of paraneoplastic immunities in Table 25.1)
Autoimmune non-paraneoplastic limbic encephalitis	VGKC (may also occur as paraneoplastic manifestation of thymoma, SCLC)
Disorders that predominantly involve the limbic system	
Neurodegenerative disorders (Alzheimer's disease, frontotemporal dementia, mild cognitive impairment)	Amnestic syndrome may predominate at early stages
Severe hypoxia	History of cardiac arrest, carbon monoxide poisoning or drug overdose
Transient global amnesia	Bitemporal hypoperfusion as shown by SPECT or abnormal diffusion-weighted MRI
Temporal lobe seizures	Abnormal FLAIR and diffusion-weighted MRI in temporal lobes following status epilepticus; hippocampal atrophy in mesial temporal sclerosis
Endocrine dysfunction (Cushing's disease, corticosteroid treatment, post-traumatic stress disorder)	Decreased hippocampal volume may be found in chronic hypercortisolism
Vitamin deficits	Wernicke–Korsakoff's encephalopathy (deficit of B_1): poor nutrition, consumption by tumor (i.e. leukemia)
Disorders that may involve the limbic system	
Head trauma	Contusion affecting inferomedial or anterior temporal lobes ("contrecoup" lesion)
Encephalitis associated with systemic autoimmune disorders:	
Lupus erythematosus	Anti-ribosomal-P antibodies
Hashimoto's encephalitis	Antibodies to thyroperoxidase/thyroglobulin
Sjögren's syndrome	SS-A, SS-B antibodies; salivary gland biopsy
Infections	Human herpes virus 6 (usually after stem cell transplantation), neurosyphilis
Tumors (gliomatosis cerebri)	Diagnostic brain biopsy
Stroke with bilateral posterior cerebral artery involvement	Amnestic syndrome often coexists with cortical blindness, prosopagnosia, apraxia of ocular movements, and other

Notes:
CSF, cerebrospinal fluid; VGKC, voltage-gated potassium channel; SCLC, small cell lung cancer; MRI, magnetic resonance imaging; SPECT, single-photon emission computed tomography; FLAIR, fluid-attenuated inversion recovery

PLE phenotype, but the accompanying neurologic symptoms and specific underlying tumors define different clinical-immunological profiles.

Anti-Hu. This is the antibody more frequently associated with PLE in patients with small cell lung cancer (SCLC) (Fig. 25.2A) (Alamowitch et al., 1997). Patients often have progression of symptoms outside the limbic system, including brainstem, cerebellum, dorsal root ganglia or autonomic nerves (paraneoplastic encephalomyelitis). In three clinically based series of patients with anti-Hu-associated encephalomyelitis, comprising 344 patients, approximately 20% presented with dominant or isolated symptoms of limbic dysfunction (Dalmau et al., 1992; Graus et al., 2001; Sillevis et al., 2002). When patients with SCLC develop pure or isolated PLE, only 50% harbor anti-Hu antibodies; these patients are less likely to improve than those without antibodies (Alamowitch et al., 1997). Some of the patients without anti-Hu antibodies that improve with immunotherapy harbor anti-VGKC antibodies (Pozo-Rosich et al., 2003).

Anti-CV2 or anti-CRMP5. This antibody can occur in patients with PLE associated with SCLC, thymoma or, less frequently, other tumors (Antoine et al., 2001). In patients with SCLC, anti-CV2 or anti-CRMP5 may occur in association with anti-Hu. The repertoire of syndromes associated with antibodies to CV2 is ample and includes encephalomyelopathy, axonal sensorimotor neuropathy and, more distinctively chorea, uveitis and optic neuritis (Antoine *et al.*, 1993; Yu *et al.*, 2001; Vernino *et al.*, 2002). For this reason, the MRI studies of patients with anti-CV2 antibodies may show typical PLE abnormalities involving the medial temporal lobes combined with FLAIR and T_2-weighted abnormalities in other areas of the CNS; those with chorea frequently show hyperintensities in the striatum and caudate (see paraneoplastic striatal encephalitis). The involvement of frontostriatal and basal ganglia circuitry may result in personality change, obsessive–compulsive behavior and cognitive deficits (Muehlschlegel *et al.*, 2005).

Other paraneoplastic antibodies. There have been infrequent reports of other antibodies in association with PLE including anti-Ri in a patient with carcinoid tumor (Harloff *et al.*, 2005), anti-amphiphysin in patients with SCLC (Dorresteijn *et al.*, 2002) and several non-characterized antibodies in patients with tumors of the thymus (D'Avino *et al.*, 2001; Fujii *et al.*, 2001). Amphiphysin, which is an autoantigen of paraneoplastic stiff-person syndrome and encephalomyelitis, is the most common of these unusual immunological associations. A patient with SCLC and anti-amphiphysin antibodies who presented with memory deficits and a Mini-Mental State Examination of 23/30 had significant neurological improvement after successful treatment of the tumor (Dorresteijn *et al.*, 2002).

Limbic encephalitis associated with anti-VGKC antibodies

Antibodies to VGKCs usually associate with non-paraneoplastic limbic encephalitis (Thieben *et al.*, 2004; Vincent *et al.*, 2004). The neuropsychological profile of these patients is characterized by marked, generalized memory deficits, although intellectual impairment and a dysexecutive syndrome can occur. Frequent clinical accompaniments include insomnia and hyponatremia. Imaging usually shows uni- or bilateral medial temporal lobe FLAIR or T_2-weighted MRI hyperintensities that rarely enhance with contrast. As previously indicated, detection of anti-VGKC antibodies should not preclude a cancer search (Buckley *et al.*, 2001; Liguori *et al.*, 2001; Pozo-Rosich *et al.*, 2003).

Patients with anti-VGKC antibodies are less likely to have CSF pleocytosis and intrathecal synthesis of IgG than those with other paraneoplastic immunities (Ances *et al.*, 2005). Anti-VGKC antibodies also occur in patients with Morvan's syndrome (Liguori *et al.*, 2001). Although 70–80% of patients with anti-VGKC associated disorders respond clinically and radiologically to corticosteroids, intravenous IgG or plasma exchange (Thieben *et al.*, 2004; Vincent *et al.*, 2004), rapid development of hyponatremia and severe seizures may be life threatening. One of our patients developed non-convulsive status epilepticus associated with a precipitous decrease in serum sodium from 122 to 110 mEq/l over a 24 hour period. The patient recovered from the hyponatremia and seizures but remains with severe impairment of memory and executive functions 3 years after presentation.

Paraneoplastic encephalitis of the limbic system, diencephalon and brainstem (Ma2 encephalitis)

Patients with Ma2 encephalitis develop symptoms of limbic encephalitis usually combined with hypothalamic and upper brainstem dysfunction (Rosenfeld *et al.*, 2001; Dalmau *et al.*, 2004). In a study of 38 patients, 34 (89%) presented with isolated or combined symptoms of limbic, diencephalic or brainstem dysfunction, and four with other syndromes. When considering the clinical and MRI follow-up, 95% of the patients developed limbic, diencephalic or brainstem encephalopathy. Figure 25.6 shows the distribution of syndromes in these patients. In a few instances, the initial symptoms resembled a pure psychiatric disorder, including obsessive–compulsive behavior, loss of self-confidence or an unexplained sense of fear (Scheid *et al.*, 2003; Dalmau *et al.*, 2004).

The hypothalamic involvement can result in endocrine deficits, excessive daytime sleepiness, diaphoresis, hyperthermia and narcolepsy–cataplexy, with low or undetectable CSF hypocretin levels (Overeem *et al.*, 2004). The upper brainstem dysfunction results in vertical ophthalmoparesis, but as the disorder progresses horizontal gaze and lower cranial nerves can be involved, along with cerebellar ataxia, nystagmus or, less frequently, opsoclonus.

Some patients develop severe hypokinesia, rigidity, hypophonia and a tendency to continuous eye closure

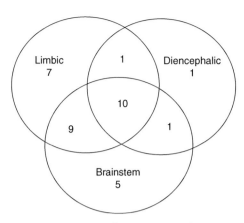

Fig. 25.6. Distribution of predominant syndromes in 34 patients with anti-Ma2 encephalitis. Twenty-one patients developed symptoms of multifocal involvement of the limbic system, diencephalon or brainstem. Thirteen patients developed unifocal involvement of these areas. (reproduced from *Brain*, [Dalmau *et al.*, 2004] with permission from Oxford University Press © 2004 Guarantors of *Brain*.)

without evidence of ptosis; despite the appearance of extreme drowsiness and minimal verbal output, they have relative preservation of comprehension and of the ability to follow simple commands (Dalmau *et al.*, 2004). Three patients became extremely hypokinetic; they stopped speaking and eating but were able to respond "thumbs up or down" with good accuracy when answering autobiographic questions.

The frequency and type of CSF inflammatory abnormalities are similar to other PND of the CNS, but patients with Ma2 encephalitis have MRI abnormalities than predominate in the medial temporal lobes, hypothalamus, thalamus, basal ganglia and upper brainstem (superior colliculi and periaqueductal region). Contrast enhancement of the lesions occurs more frequently (38% of patients) than in other PND (Fig. 25.7) (Rosenfeld *et al.*, 2001; Dalmau *et al.*, 2004).

In young male patients (< 45 years), the primary tumor is usually in the testis (Voltz *et al.*, 1999); in other patients the repertoire of tumors is varied, but the leading neoplasm is non-small-cell lung cancer. We have encountered four young patients whose testicular tumors initially escaped detection despite comprehensive evaluation, including testicular ultrasound and FDG-PET obtained in two (Dalmau *et al.*, 1999). Because of the rapid neurologic deterioration, detection of anti-Ma2 antibodies and development of subtle changes in serial ultrasound studies, they underwent orchiectomy; all four had microscopic carcinoma in situ of the testis.

All patients with Ma2 encephalitis harbor anti-Ma2 antibodies in serum or CSF; 40% have additional antibodies to Ma1. These patients are more likely to have tumors other than testicular cancer, develop ataxia and have a worse prognosis (Dalmau *et al.*, 2004).

The diagnosis of Ma2 encephalitis is often delayed. In 20% of patients, a diagnosis of Whipple's disease was initially considered and 16% had undergone duodenal biopsy, which in all instances was normal (data not published). Prompt recognition of Ma2 encephalitis is important because it differs from most PND associated with antineuronal antibodies (i.e. Hu, CV2/CRMP5) in that a significant number of patients with anti-Ma2 antibodies respond to treatment of the tumor and immunotherapy (corticosteroids, intravenous IgG, or plasma exchange). In our study of 38 patients, 33% had neurologic improvement (four patients with complete recovery), 21% long-term stabilization (median follow-up 3.5 years) and 46% deteriorated. Features associated with improvement included male gender, underlying testicular germ-cell tumors with complete response to treatment, absence of anti-Ma1 antibodies and limited involvement of the nervous system.

Paraneoplastic striatal encephalitis

Paraneoplastic mechanisms may result in hyperkinetic syndromes, such as chorea and hemi- or biballismus. Approximately 26 patients have been reported with these disorders (Batchelor *et al.*, 1998; Croteau *et al.*, 2001; Vernino *et al.*, 2002; Samii *et al.*, 2003), and approximately 50% had accompanying symptoms of PLE and diverse cognitive deficits, ranging from mild decrease of attention and constructional apraxia to severe obsessive–compulsive behavior and frank dementia (Nuti *et al.*, 2000; Tani *et al.*, 2000; Muehlschlegel *et al.*, 2005). At early stages of the disorder, MRI shows involvement of the caudate and anterior putamen, and less frequently the pallidum. The MRI can be normal, particularly when obtained several months after symptom development (Vernino *et al.*, 2002). The tumors more frequently involved are SCLC (68%), followed by lymphoma and renal cancer. The paraneoplastic antibodies more frequently detected are to CV2/CRMP5, frequently in association with anti-Hu.

The association of chorea with cognitive and psychiatric changes may suggest the diagnosis of Huntington's disease, Wilson's disease or vasculitis of the CNS. Patients with paraneoplastic chorea can improve with treatment of the tumor and symptomatic

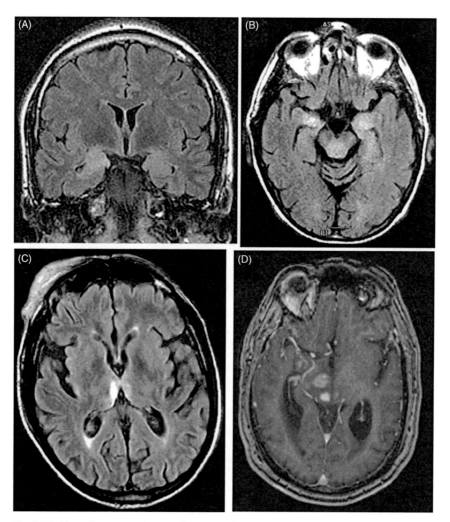

Fig. 25.7. Magnetic resonance imaging of patients with anti-Ma2 encephalitis. (A) Fluid-attenuated inversion recovery (FLAIR) sequence from a patient with testicular germ cell tumor and isolated temporal lobe seizures. Note the presence of asymmetric abnormalities in the temporal lobes; the cerebrospinal fluid was positive for oligoclonal bands and anti-Ma2 antibodies. (B,C) FLAIR sequences from a patient with severe hypokinetic syndrome, non-paretic eye closure and reduced verbal output, showing abnormalities in the mesial temporal lobes and dorsal mesencephalon (B), and medial thalami (C). (D) This T_1-weighted image of a patient with non-small cell lung cancer and anti-Ma2 encephalitis shows nodular areas of contrast enhancement in the right temporal lobe, thalamic, subthalamic and collicular regions. Biopsy of one of the lesions demonstrated perivascular and interstitial infiltrates of mononuclear cells and plasma cells. (Reproduced from *Brain* [Dalmau *et al.* 2004] with permission from Oxford University Press © 2004 Guarantors of *Brain*.)

medication (haloperidol, risperidone) (Vernino *et al.*, 2002), but the cognitive dysfunction is less responsive to treatment (Nuti *et al.*, 2000).

Paraneoplastic temporal lobe encephalitis with neuropil antibodies

Some patients with encephalitis predominantly involving the temporal lobes harbor serum or CSF antibodies to antigens expressed in the cell membrane of neurons and dendritic processes of the neuropil of the hippocampus (Ances *et al.*, 2005). There is a common clinical phenotype to all these disorders, which includes dominant behavioral and psychiatric symptoms (often obscuring the short-term memory deficits), seizures and brain MRI abnormalities that are less frequently restricted to the hippocampus than in classical PLE. Studies with FDG-PET may reveal multifocal FDG hyperactivity involving frontotemporal lobes, brainstem or cerebellum. Combining MRI and FDG-PET studies, the temporal lobes are preferentially affected. Patients are more likely to have

CSF inflammatory findings and underlying tumors (thymoma, teratoma) than those with anti-VGKC antibodies, and they do not develop hyponatremia (Ances et al., 2005).

Preliminary characterization of the autoantigens indicated that these are diverse and more concentrated in the hippocampus than the VGKC. Some autoantigens partially colocalized with synaptophysin and spinophilin, suggesting an immune-mediated pathology of hippocampal dendrites, similarly to that reported in some patients with schizophrenia and mood disorders (Lawn et al., 2003).

In contrast to patients with paraneoplastic antibodies to intracellular antigens, the encephalitis of patients with any of these collectively termed neuropil antibodies improves with immunotherapy and, if present, treatment of the associated tumor. This improvement often associates with improvement of MRI and FDG-PET abnormalities and a decrease of antibody titers (Ances et al., 2005).

Encephalitis of patients with ovarian teratoma and neuropil antibodies

Attempts to characterize each neuropil autoantigen and corresponding subsyndrome resulted in the identification of a specific immune-mediated phenotype in four patients with ovarian teratoma (Vitaliani et al., 2005). These patients presented with subacute psychiatric symptoms, short-term memory deficits, seizures, rapid decrease of level of consciousness and frequent central hypoventilation (Muni et al., 2004; Stein-Wexler et al., 2005). Because of the type of symptoms and because the disorder affects young women with an occult (sometimes benign) ovarian teratoma, the differential diagnosis often includes acute psychosis, malingering or drug abuse. A similar encephalitic syndrome has been reported in five other patients with ovarian teratoma (Nokura et al., 1997; Okamura et al., 1997; Aydiner et al., 1998; Lee et al., 2003; Fadare and Hart 2004).

Serum or CSF from these patients showed immunolabeling of antigens that were expressed at the cytoplasmic membrane of hippocampal neurons and processes, and which were readily accessed by antibodies in live neurons. Immunoprecipitation studies demonstrated that the target antigen is the NMDA receptor and that the main epitope region is contained in the extracellular domain of NR1 (Dalmau et al., 2008).

A series of 100 patients with anti-NMDA receptor encephalitis demonstrated that only 60% had tumors (usually teratomas of the ovary). The same study showed that men and children can also be affected by the same neurological syndrome. Despite the severity of the clinical features, 75% of the patients had substantial improvement after immunotherapy and, when appropriate, tumor removal. The clinical improvement is usually slow and may take several months until full recovery (Vitaliani et al., 2005; Dalmau et al., 2008).

Paraneoplastic syndromes of children with neural crest tumors
Opsoclonus–myoclonus–ataxia

Approximately 50% of children with opsoclonus–myoclonus–ataxia have an underlying neuroblastoma. The disorder usually affects infants younger than 4 years of age (median, 18 months) and associates with hypotonia and behavioral and psychomotor abnormalities (Russo et al., 1997). The ocular movement disorder and myoclonus inconsistently respond to treatment of the tumor (chemotherapy), steroids, adrenocorticotropic hormone, plasma exchange or intravenous IgG (Mitchell and Snodgrass 1990; Hammer et al., 1995; Russo et al., 1997; Yiu et al., 2001). The positive effects of immunotherapy and the frequent detection of antibodies against the CNS suggest an immune-mediated pathogenesis, but the specific autoantigens remain to be identified.

More than 70% of patients are left with behavioral abnormalities or psychomotor retardation (Koh et al., 1994; Russo et al., 1997). A recent study of 17 children with opsoclonus–myoclonus–ataxia showed that all patients had delayed or abnormal cognitive development and adaptive behavior (Mitchell et al., 2002). Speech intelligibility and output and motor abilities were frequently affected. At the early stage of the disorder, all patients had severe irritability and inconsolability, and at the later stage oppositional behavior and sleep disorders were common. The long-term outcome of cognitive functions did not differ with the type of treatment or with the initial response of the opsoclonus and fine motor and speech functions to intravenous IgG (Mitchell et al., 2002). Late cerebellar atrophy appears to be a common finding regardless of the neurologic outcome (Hayward et al., 2001).

Hypothalamic syndrome

There are a few reports of children with neural crest tumors who developed dominant hypothalamic dysfunction characterized by personality change and

389

Table 25.5. Clinical features, response to treatment, and prognosis related to type of antibody and location of antigens

	Neuronal antibodies to Hu, Ma2, CV2/CRMP5, amphiphysin, atypical (intracellular antigens)	Antibodies to VGKC (cell membrane antigens)	"Novel neuropil antibodies" (cell membrane antigens[a])
Hippocampal specificity of antibodies	No; antibodies react with neurons of any part of the neuraxis	Mild; all patients with similar pattern of antibody reactivity	Intense; different patterns (some with pure limbic reactivity)
CSF inflammatory abnormalities[b]	Frequent	Infrequent (normal CSF or with mild abnormalities)	Frequent
Intrathecal synthesis of antibodies	Frequent	Infrequent/absent	Frequent
Hyponatremia	No (except some patients with SCLC)	Frequent	No
Clinical phenotypes other than limbic encephalitis	Several according to type of antibody (Bataller and Dalmau 2004)	Neuromyotonia; Morvan's syndrome (Vincent et al., 2004)	Prominent behavioral abnormalities, psychiatric symptoms and seizures; central hypoventilation may occur (Ances et al., 2005; Dalmau et al., 2008; Lai et al., 2008)
Brain MRI	Frequent medial temporal lobe FLAIR/T_2 weighted hyperintensities (classical findings)	Frequent classical findings	Infrequent classical findings, but frequent temporal lobe involvement
Tumor association	SCLC, non-SCLC, testicular tumors, thymoma, other	Infrequent: SCLC, thymoma	Frequent: teratoma, thymoma
Response to treatment (tumor and/or immunosuppression)	Rare; except for patients with testicular tumors and Ma2 encephalitis	Frequent (corticosteroids, intravenous IgG, plasma exchange)	Frequent (tumor and/or corticosteroids, intravenous IgG, plasma exchange, rituximab)
Clinical course	Progressive until stabilization or death (Hu, CV2/CRMP5); relapses rare	Relapses may occur and are treatable	Relapses may occur and are treatable
Outcome of antibody titers	Usually detectable for months or years	Decrease or disappear in months	Decrease or disappear in months

Notes:
MRI, magnetic resonance imaging; FLAIR, fluid-attenuated inversion recovery; see Table 25.1 for other abbreviations.
[a]NMDA and AMPA receptors plus others.
[b]Pleocytosis, increased protein concentration, elevated IgG index, oligoclonal bands.
Source: From: Ances et al. (2005) reproduced with permission from Oxford University Press.

abnormal affect, hyperphagia, adipsia–hypernatremia, hypersomnia, reversal of sleep–wake cycle, abnormal thermoregulation, seizures and endocrine dysfunction (Nunn *et al.*, 1997). Similar to the encephalitic syndrome associated with ovarian teratoma (see above), children with this disorder frequently develop central hypoventilation.

Sirvent *et al.* (2003) reported two patients and reviewed five previous ones with neural crest tumors and a hypothalamic syndrome, all of whom developed central hypoventilation. Autopsy studies may show no pathology, or extensive lymphocytic infiltration of the hypothalamus and brainstem (North *et al.*, 1994; Nunn *et al.*, 1997). No paraneoplastic antibodies have been identified. Treatment should focus on removing the tumor and controlling the hypothalamic–endocrine deficits, along with a restrictive diet and regular exercise. Behavioral and psychomotor abnormalities usually do not respond to therapy.

General approach to treatment

There is no standard of care for PND. Experience from series of patients indicate that treatment of the tumor is critical to improve or stabilize the neurologic syndrome (Keime-Guibert *et al.*, 1999; Dalmau *et al.*, 2004), immunotherapy may contribute to neurologic improvement or symptom stabilization if started at early stages of the PND (Bataller *et al.*, 2001; Vernino *et al.*, 2004) and immunotherapy does not appear to favor tumor growth (Keime-Guibert *et al.*, 1999).

One study has suggested that the type of auto-antigen and its location in the neuron provides a clue for developing the treatment strategy and predicting outcome (Table 25.5) (Ances *et al.*, 2005). In general, patients with PND associated with antibodies to cytoplasmic or nuclear antigens (i.e. Hu, CV2/CRMP5, amphiphysin, Ma2) have extensive infiltrates of T-cells in the involved brain regions, with activated cytotoxic T-cells causing cell killing via granzyme or perforin (Bernal *et al.*, 2002). Therefore, in these patients, the immunotherapeutic strategies should focus on the cytotoxic T-cell response (reviewed by Bataller and Dalmau [2004]). Except for a subgroup of patients with anti-Ma2 antibodies (Dalmau *et al.*, 2004), the neurologic and oncologic outcomes of these PND are poor.

In contrast, most paraneoplastic encephalitides associated with antibodies to antigens expressed on the cell membrane (i.e. VGKC and novel neuropil antigens) respond better to IgG-depleting strategies (corticosteroids, plasma exchange, intravenous IgG) and have a better neurologic outcome (Thieben *et al.*, 2004; Vincent *et al.*, 2004; Ances *et al.*, 2005; Vitaliani *et al.*, 2005; Dalmau *et al.*, 2008; Lai *et al.*, 2008). This, and the fact that the antibody titers decrease in parallel with the clinical improvement, suggest a direct pathogenic role of the antibodies.

References

Alamowitch, S., Graus, F., Uchuya, M. *et al.* (1997). Limbic encephalitis and small cell lung cancer. Clinical and immunological features. *Brain* **120**, 923–928.

Albert, M. L., Darnell, J. C., Bender, A. *et al.* (1998). Tumor-specific killer cells in paraneoplastic cerebellar degeneration. *Nat Med* **11**, 1321–1324.

Ances, B. M., Vitaliani, R., Taylor, R. A. *et al.* (2005). Treatment-responsive limbic encephalitis identified by neuropil antibodies: MRI and PET correlates. *Brain* **128**, 1764–1777.

Antoine, J. C., Honnorat, J., Vocanson, C. *et al.* (1993). Posterior uveitis, paraneoplastic encephalomyelitis and auto-antibodies reacting with developmental protein of brain and retina. *J Neurol Sci* **117**, 215–223.

Antoine, J. C., Honnorat, J., Camdessanche, J. P. *et al.* (2001). Paraneoplastic anti-CV2 antibodies react with peripheral nerve and are associated with a mixed axonal and demyelinating peripheral neuropathy. *Ann Neurol* **49**, 214–221.

Aydiner, A., Gurvit, H. and Baral, I. (1998). Paraneoplastic limbic encephalitis with immature ovarian teratoma: a case report. *J Neurooncol* **37**, 63–66.

Bakheit, A. M., Kennedy, P. G. and Behan, P. O. (1990). Paraneoplastic limbic encephalitis: clinico-pathological correlations. *J Neurol Neurosurg Psychiatry* **53**, 1084–1088.

Bataller, L. and Dalmau, J. O. (2004). Paraneoplastic disorders of the central nervous system: update on diagnostic criteria and treatment. *Semin Neurol* **24**, 461–471.

Bataller, L., Graus, F., Saiz, A. and Vilchez, J. J. (2001). Clinical outcome in adult onset idiopathic or paraneoplastic opsoclonus-myoclonus. *Brain* **124**, 437–443.

Bataller, L., Wade, D. F., Graus, F. *et al.* (2004). Antibodies to Zic4 in paraneoplastic neurologic disorders and small-cell lung cancer. *Neurology* **62**, 778–782.

Batchelor, T. T., Platten, M., Palmer-Toy, D. E. *et al.* (1998). Chorea as a paraneoplastic complication of Hodgkin's disease. *J Neurooncol* **36**, 185–190.

Bernal, F., Graus, F., Pifarre, A. *et al.* (2002). Immunohistochemical analysis of anti-Hu-associated paraneoplastic encephalomyelitis. *Acta Neuropathol* **103**, 509–515.

Brierley, J. B., Corsellis, J. A. N., Hierons, R. and Nevin, S. (1960). Subacute encephalitis of later adult life. Mainly affecting the limbic areas. *Brain* **83**, 357–368.

Buckley, C., Oger, J., Clover, L. et al. (2001). Potassium channel antibodies in two patients with reversible limbic encephalitis. *Ann Neurol* **50**, 73–78.

Corsellis, J. A., Goldberg, G. J. and Norton, A. R. (1968). "Limbic encephalitis" and its association with carcinoma. *Brain* **91**, 481–496.

Croteau, D., Owainati, A., Dalmau, J. and Rogers, L. R. (2001). Response to cancer therapy in a patient with a paraneoplastic choreiform disorder. *Neurology* **57**, 719–722.

D'Avino, C., Lucchi, M., Ceravolo, R. et al. (2001). Limbic encephalitis associated with thymic cancer: a case report. *J Neurol* **248**, 1000–1002.

Dalmau, J., Gleichman, A. J., Hughes, E. G. et al. (2008). Anti-NMDA receptor encephalitis: case series and analysis of the effects of antibodies. *Lancet Neurol* **7**, 1091–1098.

Dalmau, J., Graus, F., Rosenblum, M. K. and Posner, J. B. (1992). Anti-Hu–associated paraneoplastic encephalomyelitis/sensory neuronopathy. A clinical study of 71 patients. *Medicine* **71**, 59–72.

Dalmau, J, Gultekin, H. S. and Posner, J. B. (1999). A serologic marker of paraneoplastic limbic and brain-stem encephalitis in patients with testicular cancer (letter). *N Engl J Med* **341**, 1475–1476.

Dalmau, J., Graus, F., Villarejo, A. et al. (2004). Clinical analysis of anti-Ma2-associated encephalitis. *Brain* **127**, 1831–1844.

Darnell, R. B. and Posner, J. B. (2003). Paraneoplastic syndromes involving the nervous system. *N Engl J Med* **349**, 1543–1554.

Dirr, L. Y., Elster, A. D., Donofrio, P. D. and Smith, M. (1990). Evolution of brain MRI abnormalities in limbic encephalitis. *Neurology* **40**, 1304–1306.

Dorresteijn, L. D., Kappelle, A. C., Renier, W. O. and Gijtenbeek, J. M. (2002). Anti-amphiphysin associated limbic encephalitis: a paraneoplastic presentation of small-cell lung carcinoma. *J Neurol* **249**, 1307–1308.

Elrington, G. M., Murray, N. M., Spiro, S. G. and Newsom-Davis, J. (1991). Neurological paraneoplastic syndromes in patients with small cell lung cancer. A prospective survey of 150 patients. *J Neurol Neurosurg Psychiatry* **54**, 764–767.

Fadare, O. and Hart, H. J. (2004). Anti-Ri antibodies associated with short-term memory deficits and a mature cystic teratoma of the ovary. *Int Semin Surg Oncol* **1**, 11.

Fadul, C. E., Stommel, E. W., Dragnev, K. H., Eskey, C. J. and Dalmau, J. O. (2005). Focal paraneoplastic limbic encephalitis presenting as orgasmic epilepsy. *J Neurooncol* **72**, 195–198.

Fujii, N., Furuta, A., Yamaguchi, H., Nakanishi, K. and Iwaki, T. (2001). Limbic encephalitis associated with recurrent thymoma: a postmortem study. *Neurology* **57**, 344–347.

Graus, F., Dalmau, J., Rene, R. et al. (1997). Anti-Hu antibodies in patients with small-cell lung cancer: association with complete response to therapy and improved survival. *J Clin Oncol* **15**, 2866–2872.

Graus, F., Keime-Guibert, F., Rene, R. et al. (2001). Anti-Hu-associated paraneoplastic encephalomyelitis: analysis of 200 patients. *Brain* **124**, 1138–1148.

Graus, F., Delattre, J. Y., Antoine, J. C. et al. (2004). Recommended diagnostic criteria for paraneoplastic neurological syndromes. *J Neurol Neurosurg Psychiatry* **75**, 1135–1140.

Gultekin, S. H., Rosenfeld, M. R., Voltz, R. et al. (2000). Paraneoplastic limbic encephalitis: neurological symptoms, immunological findings and tumour association in 50 patients. *Brain* **123**, 1481–1494.

Hammer, M. S., Larsen, M. B. and Stack, C. V. (1995). Outcome of children with opsoclonus-myoclonus regardless of etiology. *Pediatr Neurol* **13**, 21–24.

Harloff, A., Hummel, S., Kleinschmidt, M. and Rauer, S. (2005). Anti-Ri antibodies and limbic encephalitis in a patient with carcinoid tumour of the lung. *J Neurol* **252**, 1404–1405.

Hayward, K., Jeremy, R. J., Jenkins, S. et al. (2001). Long-term neurobehavioral outcomes in children with neuroblastoma and opsoclonus-myoclonus-ataxia syndrome: relationship to MRI findings and anti-neuronal antibodies. *J Pediatr* **139**, 552–559.

Jean, W. C., Dalmau, J., Ho, A. and Posner, J. B. (1994). Analysis of the IgG subclass distribution and inflammatory infiltrates in patients with anti-Hu-associated paraneoplastic encephalomyelitis. *Neurology* **44**, 140–147.

Kassubek, J., Juengling, F. D., Nitzsche, E. U. and Lucking, C. H. (2001). Limbic encephalitis investigated by [18]FDG-PET and 3D MRI. *J Neuroimaging* **11**, 55–59.

Keime-Guibert, F., Graus, F., Broet, P. et al. (1999). Clinical outcome of patients with anti-Hu-associated encephalomyelitis after treatment of the tumor. *Neurology* **53**, 1719–1723.

Koh, P. S., Raffensperger, J. G., Berry, S. et al. (1994). Long-term outcome in children with opsoclonus-myoclonus and ataxia and coincident neuroblastoma. *J Pediatr* **125**, 712–716.

Lai, M., Hughes, E. G., Peng, X. et al. (2008). AMPA receptor antibodies in limbic encephalitis alter synaptic receptor location. *Ann Neurol* in press.

Lawn, N. D., Westmoreland, B. F., Kiely, M. J., Lennon, V. A. and Vernino, S. (2003). Clinical, magnetic resonance imaging, and electroencephalographic findings in paraneoplastic limbic encephalitis. *Mayo Clin Proc* **78**, 1363–1368.

Lee, A. C., Ou, Y., Lee, W. K. and Wong, Y. C. (2003). Paraneoplastic limbic encephalitis masquerading as chronic behavioural disturbance in an adolescent girl. *Acta Paediatr* **92**, 506–509.

Liguori, R., Vincent, A., Clover, L. et al. (2001). Morvan's syndrome: peripheral and central nervous system and cardiac involvement with antibodies to voltage-gated potassium channels. Brain 124, 2417–2426.

Linke, R., Schroeder, M., Helmberger, T. and Voltz, R. (2004). Antibody-positive paraneoplastic neurologic syndromes: value of CT and PET for tumor diagnosis. Neurology 63, 282–286.

Mitchell, W. G. and Snodgrass, S. R. (1990). Opsoclonus-ataxia due to childhood neural crest tumors: a chronic neurologic syndrome. J Child Neurol 5, 153–158.

Mitchell, W. G., Davalos-Gonzalez, Y. and Brumm, V. L. (2002). Opsoclonus-ataxia caused by childhood neuroblastoma: developmental and neurologic sequelae. Pediatrics 109, 86–98.

Muehlschlegel, S., Okun, M. S., Foote, K. D. et al. (2005). Paraneoplastic chorea with leukoencephalopathy presenting with obsessive-compulsive and behavioral disorder. Mov Disord 20, 1523–1527.

Muller-Hermelink, H. K. and Marx, A. (2000). Thymoma. Curr Opin Oncol 12, 426–433.

Muni, R. H., Wennberg, R., Mikulis, D. J. and Wong, A. M. (2004). Bilateral horizontal gaze palsy in presumed paraneoplastic brainstem encephalitis associated with a benign ovarian teratoma. J Neuroophthalmol 24, 114–118.

Mut, M., Schiff, D. and Dalmau, J. (2005). Paraneoplastic recurrent multifocal encephalitis presenting with epilepsia partialis continua. J Neurooncol 72, 63–66.

Nokura, K., Yamamoto, H., Okawara, Y. et al. (1997). Reversible limbic encephalitis caused by ovarian teratoma. Acta Neurol Scand 95, 367–373.

North, K. N., Ouvrier, R. A., McLean, C. A. and Hopkins, I. J. (1994). Idiopathic hypothalamic dysfunction with dilated unresponsive pupils: report of two cases. J Child Neurol 9, 320–325.

Nunn, K., Ouvrier, R., Sprague, T., Arbuckle, S. and Docker, M. (1997). Idiopathic hypothalamic dysfunction: a paraneoplastic syndrome? J Child Neurol 12, 276–281.

Nuti, A., Ceravolo, R., Salvetti, S. et al. (2000). Paraneoplastic choreic syndrome during non-Hodgkin's lymphoma. Mov Disord 15, 350–352.

Okamura, H., Oomori, N. and Uchitomi, Y. (1997). An acutely confused 15-year-old girl. Lancet 350, 488.

Overeem, S., Dalmau, J., Bataller, L. et al. (2004). Anti-Ma2 antibodies in idiopathic and paraneoplastic hypocretin-deficient narcolepsy. Neurology 62, 138–140.

Posner, J. B. (1995). Metabolic and nutritional complications of cancer. Neurologic Complications of Cancer, Ch. 11. Philadelphia, PA: F. A. Davis, pp. 264–281.

Pozo-Rosich, P., Clover, L., Saiz, A., Vincent, A. and Graus, F. (2003). Voltage-gated potassium channel antibodies in limbic encephalitis. Ann Neurol 54, 530–533.

Rojas, I., Graus, F., Keime-Guibert, F. et al. (2000). Long-term clinical outcome of paraneoplastic cerebellar degeneration and anti-Yo antibodies. Neurology 55, 713–715.

Rosenfeld, M. R., Eichen, J. G., Wade, D. F., Posner, J. B. and Dalmau, J. (2001). Molecular and clinical diversity in paraneoplastic immunity to Ma proteins. Ann Neurol 50, 339–348.

Russo, C., Cohn, S. L., Petruzzi, M. J. and de Alarcon, P. A. (1997). Long-term neurologic outcome in children with opsoclonus–myoclonus associated with neuroblastoma: a report from the Pediatric Oncology Group. Med Pediatr Oncol 28, 284–288.

Samii, A., Dahlen, D. D., Spence, A. M. et al. (2003). Paraneoplastic movement disorder in a patient with non-Hodgkin's lymphoma and CRMP-5 autoantibody. Mov Disord 18, 1556–1558.

Scheid, R., Voltz, R., Guthke, T. et al. (2003). Neuropsychiatric findings in anti-Ma2-positive paraneoplastic limbic encephalitis. Neurology 61, 1159–1161.

Scheid, R., Lincke, T., Voltz, R., von Cramon, D. Y. and Sabri, O. (2004). Serial ^{18}F-fluoro-2-deoxy-D-glucose positron emission tomography and magnetic resonance imaging of paraneoplastic limbic encephalitis. Arch Neurol 61, 1785–1789.

Scheid, R., Voltz, R., Vetter, T., Sabri, O. and von Cramon, D. Y. (2005). Neurosyphilis and paraneoplastic limbic encephalitis: important differential diagnoses. J Neurol 252, 1129–1132.

Shavit, Y. B., Graus, F., Probst, A., Rene, R., and Steck, A. J. (1999). Epilepsia partialis continua: a new manifestation of anti-Hu-associated paraneoplastic encephalomyelitis. Ann Neurol 45, 255–258.

Sillevis, S. P., Grefkens, J., De Leeuw, B. et al. (2002). Survival and outcome in 73 anti-Hu positive patients with paraneoplastic encephalomyelitis/sensory neuronopathy. J Neurol 249, 745–753.

Sirvent, N., Berard, E., Chastagner, P. et al. (2003). Hypothalamic dysfunction associated with neuroblastoma: evidence for a new paraneoplastic syndrome? Med Pediatr Oncol 40, 326–328.

Stein-Wexler, R., Wootton-Gorges, S. L., Greco, C. M. and Brunberg, J. A. (2005). Paraneoplastic limbic encephalitis in a teenage girl with an immature ovarian teratoma. Pediatr Radiol 35, 694–697.

Stubgen, J. P. (1998). Nervous system lupus mimics limbic encephalitis. Lupus 7, 557–560.

Tanaka, K., Tanaka, M., Inuzuka, T., Nakano, R. and Tsuji, S. (1999). Cytotoxic T lymphocyte-mediated cell death in paraneoplastic sensory neuronopathy with anti-Hu antibody. J Neurol Sci 163, 159–162.

Tani, T., Piao, Y., Mori, S. et al. (2000). Chorea resulting from paraneoplastic striatal encephalitis. J Neurol Neurosurg Psychiatry 69, 512–515.

Thieben, M. J., Lennon, V. A., Boeve, B. F. *et al.* (2004). Potentially reversible autoimmune limbic encephalitis with neuronal potassium channel antibody. *Neurology* **62**, 1177–1182.

Vernino, S., Tuite, P., Adler, C. H. *et al.* (2002). Paraneoplastic chorea associated with CRMP-5 neuronal antibody and lung carcinoma. *Ann Neurol* **51**, 625–630.

Vernino, S., O'Neill, B. P., Marks, R. S., O'Fallon, J. R. and Kimmel, D. W. (2004). Immunomodulatory treatment trial for paraneoplastic neurological disorders. *Neurooncology* **6**, 55–62.

Vincent, A., Buckley, C., Schott, J. M. *et al.* (2004). Potassium channel antibody-associated encephalopathy: a potentially immunotherapy-responsive form of limbic encephalitis. *Brain* **127**, 701–712.

Vitaliani, R., Mason, W., Ances, B. *et al.* (2005). Paraneoplastic encephalitis, psychiatric symptoms and central hypoventilation: association with teratoma and hippocampal antibodies. *Ann Neurol* **58**, 594–604.

Voltz, R., Gultekin, S. H., Rosenfeld, M. R. *et al.* (1999). A serologic marker of paraneoplastic limbic and brain-stem encephalitis in patients with testicular cancer. *N Engl J Med* **340**, 1788–1795.

Yiu, V. W., Kovithavongs, T., McGonigle, L. F. and Ferreira, P. (2001). Plasmapheresis as an effective treatment for opsoclonus–myoclonus syndrome. *Pediat Neurol* **24**, 72–74.

Younes-Mhenni, S., Janier, M. F., Cinotti, L. *et al.* (2004). FDG-PET improves tumour detection in patients with paraneoplastic neurological syndromes. *Brain* **127**, 2331–2338.

Yu, Z., Kryzer, T. J., Griesmann, G. E. *et al.* (2001). CRMP-5 neuronal autoantibody: marker of lung cancer and thymoma-related autoimmunity. *Ann Neurol* **49**, 146–154.

Index

399

403

Made in the USA
Middletown, DE
20 August 2015